First Responder
A Skills Approach

Seventh Edition

Daniel Limmer, EMT-P

Paramedic, Kennebunk Fire Rescue
Kennebunk, Maine

Adjunct Faculty
Southern Maine Technical College
South Portland, Maine

Keith J. Karren, PhD

Professor, Department of Health Sciences
Brigham Young University
Provo, Utah

Brent Q. Hafen, PhD

Late of Brigham Young University
Provo, Utah

Medical Editor
Edward T. Dickinson, MD, NREMT-P, FACEP

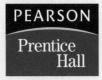

PEARSON
Prentice
Hall

Upper Saddle River, New Jersey 07458

Library of Congress Cataloging-in-Publication Data

Limmer, Daniel.
   First responder: a skills approach/Daniel Limmer, Keith
  J. Karren, Brent Q. Hafen, ; medical editor, Edward T. Dickinson. — 7th ed.
     p. ; cm.
   Includes index.
   ISBN 0-13-172048-1
     1. Medical emergencies. 2. Emergency medical technicians.
  I. Karren, Keith J. II. Hafen, Brent Q. III. Dickinson, Edward T.
IV. Title.
   [DNLM: 1. Emergencies. 2. Emergency Medical Technicians. 3. First Aid.
  WX 215 L734fa 2007] RC86.7.K365 2007
  616.02'5—dc22

                               2006019982

Publisher: *Julie Levin Alexander*
Publisher's Assistant: *Regina Bruno*
Executive Editor: *Marlene McHugh Pratt*
Senior Managing Editor for Development:
  Lois Berlowitz
Project Manager: *Jo Cepeda*
Associate Editor: *Monica Moosang*
Director of Marketing: *Karen Allman*
Executive Marketing Manager:
  Katrin Beacom
Marketing Coordinator: *Michael Sirinides*
Marketing Assistant: *Wayne Celia, Jr.*
Director of Production and Manufacturing:
  Bruce Johnson
Managing Production Editor: *Patrick Walsh*
Production Liaison: *Julie Li*
Production Editor: *Sarvesh Mehrotra*
Media Product Manager: *John Jordan*
Manager of Media Production: *Amy Peltier*
New Media Project Manager: *Tina Rudowski*

Manufacturing Manager: *Ilene Sanford*
Manufacturing Buyer: *Pat Brown*
Senior Design Coordinator:
  Cheryl Asherman
Interior Designer: *Maureen Mooney/Spiral*
  Design
Cover Designer: Blair Brown
Director, Image Resource Center:
  Melinda Reo
Manager, Rights and Permissions:
  Zina Arabia
Manager, Visual Research: *Beth Brenzel*
Manager, Cover Visual Research and
  Permissions: *Karen Sanatar*
Image Permission Coordinator: *Michelina*
  Viscusi
Composition: *Techbooks*
Printing and Binding: *The Banta*
  Company
Cover Printer: *Phoenix Color Corporation*

Pearson Education, Inc., Upper Saddle
  River, N. J.
Pearson Education LTD.
Pearson Education Singapore, Pte. Ltd
Pearson Education, Canada, Ltd

Pearson Education–Japan
Pearson Education Australia PTY, Limited
Pearson Education North Asia Ltd
Pearson Educación de Mexico, S.A. de C.V.
Pearson Education Malaysia, Pte. Ltd

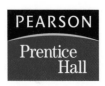

10 9 8 7 6 5 4 3 2 1
ISBN 0-13-172048-1

Dedication

To Stephanie, Sarah, and Margo. A husband and father is blessed to be surrounded by such love, beauty, support, and smiles.

DL

To the new generation, who are just beginning their life experience—specifically, to my grandchildren Joshua Keith, Kennedi, and Jackson David—and to all of the children whose educations will need excellent preparation.

KJK

In memory of Brent Q. Hafen, PhD

Brent was a man of great conviction. He was dedicated to his family, his beliefs, his students, and to the field of EMS. Early editions of this book and others authored by Brent had a tremendous influence on EMS training and education. He is deeply missed as a friend and as a co-author.

DL, KJK

Content Overview

Detailed Contents

Module 2

Airway (Chapters 6–7)

Module 4   Patient Assessment (Chapters 10–13)

Module 5

Illness and Injury (Chapters 14–25)

Module 6   Childbirth and Children (Chapters 26–27)

Module 7

Geriatric Considerations (Chapter 28)

Module 8

EMS Operations (Chapters 29–34)

Skill Summaries

(The 72 Skill Summaries that appear in this book are listed below in order of appearance.)

Preface

About FIRST RESPONDER: A SKILLS APPROACH

The role of First Responder is a unique one. Now more than ever it's considered a key position on the EMS team. While the EMS system is comprised of many talented individuals at different certification levels, you will most likely be the one who arrives on the scene of an emergency first. In addition to providing emergency medical care, you also will help your patient, bystanders, and your crew stay safe. Yours is a special responsibility, one for which you will be well trained.

This seventh edition of *First Responder: A Skills Approach* maintains the standard it set in previous editions with its easy readability and dependable coverage of essential skills and concepts. It also includes features that you'll find valuable as study aids and as enrichment:

NEW EXPANDED Media Support

- *Student CD-ROM.* Bound into the back cover of your textbook, this CD-ROM includes videos, a hazmat situation simulator, games, drag-and-drop forms, as well as multiple-choice and short-answer questions, photographs of actual injuries, and audio recordings of the pronunciation of every word in the textbook glossary.
- *Companion Website.* Offering multiple-choice questions, case studies, links to additional resources, anatomy labeling exercises, and Spanish chapter outlines, this website may be found at: www.prenhall.com/limmer

NEW UPDATED Text

- *Expanded airway coverage.* Two chapters, instead of one, now focus on airway, breathing, and ventilation.
- *CPR and ECC.* All information related to CPR and effective chest compressions has been updated to meet the American Heart Association's 2005 Guidelines.
- *Clinical updates.* The text has been reviewed especially to make sure that this new edition reflects current research findings.
- *New in-text features.* Look for the "First on Scene" and "First Responder Practice" boxes in every chapter. They offer insights from the actual practice and experience of today's First Responders.
- *Expanded case studies.* In the voice of First Responders reporting the events of an emergency call, each scenario now concludes with a model hand-off report.
- *Expanded chapter review materials.* End-of-chapter features now include "Focus on the EMS Team," "Summing Up," "Key Terms," and a "Knowledge Check" that culminates in scenario questions.

Enrichment Material

Just as in previous editions, this edition of *First Responder: A Skills Approach* meets and exceeds the knowledge and skills identified in the U.S. DOT First Responder National Standard Curriculum. Look at the objectives that introduce each chapter. Those belonging to the DOT curriculum are listed verbatim, each followed by references to textbook pages on which corresponding text appears.

In addition, the U.S. DOT acknowledges that many instructors add enrichment materials to their lessons. This is to cover topics not included in the national curriculum but necessary due to state or regional mandates and special situations.

First Responder: A Skills Approach offers an abundance of enrichment materials, including the topics listed below:

- *Circulation enrichment.* Today, the concept of automated external defibrillation extends to First Responders and to the public. The proper use of AEDs is quickly becoming an essential skill in public areas across the nation. This text offers a full chapter on the topic updated to meet the 2005 American Heart Association guidelines.
- *Airway enrichment.* Pulse oximetry and how it is used, minute volume and its effects on respiration, bag-valve-mask ventilation, oxygen therapy, special considerations related to chronic obstructive pulmonary diseases, and assisting advanced EMS providers with airway care have all been included in the two new airway chapters.

- *Medical emergencies.* A full chapter is given to two of the most frequent reasons First Responder are called—cardiac and respiratory emergencies. In another chapter, you will find coverage of diabetic emergencies, alcohol and drug emergencies, and emergencies caused by stroke, poisoning, seizures, and abdominal pain. Anaphylactic shock also receives special attention.

- *Patient assessment.* How to take a patient's vital signs including blood pressure and pulse oximetry are included in the patient assessment chapters.

- *Communications and documentation.* A full chapter is devoted to these two topics and, along with the basic facts required by the DOT curriculum, includes effective verbal and written communication, as well as the legal implications associated with the written prehospital care report.

- *Splinting.* From self-splinting an injured finger to immobilizing an injured femur, splinting is included in the chapter on musculoskeletal injuries.

- *Immobilization.* From manual stabilization to complete immobilization on a long backboard, protecting a trauma patient's spine is detailed in the spine injury chapter.

- *Water emergencies.* This chapter includes key components of scene size-up and the hazards involved in water rescues, assessing and providing care to a patient in the water, ice rescues, and diving emergencies.

Among the other enrichment topics in the book, you'll find bites and stings, psychological emergencies and crises intervention (including rape), complications of pregnancy and delivery, geriatric patients, agricultural and industrial emergencies, safety for emergency vehicles, special rescue situations, first response to terrorist incidents, and so much more. To find all the enrichment in *First Responder: A Skills Approach,* look at the list of objectives at the beginning of every chapter for the "Enrichment" topics.

We believe that you will be pleased with the seventh edition of *First Responder: A Skills Approach.* We welcome your comments, which may be mailed to:

Marketing Manager
BRADY PUBLISHING
One Lake Street
Upper Saddle River, NJ 07458

You may contact the authors via email at **danlimmer@mac.com**

American Heart Association
2005 Guidelines for CPR and ECC
Highlights and Rationales

A Greater Emphasis on Effective Chest Compressions

During cardiac arrest there is virtually no blood flow. The less that compressions are interrupted the better the circulation to the vital organs such as the brain and heart.

- Compressions should be delivered hard and fast at a rate of about 100 per minute for all patients.
- A single compression to ventilation ratio of 30:2 is recommended for all single rescuers for all patients. This was changed to increase blood flow to the heart and to simplify the skill of CPR.
- The chest should be allowed to fully recoil after each compression. It is known that incomplete recoil of the chest results in less blood flow through the heart.

Opening the Airway

Due to the importance of an open and clear airway during resuscitation, it is essential that the rescuer do whatever is necessary to ensure an open airway. When caring for trauma patients in cardiac arrest, attempt the jaw-thrust maneuver first. If unable to establish an adequate airway, then perform the head-tilt/chin-lift maneuver.

Less of an Emphasis on Rescue Breaths

Blood flow to the lungs in a cardiac-arrest patient is greatly reduced, so the need for oxygen is much less as well. In addition, time taken away from compressions to provide rescue breaths is more harmful. Therefore, rescue breaths should be given at a rate of 10 to 12 breaths per minute for an adult and 12 to 20 breaths per minute for a child or infant. Due to this reduced emphasis on ventilations, each breath should now be delivered over one second and produce visible chest rise.

When an advanced airway is in place, ventilations should be delivered at a rate of 8 to 10 per minute.

When Attempting Defibrillation

When indicated, all rescuers should deliver a single shock followed by two minutes of CPR beginning with compressions. CPR should continue for approximately two minutes (5 cycles), at which time the rescuer should recheck for signs of circulation. These changes were driven by three primary findings:

- There were long delays before rescuers were delivering the first shock.
- When using the latest AEDs, the first shock can eliminate fibrillation up to 85% of the time.
- Even when a shock eliminates fibrillation, it takes time for the heart to begin pumping again. A brief period of compressions can deliver valuable oxygen and blood to the heart muscle itself. There is no evidence to suggest that compressions following defibrillation will cause VF.

Pediatric Guidelines

Children are now defined by developmental signs and not so much by age. For purposes of CPR a child is anyone from the age of one to the onset of puberty. This can be determined by the presence of armpit hair in young males and the development of breasts in young women.

When two rescuers are present the compression ventilation ratio should be 15:2 for infants and children.

Tailor the Response to the Probable Cause

If a patient of any age has suffered cardiac arrest from a hypoxic (lack of sufficient oxygen) cause such as drowning, the lone rescuer should provide immediate CPR for two minutes before leaving the victim to activate EMS and obtain an AED.

Acknowledgments

This textbook is the result of the efforts and cooperation of many people. As authors we create a vision for our textbook, determine an organization, establish a writing style, and of course present the information. In the complex process of text development, we look to many others for assistance.

Medical Editor

We would like to express special appreciation to our medical editor, Edward Dickinson, MD, NREMT-P, FACEP, who provided essential review and advice to ensure accuracy throughout the text. He was always available for questions. His energy, dedication, and knowledge of medicine and field procedures were indispensable. Dr. Dickinson is currently Associate Professor and Director of EMS Field Operations in the Department of Emergency Medicine of the University of Pennsylvania School of Medicine in Philadelphia. He is Medical Director of the Malvern Fire Company, the Berwyn Fire Company, and the Township of Haverford paramedics in Pennsylvania. He is a residency-trained, board-certified emergency medicine physician who is a Fellow of the American College of Emergency Physicians.

Dr. Dickinson began his career in emergency services in 1979 as a firefighter-EMT in upstate New York. He has remained active in fire service and EMS for the past 26 years. He frequently rides with EMS units and has maintained his certification as a National Registry EMT-Paramedic.

He has served as medical editor for numerous Brady EMT-B and First Responder texts and is the author of *Fire Service Emergency Care* and co-author of *Emergency Care, Fire Service Edition,* and *Emergency Incident Rehabilitation.* He is co-editor of *ALS Case Studies in Emergency Care.*

Contributors

To those who contributed chapters to the seventh edition, thank you. Jon Politis and Andy Stern prepared material reflecting up-to-date standards. We are pleased to have each on our team of contributors.

Jon Politis
  Director, Emergency Medical Services
  Colonie, NY

Andy Stern
  Senior Paramedic,
  Colonie EMS Department,
  Colonie, NY

Reviewers

The following reviewers provided helpful perspective and suggestions. Our thanks to all.

David K. Anderson, BS, EMT-P
  Director, Paramedic Education
  NW Regional Training Center
  Vancouver, WA

John L. Beckman, AA
  FF/EMT-P Instructor
  Affiliated with Addison
    Fire Protection District
  Fire Science Instructor, Technology
    Center of DuPage
  Addison, IL

Cheryl Blazek, EMT-P
  EMS Training Program Coordinator
  Southwestern Community College
  Creston, IA

Jodi L. Braswell, NR, EMT-I
  Jackson, GA

Steve Brumm, MS, EMT
  Gulf Coast Community College
  Panama City, FL

Diana Cave, RN, MSN
  Portland Community College
  Institute for Health Professionals
  Portland, OR

Jerry Chaney, A.A.S., EMT-P
  Coastal Carolina Community College
  Jacksonville, NC

Mark Dixon
  FF/Paramedic Columbus Fire Dept.
  EMT Coordinator/C-Tec Adult
  Education
  Newark, OH

James W. Fox, EMT-P
  Emergency Medical Services
    Assistant Coordinator
  Des Moines Fire Department
  Des Moines, IA

Roberta S. Gearhardt, RN, BSN, EMT-P
  J & T Applications, Inc.
  Beaver Creek, OH

Janie Gunnell
  Florida State Fire College
  Fernandina Beach, FL

Christopher J. Hafley, FF/EMT-P, EMSI
  EHOVE Adult Career Center
  Public Safety Department
  Milan, OH

Elizabeth "Bunny" Hearn
  Captain, Augusta County Fire-Rescue
  Verona, VA

Lawrence W. Hepburn
  Torrington Fire Department
  Torrington, CT

Attila Hertelendy, MHSM,
    NREMT-P, CCEMT-P
  University of Mississippi
    Medical Center
  Department of Health Sciences
  Jackson, MS

Jordan J. Khoury, NREMT-B
SPCI
Taunton, MA

Ken Krupich, NREMT-P
Operations Manager
Fargo-Moorhead Ambulance Service
Fargo, ND

Jeff Och
Carver Fire & Rescue Department
Carver, MN

John L. Peters, Jr., EMT-P
Amarillo, TX

Mark W. Schooley
President, Emergency Response
Technologies, Inc.
Rives Junction, MI

John M. Slider, EMT-I
Instructor/Coordinator
Matrix Training Center, LLC
Carson City, NV

Jeff Travers
Great Oaks Institute
Cincinnati, OH

Jonathan D. Ward
Mid-Coast Maine EMS
Union, ME

Photo Acknowledgments

Photo credits are presented under individual photographs. All other photographs were taken on assignment for Brady/Prentice Hall/Pearson Education.

Organizations

We wish to thank the following organizations for their valuable assistance in creating the photo program for this edition:

American Medical Response
Eric Polan, Director of Operations
Dean Anderson, Operations
Manager
Sonoma/Marin, California

REACH Air Medical Services
Jim Adams, CEO
Santa Rosa, CA

Santa Rosa Junior College
Ken Bradford, Director of
EMC Programs
Santa Rosa, CA

Sonoma County Sheriffs Department
Sgt. Scott Dunn
Sonoma County, CA

Rincon Valley Fire Department
Chief Doug Williams
Santa Rosa, CA

Windsor Fire Department
Chief Ron Collier
Windsor, CA

Technical Advisors

Thanks to the following people for providing valuable technical support during the photo shoots:

John Martin, EMT-B
Sonoma County Search and Rescue
Sonoma County, CA

Scott R Snyder, EMT-P
Folsom, CA

Ted Williams, EMT-B
Sonoma Life Support
Santa Rosa, CA

Photo Assistant/Digital post-production: Sam Willard, Berkeley, CA

Dear Instructor:

Brady, your partner in education, is pleased to present the 7th edition of our best-selling text *First Responder: A Skills Approach*. This revision is one of the most exciting we've ever worked on and represents the efforts of many people. Our mission for this text is simple—it's about *Skills for Life*. Your role as a First Responder is an extremely important one, as you are the one who will arrive first at an emergency scene. The skills you learn through this text program may well make a critical difference in the lives of others. These are skills for life also in the sense that they represent for you a precious body of lifelong knowledge and understanding. We're proud of your decision to train as a First Responder, and we strive to provide you the strongest possible foundation to do so.

The following Walkthrough outlines the features found in each chapter. We've retained the tried-and-true and added some new ones based on what we've discovered works in educational publishing. The Walkthrough also provides information for each of our student and instructor supplements, which have been reviewed and updated extensively. We introduce several related products that can be used to make your program the best it can be. We are truly proud to be able to offer you a complete set of resources for education.

First Responder: A Skills Approach continues to offer the high-quality content and innovation you've come to know and trust from Brady. We are proud of our tradition of bringing to EMS education the highest standards of writing, development, production, and service that our customers expect and deserve.

After all, it is our responsibility to present you with….skills for life.

Sincerely,

Julie Levin Alexander
VP, Publisher

Marlene McHugh Pratt
Executive Editor

Lois Berlowitz
Senior Managing Editor

Katrin Beacom
Executive Marketing Manager

Thomas Kennally
National Sales Manager

Monica Moosang
Associate Editor

A Guide to Key Features: SKILLS FOR LIFE

*The Call

A true-to-life scenario draws students into the reading and offers a link between text content and real-life experiences. The scenario stops short of resolution, which is found in *The Call Follow-up* at the end of the chapter.

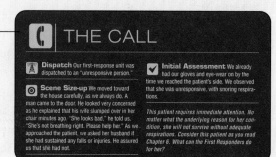

THE CALL

Dispatch Our first-response unit was dispatched to an "unresponsive person."

Scene Size-up We moved toward the house carefully, as we always do. A man came to the door. He looked very concerned as he explained that his wife slumped over in her chair minutes ago. "She looks bad," he told us. "She's not breathing right. Please help her." As we approached the patient, we asked her husband if she had sustained any falls or injuries. He assured us that she had not.

Initial Assessment We already had our gloves and eye-wear on by the time we reached the patient's side. We observed that she was unresponsive, with snoring respirations.

This patient requires immediate attention. No matter what the underlying reason for her condition, she will not survive without adequate respirations. Consider this patient as you read Chapter 6. What can the First Responders do for her?

▶▶ The Call Follow-up

At the beginning of this chapter, you read that First Responders were called to help an unresponsive adult with snoring respirations. To see how they responded to this emergency, read the following. It describes how the call was completed.

Initial Assessment *(continued)* Since it was not possible to assess the patient's airway while she was slumped in a chair, we quickly but carefully moved her to the floor. My partner, Pete, immediately performed a head-tilt/chin-lift maneuver. It eliminated the snoring sounds.

Pete suctioned the airway to remove the built up secretions. Mrs. Constantino didn't have a gag reflex, so she accepted the oropharyngeal airway well.

Our assessment of her breathing revealed minimal chest movement and slow respirations. She also was beginning to show signs of blue coloring around her lips. Realizing that Mrs. Constantino was breathing inadequately and her pulse was rapid and weak, we ventilated her using a pocket face mask with one-way valve and supplemental oxygen.

Physical Examination We believed that Mrs. Constantino had a medical problem rather than a traumatic condition, but I wanted to be sure. So I did a quick physical examination while my partner

continued to assist ventilations. There were no signs of injury on her head, neck, chest, abdomen, or extremities. Her pulse was 96 and bounding. The respiratory rate was 8 and shallow.

Patient History Mr. Constantino told us that his wife had a heart attack several years ago. She takes medications for her heart and high blood pressure. She had complained of a headache about an hour before she became unresponsive. She ate breakfast earlier. She has no allergies.

Ongoing Assessment Our primary focus was on making sure Mrs. Constantino was ventilated properly. We also checked her pulse frequently. Her pulse on our second check was 104, bounding and regular. Her respirations were about 6 and shallow, being assisted.

Patient Hand-off We had the airway under control when the paramedics arrived. The pa[tient's] color had improved. Her pulse also had [calmed] a bit. Pete gave them the hand-off report.

I saw Mr. Constantino in the grocery [store re]cently. He told me that his wife had [had a] stroke. She remained in the hospital for [days] and was eventually moved to a rehabilit[ation]. I hope she will be able to go home soo[n].

*The Call Follow-up and Hand-off Report

The Call Follow-up describes how the call was completed. A sample First Responder *Hand-off Report* for each chapter call is highlighted.

Hand-off Report

"This is Mrs. Constantino. She is 74 years old. She had a headache about an hour ago. She was found by her husband slumped over in a chair. We moved her to the floor and found that she had inadequate ventilations. We began assisting with a pocket mask and oxygen. She groans with loud verbal stimulus. Her respiratory rate was about 6, pulse 104 and bounding. She has a history of heart attack and high blood pressure. She ate breakfast. She has no allergies."

*First On Scene

New! This special feature focuses on the responsibilities of First Responders, who are the first medically trained rescuers on scene.

First on Scene

CPR is a procedure that can help circulate blood and oxygen when a patient's heart has stopped. It helps keep the patient viable until defibrillation and advanced care becomes available. Alone, it will rarely start a stopped heart. Unfortunately, not all patients can be saved. If you perform CPR on a patient who ultimately dies, remember that it is not your fault. All you can do is perform CPR to the best of your ability. If you respond to a call where a patient dies—and that will happen—be sure to talk about it with someone you trust and, if needed, seek out stress counseling.

First Responder Practice

When it comes to ventilation, more is *not* better. The American Heart Association (AHA) guidelines require ventilations to be given at about one second each and in an amount that makes the chest rise visibly. The reason is this: when ventilations are too forceful or have too much volume, air goes into the stomach. This causes gastric distention and vomiting in the patient. Vomiting causes airway problems and aspiration, which can kill the patient through infection and pneumonia.

*First Reponder Practice

New! Continuing the focus on real-life experience, this special feature highlights actual practice and experiences of today's First Responders.

A Guide to Key Features: PATIENT ASSESSMENT AND FIRST RESPONDER CARE

256 MODULE 6 | **Illness and Injury**

First on Scene

Sudden cardiac death is a death that occurs within two hours of the onset of symptoms. Unfortunately, the average time for a person to recognize symptoms and seek some sort of care is four to six hours. This means that lives could be saved by simply recognizing the problem and seeking help immediately.

and care of a patient with chest pain will be the same, no matter what the actual cause.

Patient Assessment

The general signs and symptoms of a cardiac emergency are as follows (Figure 14-3):

- Chest pain or discomfort described as heaviness or squeezing. The sensation also may radiate to the arms, shoulder, neck, or jaw.
- Difficulty breathing, shortness of breath.
- Unusual pulse (rapid, weak, slow, or irregular).
- Palpitations.
- Indigestion, nausea, vomiting.
- Sweating.
- Skin color, including mucous membranes, may be pale, gray, or cyanotic.
- Feeling of impending doom.
- History of heart problems or a previous similar experience.

Note that many patients experience a "silent" heart attack. This means that these patients do not experience the classic pain patterns. Patients who have diabetes, those who are elderly, and women may not experience pain. Instead, difficulty breathing and a feeling of weakness are the most common presenting symptoms.

As soon as you recognize a possible cardiac emergency, update the incoming EMS unit. Request advanced care if it is available in your area. Remember that a patient with chest pain will be very anxious. He may feel as if he is going to die. This requires compassion and reassurance. Make sure he understands that everything that can possibly be done is being done. Advise him and his family that further help is on the way and that he will be transported promptly to a medical facility.

Later, when you take the patient's history, use OPQRRRST as a memory aid to help you get a good description of the pain. Each letter identifies an important area of questioning:

O—*Onset.* When did the pain begin?
P—*Provocation.* Did anything cause or start the pain (exercise, an activity)?
Q—*Quality.* What is the pain like (crushing, stabbing, etc.)?
R—*Region.* Where is the pain?
R—*Radiation.* Does the pain begin in one place and then seem to travel somewhere else?
R—*Relief.* Does anything relieve the pain?
S—*Severity.* On a scale of 1–10, with 10 the worst, how bad is the pain?
T—*Time.* How long have you had the pain?

When you perform a physical exam, palpate the chest for DOTS (deformities, open injuries, tenderness, swelling). Make a note if your touch causes pain. If you are trained to do so, listen to the lungs to determine if air is moving in and out of both sides equally. ■

First Responder Care

To provide care to a patient with chest pain or discomfort, follow these steps:

1. *Place the patient in a position of comfort.* This is usually a semi-reclining or sitting position. Also have him cease all movement.
2. *Ensure adequate breathing.* See that the airway is open. If breathing is adequate, administer high-flow oxygen with a nonrebreather mask. If breathing is not adequate, assist ventilations with a BVM and supplemental oxygen.
3. *Loosen tight clothing.*
4. *Maintain body temperature* as close to normal as possible.
5. *Continually monitor the patient.* He may become unstable rapidly. Be alert for changes in the patient's mental status and be prepared to perform CPR with supplementary oxygen, if possible, and to use an AED.

Your patient may tell you that he has had heart surgery or that he has a **pacemaker** or an implanted defibrillator. (An implanted defibrillator delivers shocks to a patient but at much less power than an AED.) Treat these patients in the same way as described above. Note that a malfunctioning pacemaker may cause a slow heart rhythm. If this occurs, monitor the patient carefully. Provide oxygen and be prepared to administer CPR if necessary.

Specific Cardiac Conditions

Two problems are commonly caused by coronary artery disease. They are *angina pectoris,* sometimes called *angina,* and *myocardial infarction,* the medical term for heart attack.

---

*Patient Assessment

Discussions of patient assessment present the signs and symptoms of particular injuries or disorders. These are clearly written, with important points often bulleted.

Injuries to the Chest, Abdomen, and Genitalia | CHAPTER 20 **377**

Section 2 Injuries to the Abdomen

A wound that penetrates the skin and abdominal cavity is a dangerous one. Internal bleeding may occur. Bacteria may be introduced into the abdomen from the outside as well as from a penetrated intestine (Figure 20-10). In the presence of open wounds of the abdomen, assume that internal organs have been damaged. Closed abdominal injuries, such as a severe blow or crushing injury, can be extremely dangerous and lead to internal bleeding and shock.

(Now may be a good time to review the four quadrants of the abdomen as described in Chapter 4.)

Patient Assessment

To assess for a closed abdominal injury, have the patient lie down on his or her back. The knees should be flexed and supported. Remove or loosen clothing over the abdomen to expose it. Then look and feel for signs of injury. Look for bruising, lacerations and other open wounds, impaled objects, and protruding organs. Watch how the abdomen moves as the patient breathes. Gently feel all four quadrants. Note rigidity, pain, and tenderness. Also note any guarding, a common reaction to a painful abdomen. If the patient complains of pain in a particular area, palpate that area last. If the area is palpated first, it may prevent accurate palpation of the remaining quadrants.

Suspect abdominal injuries in patients involved in fights, falls, and car crashes. The most common symptom is pain. In addition to open wounds such as an evisceration, general signs and symptoms of an injured abdomen include:

- Distended or irregularly shaped abdomen.
- Bruising of the abdomen, back, or flanks.
- Rigid and tender abdomen.

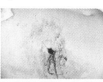

FIGURE 20-10 **A patient with an open wound to the abdomen.** *(Charles Stewart, M.D. & Associates)*

FIGURE 20-11 **Patient guarding a painful abdomen.**

- Mild discomfort progressing to intolerable pain.
- Pain radiating to a shoulder, both shoulders, or the back.
- Abdominal cramping.
- Lying still with legs drawn up (Figure 20-11).
- Rapid, shallow breathing.
- Rapid pulse, low blood pressure.
- Nausea, vomiting.
- Blood in the urine, vomiting of blood.
- Shock.
- Weakness.
- Thirst.

Remember to communicate with empathy. Your attitude toward the patient will have an impact, so put his or her needs first. Stay calm, cool, and sympathetic. ■

First Responder Care

To provide care to a patient with abdominal injuries, make your top priorities airway, breathing, and circulation. Once the ABCs are assessed and life-threats treated, update or activate EMS immediately to arrange for transport.

1. *Maintain an open airway.* Be alert for vomiting. Position the patient for adequate drainage. Be prepared to suction. Do not give the patient anything to eat or drink.
2. *If breathing is adequate, administer oxygen via nonrebreather.* If it is inadequate, assist ventilations with BVM and supplemental oxygen. Be prepared to provide basic life support, if needed.
3. *Suspect and treat for shock.* Work diligently to prevent it. Keep the patient warm, but do not overheat. Administer high-concentration oxygen, if you are allowed.
4. *Control external bleeding.* Dress open wounds with dry, sterile dressings or follow local protocol.

---

*First Responder Care

Treatment for medical and trauma emergencies is uniformly presented in step-by-step format.

---

5. *Position the patient.* The patient usually is most comfortable lying on his or her back with knees flexed. If you suspect a pelvic fracture, prevent movement. Immobilize the patient on a long backboard if possible.

If there is an abdominal evisceration, you must cover the exposed organs (Figure 20-12). Never touch exposed organs. Never try to replace them. Instead, use a thick, moist, sterile dressing to cover them completely. You should moisten the dressing with sterile saline. Never use absorbent materials as dressings, such as toilet tissue or paper towels, which can shred and cling to the organs. Gently and loosely tape the moist dressing in place. Then, loosely cover it with an occlusive dressing. Tape down the edges to help keep the first dressing moist and warm.

...e exposed organs with a

Maintain the temperature of the wound area by covering the dressing with layers of dressings such as a particle-free bath blanket or towel. They may be held loosely in place with a bandage or clean sheet. ■

Q
1. What is the most common symptom of abdominal injury?

2. What are three other signs and symptoms associated with abdominal injury?

3. What is First Responder care for a patient with abdominal injuries?

A Guide to Key Features: A SKILLS APPROACH

*Skill Summaries

These features provide a step-by-step visual presentation of how to perform skill procedures.

cessful. Deliver each thrust with the intent of relieving the obstruction. It may take as many as five or more thrusts to succeed. Continue with thrusts until the item is dislodged or the patient becomes unconscious.

Responsive Adult. If the patient is responsive, perform the Heimlich maneuver as follows (Figure 7-13):

1. *Get in position.* Stand behind the patient. Wrap your arms around his waist. Keep your elbows out, away from his ribs.

2. *Position your hands.* Make a fist with one hand. Place the thumb side of the fist on the middle of the abdomen slightly above the navel and well below the xiphoid process.

3. *Perform an abdominal thrust.* First, grasp your fist with your other hand, thumbs toward the patient. Then press your fist into the patient's abdomen with a quick inward and upward thrust.

4. If the first thrust does not dislodge the foreign body, make each new thrust separate and distinct. Continue

SKILL SUMMARY *Foreign Body Airway Obstruction—Responsive Adult*

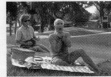

FIGURE 7-13A The universal sign of choking.

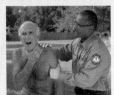

FIGURE 7-13B Determine if the patient can speak or cough by asking, "Are you choking?"

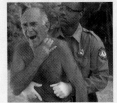

FIGURE 7-13C If so, perform the Heimlich maneuver to dislodge the object.

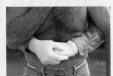

FIGURE 7-13D Hand position for Heimlich maneuver.

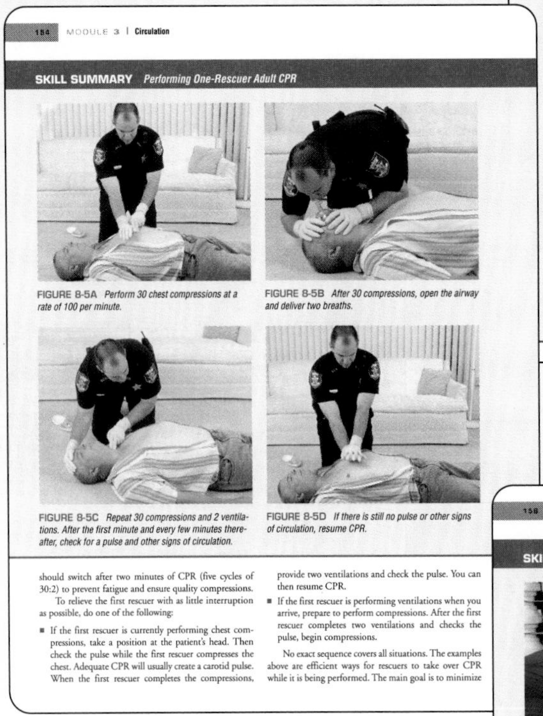

SKILL SUMMARY *Performing One-Rescuer Adult CPR*

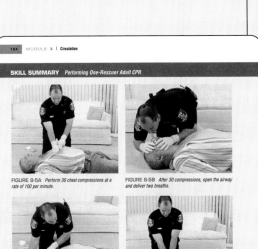

FIGURE 8-5A Perform 30 chest compressions at a rate of 100 per minute.

FIGURE 8-5B After 30 compressions, open the airway and deliver two breaths.

FIGURE 8-5C Repeat 30 compressions and 2 ventilations. After the first minute and every few minutes thereafter, check for a pulse and other signs of circulation.

FIGURE 8-5D If there is still no pulse or other signs of circulation, resume CPR.

should switch after two minutes of CPR (five cycles of 30:2) to prevent fatigue and ensure quality compressions.

To relieve the first rescuer with as little interruption as possible, do one of the following:

- If the first rescuer is currently performing chest compressions, take a position at the patient's head. Then check the pulse while the first rescuer compresses the chest. Adequate CPR will usually create a carotid pulse. When the first rescuer completes the compressions,

provide two ventilations and check the pulse. You can then resume CPR.

- If the first rescuer is performing ventilations when you arrive, prepare to perform compressions. After the first rescuer completes two ventilations and checks the pulse, begin compressions.

No exact sequence covers all situations. The examples above are efficient ways for rescuers to take over CPR while it is being performed. The main goal is to minimize

---

SKILL SUMMARY *Performing Two-Rescuer Adult CPR*

FIGURE 8-6A Two rescuers get in position, one at the head and one at the patient's side.

FIGURE 8-6B The rescuer at the side performs 30 chest compressions at a rate of 100 per minute.

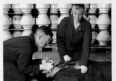
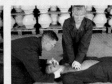

FIGURE 8-6C After every 30 compressions, the rescuer at the head delivers two breaths.

FIGURE 8-6D After the first minute of CPR and every few minutes thereafter, the rescuer at the head checks the patient's pulse. If there is no pulse or no other sign of circulation, they resume CPR.

should check the carotid artery for 5–10 seconds after two minutes of CPR and every few minutes thereafter. Note that the pulse must be checked when CPR is not in progress.

In general, CPR should be interrupted for no more than 10 seconds. One of the few exceptions to this rule applies to moving a patient. It may not be possible to perform CPR in a cramped bedroom or other small area. In that case, it is acceptable to move the patient so proper CPR can be performed. These actions must be kept as close to 10 seconds as possible.

Signs of Successful CPR

Signs of successful CPR include the following:

- Each time the sternum is compressed, you should feel a pulse in the carotid artery. It will feel like a flutter.
- Chest should rise and fall with each ventilation.
- Pupils may react or appear to be normal. (Pupils should constrict when exposed to light.)
- Heartbeat may return.
- Spontaneous gasp of breathing may occur.
- Skin color may improve or return to normal.

A Guide to Key Features: ENHANCED VISUALS

*Illustrations

Updated art and photos help to explain and enhance chapter content.

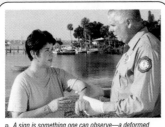

a. *A sign is something one can observe—a deformed wrist, for example.*

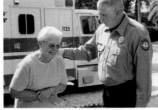

b. *A symptom is something the patient feels and describes, such as a stomach ache.*

FIGURE 12-26 Use the terms "signs" and "symptoms" correctly.

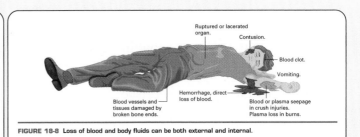

FIGURE 18-8 Loss of blood and body fluids can be both external and internal.

*Tables

Tables summarize and condense difficult or complex subjects. Some contain photos to enhance and better explain content.

TABLE 6-3 **Respiratory Status and First Responder Care**

Respiratory Status	Signs	First Responder Care	
Breathing adequately.	• Rate and depth of breathing are normal. • No abnormal breath sounds. • Air moves freely in and out of the chest. • Skin color appears to be normal.	Monitor the patient's breathing for any changes. If allowed, also administer oxygen by nonrebreather or nasal cannula.	
Breathing inadequately. Patient is moving some air in and out but breathing is slow or shallow and not enough to sustain life.	• Rate and/or depth of breathing not within normal range. • Shallow breathing. • Diminished or absent breath sounds. • Noises with breathing such as crowing, stridor, snoring, gurgling, or gasping. • Blue or gray skin color (cyanosis). • Decreased minute volume.	Assist ventilations. If allowed, also administer supplemental oxygen during ventilation by way of a pocket face mask or bag-valve mask.	
No breathing at all.	• No chest rise. • No evidence of air being moved from the mouth or nose. • No breath sounds.	Provide ventilations. If allowed, also administer supplemental oxygen during ventilation by way of a pocket face mask or bag-valve mask.	

A Guide to Key Features: EXPANDED CHAPTER REVIEW

*Focus on the EMS Team

New! Presents the chapter topic in the context of working as a team member.

*Summing Up

New! Provides students with a thorough review of chapter content.

*Key Terms

New! Will help students master new terminology.

*Knowledge Check

Expanded! Asks students to recall and apply the principles they've just learned through multiple-choice, true/false, short-answer, and matching questions.

*Scenario

New! Provides the opportunity to decide on treatment and care in real-life situations.

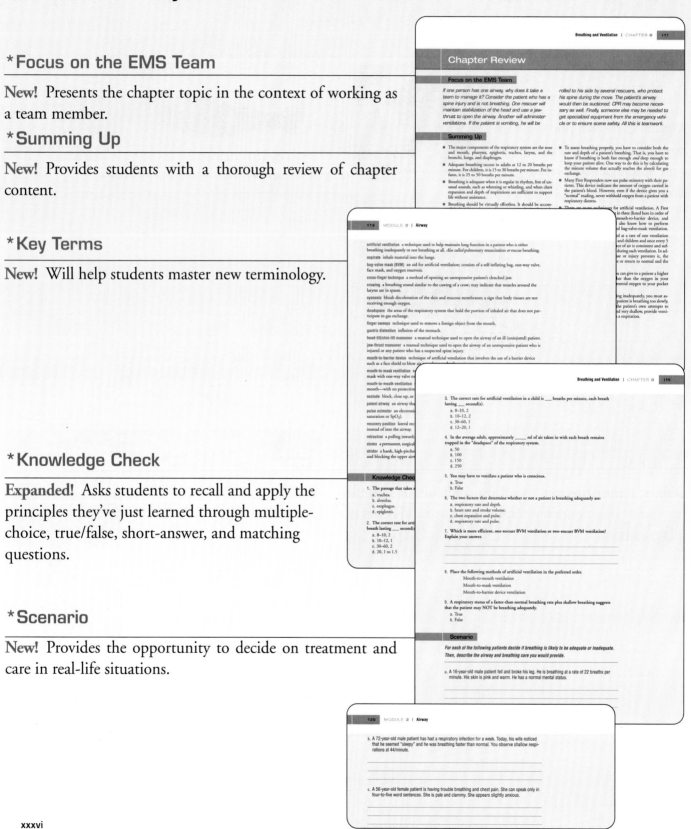

A Guide to Key Features: STUDENT CD

A **New!** Student CD contains quizzes, virtual tours, games and puzzles, scene size-up and hazmat exercise, documentation practice, and much more!

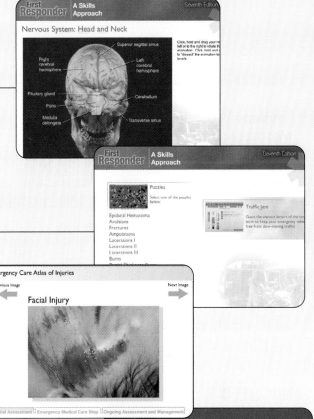

*Virtual Tours

Including airway, the nervous sytem, cardiovascular system, musculoskeletal system, and heart, these narrated tours guide you through the intricate workings of body systems in an easy-to-understand presentation.

*Games and Puzzles

Crosswords, Hangman, and Traffic Jam games make learning terminology easy and fun.

*Atlas of Injuries

Trauma photos are presented with information on assessment, care steps, and ongoing assessment.

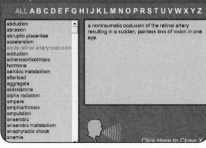

*Audio Glossary

Terms are accompanied by an audio pronunciation and text definition.

Also....

*Scene Size-up
Tests student ability by flashing scenes on screen and asking students to answer questions regarding the number of patients, resource determination, BSI precautions, scene safety, and mechanism of injury.

*Hazmat Exercise
Presents a hazmat situation. Students can zoom in on hazmat signs and access Hazmat Guidebook pages to properly identify tasks.

*Quizzes
Multiple-choice quizzes for each chapter help to reinforce knowledge.

*Documentation
Uses drag-and-drop forms that allow students to properly fill out prehospital care reports.

A Guide to Key Features: TEACHING AND LEARNING PACKAGE

FOR THE STUDENT

In addition to the **Student CD,...**

*Student Workbook

(0-13-195811-9)

Contains key ideas, multiple-choice questions, short-answer review questions, vocabulary practice, scenarios with questions, and active learning exercises.

*Companion Website

Check out the companion website at ***www.prenhall.com/limmer***. You will find resources such as chapter review quizzes with immediate scoring and feedback, anatomy and physiology labeling exercises, annotated links to appropriate EMS resources, case studies, and an audio glossary.

*For Review and Reference

Pocket Reference for BLS Providers, 3rd ed.
(0-13-173730-9)

This handy field reference is on water-resistant paper and includes skills checklists, abbreviations and acronyms, and anatomy charts. It has been updated to meet AHA 2005 Guidelines.

First Responder Achieve: Test Preparation
(0-13-198894-8)

On-line test preparation for the First Responder. Take practice quizzes and tests and immediately get results. Check it out at ***www.prenhall.com/emtachieve.***

Review Manual for the First Responder
(0-13-118439-3)

This is the resource to help students pass certification exams. All items are written and reviewed by educators and offer proven, authoritative information.

FOR THE INSTRUCTOR

*Instructor's Resource Manual

(0-13-195810-0)

Includes Transition Guides to assist instructors in moving to this 7th edition text; lecture outlines; teaching tips; media and reading references; handouts for evaluation and reinforcement.

*TestGen

(0-13-195812-7)

Thoroughly reviewed and updated. Contains hundreds of exam-style questions, as well as references to DOT objectives and text pages where answers can be found or supported.

*PowerPoints

(0-13-188901-X)

New PowerPoint slide program provides the basis of dynamic classroom presentations.

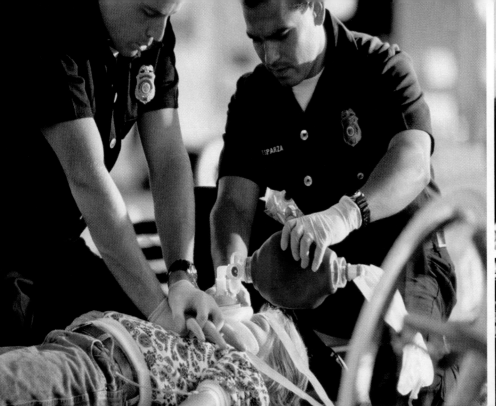
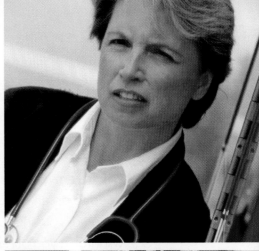
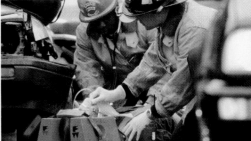

1 | Introduction to the EMS System

Objectives

From the U.S. Department of Transportation (DOT) 1995 "First Responder: National Standard Curriculum." Material that supplements the DOT curriculum is listed under "Enrichment."

Cognitive

1-1.1 ▶ Define the components of the Emergency Medical Services (EMS) systems. (p. 7)

1-1.2 ▶ Differentiate the roles and responsibilities of the First Responder from other out-of-hospital care providers. (pp. 4–6, 8–9)

1-1.3 ▶ Define *medical oversight* and discuss the First Responder's role in the process. (p. 9)

1-1.4 ▶ Discuss the types of medical oversight that may affect the medical care of a First Responder. (p. 9)

1-1.5 ▶ State the specific statutes and regulations in your state regarding the EMS system. (p. 9)

Affective

1-1.6 ▶ Accept and uphold the responsibilities of a First Responder in accordance with the standards of an EMS professional. (pp. 8–9)

1-1.7 ▶ Explain the rationale for maintaining a professional appearance when on duty or when responding to calls. (p. 9)

1-1.8 ▶ Describe why it is inappropriate to judge a patient based on a cultural, gender, age, or socioeconomic model, and to vary the standard of care rendered as a result of that judgment. (p. 9)

Psychomotor

No objectives are identified by the DOT.

Enrichment

▶ Describe the various methods by which the public can access EMS. (p. 4)

Introduction

You are about to join a vitally important profession. As a First Responder, you can make a difference. Sometimes you will perform medical techniques that save a life. Other times, your presence and reassurance will comfort your patient until the ambulance arrives. This course will help you gain the knowledge, skills, and attitudes you need to be an effective First Responder.

To begin, your instructor will describe what you can expect in the course. He or she will inform you of required immunizations and physical exams and outline your state and local certification requirements. Your instructor also will explain local policies concerning the Americans with Disabilities Act (ADA) and the implications of harassment in the classroom environment.

Section 1 Emergency Medical Services (EMS)

Since the Vietnam War, emergency medical personnel have called the time immediately after an injury the "Golden Hour." This is when lives that hang in the balance can be saved by proper emergency care. Too often those who arrive first at an emergency scene lack medical training. As a result, patients who might have been saved either suffer permanent disability or die.

The **emergency medical services (EMS) system** is a network of resources linked together for one purpose. That purpose is to provide emergency care and transport to victims of sudden illness or injury (Figure 1-1). For

THE CALL

Dispatch We were dispatched to a woman with chest pain. As a new First Responder, I felt very nervous, especially with the lights and siren on.

Scene Size-up Once we arrived on scene, my partner turned off the lights and siren. We grabbed protective gloves and, when we saw it was safe, left our rig. We kept alert for signs of danger as we got closer to the house.

Initial Assessment Inside the house, we saw our patient sitting on a chair, pale and sweaty. Immediately we began to assess her ABCs—airway, breathing, and circula-

tion. She was in serious condition. I radioed the dispatcher to update the incoming unit and requested the paramedics. My partner gave oxygen to the patient while keeping her and her husband calm.

You will encounter a wide range of calls as a First Responder. Some may be medical calls such as this one. Others may involve trauma (injury). You will learn how these First Responders handled their patient's emergency at the end of this chapter. In the meantime, think about this question: What roles and responsibilities do you think the First Responders will have in the continuing care of this patient?

SKILL SUMMARY *An EMS Call*

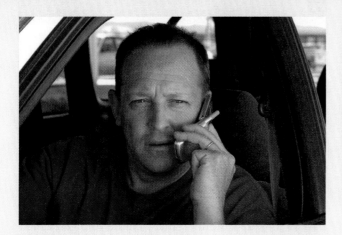

FIGURE 1-1A *A citizen recognizes an emergency and calls for help.*

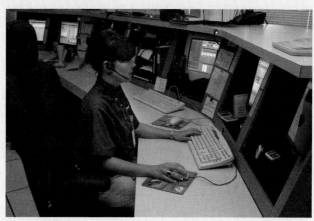

FIGURE 1-1B *In response to the 9–1–1 call, EMS dispatch sends a First Responder to the scene.*

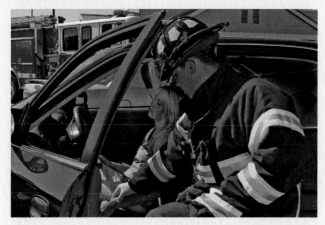

FIGURE 1-1C *When the First Responder arrives, he assesses the situation and initiates patient care.*

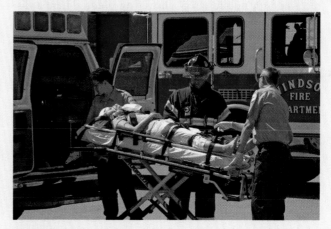

FIGURE 1-1D *Other EMS personnel respond as needed and transfer from First Responder care to EMT care takes place.*

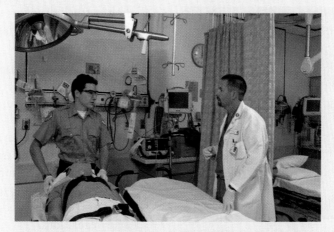

FIGURE 1-1E *The EMTs then take the patient to the appropriate medical facility's emergency department, where the medical staff takes over patient care.*

example, when an emergency occurs, a citizen at the scene recognizes it and calls for help. If the citizen has dialed 9–1–1 or another emergency number, he or she may receive patient care instructions from an EMS dispatcher. When First Responders arrive, they assess the situation and take over care. They also inform dispatch of any need for additional EMS resources. Usually, EMS personnel with higher levels of training are called to the scene. They continue care and transport the patient to the hospital. There, patient care transfers to emergency department personnel and, finally, to the in-hospital care system.

Access to EMS

There are two general systems by which the public can access EMS: **9–1–1** and **non-9–1–1.** Often called the "universal number," 9–1–1 is used in most areas to call for police, fire, rescue, and ambulance services. Such calls are received at a public safety answering point. There a dispatcher decides which service to activate and alerts that service (Figure 1-2).

Non-9–1–1 systems use regular seven-digit phone numbers. Callers must phone the specific service they need (police, fire, and so on) or, in some areas, a dispatch center. Probably the most serious drawback of a non-9–1–1 system is the delay in reaching the appropriate services.

In contrast, calling 9–1–1, the universal number, offers two main benefits. First, the public safety answering point generally is staffed by trained dispatchers. They may offer medical advice over the phone while the patient waits for rescuers to arrive. This is referred to as "emergency medical dispatching." Second,

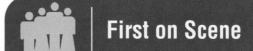

First on Scene

The First Responder is only one of the trained rescuers on the EMS team. All four nationally recognized levels of training are:

- First Responder.
- EMT-Basic.
- EMT-Intermediate.
- EMT-Paramedic.

a universal number minimizes delay. Callers do not have to look up a number, and even the youngest callers can remember it.

In addition, with **enhanced 9–1–1,** or E-9–1–1, the EMS dispatcher can see the caller's street address and phone number on a computer screen. This is valuable when a patient becomes unconscious before giving an address.

Levels of EMS Training

There are four nationally recognized levels of EMS training: First Responder, EMT-Basic, EMT-Intermediate, and EMT-Paramedic. (EMT stands for emergency medical technician.) Note that responsibilities for each level may vary from state to state. However, the U.S. Department of Transportation (DOT) publishes the minimum certification guidelines. They include:

- **First Responder** (Figure 1-3). The First Responder is the first person on scene with emergency medical training. He or she may be a police officer or firefighter, a truck driver or schoolteacher, an industrial health officer, or a community volunteer. Training includes:

  —Airway care and suctioning.
  —Patient assessment.
  —Cardiopulmonary resuscitation (CPR).
  —Bleeding control.
  —Stabilization of injuries to the spine and extremities.
  —Care for medical and trauma emergencies.
  —Use of a limited amount of equipment.
  —Assisting other EMS providers.
  —Other skills and procedures as permitted by local or state regulations.

- **EMT-Basic** (Figure 1-4). The EMT-Basic (or *EMT-B*) can do all that the First Responder does. He or she also

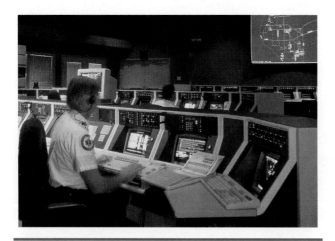

FIGURE 1-2 The emergency medical dispatcher (EMD) is an important member of the EMS team.

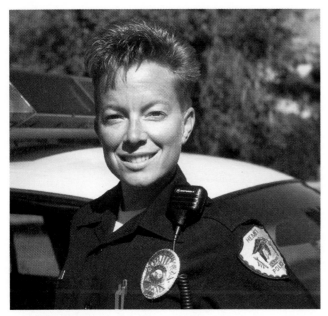

a. *First Responder—a police officer.*

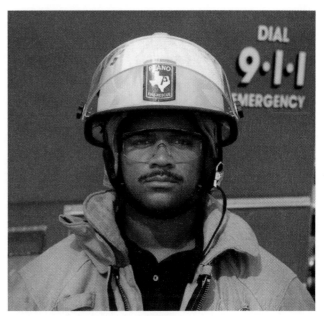

b. *First Responder—a firefighter.*

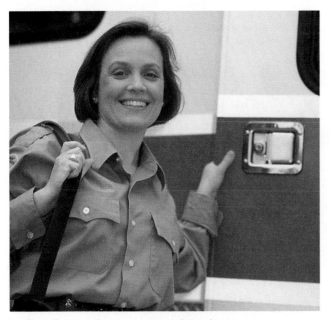

c. *First Responder—a community volunteer.*

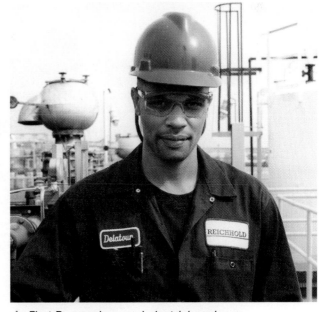

d. *First Responder—an industrial worker.*

FIGURE 1-3 First Responders may be police officers, firefighters, educators, truck drivers, industrial workers, or community volunteers.

can perform complex immobilization procedures, restrain patients, and staff and drive ambulances.

- **EMT-Intermediate** (Figure 1-5). The EMT-Intermediate (or *EMT-I*) can do all that the two previous levels do. He or she also can perform a limited number of advanced techniques and administer a few medications.

In some states, the EMT-I may be trained as a cardiac technician.

- **EMT-Paramedic** (Figure 1-6). The EMT-paramedic (or *paramedic*) has the most advanced EMS training. He or she can do all that the three previous levels do, plus administer more medications and

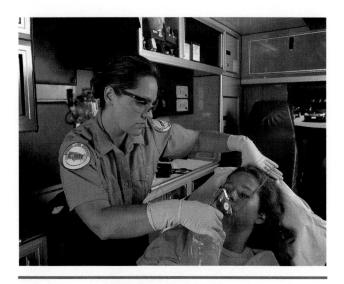

FIGURE 1-4 An EMT-Basic.

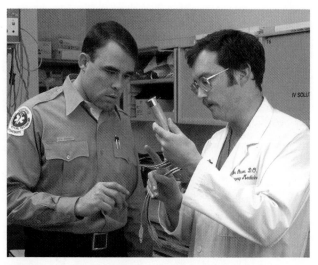

FIGURE 1-5 An EMT-Intermediate.

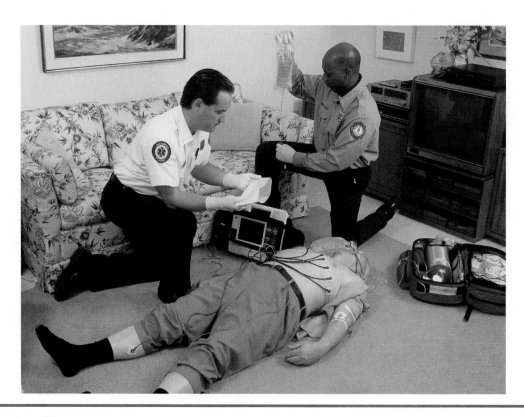

FIGURE 1-6 An EMT-Paramedic.

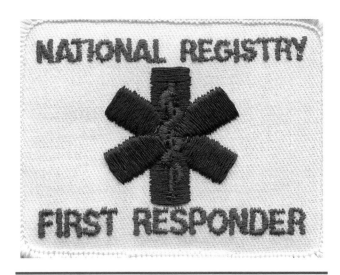

FIGURE 1-7 The National Registry First Responder patch. *(Courtesy of National Registry of Emergency Medical Technicians)*

perform more advanced techniques such as cardiac monitoring.

The National Registry of Emergency Medical Technicians (NREMT) was formed in 1970. It offers examinations for certification of First Responders and EMTs (Figure 1-7). If your state does not recognize or require national registration, certification may still be helpful if you move to another state. It also is considered desirable by private employers. Ask your instructor about getting national certification or contact:

National Registry of Emergency Medical Technicians

6610 Busch Boulevard

Columbus, OH 43229

614–888–4484

www.nremt.org

Classic Components of EMS

Each state in the United States controls its own EMS system. However, standards are set by the National Highway Traffic Safety Administration through the U.S. Department of Transportation (DOT). Those standards include 10 classic components of any EMS system:

- *Regulation and policy.* Each state must have laws, regulations, policies, and procedures that govern its EMS system. It also is required to provide leadership to local jurisdictions.

- *Resources management.* Each state must have central control of EMS resources so all patients have equal access to acceptable emergency care.

- *Human resources and training.* All personnel who staff ambulances and transport patients must be trained to at least the EMT-Basic level.

- *Transportation.* Patients must be safely and reliably transported by ground or air ambulance.

- *Facilities.* Every seriously ill or injured patient must be delivered in a timely manner to an appropriate medical facility.

- *Communications.* A system for public access to the EMS system must be in place. Communication among dispatcher, ambulance crew, and hospital also must be possible.

- *Public information and education.* EMS personnel should participate in programs designed to educate the public. The programs must focus on injury prevention and how to properly access the EMS system.

- *Medical oversight.* Each EMS system must have a physician as a medical director.

- *Trauma systems.* Each state must develop a system of specialized care for trauma patients, including one or more trauma centers and rehabilitation programs. It must also develop systems for assigning and transporting patients to those facilities.

- *Evaluation.* Each state must have a quality improvement system in place for continuing evaluation and upgrading of its EMS system.

In-Hospital Care System

First Responders and EMTs provide *prehospital care,* or emergency medical treatment, before transport to a medical facility. In some areas, the term *out-of-hospital care* is preferred. It reflects a trend toward providing care on scene with or without transport to a hospital. (Your instructor will provide information on how these terms apply to your EMS system.)

Specialized medical facilities include the trauma center, burn center, pediatric center, perinatal center, and poison center. A *trauma center* focuses on injury treatment that may exceed what a general hospital can provide. A *burn center* specializes in the treatment of burns and often offers long-term care and rehabilitation services. A *pediatric center* is devoted to the treatment of infants and children. A *perinatal center* is for high-risk pregnant patients. Finally, the *poison center* focuses on providing information and advice on how to treat poisoning victims.

The most familiar destination of EMS patients is the local hospital emergency department. There, a staff of physicians, nurses, and allied health professionals stabilize the patient and prepare him or her for further care elsewhere in the hospital.

Q: 1. To whom do First Responders provide emergency care?

2. How can the public access EMS?

3. What are the four levels of EMS training?

Section 2 The First Responder

As a First Responder, you may be called to emergencies where you are the only trained rescuer on scene. At other times, specialized rescue teams and fire personnel, as well as law enforcement, may all be involved.

Your Role

Generally, your role includes the following:

- *Protect your own safety and the safety of your crew, the patient, and bystanders.* This is your first and most important priority. Remember that you cannot help the patient if you are injured. You also do not want to endanger other rescuers by forcing them to rescue you. Once scene safety is ensured, the patient's needs become your primary concern.

- *Gain access to the patient.* In some emergencies, you may need to move one patient in order to gain access to a more critically injured one.

- *Assess the patient to identify life-threatening problems.* Always perform an initial assessment to help you identify life threats. Such problems may include a blocked airway, heart attack, or severe bleeding.

- *Alert additional EMS resources.* In cases where a patient needs medical care or transport to a medical facility, you

First on Scene

As the first to approach a scene, First Responders can face unpredictable—and occasionally dangerous—situations. Your priority will be to protect yourself and your crew, the patient, and bystanders. Do so by observing for hazards, remaining calm, not entering an unsafe scene, and requesting assistance as needed.

✓ **First Responder Practice**

In your practice as a First Responder, you will care for many patients close to death and many others who have only minor problems. In either case, do you know what they will remember after the call? It won't be the medical care you provided. It's *you.* The time you spent comforting and reassuring them is usually what they remember most.

must remain with him or her until other EMS personnel take over patient care.

- *Provide care based on assessment findings.* While you are waiting for EMS resources to arrive, you must provide patient care based on the needs you identified during patient assessment.

- *Assist other EMS personnel.* When requested, assist other EMS personnel with patient care as needed.

- *Participate in record keeping and data collection as required.* You may be required by state law or your local EMS system to document your calls, especially if a patient refuses care.

- *Act as liaison with other public safety personnel.* These may include local, state, or federal law enforcement, fire department personnel, and other EMS providers.

Your Responsibilities

The responsibilities of a First Responder vary from state to state. However, they always include ensuring scene safety and maintaining a professional attitude, appearance, and up-to-date skills. Specifically, you should:

- *Guard your personal health and safety.* Drive safely at all times. Use a seat belt whenever you drive or ride. Remove yourself from hazards such as gas leaks, fires, chemical spills, and so on, and follow the directions of specialized rescuers at those scenes. Never enter a crime scene or an angry crowd until the police have controlled the situation. Locate or create a safe area in which you can care for patients. Stay away from high-traffic areas. Redirect traffic as needed. Always wear the proper personal protective equipment (PPE) including a helmet and leather gloves, when appropriate. (See Chapter 2 for more details.)

■ *Maintain a caring attitude.* Often you will arrive at an emergency scene to find the patient, family, and bystanders in a state of panic or chaos. These are normal reactions. Reassure and comfort them. Identify yourself, assure them that you will begin to stabilize the patient, and let them know that more help is on the way.

■ *Maintain your own composure.* Many calls are routine. However, some calls involve life-threatening or emotionally charged problems. In those cases, it is critical that you stay calm so you can get an accurate picture of the scene and properly establish your priorities.

■ *Keep a neat, clean, professional appearance.* Excellent personal grooming and a crisp, clean appearance help instill confidence in patients. Being clean also helps to protect your patients from contamination from dirty hands or soiled clothing. Respond to every call in complete uniform or other appropriate dress. Portray the positive image you want to project. Remember that you are on a medical team. Your appearance can send the message that you are competent and trustworthy.

■ *Maintain up-to-date knowledge and skills.* New research often shows us better ways of doing things. Take every opportunity to continue your education, including refresher courses offered through your local EMS system.

■ *Maintain current knowledge of local, state, and national issues affecting the EMS system.* Attend conferences and read professional journals dedicated to EMS issues.

You always will be expected to accept and uphold the responsibilities of a First Responder in accordance with the standards of an EMS professional. As a First Responder, you will come in contact with people of different genders, ages, cultures, and socioeconomic backgrounds. It is your responsibility to meet the standard of care for all.

Section 3 Medical Oversight

Medical Director

A formal relationship exists between a community's EMS providers and the physician responsible for out-of-hospital emergency medical care. This physician is often referred to as the system **medical director.** He or she is legally responsible for the clinical and patient-care aspects of an EMS system.

Every EMS system *must* have a medical director. He or she must provide guidance to all EMS personnel. The medical director is also responsible for reviewing and improving the quality of care in an EMS system.

Medical Control

Two basic types of medical oversight are **direct medical control** and **indirect medical control.** Direct medical control occurs when the medical director or another physician gives instructions to an EMS rescuer at the scene of an emergency via telephone or radio or in person. This usually occurs when an EMS rescuer asks for help with a patient. Note that direct medical control is also called "on-line," "base station," or "immediate."

Indirect medical control may be called "off-line" medical oversight. It includes such things as system design and quality management. The medical director who writes **standing orders** and **protocols** is using indirect medical control. These define the accepted practice for First Responders in your area. For example, they tell you whether or not you can give oxygen to a patient or how to respond to a family who refuses your help. They also tell you how to document each call, participate in reviews, gather feedback, and maintain your skills.

The First Responder

In general, First Responders are the designated agents of the medical director. If this is true in your area, the care you render by law may be considered an extension of the medical director's authority. Your instructor will tell you what the law is in your area.

1. As a First Responder, what is your first and most important priority?

2. What should First Responder responsibilities always include, no matter what the circumstance?

1. Who is the EMS medical director?

2. What is one example of direct medical control?

3. What is one example of indirect medical control?

▶▶ The Call Follow-up

At the beginning of this chapter, you read that First Responders were caring for a patient with chest pain. They had just radioed for assistance and administered oxygen to the patient. To see what their roles and responsibilities were in the continued care of this patient, read the following. It describes how the call was completed.

Patient History The woman told us she was 67 and her name was Paula McMaster. She said she had a heavy feeling in her chest for about two hours. It radiated to her left shoulder. The pain came on while she was watching TV. The patient told us she has high blood pressure, she had two heart attacks in the past five years, and she takes blood pressure medication and a pill for diabetes. She denied any allergies. Her last meal was about two hours ago, when she had a sandwich and coffee.

Physical Examination The patient denied any injury such as an earlier fall or car crash. Because of this we did not perform a hands-on, head-to-toe exam. We did check her chest, shoulders, and arms for pain. We took her vital signs and found

that her pulse was 96, weak, and irregular. Her respirations were 20 and labored. Blood pressure was 100/56. Listening to her chest, we heard adequate air entering on both sides.

We continued to administer oxygen and made sure the paramedics were on the way.

Ongoing Assessment We remained concerned because the patient was pale, sweaty, and had some difficulty breathing. So we verified that the patient was still alert and breathing adequately. Oxygen continued to flow through a nonrebreather mask. We checked that the patient was as comfortable as she could be and tried to reassure her and her husband. We finished another set of vitals just as the ambulance pulled up.

Patient Hand-off Since my partner had responsibility for patient care during this call, he gave the paramedics the hand-off report (see below). After we made sure the paramedics didn't need us any longer, we radioed dispatch to say we were available for our next call. Then we headed back to headquarters.

Hand-off Report

"This is Mrs. McMaster. She is a 67-year-old female patient. She began having heaviness in the chest and left shoulder about two hours ago while watching TV. She is pale and sweaty with some labored breathing. Her vital signs are 100/56, pulse is 96, weak and irregular, respirations are 20 and labored. She has a history of heart attack, high blood pressure, and diabetes. We tried to make her comfortable and gave her oxygen by nonrebreather mask."

The Last Word *From the initial call received by the 9–1–1 dispatcher to EMS rescuers responding to that call, straight through to final disposition at the hospital emergency department—it takes all the resources of an EMS system working together to help a patient survive a sudden illness or injury. As the first emergency medical responder on scene, you are a valuable, vital member of that EMS system team.*

Chapter Review

Focus on the EMS Team

As a First Responder, you will play a vital role in the emergency medical care of patients experiencing a sudden illness or injury. Perhaps the most important reason your role is so crucial is that you will be responsible for the first few minutes with the patient. Other EMS personnel depend on your actions during this time to set the foundation for the remainder of the call.

During your time with the patient, correcting a breathing problem or stopping serious bleeding may actually save a life. You also will help patients who are not in critical condition when you prevent further injury, perform the proper assessments, gather a medical history, and prepare for the arrival of other rescue personnel.

Summing Up

- The EMS system is a network of resources linked together to provide emergency care and transport to victims of sudden illness or injury.

- The public can access EMS by using a 9–1–1 or a non-9–1–1 phone number. With enhanced 9–1–1, an EMS dispatcher can see the caller's street address and phone number.

- Levels of EMS training include First Responder, EMT-Basic, EMT-Intermediate, and EMT-Paramedic. The National Registry of Emergency Medical Technicians (NREMT) offers examinations for certification of First Responders and EMTs.

- The 10 classic components of EMS are regulation and policy, resources management, human resources and training, transportation, facilities, communications, public information and education, medical oversight, trauma systems, and evaluation.

- After prehospital care (out-of-hospital care), a patient may be taken to a local hospital emergency department or to a specialized medical facility. Specialized medical facilities include trauma centers, burn centers, pediatric centers, perinatal centers, and poison centers.

- First Responder roles include the following: Protect your own safety and the safety of your crew, the patient, and bystanders. Safely gain access to the patient, identify life-threatening problems, alert additional EMS resources as needed, and provide care based on assessment findings. First Responders should assist other EMS personnel when asked to do so, participate in record keeping and data collection as required, and act as liaison with other public safety personnel.

- First Responder responsibilities include the following: Guard your own health and safety. Maintain a caring attitude and your own composure. Keep a neat, clean, professional appearance. Maintain and regularly update your knowledge and skills, including your knowledge of local, state, and national issues affecting the EMS system.

- The physician responsible for out-of-hospital emergency medical care is the medical director. Every EMS system *must* have a medical director. Direct medical control occurs when the medical director or another physician gives instructions to an EMS rescuer at the scene of an emergency via telephone, radio, or in person. Indirect medical control occurs through standing orders and protocols, which define accepted practice. First Responders are the designated agents of the medical director.

Key Terms

direct medical control refers to an EMS medical director or other physician giving orders to an EMS rescuer on scene via telephone, radio, or in person.

emergency medical services (EMS) system a network of resources linked together to provide emergency care and transport to victims of sudden illness or injury.

EMT-Basic an emergency medical technician trained to the next level above the EMS First Responder. *Also called* EMT-B.

EMT-Intermediate an emergency medical technician trained to a higher level than the First Responder and EMT-Basic. *Also called* EMT-I.

EMT-Paramedic the most highly trained emergency medical technician in EMS. *Also called* EMT-P *or* paramedic.

enhanced 9–1–1 a type of 9–1–1 service in which the EMS dispatcher can see the caller's address and phone number on a computer screen. *Also called* E–9–1–1.

First Responder the first person on scene with EMS training.

indirect medical control refers to EMS system design, standing orders and protocols, education for EMS personnel, and quality management.

medical director the physician legally responsible for the clinical and patient-care aspects of an EMS system.

9–1–1 a phone number by which the public can access EMS and, in some areas, other emergency services. *Also called* universal number.

non-9–1–1 system a system that uses a regular seven-digit phone number (or numbers) for emergency services.

protocols developed by the medical director, these are lists of steps to be taken in certain situations.

standing orders a policy issued by a medical director that authorizes EMS personnel to perform particular skills in certain situations.

Knowledge Check

1. **Which one of the following is NOT one of the four levels of EMS training?**
   a. EMT-Basic
   b. EMT-Paramedic
   c. EMT-Instructor
   d. First Responder

2. **Which one of the following is NOT the First Responder's responsibility?**
   a. providing a medical diagnosis to the patient
   b. ensuring the safety of the crew and patients
   c. maintaining up-to-date knowledge and skills
   d. keeping a neat, clean, professional appearance

3. **The ___ 9–1–1 phone system allows the EMS dispatcher to see the address and phone number of the caller.**
   a. non-
   b. enhanced
   c. emergency
   d. off-line

4. **The physician legally responsible for the clinical and patient-care aspects of an EMS system is the:**
   a. captain or chief of a squad or department.
   b. nearest emergency department physician.
   c. most experienced EMT-paramedic.
   d. medical director.

5. **A standing order or protocol that spells out how a First Responder should use an automated external defibrillator is an example of ___ medical control.**
   a. on-line
   b. off-line
   c. immediate
   d. base station

6. According to the standards set by the U.S. DOT for the EMS system, each state must manage EMS resources so that:
    a. it can decide if rural or urban areas get the best equipment.
    b. all patients have equal access to acceptable emergency medical care.
    c. the public can focus on the prevention of injuries.
    d. all EMS systems have access to air ambulances.

7. One of the benefits of using a "universal number" to access police, fire, and rescue is:
    a. there is no need for a dispatcher to answer a call.
    b. the caller does not need to give a name or address.
    c. it can notify the patient's personal physician.
    d. even the youngest caller can remember and dial it.

8. As a First Responder, safety is:
    a. NOT your responsibility.
    b. your first and most important responsibility.
    c. a priority only if no police are on scene.
    d. addressed only after the medical care of a patient.

9. The First Responder level of certification prepares students to be in charge of an ambulance crew.
    a. True
    b. False

10. As a First Responder, you will assess patients to determine what emergency medical care is appropriate.
    a. True
    b. False

11. Why should a First Responder seek training after completing the initial certification course? Write at least one reason.

_____

_____

12. Explain the difference between on-line and off-line medical direction.

_____

_____

13. Write a list of at least three actions considered part of your role as a First Responder.

_____

_____

_____

14. Write a list of three types of specialty hospitals or specialty medical facilities.

_____

_____

_____

Scenario

An elderly member of your family was walking to the store when she tripped and fell on the sidewalk. She is sitting there, feeling a bit embarrassed, and just about ready to get back up onto her feet when a First Responder approaches. What would you want him to say to your family member? Write three short examples.

_____

_____

_____

_____

_____

_____

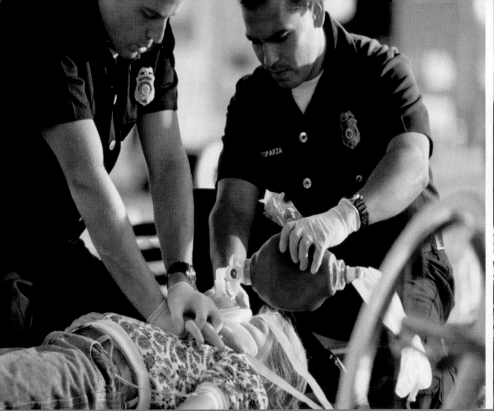
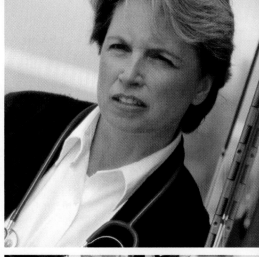
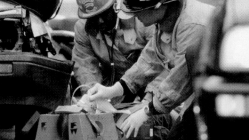

2 | Well-Being of the First Responder

Objectives

From the U.S. Department of Transportation (DOT) 1995 "First Responder: National Standard Curriculum."

Cognitive

1-2.1 ▸ List possible emotional reactions that the First Responder may experience when faced with trauma, illness, death, and dying. (pp. 25-29)

1-2.2 ▸ Discuss the possible reactions that a family member may exhibit when confronted with death and dying. (p. 26)

1-2.3 ▸ State the steps in the First Responder's approach to the family confronted with death and dying. (pp. 26-27)

1-2.4 ▸ State the possible reactions that the family of the First Responder may exhibit. (p. 28)

1-2.5 ▸ Recognize the signs and symptoms of critical incident stress. (pp. 28-29)

1-2.6 ▸ State possible steps that the First Responder may take to help reduce/alleviate stress. (pp. 27-29)

1-2.7 ▸ Explain the need to determine scene safety. (pp. 23-25)

1-2.8 ▸ Discuss the importance of body substance isolation (BSI). (pp. 18-21)

1-2.9 ▸ Describe the steps the First Responder should take for personal protection from airborne and bloodborne pathogens. (pp. 18-22)

1-2.10 ▸ List the personal protective equipment necessary for each of the following situations: hazardous materials, rescue operations, violent scenes, crime scenes, electricity, water and ice, exposure to bloodborne pathogens, and exposure to airborne pathogens. (pp. 23-25)

Affective

1-2.11 ▸ Explain the importance of serving as an advocate for the use of appropriate protective equipment. (pp. 20-21)

1-2.12 ▸ Explain the importance of understanding the response to death and dying and communicating effectively with the patient's family. (pp. 25-29)

1-2.13 ▶ Demonstrate a caring attitude towards any patient with illness or injury who requests emergency medical services. (pp. 25-29)

1-2.14 ▶ Show compassion when caring for the physical and mental needs of patients. (pp. 25-29)

1-2.15 ▶ Participate willingly in the care of all patients. (p. 18)

1-2.16 ▶ Communicate with empathy to patients being cared for, as well as with family members, and friends of the patient. (pp. 25-29)

Psychomotor

1-2.17 ▶ Given a scenario with potential infectious exposure, the First Responder will use appropriate personal protective equipment. At the completion of the scenario, the First Responder will properly remove and discard the protective garments. (pp. 18-21)

1-2.18 ▶ Given the above scenario, the First Responder will complete disinfection/cleaning and all reporting documentation. (pp. 19-22)

Introduction

Most basic training programs teach how to react safely to a variety of threats, such as fire and hazardous materials. But the most common threat to a rescuer is likely to be as simple as oncoming traffic. This chapter outlines the many elements that make up rescuer safety and covers the basic steps you should take to maintain your well-being. It includes how to protect yourself against infection and how to anticipate and handle the emotional aspects of emergencies. It also introduces you to scene safety.

Section 1 Preventing Disease Transmission

As a First Responder, you will come in contact with patients who are sick. If you are worried about "catching" their diseases, you are justified. But don't despair. The following section will explain how diseases are transmitted and describe the ones of most concern to EMS personnel. It also outlines proven ways for you to protect yourself.

How Diseases Are Transmitted

Diseases are caused by **pathogens,** microorganisms such as bacteria and viruses. An **infectious disease** spreads from one person to another (Figure 2-1). It can spread *directly* through blood-to-blood contact (bloodborne), contact with open wounds or exposed tissues, and contact with the mucous membranes of the eyes and mouth. An infectious disease also can spread *indirectly* by way of a contaminated object, such as a needle, or by

HOW INFECTIOUS DISEASES CAN SPREAD

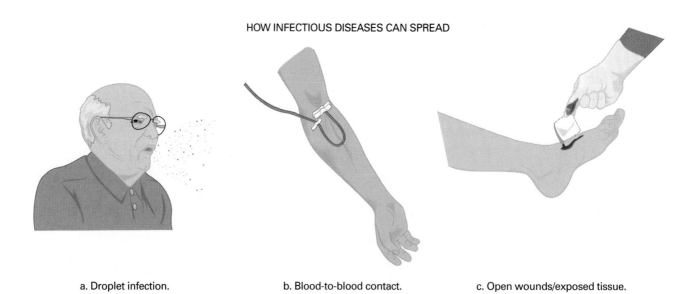

a. Droplet infection.　　　　b. Blood-to-blood contact.　　　　c. Open wounds/exposed tissue.

FIGURE 2-1 Infectious diseases can spread from one person to another

THE CALL

Dispatch My partner and I are community volunteers associated with the fire department. We were on the 3-to-12 shift, and it was just about time to quit when dispatch called. There was a person bleeding at 1433 Magnolia. We got in our unit. It was my partner's turn to drive. I got out the town map and located the residence. On the way, I mentally went over the procedures for body substance isolation and bleeding control.

Scene Size-up We arrived at the patient's house in about four minutes. We

approached carefully. When we got to the door, we waited a second and listened. Men were yelling, and I heard glass breaking. Loud thumps and scuffling made it obvious that people were fighting in there.

Caution will help you to recognize potential dangers at an emergency scene. But is violence the only kind of danger you may face? What precautions would you take in the situation described above? Consider your answers as you read Chapter 2.

way of infected droplets breathed into the respiratory tract (airborne).

Some pathogens are transmitted easily, such as the viruses that cause the common cold. Others need specific routes of contact. Tuberculosis bacteria, for example, are transmitted by droplets from a cough or sneeze of an infected patient. Poor nutrition, poor hygiene, crowded or unsanitary living conditions, and stress all make infection from any disease easier. To protect yourself, *always* use appropriate personal protective equipment. That includes wearing protective gloves and using a barrier device such as a pocket face mask *every time* you ventilate a patient (Figure 2-2). Make sure the device has a one-way valve that prevents fluid from backing up.

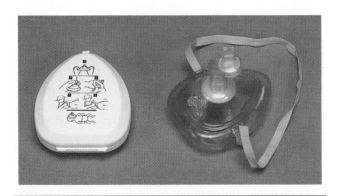

FIGURE 2-2 A pocket face mask with one-way valve and carrying case.

Diseases of Concern

As a First Responder, you can be exposed to infectious diseases whenever you treat a patient. Three diseases of most concern are hepatitis, tuberculosis, and AIDS.

Hepatitis

These are several hepatitis viruses that directly affect the liver. In some cases, viral hepatitis—especially hepatitis B—can be fatal. Viral hepatitis is contracted through blood and body fluids. A major source of the virus is the "chronic carrier." This person can carry the virus for years. He or she usually has no signs or symptoms and often is unaware of being ill. When signs and symptoms do appear, they may include:

- Nausea, loss of appetite.
- Abdominal pain.
- Headache.
- Fever.
- Yellowish color of the skin and whites of eyes.

The most effective way to deal with the hepatitis B virus is prevention through the use of personal protective equipment and vaccination. If you suspect you have been exposed to hepatitis, report the incident to your supervisor. Immediately contact a physician or your local public health agency for care. Care may include injections of HBIG (hepatitis B immunoglobulin). You also may receive a vaccination if you have not already had one. Medical authorities strongly recommend the hepatitis B vaccine. Employers and most agencies offer it free of charge.

As previously mentioned, there are several types of hepatitis. Hepatitis B is of primary concern for EMS providers because it survives outside the body and can be transmitted much easier than the HIV (AIDS) virus. Another type of hepatitis—hepatitis C—raises concerns because it is spread much like hepatitis B, but there is no vaccine for hepatitis C. Fortunately, all diseases, including hepatitis C, can be prevented by taking the appropriate body substance isolation (BSI) precautions. (These precautions are described later in the chapter.)

Tuberculosis

Tuberculosis (TB) almost vanished once, but it's back. In fact, researchers are worried because new drug-resistant strains are developing. The pathogen that causes TB is found in the lungs and other tissues of the infected patient. You can be infected from droplets in a patient's cough or from infected sputum. The main signs and symptoms of TB include:

- Fever.
- Cough.
- Night sweats.
- Weight loss.

The U.S. Occupational Safety and Health Administration (OSHA) has adopted standards for rescuer protection against TB. They include the use of special masks. One type of mask is called the **N-95 respirator** (Figure 2-3). Another type is called the *high efficiency particulate air respirator*, or the **HEPA respirator.** Wear one whenever you suspect TB.

Acquired Immune Deficiency Syndrome (AIDS)

Fortunately, AIDS is not spread through casual contact. It cannot be spread by touching the skin, coughing, sneezing, sharing eating utensils, or other indirect ways. *Transmission requires intimate contact with the body fluids of infected persons.* Infection may occur in these ways:

- Sexual contact involving the exchange of semen, saliva, blood, urine, or feces.
- Infected needles.
- Infected blood or blood products.
- Mother to child during pregnancy, birth, or breastfeeding.

Simply stated, the human immunodeficiency virus (HIV) knocks out the body's ability to fight infection. HIV

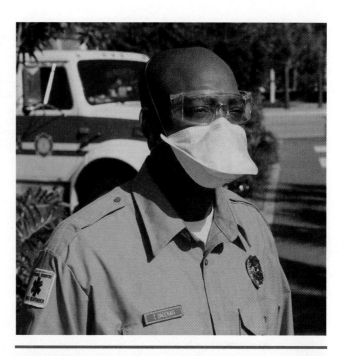

FIGURE 2-3 An N-95 respirator. Always use OSHA-approved masks and respirators with your patients.

can lead to AIDS. AIDS victims get infections caused by viruses, bacteria, parasites, and fungi. These are serious illnesses that do not occur (or occur only mildly) in people with healthy immune systems. They involve many organs of the body, causing a wide array of signs and symptoms.

Although not everyone infected by HIV has developed AIDS, people who carry HIV can still spread the infection to others. So, because any patient could be infected with HIV—or any other disease–follow all the precautions described below at all times and with all patients.

Body Substance Isolation (BSI)

For many years, OSHA guidelines required EMS personnel to take steps to protect themselves against diseases transmitted by way of blood. They were called "universal precautions." In the late 1980s, the Centers for Disease Control (CDC) published guidelines that set a new standard: *Assume all blood and body fluids are infectious.* This requires EMS personnel to practice a strict form of infection control called **body substance isolation** (BSI) with *all* patients.

BSI precautions help you to care for all patients safely, even those with infectious diseases. BSI precautions include handwashing; properly cleaning, disinfecting, or sterilizing equipment; and use of personal protective equipment (PPE).

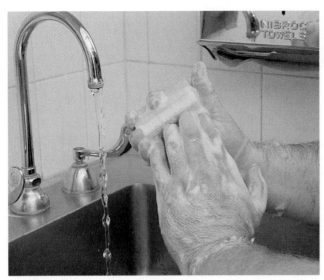

a. *Wash your hands thoroughly with soap and water after each call.*

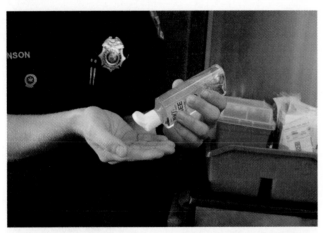

b. *If water is not available, use a foam or liquid alcohol-based washing agent.*

FIGURE 2-4 **The first line of protection against infectious disease is handwashing.**

Handwashing

Handwashing is the single most important thing you can do to prevent the spread of infection. According to the U.S. Public Health Service, most contaminants can be removed from the skin with 10 to 15 seconds of vigorous lathering and scrubbing with plain soap.

Always wash your hands after caring for a patient, *even if you were wearing gloves.* For maximum protection, begin by removing all jewelry from your hands and arms. Then lather up and rub together all surfaces of your hands. Pay attention to creases, crevices, and the areas between your fingers. Use a brush to scrub under and around your fingernails (Figure 2-4). (It is a good idea

for you to keep your nails short and unpolished.) If your hands are visibly soiled, spend more time washing them. Wash your wrists and forearms, too. Rinse thoroughly under a stream of water and dry well. Use a disposable towel if possible.

When no water is available to wash up, use a foam or liquid alcohol-based washing agent. Make sure you have this type of cleaner available in your rescue vehicle or first-in kit at all times. As soon as you can, wash your hands again with soap and water using the procedure described above.

Cleaning Equipment

Cleaning, disinfecting, and sterilizing are related terms. **Cleaning** is simply the process of washing a soiled object with soap and water. **Disinfecting** is cleaning plus using a chemical such as alcohol or bleach to kill many of the microorganisms on an object. **Sterilizing** is a process in which a chemical or other substance (such as superheated steam) kills all of the microorganisms on an object.

Generally, disinfect items that contact the intact skin of a patient. Items that contact open wounds or mucous membranes should be sterilized.

Whenever possible, use disposable equipment. *Never reuse disposable items.* Instead, place them in a plastic bag that is clearly labeled "infectious waste" (Figure 2-5). Then seal the bag. Disposable items used with patients who have hepatitis B or HIV should be double-bagged.

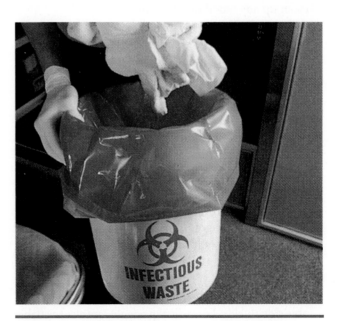

FIGURE 2-5 **Be sure to discard contaminated items properly.**

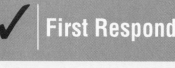

First Responder Practice

Your personal protective equipment (PPE) is the barrier between you and a patient's body fluids. Use PPE appropriately. Here are examples of PPE for common emergency situations:

Situation	Personal Protective Equipment
Minor bleeding	Gloves
Bleeding from face or other serious bleeding	Gloves and face shield (or protective eyewear and mask)
Suctioning, splashing fluids, spitting	Gloves and face shield (or protective eyewear and mask)
Childbirth or severe bleeding (multiple trauma, arterial bleeding)	Gloves, face shield (or protective eyewear and mask), gown

Remember to protect the mucous membranes of your face (eyes, nose, and mouth). Face shields or protective eyewear and mask are necessary even if only the potential exists for airborne contamination.

After each use, clean nondisposable equipment. Wash off all blood, mucus, tissue, and other residue. Be sure to wear a good pair of utility gloves while doing so. Then disinfect or sterilize equipment according to local protocols.

Wash items that do not normally touch the patient. Rinse them with clear water and dry thoroughly. Clean walls or window coverings in an ambulance or rescue vehicle when they get soiled. Then use a hospital-grade disinfectant or a solution of household bleach and water to clean up any blood or body fluids.

If your clothes get soiled with body fluids, you must remove, bag, and label them. Wash them in hot, soapy water for at least 25 minutes. Take a hot shower yourself and be sure to rinse thoroughly.

Personal Protective Equipment (PPE)

Always use **personal protective equipment** (PPE) as a barrier against infection. Such items will keep you from coming into contact with a patient's blood and body fluids. They include eye protection, gloves, gowns, and masks.

- *Eye protection* (Figure 2-6). Use eye shields to keep blood and body fluids from splashing into your eyes. Several types are available. Clear plastic shields cover the eyes or the whole face. Safety glasses have side shields. If you wear prescription glasses, attach removable side shields. Form-fitting goggles are also available but are not required.

- *Gloves* (Figure 2-7). Wear high-quality vinyl or latex gloves whenever you care for a patient. Never reuse them. Put on a new pair for each patient to avoid

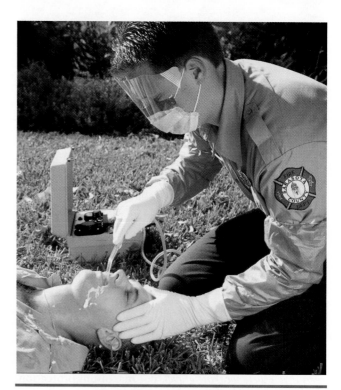

FIGURE 2-6 In addition to eye protection, personal protective equipment (PPE) includes face mask or shield, gown or apron, gloves, cap, and shoe coverings.

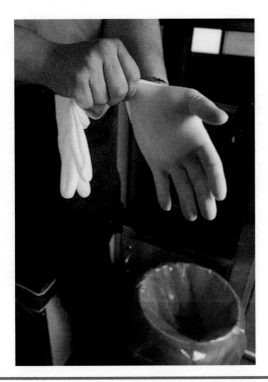

FIGURE 2-7 Wear protective gloves whenever you care for a patient.

exposing one patient to another's infection. Change soiled gloves as soon as it is practical to do so. If a glove accidentally tears, remove it as soon as you can do so safely. Then wash your hands and replace the torn glove with a new one.

- *Gowns.* Wear a gown when there might be significant splashing of blood or body fluids. Generally, you will need a gown during childbirth or major injury. Whenever possible, use a disposable one. It also is recommended that you change your clothes if the gown gets soiled.
- *Masks.* Wear a disposable surgical-type face mask to protect against possible splatter of blood or body fluids. An N-95 or HEPA respirator is recommended for use with suspected tuberculosis patients.

Use personal protective equipment yourself and be sure to remind other EMS personnel at the scene to wear it, too. Make gloves and other PPE available to others who arrive to help.

Removing Gloves

Much attention is given to donning gloves to prevent spread of disease. Removing them safely is also important. When you finish care—or change gloves because they are soiled, follow these guidelines (Figure 2-8):

1. *Remove the first glove.* With one hand, pinch an area of the glove on your other hand near the cuff. Do not touch your skin. Pull this glove off inside out. While doing this, hold the gloves away from your body. Do not "snap" the glove or allow substances that may be on it to spray. Leave the glove just removed inside out in the hand that removed it.

2. *Remove the second glove.* With the hand that is now free, carefully find a non-contaminated area of the remaining glove and pull it off inside out. The glove removed first will end up inside the second glove.

3. *Dispose of the gloves properly.*

4. *Wash your hands immediately.*

Immunizations

Before you start active duty, have a physician make sure you are adequately protected against common infectious diseases. The following immunizations are recommended for active-duty First Responders:

- Tetanus prophylaxis (every 10 years).
- Hepatitis B vaccine.
- Influenza vaccine (every year).
- Polio.
- Rubella (German measles).
- Measles.
- Mumps.

Because some immunizations offer only partial protection, have your physician verify your immune status against rubella, measles, and mumps. Remember to *always* practice BSI precautions—even after being vaccinated.

Have a tuberculin skin (PPD) test at least once every year you are on duty. It will tell you if you have been exposed to TB. Your agency's medical director or your physician can advise you.

Reporting Exposures

Report any suspected exposure to blood or body fluids. Report the incident as soon as possible to your supervisor and to medical control. Be especially diligent in reporting if the patient is HIV-positive, has hepatitis, or is in a high-risk category for infection. Include in your report the date and time of the exposure, the type of body fluid involved, the amount, and details of the incident. State laws vary. Follow all local protocols.

The Ryan White CARE Act is a federal act that sets a procedure by which emergency personnel can find out if

SKILL SUMMARY *Removing Used Gloves*

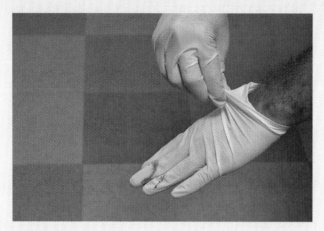

FIGURE 2-8A *With one gloved hand, pinch an area of the glove on your other hand near the cuff. Do not touch your skin.*

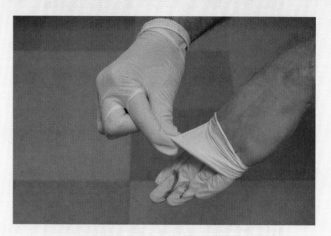

FIGURE 2-8B *Pull this glove off inside out.*

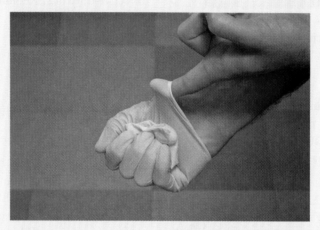

FIGURE 2-8C *Carefully find a non-contaminated area of the remaining glove and pull it off inside out. The first glove should end up inside the second glove.*

they have been exposed to a potentially life-threatening disease. If you were exposed to blood or body fluids prior to this act, you had no set way to find out if a patient had an infectious disease. Highlights of the Ryan White CARE Act include:

- Notification systems for airborne and bloodborne disease exposure.
- Requirements for each agency to have a "designated officer" who gathers facts and communicates information about the exposure to the appropriate people.
- Your right to know if a patient you were exposed to has an infectious disease (airborne or bloodborne).

NOTE: The act does not force patients to be tested, but it allows hospitals to share information on the disease status of patients who have this information in their medical records.

1. How can a disease be spread "directly"?

2. How can a disease be spread "indirectly"?

3. What precautions are included in the standard called "body substance isolation"?

4. What immunizations are recommended for First Responders?

First on Scene

Don't become another casualty someone else has to rescue. Take proper precautions to avoid the problems that affect your patients and the dangers of an emergency scene. If you, too, become a victim, you won't help your patient. And you may place other EMS personnel in jeopardy as well.

Section 2 Scene Safety

Always protect yourself at emergency scenes (Figure 2-9). In general, as you approach a scene—whether you are walking or driving—take a good look at the environment you are about to enter. If you are driving an emergency vehicle, do not park directly in front of the call address. This is so you can size up the scene unnoticed and save a place for the ambulance to park.

Then decide whether or not it is safe to approach the patient. If any of the following exists on scene, you may need to call for help:

- Motor-vehicle or airplane crashes.
- Presence of toxic substances or low levels of oxygen.
- Crime scenes.
- Presence of a weapon of any kind.
- Possible drug or alcohol use.
- Arguing, threats, violent behavior, broken glass, over-turned furniture.
- Unstable surfaces, such as water and ice.

Although each emergency scene is unique, a general rule applies to all. *If the scene is unsafe, make it safe before you enter.* Otherwise, wait for help to arrive. Specialized personnel have the training, equipment, and protective gear needed to enter an unstable scene safely.

Once a scene is secure, take measures to protect the patient from hazards. That includes fire, structural instability, gasoline leaks, chemical spills, oncoming traffic, and extremes in temperature. Bystanders also should be protected from risk of illness or injury.

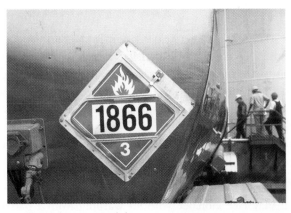

a. *Hazardous materials.*

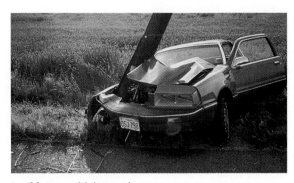

b. *Motor-vehicle crash.* (Robert J. Bennett)

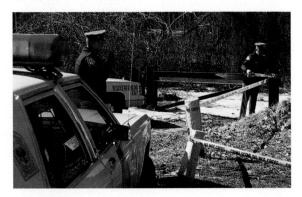

c. *Crime scene.*

FIGURE 2-9 Always be alert to potential hazards when you approach an emergency scene.

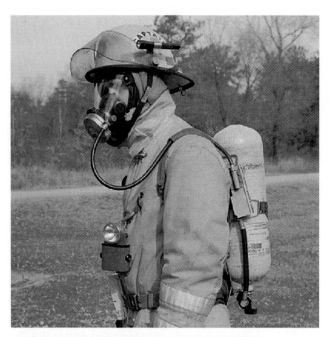

a. *Self-contained breathing apparatus (SCBA).*

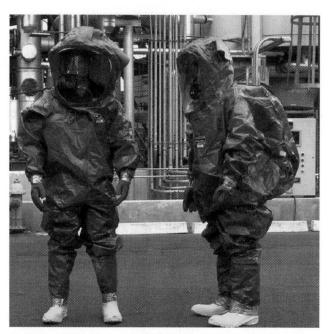

b. *Typical hazardous materials protective suit.*

FIGURE 2-10 Never enter a hazardous materials scene. Call for rescuers who have the proper protective equipment.

Hazardous Materials

Do not enter a hazardous-materials scene. Call a specialized team of rescuers to secure the scene first. Provide emergency care only after the scene is safe and patient contamination is limited. In general, rescuers should wear protective clothing such as a self-contained breathing apparatus and a "hazmat" suit (Figure 2-10). Check with your instructor about the availability of training for hazmat situations. Also learn how to access your local hazmat team. (See Chapter 30.)

Motor-Vehicle Crashes

Some car crashes lead to situations that threaten the lives of patients and rescuers. For example, crashes can lead to:

- Downed power lines or other potential sources of electrocution.
- Fire or the potential for fire such as leaking gasoline.
- Explosion or the potential for explosion.
- Hazardous materials spills or leaks.
- Oncoming traffic hazards.

When there is life-threatening danger on scene, call for specially trained personnel before you enter. Also call for special teams when a complex or extensive rescue is needed. Once a scene is safe, make sure you are wearing the proper personal protective equipment before you enter. That may include turnout gear, puncture-proof gloves, helmet, and eye protection (Figure 2-11). Follow local protocols.

Many traffic emergencies occur in the dark or in bad weather. So be sure to wear reflective clothing in those conditions. Depending on the scene, you might also consider waterproof boots and slip-resistant gloves in wet weather. Wear gloves, a warm hat, and long underwear when it is cold. An impact-resistant helmet with reflective tape and a chin strap is also useful when there is risk of falling debris.

Violence

You may face violence without warning from a patient, bystander, or perpetrator of a crime. If you suspect potential violence, *call law enforcement before you enter the scene.* Never enter to give patient care until the scene has been adequately controlled by the police.

Always call for law enforcement in cases of domestic disputes, street or gang fights, bar fights, or potential suicide. Call them for any type of crime scene and for scenes that involve angry family or bystanders.

Some EMS providers consider wearing **body armor** (Figure 2-12). It is made of Kevlar™ or other synthetic materials that resist penetration by bullets. The amount of protection armor offers depends on the tightness of the weave and the number of layers. Although it will protect you, body armor will not make you invincible. You are still vulnerable in the areas of your body that are not covered and by high-powered bullets that can penetrate the west.

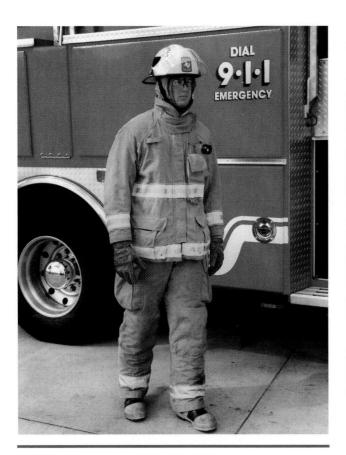

FIGURE 2-11 Turnout gear plus helmet, eye wear, puncture-proof gloves, and boots.

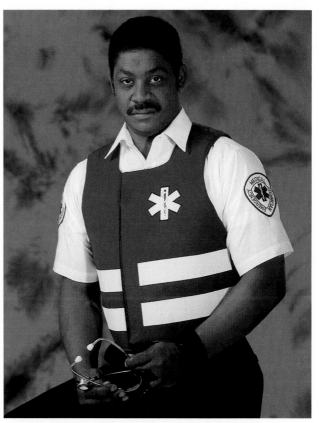

FIGURE 2-12 Body armor, or bullet-proof vest.
(Second Chance Body Armor)

The blunt force of a bullet can still kill you, even if it does not penetrate the armor. Never take chances you would normally avoid just because you are wearing armor.

If you need to care for patients at a crime scene, you must make every reasonable effort to preserve the chain of evidence needed for investigation and prosecution. A general rule is to avoid disturbing the scene unless absolutely necessary for medical care. Basic guidelines include:

■ Never wipe away blood. It can be used as evidence.

■ Touch only what you need to touch to provide patient care.

■ Move only what you need to move to protect the patient and to provide proper care.

■ Do not use a telephone unless the police give you permission to do so.

■ Observe and document anything unusual at the scene.

■ Do not cut through holes in the patient's clothing that could have been caused by bullets or other penetrating weapons.

■ Do not cut through any knot in a rope or tie. Knots are used as evidence. Cut the rope or tie somewhere away from the knot.

■ If the crime is rape, do not wash the patient or allow the patient to wash. Do not allow the patient to change clothing, use the bathroom, or take anything by mouth. Any of these actions could damage valuable evidence.

1. Under what conditions might a First Responder need to call for specialized assistance on scene?

2. What are some hazards associated with a car crash that can threaten the lives of patients and rescuers?

3. What are the limitations of body armor?

Section 3 Emotional Aspects of Emergency Medical Care

By their very nature, emergencies are emotional situations. Common emotions include the stress you feel as a rescuer, the panic and pain patients feel, and the occasional helpless and angry emotions of the patient's family. This section will help you understand some of the stressful issues related to critical incidents and the death of patients.

Death and Dying

Death and dying are inherent parts of emergency medical care. When your patient is dying, you must care for his or her emotional needs as well as the injury or illness. If the patient dies suddenly, help the family or bystanders deal with their grief.

Grieving Process

Dying patients—and those close to them—may experience five general stages of grief referred to as the **grieving process.** Each person progresses through the stages at his or her own rate and in his or her own way.

Patients with nonfatal emergencies also may go through a grieving process. For example, a patient who loses both legs in a factory accident will grieve the loss of his limbs.

As a First Responder, you will not witness all five stages. A critically injured patient who is aware that death is imminent may just begin the process. A terminally ill patient who is more prepared may be at the final stage. The key is to accept all emotions as real and necessary. Respond accordingly.

The stages of the grieving process occur as follows:

- *Denial ("Not me!").* At first the patient may refuse to accept the idea that death is near. This refusal creates a buffer between the shock of approaching death and the need to deal with the illness or injury. Families of dying patients often are at the denial stage.

- *Anger ("Why me?").* Watch out. You may be the target of this anger. But remember that it is a normal part of the grieving process. Do not take it personally. Be tolerant, and try to understand. Use your best listening and communication skills.

- *Bargaining ("Okay, but first let me . . .").* In the patient's mind, a bargain or agreement of sorts will postpone death. For example, a patient may mentally determine that if he is allowed to live, he will patch up a long-standing break with his parents.

- *Depression ("Okay, but I haven't . . .").* As reality settles in, the patient may become silent, distant, withdrawn, and sad. He usually is thinking about those he leaves behind and all the things left undone.

- *Acceptance ("Okay, I am not afraid").* Finally, the patient may appear to accept the fact that he is dying, though he is not happy about it. At this stage, the family may need more support than the patient does.

Dealing with the Dying Patient

It is one of your jobs to help a patient and his or her family through the grieving process. Keep in mind that they may progress through the stages of grief at different rates. What-

ever stage they are in, their needs include dignity, respect, sharing, communication, privacy, and control. To help reduce their emotional burden, consider the following:

- *Do everything possible to maintain the patient's dignity.* Avoid negative statements about the patient's condition. Even an unresponsive patient may hear what you say and feel the fear in your words. Talk to the patient as if he is fully alert. Explain the care you are providing.

- *Show the greatest possible respect for the patient.* Do this especially when death is imminent. Families are extra sensitive at this time. Even attitudes and unspoken messages are perceived. So explain what you are doing. Assure family members that you are making every possible effort to help the patient. It is important for them to know with certainty that you never simply "gave up."

- *Communicate.* Help the patient become oriented to the surroundings. If necessary, explain several times what happened and where. Explain who you are and what you and others are planning. Assure the patient that you are doing everything possible and that you will see that he gets to a hospital as quickly as possible. Without interrupting care, communicate the same message to the family. Explain any procedure you need to carry out. Answer their questions. Do not guess. Report only what you know to be true.

- *Allow family members to express rage, anger, and despair.* They should be able to scream, cry, or vent grief but in a way not dangerous to you or others. Be tolerant. If they vent their anger at you, do not get angry or hostile.

- *Listen with empathy.* Many dying people want messages delivered to survivors. Take notes. Assure the patient that you will do whatever you can to honor his requests. Then follow through on your promise. If possible, stay with the family to listen to their concerns and answer their questions.

- *Do not give false assurances but allow for hope.* Be honest but tactful. If the patient asks if he is dying, do not confirm it. Patients who do the most poorly are often the ones who feel hopeless. Instead, say something like "We are doing everything we can. We need you to help us by not giving up." If the patient insists that death is imminent, say, "That might be possible, but we can still try our best, can't we?"

- *Use a gentle tone of voice.* Be kind to both the patient and the family. Explain the scope of the injury, your medical care, and when necessary, the suspected cause of death to the best of your ability. Do so as gently and kindly as you can in terms they will understand.

- *Let the patient know that everything that can be done will be done.* Emphasize that you are not going to give up.

Say that you are doing everything possible and you will see that the patient gets to a hospital as quickly as possible for further care.

- *Use a reassuring touch, if appropriate.* In addition, if family members want to touch or hold the body after death, and local protocol allows it, arrange for it. Do what you can to improve the appearance of the body. If the body is mutilated, warn the family first. Tell them you covered the badly injured parts.

    Note: At a possible crime scene, *never* clean the patient or remove any blood from the patient or the scene.

- *Do what you can to comfort the family.* Arrange for them to briefly see or talk to the patient. However, do not interrupt your emergency care or delay transport. If the patient is deceased and the family asks you to pray with them, do so. Stay with the family until the medical examiner or coroner arrives.

Stress Management

Many First Responders expose themselves to a great deal of stress in order to meet the needs of their patients. They feel completely responsible for everything that happens at the scene, even things clearly out of their control. Some become so involved that they base their self-image on job performance.

Chronic stress at work plus an emotionally charged environment can lead to a state of exhaustion and irritability. Beware. That state can markedly decrease your effectiveness. Even some of the very best EMS workers have had to leave the system because of it.

Recognize Warning Signs

One of the best ways to manage chronic stress and prevent burnout is to be aware of the warning signs. The earlier they are spotted, the easier they are to remedy. The warning signs include (Figure 2-13):

- Irritability with coworkers, family, and friends.
- Inability to concentrate.
- Difficulty sleeping, nightmares.
- Anxiety.
- Inability to make decisions.
- Guilt.
- Loss of appetite.
- Loss of sexual desire.
- Isolation.
- Loss of interest in work.

In addition, the following general signs and symptoms have been identified with stress:

- *Cognitive*—confusion, inability to make judgments or decisions, loss of motivation, memory problems, loss of objectivity.
- *Psychological*—depression, excessive anger, over-reacting, negativism, hostility, defensiveness, mood swings, feelings of worthlessness.
- *Physical*—constant exhaustion, headaches, stomach problems, dizziness, pounding heart.
- *Behavioral*—overeating, increased use of drugs or alcohol, grinding teeth, hyperactivity, lack of energy.

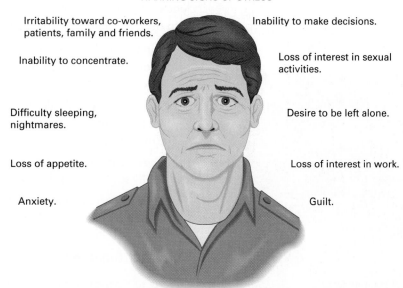

WARNING SIGNS OF STRESS

Irritability toward co-workers, patients, family and friends.

Inability to concentrate.

Difficulty sleeping, nightmares.

Loss of appetite.

Anxiety.

Inability to make decisions.

Loss of interest in sexual activities.

Desire to be left alone.

Loss of interest in work.

Guilt.

FIGURE 2-13 Beware! Chronic stress can lead to burnout.

■ *Social*—frequent arguments, decreased ability to relate to patients.

Make Lifestyle Changes

Certain lifestyle changes can be helpful in dealing with chronic stress. One change you can make is in your diet. Certain foods increase the body's response to stress. So cut down on sugar, caffeine, and alcohol. Avoid fatty foods, and eat more low-fat carbohydrates. While at work, eat often but in small amounts.

Avoid alcohol and other kinds of self-medication. Reaching for a drink or pills will not help you cope with stress. In fact, they increase stress. Remember, problems will still be there when you wake from your stupor. They may even be worse, because you did not act on them right away.

Exercise often (Figure 2-14). It has all kinds of benefits, including release for pent-up emotions.

Finally, learn to relax. Meditation and visual imagery are helpful techniques. You also may want to try to cut loose a little bit. Watch a funny movie, read a good book, or go dancing or to a concert.

Keep Balance in Your Life

One way to balance work, recreation, family, and health is to assess your priorities. Take a few minutes to list all your activities on paper. Write "1" beside your first priority. Write "2" beside your second, and so on. Then perform those activities—all of them—in the order you assigned.

Be sure to share your worries with someone else. Talk to someone you trust and respect. It can help relieve stress and help you discover alternatives. A good confidante listens well and asks questions that help you explore your ideas honestly.

Still another way to help keep balance in your life is to accept the fact that you will sometimes make mistakes. Admit to yourself that no one is right all the time. Understand that a mistake does not reduce your value. You do not have to be perfect to do a good job.

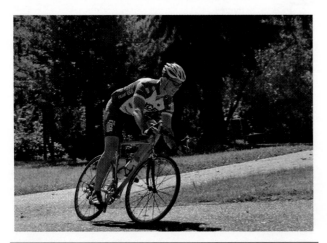

FIGURE 2-14 Safeguard your own health with regular exercise.

The support of your family and friends is essential to helping you manage stress. Keep in mind, though, that they also suffer from stress related to your job. Their stress factors include the following:

■ *Lack of understanding.* Families typically have little if any knowledge about prehospital emergency care.

■ *Fear of separation or of being ignored.* Long hours can take their toll and increase your family's distress over your absences. You may hear, "Your job is more important to you than your family!"

■ *Worry about on-call situations.* Stress at home may increase when your family focuses on the danger you face when you respond to emergency calls.

■ *Frustrated desire to share.* It may be too difficult for you to talk about what happened on certain calls. Even if your family and friends understand this, they may still feel frustrated in their desire to help and support you.

If at all possible, you can help to keep balance in your life by changing your work environment. Request work shifts that allow more time to relax with family and friends. Ask for a rotation of duty to a less stressful assignment. Take periodic breaks to exercise and to support and encourage coworkers.

Seek Professional Help

Mental-health professionals, social workers, and clergy can help you realize that your reactions are normal. They can also mobilize your best coping strategies and suggest more effective ways to deal with stress.

Respond to On-Scene Stress

A rescuer's emotional responses to stressful scenes may include weakness, nausea, vomiting, or fainting. You can help avoid these reactions by using the following techniques:

■ Remind yourself that the patient desperately needs you and your skills. You must be in control to give the best emergency care.

■ Close your eyes and take several long, deep breaths. Focus on counting each breath. When you feel more in control, return to giving emergency care.

■ Change your thought patterns. Very quietly hum or mentally sing a peaceful song.

■ Eat properly to maintain your blood sugar levels. Low blood sugar can add to a fainting problem.

Stressful Incidents

Working in emergency conditions is stressful. That's a fact. Fortunately, there are proven methods of dealing with it. Some particularly stressful incidents you may encounter include serious injury or death of a rescuer in the line of duty;

multiple-casualty incident; suicide of an emergency worker; an event that attracts media attention; injury or death of someone you know; injury or death of a child; child abuse; an incident with distressing sights, sounds, or smells.

Fortunately, those calls are pretty rare. When they do occur, responders at the scene often deal with them differently. Some are not seriously affected; others may feel anything from anxiety to sadness to anger. Each response is different. Each response is normal.

To deal with feelings from a stressful incident, maintain as normal a schedule or routine as possible. Do not focus on media reports of the event. Avoid using food, alcohol, or medications in excess. Finally, seek professional help if you have persistent stress, depression, or other ongoing problems you believe are related to the incident.

Remember, *each person reacts differently.* Some feel the stress. Others wonder if they are okay because they do not feel any stress at all. It is not a sign of weakness to seek professional help. Rather, it is wise and often covered under your agency's insurance or worker's compensation.

One theory of dealing with stress is called *critical incident stress management (CISM)*. This theory was widely practiced in EMS until recently. Some medical directors, EMS agencies, and public health authorities have begun to speak out against some of its practices and are in the process of researching other methods of dealing with stress. Ask your instructor, medical director, or agency head about current research. Some locations practice CISM and it may be on your examination; therefore, it is presented in this chapter.

There are two basic critical incident stress management techniques: *defusing* and *debriefing.* NOTE: Although some disagree with the specific methods of defusing and debriefing, all agree that seeking help from a trained, professional counselor, social worker, or psychologist for ongoing symptoms of stress is a wise thing to do.

A *critical incident* is any event that causes unusually strong emotions that interfere with your ability to function either during the incident or later. This type of stress requires aggressive and immediate management, including pre-incident stress education, on-scene peer support, one-on-one support, disaster support services, follow-up services, spouse and family support, community outreach programs, and other general health and welfare programs, such as wellness programs.

Debriefing

The cornerstone of most CISM programs is a *critical incident stress debriefing (CISD).* It combines a team of peer counselors with mental-health professionals (Figure 2-15). The debriefing is meant to help rescuers vent their feelings quickly. Its nonthreatening environment also encourages rescuers to feel free to air their concerns and reactions.

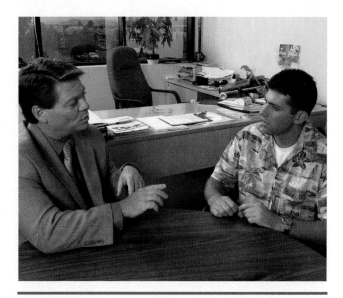

FIGURE 2-15 Seek help if you feel the effects of stress from a critical incident or from your job as an EMS responder.

CISD includes anyone involved in an incident—police, firefighters, EMS personnel, dispatchers, doctors, and so on. In some cases, it may also include their families.

Ideally, the debriefing is held within 24 to 72 hours of a critical incident. It is not an investigation or an interrogation. Everything said at a debriefing is confidential. Rescuers are urged to explore any physical, mental, or emotional symptoms they are having. CISD counselors and mental-health professionals then evaluate the information and offer suggestions on how to cope with the stress resulting from the incident. After multiple-casualty incidents (such as explosions or earthquakes), a number of CISD meetings may be needed.

Defusing

Much shorter and less formal than a debriefing, a defusing is usually held within hours of a critical incident. It is attended only by those most directly involved and lasts only 30 to 45 minutes. A defusing gives rescuers a chance to vent their feelings and gather information they may need before the larger group meets. It may either eliminate the need for a formal debriefing, or it may enhance a later debriefing.

Q:
1. What is the grieving process?

2. What are the stages of the grieving process?

3. Briefly, what are some positive steps a First Responder can take to manage stress?

The Call Follow-up

At the beginning of this chapter, you read that First Responders were at a violent and potentially dangerous scene. To find out what precautions the First Responders took to protect themselves, read the following. It describes how the call was completed.

Scene Size-up *(continued)* When we realized that the loud sounds we were hearing were people fighting, my partner and I looked at each other, returned to our vehicle, and immediately called the police. I'm glad we did. We might have been right in the middle of it if we hadn't.

We moved our vehicle out of sight and waited. When the police arrived, we reported what we knew and they went in. After a few minutes, they radioed to tell us the scene was secure. But we still approached cautiously.

The officers told us that two brothers had been in a fist fight. One of the brothers said his hands went through a window. Both of the brothers appeared to be intoxicated.

Initial Assessment After we put on eye protection and gloves, we introduced ourselves to Mike, the brother who needed medical help. He seemed calm. Mike had moderate bleeding from his right forearm. His airway and breathing were good. He denied any other injuries or falls.

Physical Examination Even though Mike denied other injuries, we decided to do a physical exam anyway. Sometimes people get into fights and get so excited, they don't know they're hurt. Since there were two of us, my partner controlled the bleeding while I checked Mike's head, neck, chest, back, abdomen, and extremities.

While we waited for an ambulance, Mike's brother became loud and abusive to the police. We had the patient walk outside with us to get away from the potential danger. There we checked his pulse and respirations.

Patient History Mike admitted to drinking six or eight cans of beer before the fight started. He told us that he had asthma, but wasn't feeling any respiratory distress or problems. He took an inhaler for his asthma, but didn't have one with him. He continued to deny any injuries other than the cut to his forearm.

Ongoing Assessment We rechecked Mike's airway and breathing. They were okay. Mike showed no changes in mental status. The bleeding was controlled and the bandages were secure. We didn't get to recheck the vitals before the ambulance arrived.

Patient Hand-off Since I was in charge of the patient's care, I reported to the EMTs (see below). After we transferred patient care to the EMTs, we asked the police if there were any more injuries on scene. They told us no, they were all set. So, we returned to service.

 ## Hand-off Report

"The patient's name is Mike. He's a 22-year-old male who had sustained a laceration to his right forearm from going through a window. The wound has been dressed and bandaged. The bleeding was moderate and easily controlled. Mike has been drinking but has been alert and oriented throughout the call. His airway and breathing are good. He denies any other injuries. He has a history of asthma and uses an inhaler. The physical exam was negative for injuries anywhere other than his arm. His pulse is 88, strong, and regular. His respirations are 18 and adequate. We were about to recheck his vitals as you pulled up."

The Last Word *Your safety and well-being are your top priorities. Without them, you cannot be an effective First Responder. Throughout this textbook, you will find reminders about taking BSI and other safety precautions. Make note of them.*

Chapter Review

Focus on the EMS Team

Television has led us to believe that it is okay to rush into calls without regard for our own well-being. Not true! That isn't real life. The fact is if rescuers become ill or injured, they will not be able to perform what they set out to do—help patients.

One of the most important factors to consider in the first 10 minutes of a call is safety. Absolutely be sure to practice body substance isolation (BSI) precautions on every call. And always remain alert to the potential for violence, hazardous materials,

and other unsafe conditions. Do this for your own sake, as well as for your partner, your EMS team members, and your patient.

It is easy to understand that all you want to do so early in your career is focus on learning about illness and injury. However, do not underestimate the importance of the information in this chapter. Just to make sure you realize how critical it is, there will be reminders about safety in every chapter in this book.

Summing Up

- An infectious disease spreads from one person to another directly (through contact with blood or other body fluids) or indirectly (by way of a contaminated object or by contaminated droplets that are coughed into the air).

- BSI precautions assume that all blood and body fluids are infectious. When the First Responder takes body substance isolation (BSI) precautions, it is possible to take care of all patients safely, even those with infectious diseases.

- BSI precautions include handwashing; properly cleaning, disinfecting, or sterilizing equipment; and using personal protective equipment (PPE).

- Personal protective equipment (PPE) for the First Responder includes eye protection, gloves, gowns, surgical masks, and the N-95 or HEPA respirator.

- Immunizations recommended for active-duty First Responders include hepatitis B, influenza, polio, rubella, measles, and mumps. A tuberculin skin (PPD) test is also recommended.

- The First Responder must report any suspected exposure to blood or body fluids as soon as possible to a supervisor and to medical control. Follow all local protocols in this matter.

- This general rule applies to all emergency scenes: If the scene is unsafe, make it safe before you enter. Otherwise, call for and then wait for help to arrive.

- Once a scene is secure, take measures to protect the patient from hazards such as fire, structural instability, gasoline leaks, chemical spills, oncoming traffic, and extremes in temperature. Bystanders also should be protected.

- A First Responder may need to call for help when the emergency involves a motor-vehicle or airplane crash; the presence of toxic substances or low levels of oxygen; a crime scene; the presence of a weapon of any kind; possible drug or

alcohol use; arguing, threats, violent behavior, broken glass, overturned furniture; and unstable surfaces such as water and ice.

- Depending on the scene hazard, First Responders may need equipment such as turnout gear, puncture-proof gloves, impact-resistant helmet with reflective tape and chin strap, reflective clothing, waterproof boots and slip-resistant gloves, body armor, or even a warm hat and long underwear.

- While caring for patients at a crime scene, preserve the chain of evidence by not disturbing the scene unless absolutely necessary for medical care.

- Death and dying are inherent parts of emergency medical care. When your patient is dying, you must care for his or her emotional needs as well as the injury or illness.

- The stages of the grieving process are denial, anger, bargaining, depression, and acceptance.

- To help a patient and his or her family through the grieving process, keep in mind that their needs will include dignity, respect, sharing, communication, privacy, and control.

- Incidents especially stressful to First Responders include serious injury or death of a rescuer in the line of duty; multiple-casualty incident; suicide of an emergency worker; an event that attracts media attention; injury or death of someone you know; injury or death of a child; child abuse; an incident with distressing sights, sounds, or smells.

- One of the best ways for a First Responder to manage chronic stress is to be aware of the warning signs of burnout, such as difficult sleeping, loss of interest in work, and so on.

- Certain lifestyle changes can be helpful in dealing with chronic stress, such as a healthy diet, exercising, and making time for relaxation.

■ In some areas, critical incident stress management (CISM) is recommended for handling particularly stressful emergencies. It offers pre-incident stress education, on-scene peer support, one-on-one support, disaster support services, follow-up serv-ices, spouse and family support, community outreach pro-grams, and other general health and welfare services, such as wellness programs.

Key Terms

body armor a garment made up of a synthetic material that resists penetration by bullets.

body substance isolation (BSI) a strict form of infection control based on the premise that all blood and body fluids are infectious.

cleaning the process of washing a soiled object with soap and water.

disinfecting the process of cleaning plus using a chemical such as alcohol or bleach to kill many of the microorganisms on an object.

grieving process the process by which people cope with death and dying.

HEPA respirator a high-efficiency particulate air respirator; a mask designed to filter out small parti-cles in the air, including bacteria.

infectious disease a disease that can spread from one person to another.

N-95 respirator a mask used by medical personnel to filter out harmful bacteria.

pathogens microorganisms such as bacteria and viruses.

personal protective equipment (PPE) equipment used by a rescuer to protect against injury and the spread of disease.

sterilizing a process in which a chemical or other substance, such as superheated steam, kills all microorganisms on an object.

Knowledge Check

1. Which one of the following is NOT a stage of the grieving process?
   a. denial
   b. acceptance
   c. bargaining
   d. lingering

2. For which one of the following diseases is a preventative vaccine available?
   a. tuberculosis
   b. hepatitis B
   c. hepatitis C
   d. HIV/AIDS

3. As a First Responder, your first scene priority is:
   a. medical intervention.
   b. patient consent.
   c. scene safety.
   d. handwashing.

4. Which one of the following statements about stressful incidents is TRUE?
   a. Everyone feels stress at about the same time and at about the same level.
   b. Some responders are stressed little or not at all by medical emergencies.
   c. Anyone can predict what call will affect which responder the most.
   d. Responders should seek professional help to make sure they have no signs of stress.

5. Family members of a dying patient should be allowed to express emotions, even anger and despair.
    a. True
    b. False

6. Stress is sometimes caused when family members do not understand what the First Responder does in EMS.
    a. True
    b. False

7. Handwashing is the single most important thing you can do to prevent the spread of infection.
    a. True
    b. False

8. Why is scene safety the first priority on any call?

_____

_____

_____

9. If you have been immunized against hepatitis B, why is it necessary to take BSI precautions on calls?

_____

_____

_____

10. What are the five stages of the grieving process?

_____

_____

_____

_____

11. What three things can you do to preserve evidence at a crime scene?

_____

_____

_____

Scenario

As you approach the emergency scene, your general impression is of an intoxicated patient who has a cut lip with minor bleeding. Every time he yells, blood and saliva spray from his mouth. Before entering the scene, which BSI precautions would be most appropriate to take?

_____

_____

_____

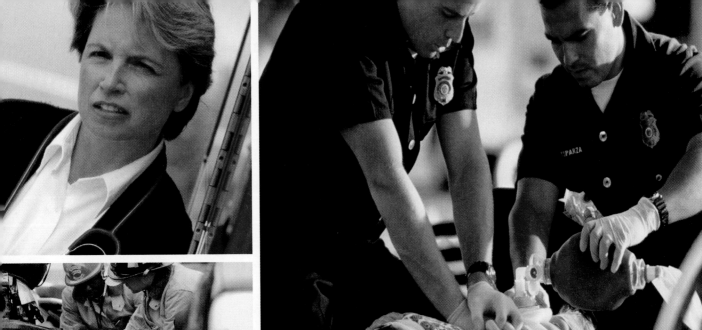

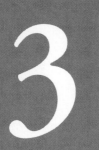

3 | Legal and Ethical Issues

Objectives

From the U.S. Department of Transportation (DOT) 1995 "First Responder: National Standard Curriculum." Material supplemental to the DOT curriculum is listed under "Enrichment."

Cognitive

1-3.1 ▶ Define the First Responder scope of care. (p. 35)

1-3.2 ▶ Discuss the importance of Do Not Resuscitate [DNR] (advance directives) and local or state provisions regarding EMS application. (p. 37)

1-3.3 ▶ Define consent and discuss the methods of obtaining consent. (pp. 36–39)

1-3.4 ▶ Differentiate between expressed and implied consent. (p. 36)

1-3.5 ▶ Explain the role of consent of minors in providing care. (pp. 36–37)

1-3.6 ▶ Discuss the implications for the First Responder in patient refusal of transport. (pp. 37–39)

1-3.7 ▶ Discuss the issues of abandonment, negligence, and battery and their implications to the First Responder. (pp. 39, 41–42)

1-3.8 ▶ State the conditions necessary for the First Responder to have a duty to act. (pp. 39, 41)

1-3.9 ▶ Explain the importance, necessity, and legality of patient confidentiality. (p. 41)

1-3.10 ▶ List the actions that a First Responder should take to assist in the preservation of a crime scene. (p. 42)

1-3.11 ▶ State the conditions that require a First Responder to notify local law enforcement officials. (p. 42)

1-3.12 ▶ Discuss issues concerning the fundamental components of documentation. (p. 42)

Affective

1-3.13 ▶ Explain the rationale for the needs, benefits, and usage of advance directives. (p. 37)

1-3.14 ▶ Explain the rationale for the concept of varying degrees of DNR. (p. 37)

Psychomotor

No objectives are identified by the DOT.

Enrichment

▶ Explain the "Good Samaritan" laws and how they affect First Responders. (pp. 41–42)

▶ Describe a First Responder's role in the process of organ retrieval. (p. 43)

Introduction

Legal and ethical issues are vital elements of a First Responder's life, both on and off duty. You may already have questions. For example, should you stop to treat an accident victim when you are off duty? May a child be treated without a parent's consent? This chapter will help you answer these and other questions. It describes your scope of care and what it means to have a duty to act. It defines patient consent and explains advance directives. It also gives you an overview of various other legal issues that will affect you in the field.

Section 1 Scope of Care

Emergency care has changed a lot since its early days. One improvement has been in the quality of EMS training. People have come to expect a competent First Responder, one who understands and accepts his or her responsibilities to patients and to the public.

Legal Duties

Each state defines a First Responder's **scope of care** (actions that are legally allowed). All First Responders must provide for the well-being of their patients as outlined in the scope of care. For example, providing CPR when needed is within your scope of care. However, stitching up a deep wound is not, and for you, it is illegal.

State law is enhanced by your local medical director. In fact, your legal right to act as a First Responder depends on medical oversight. State law is further enhanced by the "First Responder: National Standard Curriculum," established by the U.S. Department of Transportation (DOT).

When providing medical care, you should:

■ Follow standing orders and protocols as approved by medical direction.

■ Consult medical direction via phone or radio any time there is a question about the scope of care.

■ Communicate clearly and completely with medical direction.

■ Follow orders the medical director gives.

Ethical Responsibilities

A *code of ethics* is a list of rules for ideal conduct. Basically, if you place the welfare of a patient above all else during emergency care, you rarely will do anything unethical. Your ethical responsibilities are:

■ Make the physical and emotional needs of the patient a priority. Serve those needs with respect for human dignity and with no regard to nationality, race, gender, creed, or status.

■ Practice your skills to the point of mastery. Show respect for the competence of other medical workers.

■ Continue your education and take refresher courses. Stay on top of changes in EMS. Help define and uphold professional standards.

■ Critically review your performance. Seek ways to improve response time, patient outcome, and communication.

■ Report with honesty. Hold in confidence all information obtained in the course of your work, unless required by law to share it.

■ Work in harmony with other First Responders, EMTs, and other members of the health-care team.

 Q:

1. How can a First Responder be sure to act within his or her scope of care?

2. What are the ethical responsibilities of a First Responder?

THE CALL

Dispatch Our first response unit was dispatched to a child who fell. I remember thinking how calls involving kids get to me. I hoped we could help this child.

Scene Size-up We arrived to find the patient sitting up and crying. It appeared that he had fallen from his bike when it hit a tree. The bike's front tire was flat, the front end was bent in, and there were several yards of obvious skid marks. The patient had been wearing a helmet.

A police officer was kneeling and talking to the boy quietly. The officer motioned us to approach. He said, "A dog jumped onto the path.

Mark, here, did his best to avoid hitting it. But then that darn tree got in the way."

We introduced ourselves to the patient. He said he was nine years old. While my partner began an initial assessment, I spoke to the police officer to see if contact had been made with the boy's parents.

Why are they looking for the child's parents? Can't they just care for the child's injuries and let him be on his way? These questions revolve around the issue of consent—one of many legal and ethical issues you will face as a First Responder. As you read Chapter 3, consider how you might answer them.

Section 2 Patient Consent and Refusal

Patient Competence

A **competent** adult is one who is lucid and able to make an informed decision about medical care. He understands your questions. He also understands the implications of decisions made about medical care. A patient must be competent in order to refuse treatment. Therefore, you must determine competence in every adult you want to treat.

Generally, consider an adult *incompetent* if he or she:

- Is under the influence of alcohol or drugs.
- Has an altered mental status.
- Has a serious illness or injury that could affect judgment.
- Is mentally ill or mentally retarded.

Patient Consent

By law, you must get a patient's **consent**, or permission, before you can provide emergency care. For that consent to be valid, the patient must be competent and the consent must be informed. It is your responsibility, therefore, to fully explain the care you plan to give, as well as the related risks.

There are two general types of consent: **expressed consent** and **implied consent.**

Expressed Consent

Expressed consent may consist of oral consent, a nod, or an affirming gesture from a competent adult. To get it you must explain your plan for emergency care *in terms the patient can understand*. Include the risks, too. In other words, in order to make an informed decision, the patient needs a clear idea of all factors that would affect a reasonable person to either accept or refuse treatment.

Implied Consent

In an emergency when an unresponsive patient is at risk of death, disability, or deterioration of condition, the law assumes that he would agree to care. This is called *implied consent*. It applies when you assume that a patient who cannot consent to life-saving care, would if he were able to.

Implied consent also applies to a patient who refuses care and then becomes unresponsive, and to a patient who is not competent to refuse care.

Children and Mentally Incompetent Adults

Depending on state law, a **minor** usually is any person under the age of 18 or 21. A parent or legal guardian must

First Responder Practice

Consider this scenario: You walk into a house and find a patient lying on a couch. The relative who meets you says, "I think he's dead. He's had cancer, and we got this paper from his doctor so he can die in peace." Picture it. You have a patient who needs CPR and a relative who presents you with some type of form. Every second you spend trying to figure it out could be used to help the patient, and the seconds are ticking by.

This does not have to happen to you. Learn well the regulations that affect your duties as a First Responder, before you find yourself in a situation like this.

give consent before you can treat a minor. The same is true for a mentally incompetent adult. However, if a life-threatening condition exists and the parent or guardian is not available, provide emergency care under the principle of implied consent.

An **emancipated minor** is one who is married, pregnant, a parent, a member of the armed forces, or financially independent and living away from home with permission of the courts. You do not need the consent of a parent or legal guardian to treat this patient. You only need the patient's consent.

Advance Directives

There may be a time when you are called to treat a terminally ill patient. He may ask you to let him die when his heart or lungs stop working. Legally, if the patient is competent, he or she has the right to make this request.

An **advance directive** is written in advance of an emergency. It must be signed by both the patient and a physician. An example of an advance directive is a **Do Not Resuscitate (DNR) order** (Figure 3-1). Often, it will document the chronically or terminally ill patient's wish not to be resuscitated. It also may allow the First Responder to withhold resuscitation legally.

When you are given an advance directive, you must determine to the best of your ability if it is valid. Usually it is accompanied by a doctor's written instructions. Check to see that they are written clearly and concisely. They also should be typed or written legibly on professional letterhead. Phrases like "no heroics" or "no extraordinary treatment" are *not* clear enough to be legal.

In many areas, a standard form is used for a DNR order. In states, the law also requires that patients wear some

sort of DNR insignia on their bodies where emergency personnel will be sure to find it.

By its very nature, a DNR order is best suited to a hospital or nursing home. There, all personnel know the patient and his or her physician. The DNR order, if needed, can be quickly found and verified. However, problems may arise in the field. In many areas, for example, a second physician must verify the patient's condition. This can be difficult in an emergency situation, even if the DNR order is on hand. Another problem is the time it takes to verify a DNR order. Precious, life-saving moments can be lost.

There are varying degrees of DNR orders. For example, one may explain that a patient allows all medical care except long-term life support. Another might say that the patient specifically does not allow the use of a respirator.

If you are ever in doubt about the validity of an advance directive, you must begin full resuscitation immediately. However, always consult your medical director or the hospital emergency department physician before you decide to either follow or put aside a DNR order.

Be sure to review all state law and local protocols on this issue.

Patient Refusal

A competent adult has the right to refuse treatment for himself or his child. Under the law, he must first be informed of the treatment, fully understand it, and completely comprehend the risks involved in refusing it. He may refuse verbally, by pulling away, shaking his head, gesturing, or pushing you away.

A competent adult has the right to withdraw from treatment after it has started. This is true for a patient who initially gave consent but then changes his mind. It is also true for the patient who at first was unresponsive, but then wakes and asks you to stop.

A patient's legal refusal of treatment or transport must follow the rules of expressed consent. That is, the patient must be mentally competent and of legal age. The

First on Scene

When a patient (or guardian, if the patient is a child) refuses First Responder care, make every reasonable effort to persuade him to give consent. If he still refuses, remain calm and professional, but insist that the incoming EMTs or paramedics evaluate him. They have more training and may be better able to assess the emergency, explain it to the patient, and obtain consent.

PREHOSPITAL DO NOT RESUSCITATE ORDERS

<u>ATTENDING PHYSICIAN</u>

In completing this prehospital DNR form, please check part A if no intervention by prehospital personnel is indicated. Please check Part A and options from Part B if specific interventions by prehospital personnel are indicated. To give a valid prehospital DNR order, this form must be completed by the patient's attending physician and must be provided to prehospital personnel.

A) _____**Do Not Resuscitate (DNR)**:
No Cardiopulmonary Resuscitation or Advanced Cardiac Life Support be performed by prehospital personnel

B) _____**Modified Support:**
Prehospital personnel administer the following checked options:
_____Oxygen administration
_____Full airway support: intubation, airways, bag/valve/mask
_____Venipuncture: IV crystalloids and/or blood draw
_____External cardiac pacing
_____Cardiopulmonary resuscitation
_____Cardiac defibrillator
_____Pneumatic anti-shock garment
_____Ventilator
_____ACLS meds
_____Other interventions/medications (physician specify)
_____

Prehospital personnel are informed that (print patient name)_____
should receive no resuscitation (DNR) or should receive Modified Support as indicated. This directive is medically appropriate and is further documented by a physician's order and a progress note on the patient's permanent medical record. Informed consent from the capacitated patient or the incapacitated patient's legitimate surrogate is documented on the patient's permanent medical record. The DNR order is in full force and effect as of the date indicated below.

_____   _____
Attending Physician's Signature   _____

_____   _____
Print Attending Physician's Name   Print Patient's Name and Location
                                                                         (Home Address or Health Care Facility)

_____
Attending Physician's Telephone

_____   _____
Date   Expiration Date (6 Mos from Signature)

FIGURE 3-1 Example of a "do not resuscitate" order.

---

patient also must be informed of all the risks *in terms he or she can fully understand.* When in doubt, always err in favor of providing care.

Complete and accurate records are key to protecting yourself from liability (legal responsibility). So before you leave the scene:

- *Have the ambulance continue to the scene* to assist in patient assessment. EMTs or paramedics will be able to help convince the patient to accept care and to document refusal if necessary.

- *Try again to persuade the patient to accept emergency care or transport.* Tell him clearly why it is essential. Be especially clear when you explain what could happen if he refuses care. Write down what you tell him. Then have the patient read it aloud to see if he understands.

REFUSAL OF TREATMENT AND TRANSPORTATION

I, THE UNDERSIGNED HAVE BEEN ADVISED THAT MEDICAL ASSISTANCE ON MY BEHALF IS NECESSARY AND THAT REFUSAL OF SAID ASSISTANCE AND TRANSPORTATION MAY RESULT IN DEATH, OR IMPERIL MY HEALTH. NEVERTHELESS, I REFUSE TO ACCEPT TREATMENT OR TRANSPORT AND ASSUME ALL RISKS AND CONSEQUENCES OF MY DECISION AND RELEASE GOLD CROSS AMBULANCE COMPANY AND ITS EMPLOYEES FROM ANY LIABILITY ARISING FROM MY REFUSAL.

_____
SIGNATURE OF PATIENT

_____
WITNESSED BY

_____
DATE SIGNED

FIGURE 3-2 Example of a patient refusal statement.

- *Be sure the patient is able to make a rational, informed decision.* Note that a patient who is seriously ill or injured may only appear competent. Such a patient may be emotionally, intellectually, or physically impaired and may not be able to absorb all the information you give.

- *Consult medical direction as required by local protocol.*

- *Have the patient sign a refusal or "release from liability" form* (Figures 3-2 through 3-4). It must be signed by the patient and a witness. If the patient refuses to sign, indicate that on the form and have a witness sign it. Many areas use official documents for patients to sign. Check local protocols.

- *Before you leave, encourage the patient to seek help if certain symptoms develop.* Be specific. Avoid using terms the patient may not understand. For example, you might tell a patient to go to the hospital emergency department "if you get a burning pain in your stomach" or "if you start having shortness of breath." Then document the fact that you did.

- *Advise the patient to call EMS again immediately if he changes his mind.*

1. How can you recognize a "competent" adult?

2. When would you consider an adult "incompetent"?

3. How is "expressed consent" different from "implied consent"?

4. When may a patient refuse First Responder care?

Section 3 Other Legal Aspects of Emergency Care

Assault and Battery

There is no single definition of assault and battery. Traditionally, threatening physical harm is **assault.** Actual unlawful physical contact is **battery.** In the context of emergency medical care, you can be charged with assault and battery if you touch a patient's body or clothing without first getting consent.

Abandonment and Negligence

Simply stated, **abandonment** means you stopped providing care for a patient without making sure that the same or better care would be continued. Under the law, once you start giving emergency care to a patient, you must continue until another health-care professional with at least as much expertise as you takes over or until the police order you to leave the scene.

Negligence is defined as carelessness, inattention, disregard, inadvertence, or oversight that was accidental but avoidable. You may be charged with negligence if your care deviates from the accepted standard of care and results in further injury to the patient.

To establish negligence, the court must decide that all four of the following are true:

- *The First Responder had a duty to act.* The term **duty to act** refers to your contractual or legal obligation to provide care. That is, while you are on duty, you must care for a patient who needs it and consents to it.

EMS PATIENT REFUSAL CHECKLIST

PATIENT's NAME: _____ AGE: _____

LOCATION OF CALL: _____ DATE: _____

AGENCY INCIDENT #: _____ AGENCY CODE: _____

NAME OF PERSON FILLING OUT FORM: _____

I.   ASSESSMENT OF PATIENT (Check appropriate response for each item)

   1.   Oriented to: Person? ☐ Yes ☐ No
                   Place?   ☐ Yes ☐ No
                   Time?   ☐ Yes ☐ No
                   Situation? ☐ Yes ☐ No

   2.   Altered level of consciousness? ☐ Yes ☐ No

   3.   Head injury? ☐ Yes ☐ No

   4.   Alcohol or drug ingestion by exam or history? ☐ Yes ☐ No

II.   PATIENT INFORMED (Check appropriate response for each item)

☐ Yes ☐ No   Medical treatment/evaluation needed

☐ Yes ☐ No   Ambulance transport needed

☐ Yes ☐ No   Further harm could result without medical treatment/evaluation

☐ Yes ☐ No   Transport by means other than ambulance could be hazardous in light of patient's illness/injury

☐ Yes ☐ No   Patient provided with Refusal Information Sheet

☐ Yes ☐ No   Patient accepted Refusal Information Sheet

III.   DISPOSITION

☐ Refused all EMS assistance

☐ Refused field treatment, but accepted transport

☐ Refused transport, but accepted field treatment

☐ Refused transport to recommended facility

☐ Patient transported by private vehicle to_____

☐ Released in care or custody of self

☐ Released in care or custody of relative or friend

   Name:_____ Relationship:_____

☐ Released in custody of law enforcement agency

   Agency:_____ Officer:_____

☐ Released in custody of other agency

   Agency:_____ Officer:_____

IV.   COMMENTS: _____

_____

_____

_____

FIGURE 3-3 Sample patient refusal checklist from Spokane County EMS, Washington State. Such checklists are designed to ensure the patient is competent and properly informed.

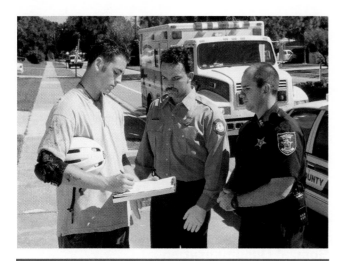

FIGURE 3-4 A refusal must be signed by the patient and a witness.

- *There was a breach of duty.* A breach of duty exists when a First Responder either fails to act or fails to act appropriately. That is, the First Responder violated the standard of care reasonably expected of a First Responder with similar background and training.
- *The patient was injured physically or psychologically.*
- *The First Responder caused the injury.* It must be proven that the First Responder's breach of duty caused or contributed to the patient's injury.

Note that your duty to act also means that you must render care to a patient to the best of your ability. You must follow accepted guidelines for care and act as any other prudent person would in the same situation.

In some cases, a duty to act refers to an implied contractual or legal obligation. For example, a patient may call for EMS. The dispatcher confirms that help will be sent. All EMS members who respond—including First Responders—then have a legal obligation to provide treatment to the patient.

In most states, you do not have a duty to act when you are off duty or driving an emergency vehicle outside your agency's service area. (Check your state laws.) However, you may feel a certain moral or ethical obligation to help. In such cases, take extra steps to protect yourself against legal risk. Carefully document all aspects of the call and treatment you give, including a patient's refusal of care.

In general, your best defense against negligence is to have a professional attitude, to provide a consistently high standard of care, and to correctly and completely document the care you provide.

Confidentiality

A patient's history, condition, and emergency care are confidential. To release this information, you must have a written form signed by the patient or legal guardian. Never release any patient information on request unless you are authorized to do so in writing.

By law, you are allowed to release information without a patient's or guardian's permission only if:

- Another health-care provider needs it in order to continue medical care.
- You are requested by the police to provide it as part of a crime investigation. State laws, for example, require the reporting of rape, abuse, gunshot wounds, and certain other crimes.
- You are required by legal subpoena to provide it in court (Figure 3-5).

You may have heard of a federal regulation called HIPAA (Health Insurance Portability and Accountability Act). You have probably already encountered it, when your own physician or pharmacologist asked you to sign a form indicating that you were given a copy of their privacy practices. That is a HIPAA requirement. It provides strict guidance on how patient information may be used and distributed. Violation can result in severe penalties. NOTE: Not all agencies are bound by HIPAA.

Good Samaritan Laws

Many states have "Good Samaritan" laws. The first of these laws was enacted in 1959 in California. It was designed to protect doctors who render emergency care from civil malpractice suits. Most states now have laws of their own,

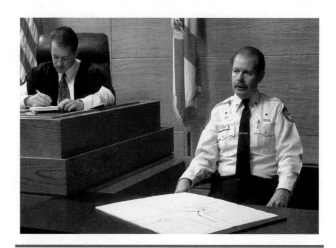

FIGURE 3-5 First Responders may be asked to testify in court.

some of which cover EMS personnel. Be sure to learn your local laws.

Generally, these laws protect an off-duty First Responder from liability for acts performed in good faith unless those acts are grossly negligent. Under these laws, the person suing must prove that emergency care was markedly below the **standard of care**. Standard of care is defined as the care expected to be provided to the same patient under the same conditions by another First Responder who had received the same training. (This is referred to as the "reasonable man" test.)

If you are sued and the case goes to court, a *tort* proceeding will be held. This is a civil court action, not a criminal one. It determines whether or not the natural rights of an individual have been violated. In a tort proceeding, it must be proven that you are guilty of **gross negligence.**

A Good Samaritan law does not prevent you from being sued. But it may give you some protection against losing the lawsuit if you have performed according to the standard of care for a First Responder. So while on and off duty, your best defense against lawsuits is prevention. Always render care to the best of your ability. Do no more or less than your scope of care allows. If you keep your patient's best interests in mind, you will seldom—if ever—go wrong.

Preservation of Evidence

Whenever a First Responder is called to a potential crime scene, dispatch should also notify the police. In general, a potential crime scene is any scene that may require police support. That includes a potential or actual suicide, homicide, drug overdose, domestic dispute, abuse, hit-and-run, riot, robbery, or any scene involving gunfire or a weapon.

Your first concern should always be your own safety. *If you suspect that a crime is in progress or a criminal is active at the scene, do not try to provide care to any patient.* Wait until the police arrive and tell you that the scene is safe. Once the scene is safe, your priority is patient care.

When on scene, do not disturb any item that may be evidence. Basic guidelines include:

- Observe and document anything unusual at the scene.
- Touch only what you need to touch.
- Move only what you need to move to protect the patient and provide emergency care.
- Do not use the telephone unless the police give you permission to do so. They may wish to find out who the last caller was.

- Move the patient only if he or she is in danger or must be moved in order for you to provide emergency care.
- If possible, do not cut through holes in the patient's clothing. They may have been caused by bullets or stabbing.
- Do not cut through any knot in a rope or tie. Knots are often used as evidence.
- If the crime is rape, do not wash the patient or allow the patient to wash. Ask him or her not to change clothing, use the bathroom, or take anything by mouth. Doing any of these things could destroy evidence.

Special Documentation

In general, physicians must report suspected child, elder, and spouse abuse. Some states require others—such as teachers and EMS first responders—to report them as well. Related state laws often grant immunity from liability for libel, slander, or defamation of character as long as the report is made in good faith.

EMS personnel may be required to report an injury that may be the result of a crime. That includes gunshot wounds, knife wounds, and poisonings. Your state may also want you to report any injury that you suspect was caused by sexual assault.

In some areas, EMS workers must report all suspected infectious disease exposure. That includes TB, hepatitis B, and AIDS. Other situations to report may include use of restraints on a patient, attempted suicides, and dog bites. Learn your local and state requirements.

All of these situations require written documentation. When doing so, remember to stay objective. Document only what you have personally seen, not opinions or anything other than facts. If you document something another person has said, place the statement in quotes: "It was Billy who stabbed me" or "He rarely takes his medications when he is suppose to."

(More information on documentation may be found in Chapter 13.)

Special Situations

Medical Identification Tags

Some patients may wear or carry a medical identification tag (Figure 3-6). Such tags may be found on bracelets, necklaces, or cards carried in a wallet. They identify a specific medical condition such as an allergy, epilepsy, or diabetes. Look for them whenever you examine a patient. Many list a phone number you can call for detailed information.

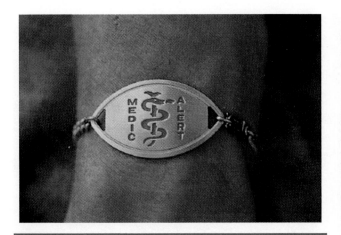

FIGURE 3-6 Example of a medical identification tag.

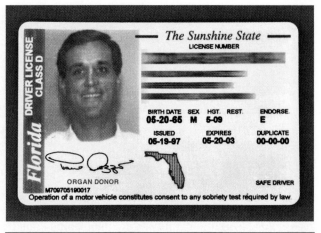

FIGURE 3-7 Example of an organ donor sticker on a driver's license. *(Don Hall Productions)*

Donor and Organ Harvesting

In general, organs may be donated only if there is a signed document giving permission to harvest them. A signed donor card is a legal document. So is the sticker on the reverse side of some driver licenses. (See Figure 3-7.)

Treat a potential organ donor the same as you would treat any other patient. Remember, the person is a patient first, an organ donor last. So, in addition to providing the appropriate emergency medical care, you can:

■ *Identify the patient as a potential donor.* Patients who are about to die or who have died within hours may be organ donors. In each case, the hospital staff and the patient's family must make the ultimate decision.

■ *Provide life-saving emergency care,* such as CPR. It will help to maintain vital organs. This is best accomplished by treating every patient equally well.

 Q:

1. In EMS, how are the terms "abandonment" and "negligence" defined?

2. When does a First Responder have a duty to act?

3. When may a First Responder release information without a patient's or guardian's permission?

4. What may you move or disturb at the scene of a crime?

The Call Follow-up

At the beginning of this chapter, you read about a nine-year-old patient who had fallen from his bike. To see how chapter information applies to this emergency, read the following. It describes how the call was completed.

Initial Assessment My partner confirmed that the patient's ABCs—airway, breathing, and circulation—were adequate. There was no obvious external bleeding. Our initial impression was that a nine-year-old boy had hit a tree with his bike. He complained of pain to his arm.

   Just then, Mark's mother arrived on scene. She gave consent for his care, and my partner continued his assessment.

Physical Examination The mother's presence calmed the boy. We checked Mark carefully. We examined his head, neck, chest, abdomen, back, pelvis, and extremities. The only sign of injury was to Mark's arm. He wasn't thrown from the bike, so we did not suspect spinal injuries. His pulse was 88, strong and regular, and his respirations were 18 and adequate. My partner manually stabilized the arm to prevent further injury. I spoke to Mark's mother about his medical history.

Patient History I was told that Mark was basically healthy. He had a heart murmur since birth,

but no related problems or complications. He takes no medications. He had a full lunch consisting of spaghetti and meatballs. He has no allergies.

Ongoing Assessment Mark continued to be responsive. He responded to his mother well, which is an important sign in a child, asking her if he was going to have a cast on his arm for his friends to sign. His ABCs were still fine. His pulse, respirations, and skin color and temperature were unchanged.

Patient Hand-off We introduced Mark and his mom to the EMTs who would be taking him to the hospital. We told the EMTs that Mark hit a tree with his bicycle and fell. Then we gave our report (see below).

   The EMTs thanked us and took over care. My partner was asked to stay, since Mark felt comfortable with him. I manually stabilized Mark's arm while the EMT applied a splint. Mark's mom thanked us as she climbed into the ambulance with her son.

   Mark did indeed need a cast for his broken arm, but he is expected to heal completely. While this might not have been a critical emergency, just by stabilizing Mark's arm, we prevented further injury and problems that could have been with him his whole life.

 ## Hand-off Report

"The patient's name is Mark. He complains of pain to his right arm, which we are now stabilizing. He was wearing a helmet. He does not complain of neck or back problems. Mark never lost consciousness and has no other complaints. His pulse is 88, respirations 18. He had spaghetti and meatballs for lunch. He has a heart murmur but no problems with it. No meds, no allergies."

The Last Word *Remember, consent is one of many legal and ethical issues you will face as a* *First Responder. Learn the laws related to you and your EMS system now.*

Chapter Review

Focus on the EMS Team

Did you know that the most common lawsuits against EMS involve patient refusal situations and motor-vehicle collisions? Though lawsuits against EMS personnel are rare, always protect yourself from liability by providing the level of *emergency care you are trained and authorized to provide. Give your patients quality care. Treat them with compassion. And document thoroughly all the emergency medical care you provide.*

Summing Up

- All First Responders are to provide for the well-being of their patients as outlined in the scope of care.

- A First Responder's scope of care is defined by state law, enhanced by the medical director, and further enhanced by the U.S. DOT's "National Standard Curriculum."

- If you place the welfare of a patient above all else during emergency care, you rarely will do anything unethical.

- A competent adult is one who is lucid and able to make an informed decision about medical care. You must determine competence in every adult you want to treat.

- By law, you must get a patient's consent before you can provide emergency care. For that consent to be valid, the patient must be competent and the consent must be informed.

- Expressed consent may consist of oral consent, a nod, or an affirming gesture from a competent adult. To get it, you must explain your plan for emergency care *in terms the patient can understand.*

- Implied consent applies when a patient is at risk of death, disability, or deterioration of condition. The law assumes that in this case he would agree to care.

- A legal guardian must give consent before emergency care may be given to a minor or mentally incompetent adult.

- When you are given an advance directive such as a Do Not Resuscitate (DNR) order, you must determine to the best of your ability if it is valid. If you are in doubt, begin full resuscitation immediately.

- Always consult your medical director or the hospital emergency department physician before you decide to follow or put aside a DNR order.

- A competent adult has the right to refuse treatment for himself or his child. However, he must first be informed of the treatment, fully understand it, and completely comprehend the risks involved in refusing it.

- A competent adult has the right to withdraw from treatment after it has started.

- If a competent adult has refused care, do your reasonable best to change his mind. If you cannot do that, consult medical direction and have the patient sign a refusal or "release from liability" form.

- A First Responder who touches a patient's body or clothing without first getting consent may be charged with assault and battery.

- A First Responder who stops providing emergency care without making sure that the same or better care is provided may be guilty of abandonment.

- A First Responder may be charged with negligence if emergency care deviates from the accepted standard of care and results in further injury to the patient.

- To release information about a patient's history, condition, or emergency care, you must have a written form signed by the patient or legal guardian.

- You may release the patient's confidential information without permission only if another health-care provider needs it to continue medical care; the police ask you to provide it as part of a crime investigation; or you are required by legal subpoena to provide it in court.

- Good Samaritan laws may protect a First Responder from liability for acts performed in good faith, unless those acts are grossly negligent.

- A First Responder should do his best to preserve evidence at a crime scene.

- Learn your state requirements for reporting incidents such as suspected child, elder, or spouse abuse; any injury that may be the result of a crime; and all suspected infectious disease exposure.

- Medical identification tags inform responders about the patient's specific medical conditions. The tags may be found on bracelets, necklaces, or cards carried in a wallet. Look for them whenever you examine a patient.

- A potential organ donor should be treated in the same way as any other patient.

Key Terms

abandonment refers to discontinuing medical care without making sure that another health-care professional with equal or a higher level of training has taken over patient care.

advance directive a patient's instructions, written in advance, regarding the kind of resuscitation efforts that should be made in a life-threatening emergency.

assault an act that unlawfully places a person in apprehension of immediate bodily harm without his consent.

battery the unlawful touching of another individual without his consent.

competent a competent adult is one who is lucid and able to make an informed decision about medical care.

consent permission to provide medical care. See *expressed consent* and *implied consent*.

do not resuscitate (DNR) order a document that relates the chronically or terminally ill patient's wish not to be resuscitated.

duty to act the legal obligation to provide emergency care to a patient who requires it.

emancipated minor a minor who is married, pregnant, a parent, in the armed forces, or financially independent and living away from home with the permission of the courts.

expressed consent permission that must be obtained from every responsive, competent adult patient before medical care may be rendered.

gross negligence willful and wanton misconduct.

implied consent the assumption that in an emergency a patient who cannot give permission for medical care would give it if he or she could.

minor any person under the legally defined age of an adult; usually under age 18 or 21.

negligence carelessness, inattention, disregard, inadvertence, or oversight that was accidental but avoidable; emergency care that deviates from the accepted standard of care and results in further injury to the patient.

scope of care actions the First Responder may legally provide.

standard of care the care expected to be provided to the same patient under the same circumstances by another First Responder who had received the same training.

Knowledge Check

1. **The legal term "abandonment" is best defined as the result of a First Responder:**
   a. allowing a patient to refuse emergency medical care.
   b. performing a skill that he or she is not allowed to perform.
   c. leaving a patient without ensuring continued care at the same level.
   d. treating a patient who is younger than 18 without parent present.

2. **For a First Responder, the term "scope of care" is best defined as the:**
   a. set of actions he or she is legally allowed to perform.
   b. skills allowed when contacting medical direction.
   c. DOT's "National Standard Curriculum."
   d. care requested by the patient or the patient's family.

3. **You respond to a call and find an unconscious adult patient. As a First Responder, your authority to begin care of this patient is due to the concept of:**
   a. expressed consent.
   b. implied consent.
   c. consent of minors.
   d. consent by habeas corpus.

4. Which one of the following is NOT a proof of negligence?
   a. The First Responder had a duty to act.
   b. A physical or psychological injury was caused.
   c. The First Responder's action or inaction caused injury.
   d. The First Responder acted within his or her scope of care.

5. A patient's medical or personal information may be released by the First Responder:
   a. by court order or subpoena.
   b. at the request of a bona fide press agency.
   c. in accordance with the Good Samaritan laws.
   d. to warn other EMS providers of an infection risk on subsequent calls.

6. If a competent patient refuses care, the First Responder should:
   a. ridicule the patient's religious reasons for refusing.
   b. force the patient to stay on scene until the EMTs arrive.
   c. follow the Good Samaritan laws and provide care anyway.
   d. ask the patient to read and sign a "refusal" form.

7. You have a patient who appears to be intoxicated. However, he knows what time it is, where he is, and today's date. It is acceptable to allow this patient to refuse transportation.
   a. True
   b. False

8. It is possible that you will be called to court to testify about a call many years after the call occurred.
   a. True
   b. False

9. List the four components required for a successful negligence lawsuit.

_____

_____

_____

_____

10. Define "standard of care."

_____

_____

_____

11. You have assessed a patient, provided emergency care, and handed the patient over to EMTs. You then leave the scene before the EMTs leave for the hospital. Have you abandoned the patient? Why or why not?

_____

_____

_____

12. This chapter states that patients must understand the risks of refusing care. How would you present these risks to a patient? How could you be sure the patient understood?

_____

_____

_____

13. You begin care of an unconscious patient. Suddenly, he wakes and tells you to stop what you are doing. May he legally refuse your care? What are the risks to you—and to the patient—if he refuses both care and transportation?

_____

_____

_____

14. Twenty-two-year-old Cora and her mother were hiking on Patriot's Path when Cora tripped and hurt her ankle. Their guide, a trained First Responder, offered assistance. The mother insisted on it, but Cora refused. Should the First Responder provide care? Explain your answer.

_____

_____

_____

Scenario

Your patient is an adult male, who is probably in his 40s. He was found slumped over on a park bench, with drug paraphernalia attached to his arm and an empty syringe in his lap. The patient is conscious, but his words are slurred and he doesn't respond appropriately to simple questions, such as "What is your name?" and "Do you know what day this is?" When you ask for his consent to treatment, he refuses it. May you provide emergency care? Explain your answer.

_____

_____

_____

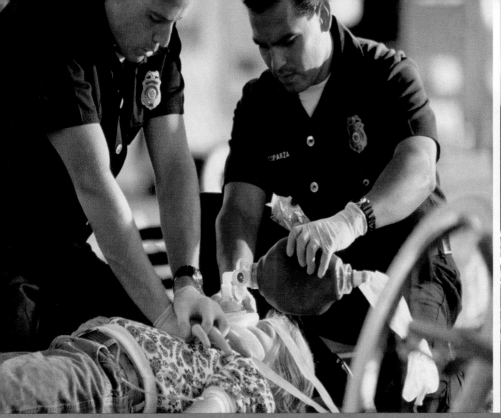
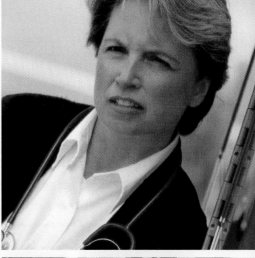
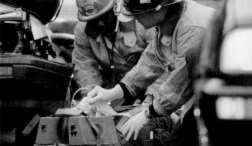

4 | The Human Body

Objectives

From the U.S. Department of Transportation (DOT) 1995 "First Responder: National Standard Curriculum." Material supplemental to the DOT curriculum is listed under "Enrichment."

Cognitive

1-4.1 ▶ Describe the anatomy and function of the respiratory system. (pp. 56–58, 59)

1-4.2 ▶ Describe the anatomy and function of the circulatory system. (pp. 58, 60)

1-4.3 ▶ Describe the anatomy and function of the musculoskeletal system. (pp. 53–56, 57)

1-4.4 ▶ Describe the components and function of the nervous system. (pp. 59, 61, 64–65)

Affective

No objectives are identified by the DOT.

Psychomotor

No objectives are identified by the DOT.

Enrichment

▶ Use anatomical terms correctly, including terms of position, direction, and location. (pp. 50–53)

▶ Describe the main body cavities. (p. 52)

▶ Describe skin and its components. (pp. 61, 66)

▶ Describe the digestive system and its components. (pp. 61–62, 66)

▶ Describe the urinary system and its components. (pp. 62, 67)

▶ Describe the endocrine system and its components. (p. 62)

▶ Describe the reproductive system and its components. (pp. 63, 67)

Introduction

As a First Responder, you must be able to recognize illness and injury and know how to care for each. You also must be able to tell other medical personnel about a patient's problem quickly and accurately. To do all this, you need a solid foundation of basic knowledge. In this chapter, you will study **anatomy** (the structure of the body) and **physiology** (how the body works). You also will be introduced to common anatomical terms.

Section 1 Anatomical Terms

As a First Responder, you will often have to describe a patient's position, direction, and location to other EMS personnel. Using correct terms will help you communicate the extent of a patient's injury quickly and accurately.

Terms of position include the following (Figure 4-1):

- **Anatomical position.** In this position, a patient's body stands erect with arms down at the sides, palms front. "Right" and "left" refer to the patient's right and left, not yours.
- **Supine position.** The patient is lying face up on his or her back.
- **Prone position.** The patient is lying face down on his or her stomach.
- **Lateral recumbent position.** In this position, the patient is lying on the left or right side. This is also known as the *recovery position.*

Terms of direction and location include the following:

- **Superior** means toward, or closer to, the head. **Inferior** means toward, or closer to, the feet.
- **Anterior** is toward the front. **Posterior** is toward the back.

First on Scene

Whenever you document patient care or transfer a patient to ambulance personnel, you will use the terms included in this chapter. Your ability to do so will take you from the role of bystander to rescuer and active contributor to the EMS team.

- **Medial** means toward the midline, or center of the body. **Lateral** refers to the left or right of the midline.
- **Proximal** means close, or near the point of reference. **Distal** is distant, or far away from the point of reference. For both proximal and distal, the point of reference is usually the torso. For example, a wound of the forearm is proximal to the wrist because it is closer to the torso than the wrist. That same wound is distal to the elbow because it is farther away from the torso than the elbow.
- **Superficial** is near the surface. **Deep** is remote, or far from the surface.
- **Internal** means inside. **External** means outside.

Anatomical regions and topography are the internal and external landmarks of the body (Figures 4-2 and 4-3).

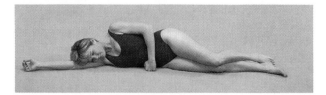

a. *Supine position.*

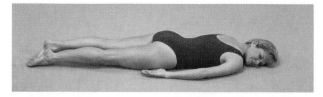

b. *Prone position.*

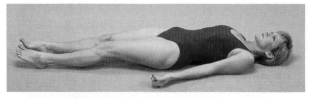

c. *Right lateral recumbent position.*

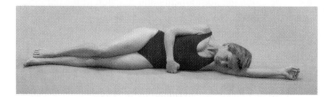

d. *Left lateral recumbent position.*

FIGURE 4-1 Terms of position.

Dispatch My first response unit was called to the mall for a "person injured." A woman missed a step on an escalator, fell, and hurt her left leg.

Scene Size-up We scanned the small crowd as we approached, making sure there were no problems. Then we saw that the patient was clear of the escalator. She was sitting on the floor, holding her left leg. Did she fall just a step or two, or did she fall down the whole flight, I wondered.

Initial Assessment The woman was responsive and alert. She denied passing out or injuring her head or spine. She had no breathing problems and no obvious bleeding. She told us that her left shin hurt near her ankle.

Knowing the basic anatomy and physiology of the human body is key to this course. It is the foundation on which you will build all your skills. Consider the patient in this scenario as you read Chapter 4. How would you communicate her condition to the responding EMTs?

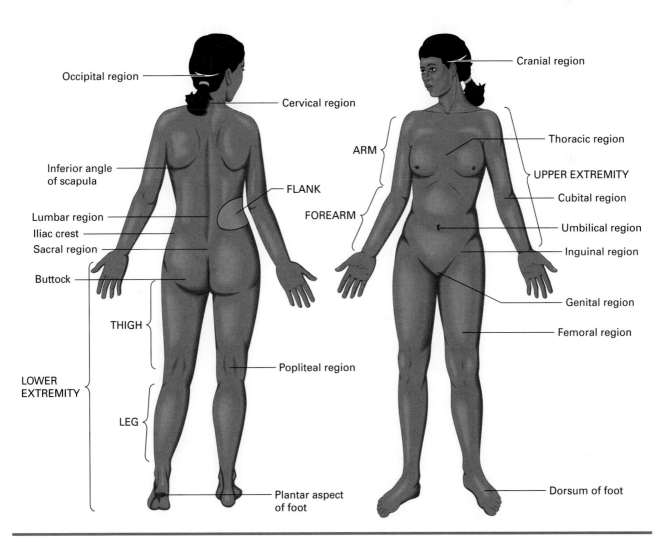

FIGURE 4-2 Anatomical regions.

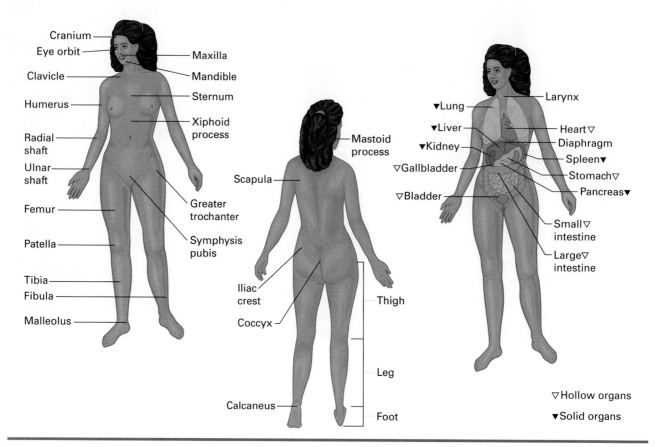

FIGURE 4-3 Topographic anatomy.

During patient assessment, refer to these landmarks. They will help make the description of a patient's condition clear to others, particularly when you use a radio.

The organs of the body are located in certain body cavities (Figure 4-4). The main body cavities include:

- **Thoracic cavity.** Also called the *chest cavity*, the lungs and heart are found here. The *diaphragm*, a muscle that moves up and down during respiration, separates this cavity from the abdomen. (See Figure 4-5.)

- **Abdominal cavity.** Containing the organs of digestion and excretion, it includes the liver, gallbladder, spleen, pancreas, kidneys, stomach, and intestines.

- **Pelvic cavity.** This cavity is bounded by the lower part of the spine, the hip bones, and the pubis. It protects the lower abdomen, including the bladder, rectum, and internal female organs.

When you think of the abdominal cavity, think of it as being divided into four parts or *quadrants*. Health-care workers often refer to it that way. The quadrants are formed by imaginary lines. One line is drawn horizontally through the navel. The other line is drawn vertically through the midline of the body. (See Figure 4-6.)

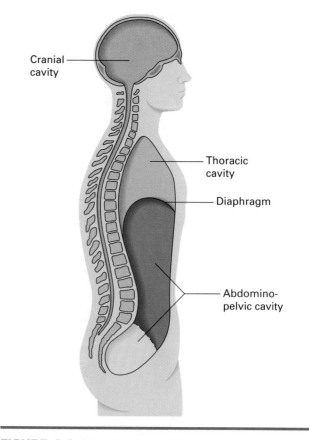

FIGURE 4-4 Main body cavities.

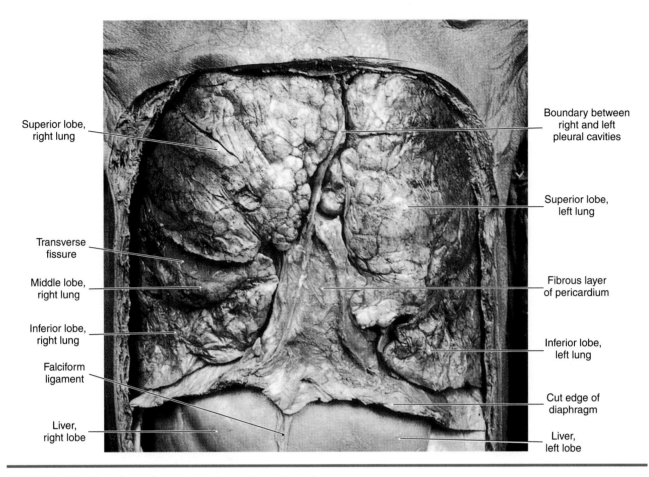

Superior lobe, right lung

Transverse fissure

Middle lobe, right lung

Inferior lobe, right lung

Falciform ligament

Liver, right lobe

Boundary between right and left pleural cavities

Superior lobe, left lung

Fibrous layer of pericardium

Inferior lobe, left lung

Cut edge of diaphragm

Liver, left lobe

FIGURE 4-5 **The thoracic cavity.** *(Ralph T. Hutchings)*

Q:

1. What are four positions in which a patient may be found? Briefly describe each one.

2. What are three terms of direction or location? Use each one in a sentence to describe a body part.

3. What are the three main body cavities? Name an organ that can be found in each one.

Section 2 Body Systems

Musculoskeletal System

The musculoskeletal system is made up of the skeleton and muscles. Each helps give the body shape and protects internal organs. The muscles also provide for movement.

The Skeleton

The human body is shaped by a bony framework (Figure 4-7). Bone is composed of both living cells and nonliving matter. The nonliving matter contains calcium compounds that help make bone hard and rigid. Without bones, the body would collapse.

The adult skeleton has 206 bones. It must be strong to support and protect, jointed to permit motion, and flexible to withstand stress. It is held together mainly by

 First Responder Practice

Your knowledge of anatomy is more than a building block. It is a keystone for the rest of your training and practice. For example, when you find a person with a broken lower leg, you will know that of the two bones there (tibia and fibula), one or both may be injured. Since you will be familiar with the adjoining areas, you will also know to examine above the injury site—both the patella and femur—and below the injury site—the tarsals and metatarsals.

ABDOMINAL QUADRANTS

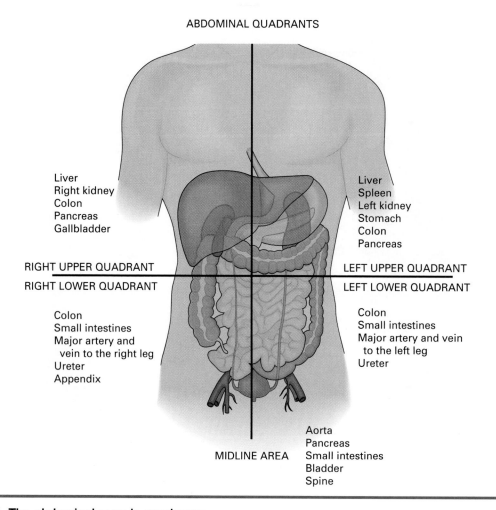

Liver
Right kidney
Colon
Pancreas
Gallbladder

Liver
Spleen
Left kidney
Stomach
Colon
Pancreas

RIGHT UPPER QUADRANT

LEFT UPPER QUADRANT

RIGHT LOWER QUADRANT

LEFT LOWER QUADRANT

Colon
Small intestines
Major artery and
  vein to the right leg
Ureter
Appendix

Colon
Small intestines
Major artery and vein
  to the left leg
Ureter

MIDLINE AREA

Aorta
Pancreas
Small intestines
Bladder
Spine

FIGURE 4-6 **The abdominal area in quadrants.**

ligaments, tendons, and layers of muscle. (*Ligaments* connect bone to bone. *Tendons* connect muscle to bone.) Bone ends fit into each other at joints. The three kinds of joints are: immovable like the skull, slightly movable like the spine, and freely movable like the elbow or knee (Figure 4-8).

The major areas of the skeleton include the following:

■ The *skull* has broad, flat bones that form a hollow shell. The top (including the forehead), back, and sides of the shell make up the *cranium*. It houses and protects the brain. There are several small bones of the face. They give shape to the face and permit the jaw to move. The major features of the face are the nose, ears, eyes, cheeks, mouth, and jowls.

■ The *spinal column* houses and protects the spinal cord. The spinal column is the central supportive bony structure of the body. It consists of 33 bones known as *vertebrae.* The spine is divided into five sections: the

cervical spine (the neck, formed by 7 vertebrae) the *thoracic spine* (the upper back, formed by 12 vertebrae), the *lumbar spine* (the lower back, formed by 5 vertebrae), the *sacrum* (the lower part of the spine, formed by 5 fused vertebrae), and the *coccyx* (the tail bone, formed by 4 fused vertebrae).

■ The *thorax,* or rib cage, protects the heart and lungs—vital organs of the body. They are enclosed by 12 pairs of ribs that are attached at the back to the spine. The top 10 are also attached in front to the **sternum,** or breastbone. The lowest portion of the sternum is called the xiphoid process.

■ The *pelvis,* or hip bones, consists of the ilium, pubis, and ischium. Iliac crests form the "wings" of the pelvis. The pubis is the anterior portion of the pelvis. The ischium is in the posterior portion.

■ The *shoulder girdle* consists of the *clavicle* (the collarbone) and the *scapulae* (shoulder blades).

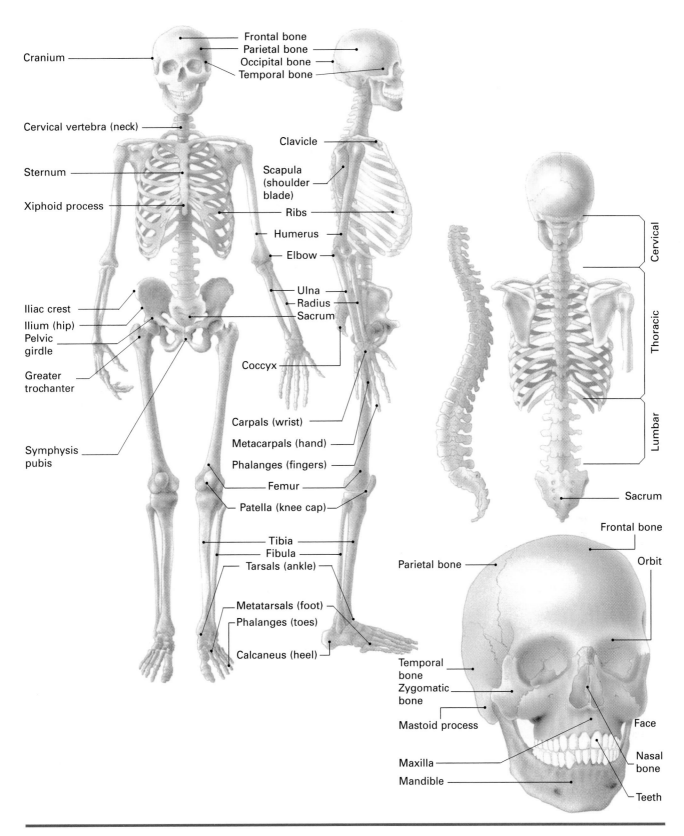

FIGURE 4-7 The skeletal system.

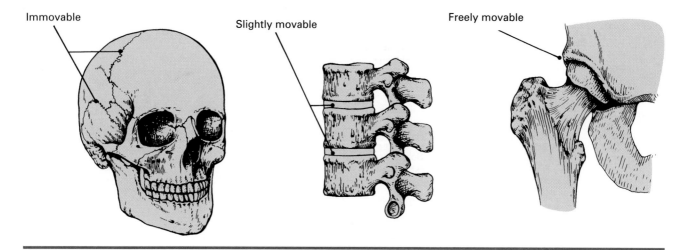

FIGURE 4-8 Three types of joints.

- The *extremities* are referred to as the upper or lower extremities. The upper extremities extend from the shoulders to the fingertips. The *arm* (shoulder to elbow) has one bone known as the *humerus*. The bones in the *forearm* are the *radius* and *ulna*. The lower extremities extend from the hips to the toes. The bone in the thigh, or upper leg, is known as the *femur*. The bones in the lower leg are the *tibia* and *fibula*. The knee cap is called the *patella*.

The Muscles

Body movement depends on work performed by the muscles. Muscles have the ability to contract (become shorter and thicker) when stimulated by a nerve impulse. Each muscle is made of long threadlike cells called *fibers,* which are closely packed or bundled. Overlapping bundles are bound by connective tissue (Figure 4-9).

There are three basic kinds of muscles (Figure 4-10):

- *Skeletal muscle,* or voluntary muscle, makes possible all deliberate acts such as walking and chewing. It helps shape the body and form its walls. In the trunk, this type of muscle is broad, flat, and expanded. In the extremities, it is long and rounded.

- *Smooth muscle,* or involuntary muscle, is made of longer fibers. It is found in the walls of tube-like organs, ducts, and blood vessels. It also forms much of the intestinal wall. A person has little or no control over this type of muscle.

- *Cardiac muscle* makes up the walls of the heart. It can stimulate itself into contraction, even when disconnected from the nervous system.

Respiratory System

The body can get enough nutrition from food to last for several weeks. It can store water to last for several days. But it can store oxygen for only a few minutes. The body depends on a constant supply of oxygen.

The respiratory system delivers oxygen to and removes carbon dioxide from the body. The passage of air into and out of the lungs is called **respiration.** Breathing in is called *inspiration* or inhaling. Breathing out is called *expiration* or exhaling.

During inspiration, the muscles of the thorax contract, moving the ribs outward and up, and the *diaphragm* contracts and lowers. These movements expand the chest cavity and cause air to flow into the lungs. During expiration the opposite happens. The muscles of the chest relax, causing the ribs to move inward, and the diaphragm relaxes and moves up.

The respiratory system consists of the organs that let us breathe (Figure 4-11). When air enters the body, it does so through the mouth and nose. The area posterior to the mouth and nose is called the **pharynx,** which is divided into the *oropharynx* and *nasopharynx.* Air travels from there down through the **larynx** (voice box) and into the **trachea** (windpipe). The trachea is the air passageway to the lungs. It is made of cartilage rings and is visible in the anterior portion of the neck. The **epiglottis** is a leaf-shaped structure that prevents foreign objects from entering the trachea during swallowing. The trachea splits into two *bronchi.* These air passages gradually become smaller and smaller until they reach the *alveoli,* where carbon dioxide and oxygen are exchanged with blood.

Always keep in mind that the respiratory structures of infants and children differ from those of adults. The

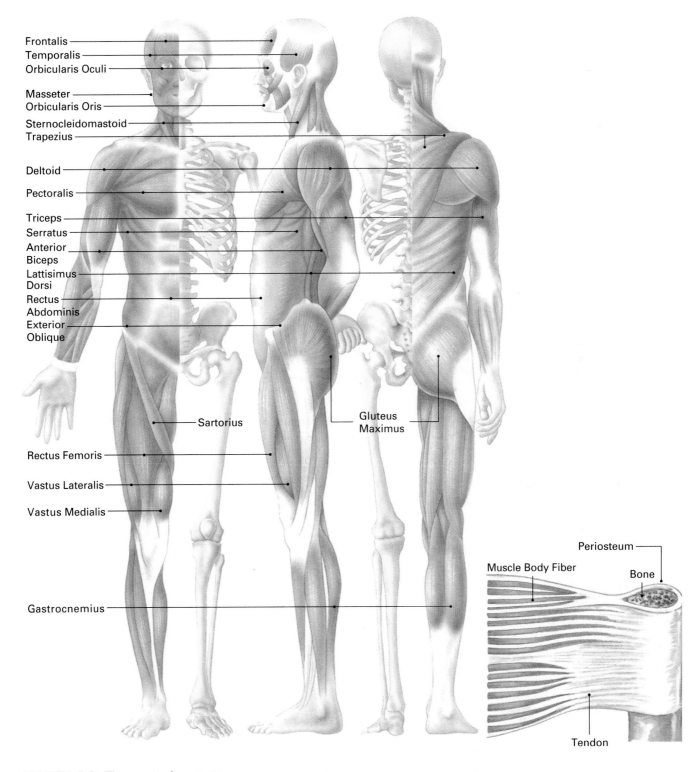

FIGURE 4-9 The muscular system.

structures have the same names but are usually smaller or less developed in infants and children. The following differences are very important to First Responder care:

In an infant or child:

■ All structures, including the mouth and nose, are smaller. They are more easily obstructed by small objects,

blood, or swelling. Pay extra attention to an infant or child to be sure the airway stays open.

■ The tongue takes up proportionally more space in the pharynx than the tongue of an adult. As a result, it can block an infant's or child's airway more easily.

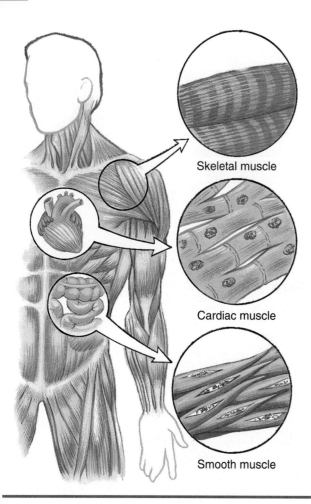

FIGURE 4-10 Three types of muscles.

- Skeletal muscle
- Cardiac muscle
- Smooth muscle

- The trachea is narrower, softer, and more flexible. Tipping the head too far back or allowing the head to fall forward can close the trachea. Whenever needed, place a folded towel or similar item under the infant's or child's shoulders to keep the airway aligned and open.

- The primary cause of cardiac arrest in infants and children is an uncorrected respiratory problem. Because the chest wall is softer, they tend to rely more heavily on the diaphragm for breathing. So watch for excessive movement of the diaphragm. It can alert you to respiratory distress in these patients.

When needed, provide oxygen and artificial ventilation promptly to infants and children. Don't delay. These interventions will make a difference.

Circulatory System

The circulatory system delivers oxygen and nutrients to the body's tissues and removes waste products via the bloodstream. It consists of the heart, blood vessels, and blood (Figure 4-12).

The heart is a muscular organ that is responsible for pumping blood through the body (Figure 4-13). The adult heart contracts between 60 and 80 times per minute when at rest and faster when under stress. Problems with the heart account for many of the emergencies you will encounter as a First Responder.

The heart is divided into four chambers. The upper chambers are called *atria*. The lower chambers are called *ventricles*. The heart has a left and right side, each of which has an atrium and a ventricle. The right side of the heart receives blood from the body and pumps it to the lungs. The left side of the heart receives oxygenated blood from the lungs and pumps it to the body.

When the heart pumps blood from the left ventricle, blood enters the arteries. This pumping action causes a wave of pressure that can be felt as a *pulse*. Among the many points where a pulse can be felt in the body, the most common are:

- **Carotid pulse point,** felt on either side of the neck.
- **Brachial pulse point,** felt on the inside of the arm between the elbow and the shoulder.
- **Radial pulse point,** felt on thumb side of wrist.
- **Femoral pulse point,** felt in the area of the groin in the crease between the abdomen and thigh.

The *blood vessels* are a closed system of tubes through which blood flows. **Arteries** and *arterioles* take blood away from the heart. The **capillaries** are distributors. They are the smallest vessels through which the exchange of fluid, oxygen, and carbon dioxide takes place between blood and tissue cells. The **veins** and *venules* carry blood back to the heart from the rest of the body. (See Figures 4-14 and 4-15.)

 First Responder Practice

The human body is made up of many systems that interact constantly. Imagine that interaction: Someone is threatened. His nervous system detects the threat. The endocrine system then releases hormones that increase his performance. The heart and lungs increase activity to provide oxygen and energy to the musculoskeletal system, which then provides the motion to flee the danger.

Think of the body's systems as working individually and together to keep us functioning, safe, and healthy.

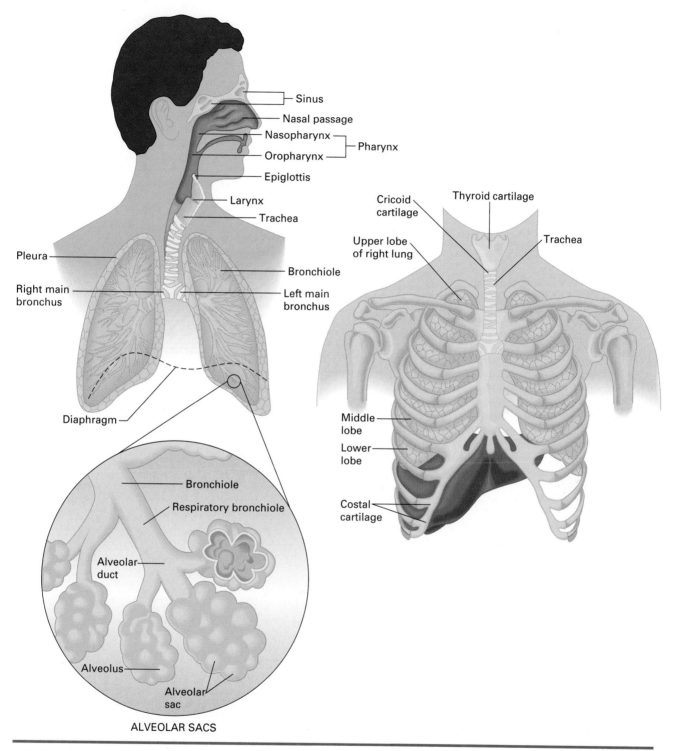

FIGURE 4-11 The respiratory system.

Nervous System

The nervous system is composed of the brain, the spinal cord, and nerves (Figure 4-16). It lets a person be aware of and react to the environment. It coordinates the body's responses to stimuli and keeps body systems working together.

The nervous system has two main parts—the **central nervous system** and the **peripheral nervous system.** The central nervous system consists of the brain and spinal cord. The peripheral nervous system consists of the nerves that carry information back and forth from the body to the spinal cord and brain.

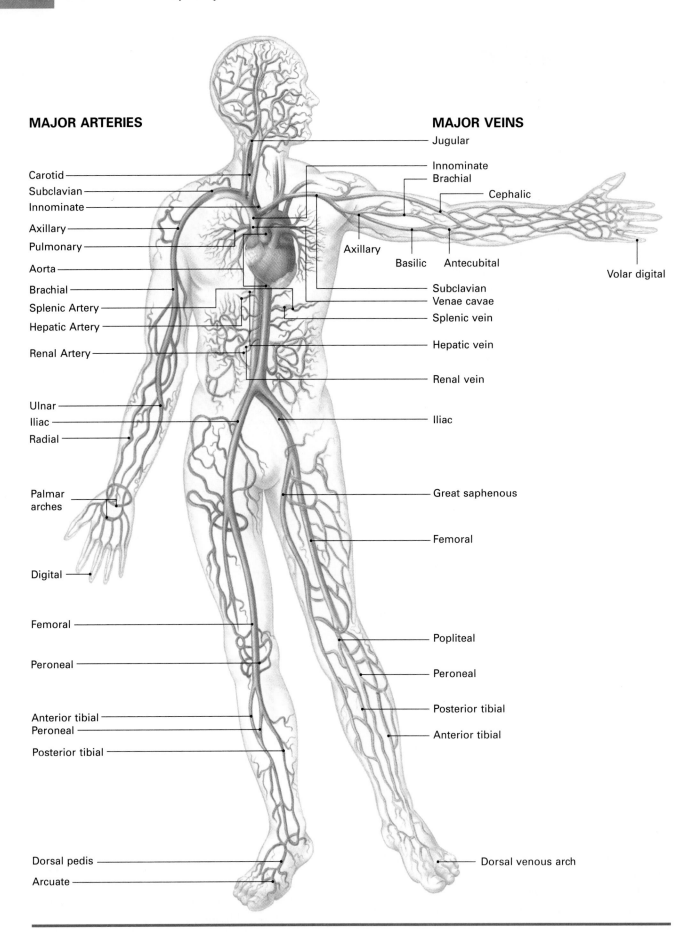

MAJOR ARTERIES

MAJOR VEINS

- Jugular
- Innominate
- Brachial
- Cephalic
- Carotid
- Subclavian
- Innominate
- Axillary
- Pulmonary
- Axillary
- Aorta
- Basilic
- Antecubital
- Volar digital
- Brachial
- Splenic Artery
- Subclavian
- Venae cavae
- Hepatic Artery
- Splenic vein
- Renal Artery
- Hepatic vein
- Renal vein
- Ulnar
- Iliac
- Radial
- Iliac
- Palmar arches
- Great saphenous
- Femoral
- Digital
- Femoral
- Popliteal
- Peroneal
- Peroneal
- Anterior tibial
- Peroneal
- Posterior tibial
- Posterior tibial
- Anterior tibial
- Dorsal pedis
- Arcuate
- Dorsal venous arch

FIGURE 4-12 The circulatory system.

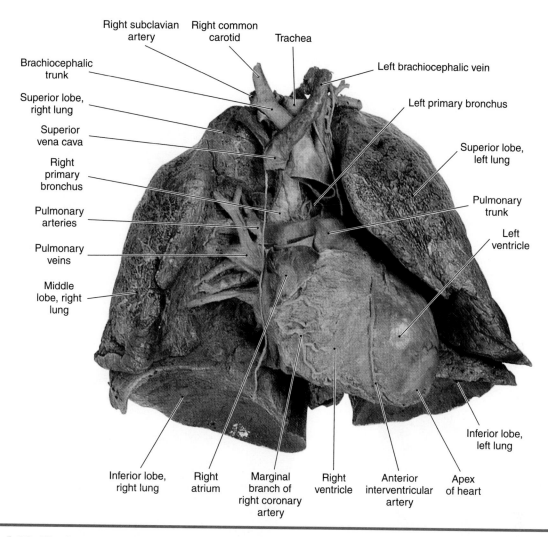

Right subclavian artery — Right common carotid — Trachea — Left brachiocephalic vein

Brachiocephalic trunk

Superior lobe, right lung — Left primary bronchus

Superior vena cava — Superior lobe, left lung

Right primary bronchus

Pulmonary arteries — Pulmonary trunk

Pulmonary veins — Left ventricle

Middle lobe, right lung

Inferior lobe, left lung

Inferior lobe, right lung — Right atrium — Marginal branch of right coronary artery — Right ventricle — Anterior interventricular artery — Apex of heart

FIGURE 4-13 The lungs, heart, and great vessels. *(Ralph T. Hutchings)*

The nervous system may also be broken down by function, or voluntary and involuntary components. Voluntary components are under our control. They are responsible for activities such as movement. Involuntary components are handled by the *autonomic nervous system.* This system is a network of nerve tissue that regulates functions we normally pay no attention to, such as how quickly or slowly the heart beats.

The Skin

The skin separates the human body from the outside world. It protects the deep tissues from injury, drying out, and invasion by bacteria and other foreign bodies. The skin helps to regulate body temperature. It aids in getting rid of water and various salts, and it helps to prevent dehydration. Finally, it acts as the receptor organ for touch, pain, heat, and cold (Figure 4-17).

The *epidermis* is the outermost layer of skin. It contains cells that give the skin its color. The *dermis,* or second layer, contains a vast network of blood vessels, hair follicles, sweat and oil glands, and sensory nerves. Just below the skin is a layer of fatty tissue, which varies in thickness (it is extremely thin in the eyelids, for example, but thick over the buttocks).

Digestive System

The digestive system is composed of the *alimentary tract* (food passageway) and accessory organs (Figure 4-18). Its main functions are to ingest food and get rid of waste. Digestion consists of two processes—mechanical and chemical. The mechanical process includes chewing, swallowing, the rhythmic movement of matter through the tract, and *defecation* (the elimination of

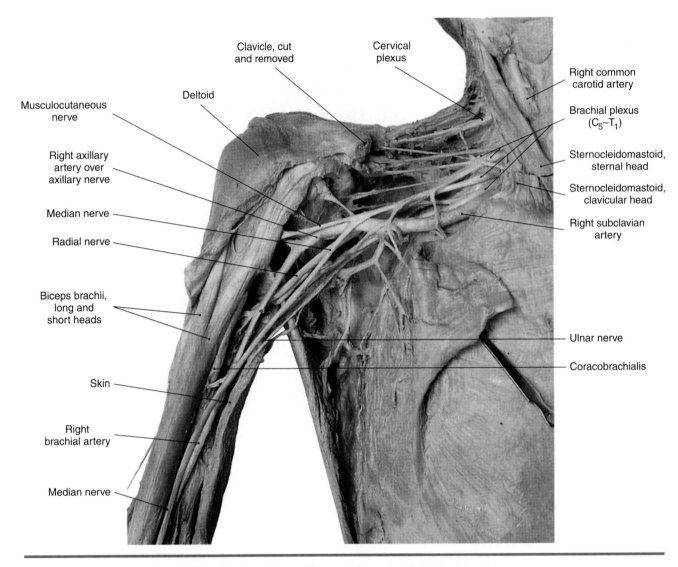

Clavicle, cut and removed

Cervical plexus

Right common carotid artery

Deltoid

Brachial plexus (C$_5$–T$_1$)

Musculocutaneous nerve

Sternocleidomastoid, sternal head

Right axillary artery over axillary nerve

Sternocleidomastoid, clavicular head

Median nerve

Right subclavian artery

Radial nerve

Biceps brachii, long and short heads

Ulnar nerve

Coracobrachialis

Skin

Right brachial artery

Median nerve

FIGURE 4-14 **Major structures in the right axillary region.** *(Ralph T. Hutchings)*

waste). The chemical process consists of breaking food into simple components that can be absorbed and used by the body.

Except for the mouth and *esophagus,* the organs of this system are in the abdomen. They include the stomach, pancreas, liver, gallbladder, small intestine, and large intestine.

Urinary System

The urinary system helps the body maintain the delicate balance of water and chemicals needed for survival. During the process of urine formation, wastes are removed and useful products are returned to the blood. It consists of two kidneys, two ureters, one urinary bladder, and one urethra (Figure 4-19). The

ureters take urine from the kidneys to the next part of the system, the bladder. The bladder stores urine until it is passed through the urethra and excreted from the body.

Endocrine System

The endocrine glands regulate the body by secreting *hormones* directly into the bloodstream. They affect physical strength, mental ability, stature, reproduction, hair growth, voice pitch, and behavior. How people think, act, and feel depends largely on these tiny secretions. Each gland produces one or more hormones. The glands include the pituitary, thyroid, parathyroids, adrenals, ovaries, testes, and the islets of Langerhans within the pancreas.

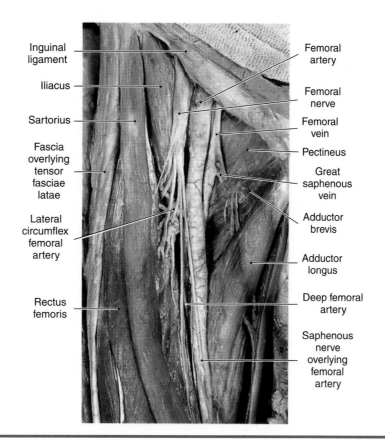

Inguinal ligament

Iliacus

Sartorius

Fascia overlying tensor fasciae latae

Lateral circumflex femoral artery

Rectus femoris

Femoral artery

Femoral nerve

Femoral vein

Pectineus

Great saphenous vein

Adductor brevis

Adductor longus

Deep femoral artery

Saphenous nerve overlying femoral artery

FIGURE 4-15 **Major structures of the thigh.** *(Ralph T. Hutchings)*

Reproductive System

The reproductive system of the male includes two testes, a duct system, accessory glands, and the penis. The reproductive system of the female consists of two ovaries, two fallopian tubes, the uterus, vagina, and external genitals. (See Figure 4-20.)

Q: 1. What are the names of the bones in the forearm? In the lower leg?

2. How does air move through the body to enter the bloodstream? Describe the path it takes.

3. How does blood move through the heart and lungs? Briefly describe the process.

4. What is the nervous system composed of? What are its functions?

THE BRAIN

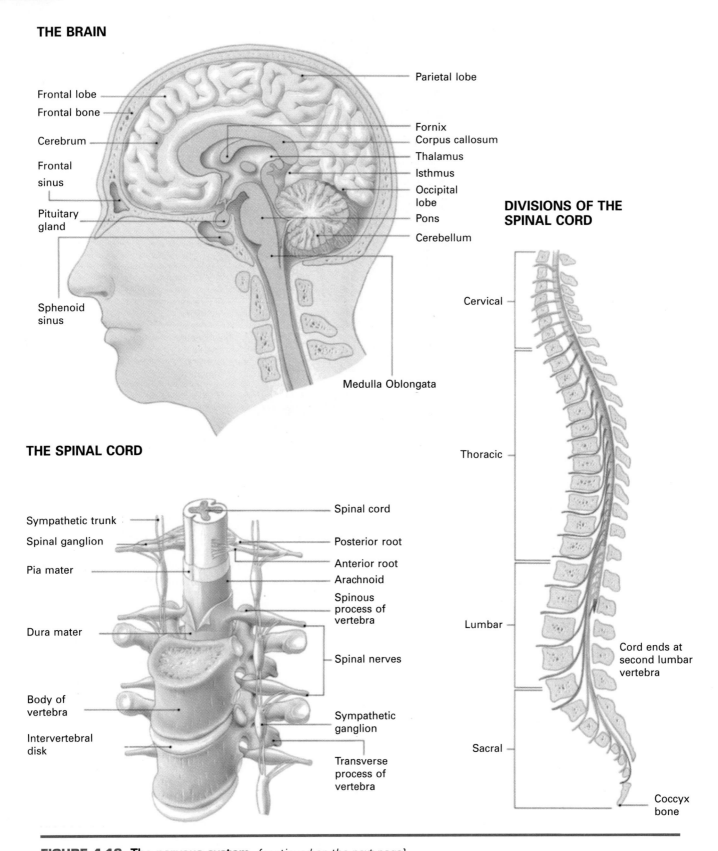

THE SPINAL CORD

DIVISIONS OF THE SPINAL CORD

FIGURE 4-16 The nervous system. *(continued on the next page)*

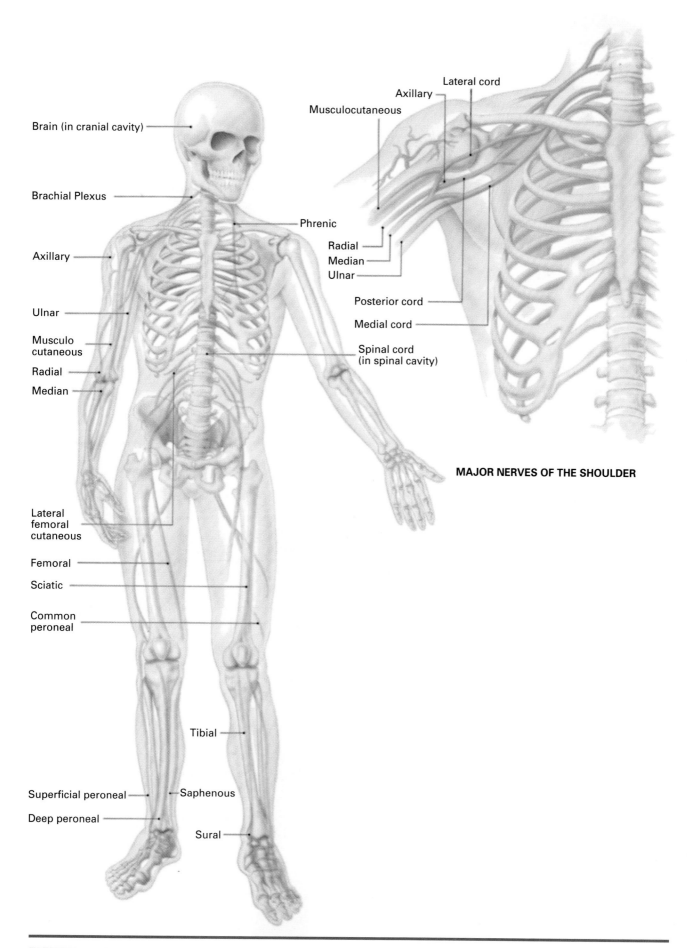

Brain (in cranial cavity)

Brachial Plexus

Axillary

Ulnar

Musculo cutaneous

Radial

Median

Lateral femoral cutaneous

Femoral

Sciatic

Common peroneal

Tibial

Superficial peroneal

Deep peroneal

Saphenous

Sural

Phrenic

Spinal cord (in spinal cavity)

Lateral cord

Axillary

Musculocutaneous

Radial

Median

Ulnar

Posterior cord

Medial cord

MAJOR NERVES OF THE SHOULDER

FIGURE 4-16 *(continued)*

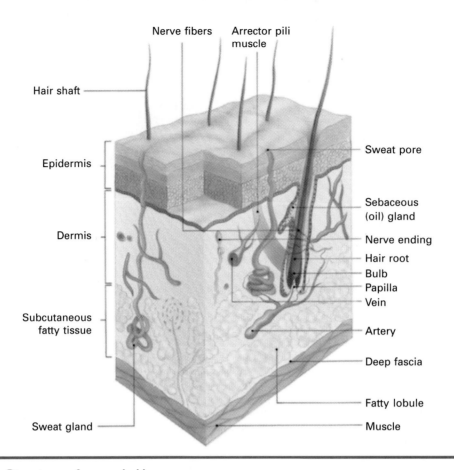

FIGURE 4-17 Structure of normal skin.

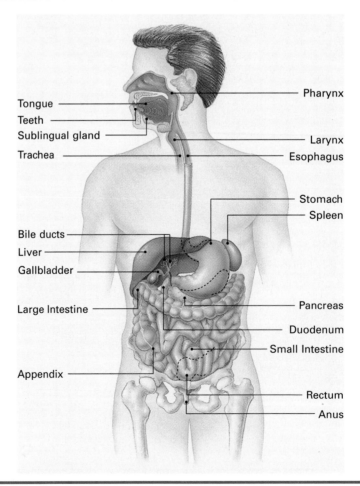

FIGURE 4-18 The digestive system.

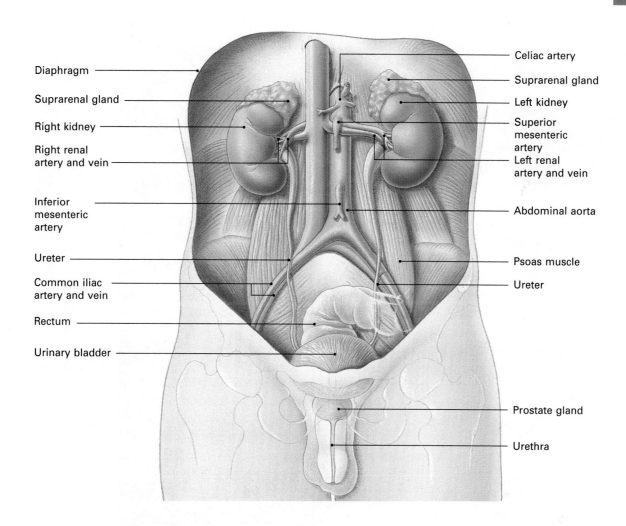

Diaphragm

Suprarenal gland

Right kidney

Right renal artery and vein

Inferior mesenteric artery

Ureter

Common iliac artery and vein

Rectum

Urinary bladder

Celiac artery

Suprarenal gland

Left kidney

Superior mesenteric artery

Left renal artery and vein

Abdominal aorta

Psoas muscle

Ureter

Prostate gland

Urethra

FIGURE 4-19 The urinary system.

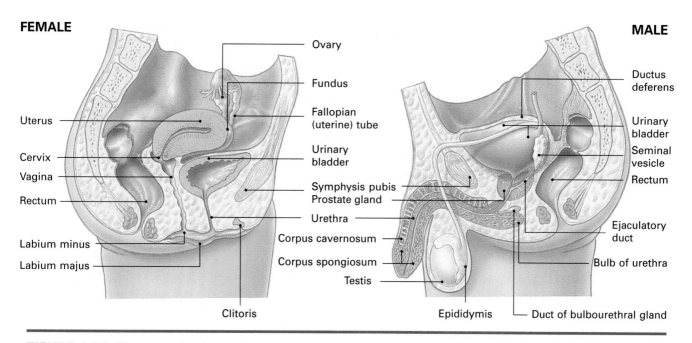

FEMALE

MALE

Uterus

Cervix

Vagina

Rectum

Labium minus

Labium majus

Clitoris

Ovary

Fundus

Fallopian (uterine) tube

Urinary bladder

Symphysis pubis

Prostate gland

Urethra

Corpus cavernosum

Corpus spongiosum

Testis

Ductus deferens

Urinary bladder

Seminal vesicle

Rectum

Ejaculatory duct

Bulb of urethra

Epididymis

Duct of bulbourethral gland

FIGURE 4-20 The reproductive system.

The Call Follow-up

At the beginning of this chapter, you read that First Responders had just started to assess a patient who was injured in a fall from an escalator. Their initial assessment found no life-threatening injuries. To see how the information you learned in this chapter applies to the emergency, read the following. It describes how the call was completed.

Physical Examination We conducted a head-to-toe exam and found no injuries other than the left lower leg. It was deformed and swollen, but we observed no bleeding. We stabilized the leg manually to prevent further damage. Then we took her vitals and checked to make sure she had a pulse, movement, and sensation below the injury site.

Patient History I asked the patient to describe what happened. She said she misstepped as she was getting off the escalator. She didn't fall its entire length. She said that when she put her weight on her left leg, she felt a twisting and then a sudden pain in the lower part of the leg. Upon further questioning, she told us that she doesn't take any medications or have any medical problems. She denied allergies. And about an hour ago, she ate a burger for lunch at the mall's food court.

Ongoing Assessment We rechecked her pulse, movement, and sensation below the injury site. They were all present and the same as the first time we checked. We repeated her vital signs. Pulse was 84, strong, and regular. Respirations were 16, regular, and deep. Blood pressure was 114/78. We made sure she was comfortable and continued to monitor her carefully.

Patient Hand-off When the EMTs arrived, my partner gave them the hand-off report (see below). While the EMTs immobilized the patient's leg in a splint, we helped keep onlookers from invading the patient's privacy. It wasn't long before the EMTs were able to move the patient to the ambulance. We walked with them to make sure the way was clear. Then, at the ambulance, we helped load the stretcher. It was a good night. We were glad that everyone turned out to be okay.

 Hand-off Report

"This is Ellen Levine, who is 43 years old. She was getting off the escalator and misstepped. She felt a twisting in her left lower leg. She never lost consciousness and denies any other injury from the fall. She has pain, swelling, and deformity in the distal third of her tib/fib. There is adequate pulse, motor function, and sensation distal to the injury. The remainder of the physical exam was negative. We've held manual stabilization on the injured leg. Ellen's vital signs are pulse 84, strong and regular; respirations 16, regular and deep; blood pressure 114/78."

The Last Word *It is of the utmost importance that you have a basic knowledge of the human body. It is just as important for you to be able to use that knowledge to communicate a patient's condition to other health-care professionals. Learn the language. Speak it and write it every chance you get. You will need it throughout this course and in the field.*

Chapter Review

Focus on the EMS Team

It may seem obvious that a solid knowledge of the human body is necessary to your work as a First Responder. Your patients will certainly rely on it to help them through their emergencies. But did you know that the EMS dispatcher, EMTs and paramedics, and even hospital personnel will rely on your knowledge, too? The EMS dispatcher will rely on it to help him decide on what assistance to send to the scene. The EMTs and paramedics will rely on it to tell them what equipment to prepare

for your patient. Hospital personnel also will rely on it to help them determine the patient's best treatment plan.

Remember, you are an important member of the EMS team. Your knowledge about the human body is one aspect of that team dynamic. But it is your commitment to excellence—to learn what is required in your course and then to maintain and refresh that knowledge on a regular basis—that will make your contribution truly valuable.

Summing Up

- When a patient is standing with arms down at the sides, palms front, he is in the anatomical position.

- The directional terms "right" and "left" always refer to the patient's right and left.

- Other directional terms include supine position (lying face up on the back), prone position (lying face down on the stomach), and lateral recumbent position (lying on the left or right side).

- Superior means toward, or closer to, the head; inferior means toward, or closer to, the feet. Anterior is toward the front; posterior is toward the back. Medial means toward the midline, or center of the body; lateral refers to the left or right of the midline. Proximal means close, or near the point of reference; distal is distant, or far away from the point of reference. Superficial is near the surface; deep is remote, or far from the surface. Internal means inside; external means outside.

- The main body cavities are the thoracic cavity, abdominal cavity, and pelvic cavity.

- The musculoskeletal system gives the body shape and protects internal organs. Major areas of the skeleton include the skull, spinal column, thorax, pelvis, shoulder girdle, and the extremities. The three basic kinds of muscle are skeletal muscle, smooth muscle, and cardiac muscle.

- The respiratory system delivers oxygen and removes carbon dioxide from the body. It consists of the organs that let us breathe: pharynx, larynx, trachea, epiglottis, lungs. The trachea splits into two bronchi, which split again and again until they reach the alveoli, where carbon dioxide and oxygen are exchanged with the blood.

- The circulatory system delivers oxygen and nutrients to the body and removes waste products. It consists of the heart, blood vessels, and blood. The heart's pumping action causes a wave of pressure called a pulse. The most common points on the body where a pulse can be felt are the carotid, brachial, radial, and femoral pulse points.

- The nervous system has two functions—communication and control. The central nervous system consists of the brain and spinal cord. The peripheral nervous system consists of the nerves.

- The skin protects the deep tissues from injury, drying out, and invasion by bacteria and other foreign bodies. It also helps the body regulate its temperature and get rid of water and certain salts, and it acts as the receptor organ for touch, pain, heat, and cold.

- The digestive system consists of the mouth, esophagus, stomach, pancreas, liver, gallbladder, and the small and large intestines.

- The urinary system consists of two kidneys, two ureters, one urinary bladder, and one urethra.

- The endocrine system produces hormones. It consists of glands, including the pituitary, thyroid, parathyroids, adrenals, ovaries, testes, and islets of Langerhans within the pancreas.

- The reproductive system of the male includes two testes, a duct system, accessory glands, and the penis. In the female it consists of two ovaries, two fallopian tubes, the uterus, vagina, and external genitals.

Key Terms

abdominal cavity   the space below the diaphragm and continuous with the pelvic cavity.

anatomical position   the position in which a patient is standing erect with arms down at sides and palms front.

anatomy   the structure of the body.

anterior   toward the front.

arteries   blood vessels that take blood away from the heart.

brachial pulse point   the location where an arterial pulse can be felt on the inside of the arm between the elbow and the shoulder.

capillaries   the smallest blood vessels through which the exchange of fluid, oxygen, and carbon dioxide takes place between the blood and tissue cells.

carotid pulse point   the location where an arterial pulse can be felt on either side of the neck.

central nervous system   the brain and the spinal cord.

cervical spine   the neck; formed by the first seven vertebrae.

deep   remote, or far from the surface. Opposite of *superficial.*

distal   distant, or far away from the point of reference, which is usually the torso. Opposite of *proximal.*

epiglottis   a leaf-shaped structure that prevents foreign objects from entering the trachea during swallowing.

external   outside. Opposite of *internal.*

extremities   the limbs of the body.

femoral pulse point   the location where an arterial pulse can be felt in the groin area in the crease between the abdomen and thigh.

inferior   toward, or closer to, the feet. Opposite of *superior.*

internal   inside. Opposite of *external.*

larynx   the voice box.

lateral   toward the left or right of (away from) the midline of the body.

lateral recumbent position   position in which the patient is lying on the left or right side.

medial   toward the midline of the body.

pelvic cavity   space bound by the lower part of the spine, the hip bones, and the pubis.

pelvis   the hip bones.

peripheral nervous system   the nerves; portion of the nervous system located outside the brain and spinal cord.

pharynx   the throat.

physiology   the study of how the body works.

posterior   toward the back. Opposite of *anterior.*

prone position   a position in which patient is lying face down on his or her stomach.

proximal   close to or near the point of reference, which is usually the torso. Opposite of *distal.*

radial pulse point   the location where an arterial pulse can be felt on the palm side of the wrist.

respiration   passage of air into and out of the lungs.

shoulder girdle   the clavicles (the collarbones) and the scapulae (shoulder blades) that attach the upper extremities to the skeleton.

sternum   the breastbone.

superficial   near the surface. Opposite of *deep.*

superior   toward or closer to the head. Opposite of *inferior.*

supine position   position in which the patient is lying face up on his or her back.

thoracic cavity   space above the diaphragm and within the walls of the thorax. *Also called* chest cavity.

thorax the rib cage. *Also called* the chest.

trachea the windpipe.

veins blood vessels that carry blood back to the heart from the rest of the body.

xiphoid process lowest portion of the sternum.

Knowledge Check

1. A patient who is in the left lateral recumbent position is:
   a. sitting down with left leg and left arm extended.
   b. in a semi-sitting position and leaning to the left.
   c. lying on the left side with the head on the left arm.
   d. lying flat on the back with arms down and palms front.

2. You will learn that to perform CPR correctly, your patient must be in a supine position on a flat, hard surface. This means the patient must be lying:
   a. face down on his stomach.
   b. face up on his back.
   c. on his right side.
   d. on his left side.

3. The term "inferior" refers to a position that is toward or closer to the:
   a. feet.
   b. head and neck.
   c. midline.
   d. back.

4. A patient has a small bruise to the forearm halfway between the wrist and the elbow. Its location is best described as ___ to the wrist.
   a. distal
   b. prone
   c. external
   d. proximal

5. Your patient has an injury to the back of his upper leg about few inches above his knee. This injury may best be described as on the ___ thigh ___ to the knee.
   a. posterior, proximal
   b. anterior, proximal
   c. posterior, distal
   d. anterior, distal

6. Which one of the following is NOT a pulse point?
   a. radial
   b. femoral
   c. carotid
   d. sternal

7. The body system that secretes hormones and affects strength and growth is the ___ system.
   a. musculoskeletal
   b. circulatory
   c. endocrine
   d. nervous

8. The body system composed of the brain, the spinal cord, and nerves is called the ___ system.
   a. nervous
   b. epidermal
   c. circulatory
   d. respiratory

9. A bone in the upper leg, or thigh, is the largest bone in the body. Which one of the following is it?
   a. humerus
   b. sternum
   c. femur
   d. tibia

10. The anatomical region of the neck is called the ___ region.
    a. femoral
    b. cervical
    c. thoracic
    d. occipital

11. The bones of the spine are known as the:
    a. ventricles.
    b. vertebrae.
    c. voluntary.
    d. venules.

12. Which one of the following is the outermost layer of skin?
    a. atria
    b. fibula
    c. follicles
    d. epidermis

13. The ___ are the smallest vessels through which the exchange of fluid, oxygen, and carbon dioxide takes place between blood and tissue cells.
    a. bronchioles
    b. capillaries
    c. alveoli
    d. veins

14. The xiphoid process is a leaf-shaped structure that prevents foreign objects from entering the trachea during swallowing.
    a. True
    b. False

15. The peripheral nervous system consists of the nerves, which carry information back and forth from the body to the spinal cord and brain.
    a. True
    b. False

16. The skeleton is composed of both living cells and nonliving matter.
    a. True
    b. False

17. The term "occipital region" refers to the posterior skull.
    a. True
    b. False

18. The esophagus, pancreas, liver, and gallbladder are all part of the digestive system.
    a. True
    b. False

19. The esophagus is the passageway to the lungs. The trachea is the passageway to the stomach.
    a. True
    b. False

Matching

Match the common names to the anatomical names. Write the letter of the anatomical names on the lines provided.

COMMON NAMES

_____ collar bone

_____ shoulder blade

_____ forearm bone

_____ thigh bone

_____ shin bone

_____ breastbone

_____ knee cap

_____ ankle

_____ wrist

_____ arm bone

ANATOMICAL NAMES

A. femur

B. sternum

C. tibia

D. tarsals

E. carpals

F. patella

G. clavicle

H. ulna

I. scapula

J. humerus

SCENARIO

You are caring for a patient who was involved in a motor-vehicle collision. She was the front-seat passenger. Impact was directly into her door. Which of the patient's abdominal organs may have been injured?

_____

_____

_____

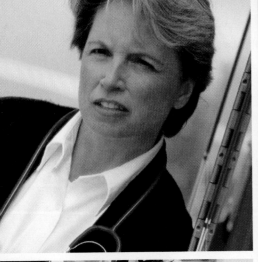
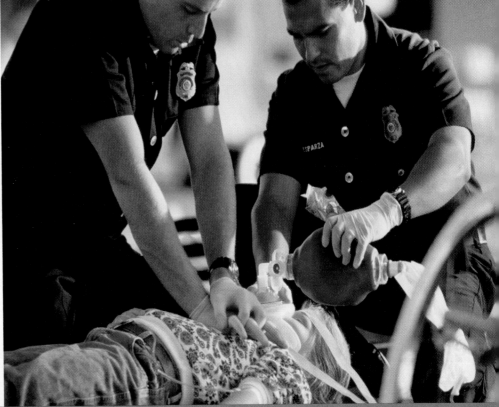
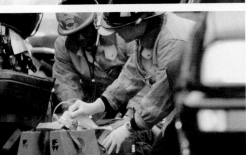

5 | Lifting and Moving Patients

Objectives

From the U.S. Department of Transportation (DOT) 1995 "First Responder: National Standard Curriculum." Material supplemental to the DOT curriculum is listed under "Enrichment."

Cognitive

1-5.1 ▸ Define body mechanics. (pp. 75–76)

1-5.2 ▸ Discuss the guidelines and safety precautions that need to be followed when lifting a patient. (pp. 75–78)

1-5.3 ▸ Describe the indications for an emergency move. (pp. 78–79)

1-5.4 ▸ Describe the indications for assisting in non-emergency moves. (p. 79)

1-5.5 ▸ Discuss the various devices associated with moving a patient in the out-of-hospital arena. (pp. 83–88)

Affective

1-5.6 ▸ Explain the rationale for properly lifting and moving patients. (pp. 75–76)

1-5.7 ▸ Explain the rationale for an emergency move. (pp. 78–79)

Psychomotor

1-5.8 ▸ Demonstrate an emergency move. (pp. 78–79, 80–81, 82)

1-5.9 ▸ Demonstrate a non-emergency move. (pp. 79–83, 84)

1-5.10 ▸ Demonstrate the use of equipment utilized to move patients in the out-of-hospital arena. (pp. 83–88)

Enrichment

▸ Describe the power lift and the power grip. (pp. 76–77)

▸ Explain how good posture and physical fitness can contribute to your well-being as an EMS provider. (pp. 77–78)

▸ Describe additional types of emergency moves, such as the piggyback carry, one-rescuer crutch, one-rescuer cradle carry, and firefighter's drag. (pp. 79, 80–82)

Introduction

Even if you don't routinely transport patients to a hospital, in an emergency you may have to reposition patients, move them to safety, or assist other EMS providers in moving them. While doing so, you are responsible for seeing that the patient is not subjected to further injury or unnecessary pain and discomfort. Knowledge in this area will help you avoid injuring yourself as well.

Section 1 Body Mechanics

Basic Principles

As a First Responder, you may be asked to lift and carry patients and heavy equipment. If you do it incorrectly, you could cause yourself injury, strain, and life-long pain. With planning, good health, and skill, you can do your job with minimum risk to yourself. So, apply the principles of proper lifting and moving every day. Practice enough for them to become automatic. Make them a habit that increases your safety and performance, even in the most stressful emergency situations.

The term **body mechanics** refers to the safest and most efficient methods of using your body to gain a mechanical advantage. Good body mechanics include the following:

- *Position your feet properly* on a firm, level surface.
- *Use your legs to lift, not your back.* To move a heavy object, use the muscles of your legs, hips, and buttocks, plus the contracted muscles of your abdomen. These muscles let you safely generate a lot of power. Never use the muscles in your back to help you move or lift a heavy object.

- *Keep the weight of the object as close to your body as possible.* Reach only a short distance to lift a heavy object (Figure 5-1). Back injury is much more likely to occur when you reach a long distance to lift an object.
- *Align shoulders, hips, and feet.* That is, visualize your shoulders stacked on top of your hips, and your hips on top of your feet. Then move as a unit. If you are out of alignment, you could create twisting forces that harm your lower back.
- *Reduce the height or distance you need to move the object.* Get closer to the object, or reposition it before you try to lift. Lift in stages if you need to.

Reaching, pushing, and pulling also can cause injury. In these cases, take the following precautions: Do not twist while reaching. Avoid reaching more than 15 to 20 inches in front of your body. Push rather than pull whenever possible. If the weight is below your waist, reach, push, or pull from a kneeling position. Do not push or pull items that are over your head.

Back injuries are a leading cause of injury and permanent disability for First Responders. To help prevent them, always use safe and appropriate lifting techniques when lifting patients and equipment. Remember, back

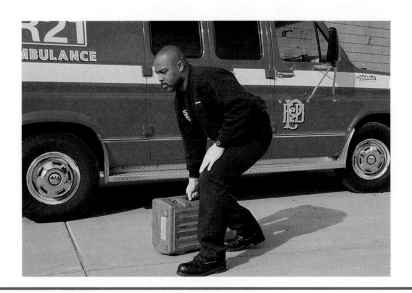

FIGURE 5-1 Keep weight close to the body as you lift.

☎ THE CALL

📡 Dispatch My partner and I were in our first-response vehicle, returning from a call, when we saw the scene of a car crash. It really took us by surprise. At least when we're dispatched, we have a little time to prepare.

◎ Scene Size-up We parked a safe distance away from the scene. As we were about to exit our vehicle, we saw smoke billow out from under the hood of the car. The fire must have been fueled by grease. We called the dispatcher to notify the fire department.

We had turnout gear on, so we carefully approached the car. A woman was in the driver's seat. She seemed dazed. The smoke was filling the car, and the windshield was turning black. Then we saw flames. We were sure the passenger compartment would soon be on fire.

Lifting and moving patients are important responsibilities. Many lifts and moves are routine, while others require quick thinking and skill. This patient needs help. Is it within the First Responders' scope of care to move her? If so, how can they do it without causing further injury? Consider her situation as you read Chapter 5.

injuries can occur at any time—not just when the object or patient is heavy. Apply the principles of body mechanics when you lift, carry, move, reach, push, and pull. Key to preventing injury during all those tasks is correct alignment of the spine. Maintain a normal inward curve in the lower back. Keep wrists and knees in normal alignment, too. Whenever possible, use equipment to do the work for you.

Lifting and moving takes teamwork. All members of a team should be trained in proper techniques. You should also avoid problems that can occur when partners are greatly mismatched. For example, if a weaker partner fails to lift, the stronger one can be injured. So can the weaker

one if he tries to do too much. Ideally, partners in lifting and moving should have adequate and equal strength and height. Know your physical abilities and limitations. Respect them. Consider the weight of the patient or equipment, and recognize the need for help.

Team members also need to communicate during a task, clearly and frequently. Use commands that are easy for team members to understand. Verbally coordinate each lift from beginning to end.

The Power Lift

The **power lift** technique offers you the best defense against injury. It also protects the patient on a stretcher by providing a safe and stable move. It is especially useful for rescuers who have weak knees or thighs. When you perform the power lift, remember to keep your back locked and avoid bending at the waist.

To perform the power lift, follow these steps (Figure 5-2):

1. *Position your feet.* Place them on a firm surface and a comfortable distance apart. (For the average-size person, this is usually about shoulder width. Taller rescuers might prefer a little wider stance.) Then turn your feet slightly outward. Most people find this helps them feel more comfortable and stable.

First on Scene

In an emergency, teamwork is essential. Just as a football coach positions players according to ability, rescuers should, too. It can help capitalize on your abilities—and the abilities of your partner and other EMS team members—to ensure the best outcome in any emergency.

SKILL SUMMARY   *Performing a Power Lift*

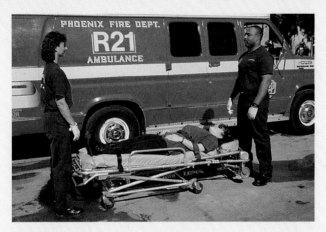

FIGURE 5-2A *Get in position.*

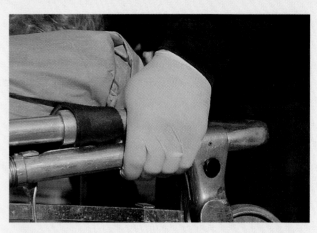

FIGURE 5-2B *Use the power grip to grasp the object.*

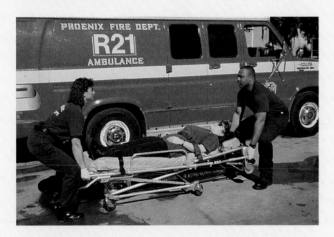

FIGURE 5-2C *Lift in unison, keeping your back locked and feet flat.*

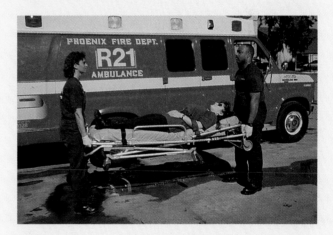

FIGURE 5-2D *Stand, making sure your back remains locked.*

2. *Bend your knees* to bring your center of gravity closer to the object. As you do so, you should feel as though you are sitting down, not falling forward.

3. *Tighten the muscles of your back and abdomen* to splint the vulnerable lower back. Your back should remain as straight as you can comfortably manage, with your head facing forward in a neutral position. Do not turn or twist.

4. *Check your stance.* Be sure your feet are flat and your weight is evenly distributed and just forward of the heels.

5. *Position your hands.* They should be a comfortable distance from each other to provide balance to the object as it is lifted. This is usually at least 10 inches apart.

6. *Perform a* **power grip**. It will help you get maximum force from your hands. In a power grip, your palms

and fingers should come in complete contact with the object and all fingers should be bent at the same angle.

7. *Lift the weight.* As lifting begins, keep your back locked as the force is driven through the heels and arches of your feet. Your upper body should come up before the hips do.

8. *To lower weight, reverse the steps.*

Posture and Fitness

Posture is a much overlooked part of body mechanics. When people spend a great deal of time sitting or standing, poor posture can easily tire back and stomach muscles. This makes back injury much more likely. One extreme of poor posture is the *swayback*. In it, the stomach

SKILL SUMMARY *Maintaining Good Posture*

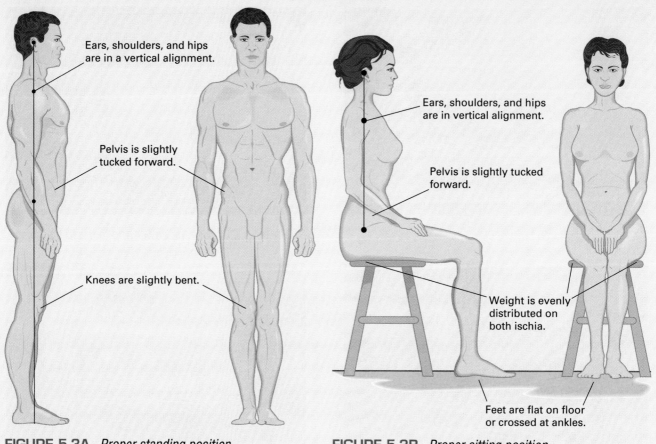

Ears, shoulders, and hips are in a vertical alignment.

Pelvis is slightly tucked forward.

Knees are slightly bent.

FIGURE 5-3A *Proper standing position.*

Ears, shoulders, and hips are in vertical alignment.

Pelvis is slightly tucked forward.

Weight is evenly distributed on both ischia.

Feet are flat on floor or crossed at ankles.

FIGURE 5-3B *Proper sitting position.*

is too far forward and the buttocks too far back, causing extreme stress on the lower back. Another extreme is the *slouch*. In it, the shoulders roll forward, putting increased pressure on every region of the spine.

Be aware of your own posture (Figure 5-3). While standing, keep your ears, shoulders, and hips in vertical alignment. Your knees should be slightly bent, and your pelvis slightly tucked forward. When sitting, your weight should be evenly distributed on both *ischia* (the lower portion of your pelvic bones). Keep your ears, shoulders, and hips in vertical alignment. Your feet should be flat on the floor or crossed at the ankles. If possible, your lower back should be in contact with the support of the chair.

Finally, proper body mechanics will not protect you if you are not physically fit. A proactive, well-balanced physical fitness program should include flexibility training, cardiovascular conditioning, strength training, and nutrition.

Q:
1. What are three rules of proper lifting and moving?

2. What are two requirements for building a safe and effective lifting and moving team?

3. What is the power grip? Describe it.

Section 2 Principles of Moving Patients

Emergency Moves

The top priority in emergency care is to maintain a patient's airway, breathing, and circulation. However, if the scene is unstable or poses an immediate threat, you may have to move the patient first. (Follow local protocols.) In general, when there is no threat to life, provide emergency medical care and wait for the EMTs to move the patient. Make an **emergency move** only when there is an immediate danger to the patient.

Examples of situations in which you may make an emergency move are:

- *Fire or threat of fire.* Fire should always be considered a grave threat, not only to patients but also to rescuers.

- *Explosion or the threat of explosion.*

- *Inability to protect the patient from other hazards at the scene.* Examples of hazards include an unstable building, an overturned car, spilled gasoline and other hazardous materials, an unruly or hostile crowd, and extreme weather conditions.

- *Inability to gain access to other patients who need life-saving care.* For example, this may occur at the scene of a car crash involving two or more patients.

- *When life-saving care cannot be given because of the patient's location or position.* For example, a patient in cardiac arrest must be supine on a flat, hard surface for you to perform CPR properly. If that patient is sitting on a chair, an emergency move must be made for you to provide life-saving care.

The greatest danger in an emergency move is the possibility of making a spine injury worse. To provide as much protection to the spine as possible, pull the patient in the direction of the long axis of the body.

It is impossible to move a patient from a vehicle quickly and, at the same time, protect the spine. So, move a patient from a vehicle immediately only if one of the five conditions described above exists.

If the patient is on the floor or the ground, use one of the following emergency moves (Figure 5-4). If you have time, you may wish to bind the patient's wrists together with a cravat or gauze. This will make the patient easier to move and will help protect the hands and arms from injury. Finally, never pull the patient's head away from the neck and shoulders.

Shirt Drag

To perform a shirt drag (Figure 5-4a), do the following. First, fasten the patient's hands or wrists loosely with a cravat or gauze to protect them during the move. Then, grasp the shoulders of the patient's shirt (not a tee shirt). Pull the shirt under the patient's head to form a support. Next, using the shirt as a "handle," pull the patient toward you. Be careful not to strangle the patient. Pulling should engage the patient's armpits, not the neck.

Blanket Drag

To perform a blanket drag (Figure 5-4b), do the following. First, spread a blanket alongside the patient. Gather half of it into lengthwise pleats. Roll the patient away from you onto his side, and tuck the pleated part of the blanket as far under him as you can. Then roll the patient onto the center of the blanket, preferably onto his back. Wrap the blanket securely around the patient. Grabbing the part of the blanket under the patient's head, drag the patient toward you.

If you do not have a blanket, you can use a coat in the same way.

Shoulder or Forearm Drag

To perform a shoulder drag (Figure 5-4c), do the following. First, stand at the patient's head. Next, slip your hands under the patient's armpits from the back. If you must drag the patient a long distance and need a better grip, perform a forearm drag. That is, position yourself as you would in a shoulder drag. After you slip your hands under the patient's armpits, grasp the patient's forearms and drag the patient toward you. Use your own forearms as a support to keep the patient's head, neck, and spine in alignment.

Other Emergency Moves

Other emergency moves include the piggyback carry, one-rescuer crutch, one-rescuer cradle carry, firefighter's drag, and others. (See Figure 5-4d through 5-4h and Figure 5-5.)

Non-Emergency Moves

A **non-emergency move,** or non-urgent move, is generally performed with other rescuers. It requires no equipment and may take less time than moves such as a blanket drag. However, do not use a non-emergency move with possible spine-injured patients, since it offers no spinal protection.

Non-emergency, or non-urgent, moves include the direct ground lift and extremity lift.

 First Responder Practice

Do lifting and moving involve strong muscles? No, they do not. Lifting and moving patients and other heavy objects involve practice, planning, and the correct use of your body. Remember to always use good body mechanics to remain safe and injury free.

SKILL SUMMARY   *Performing Emergency Moves*

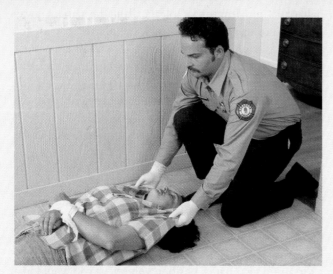

FIGURE 5-4A *Shirt drag.*

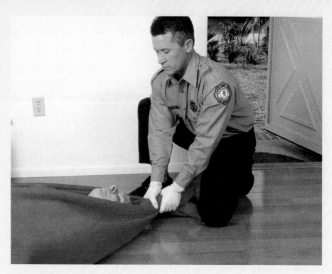

FIGURE 5-4B *Blanket drag.*

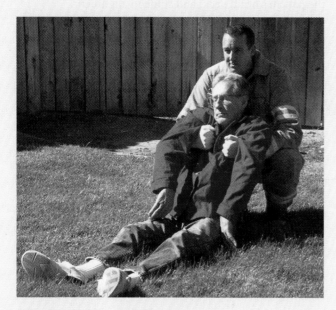

FIGURE 5-4C *Shoulder drag.*

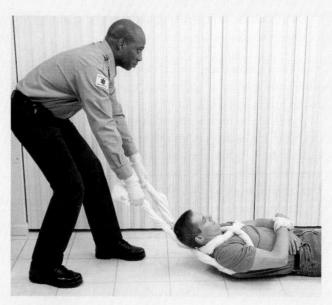

FIGURE 5-4D *Sheet drag.*

Direct Ground Lift

The direct ground lift requires two or three rescuers (Figure 5-6). It is valuable when the patient cannot sit in a chair and when a stretcher cannot be brought close to the patient. If the patient weighs more than 180 pounds, is on the ground or some other low surface, or is uncooperative, a direct ground lift is difficult to perform.

Position the stretcher as close to the patient as possible. Undo the stretcher straps, lower the railings, and clear any equipment off the mattress. Tell the patient what you are going to do. Next, warn him that he must remain still to protect your balance. Place the patient's arms on his chest, if possible. Then, follow these steps:

1. *Get in position.* Line up on one side of the patient. If at all possible, choose the least injured side. Next, rescuers kneel on one knee, preferably the same knee for all.

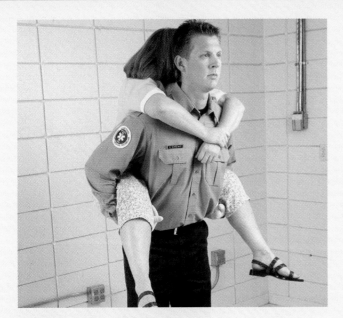

FIGURE 5-4E *Piggyback carry.*

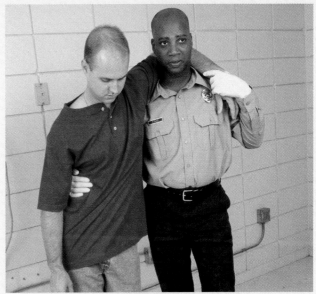

FIGURE 5-4F *One-rescuer crutch.*

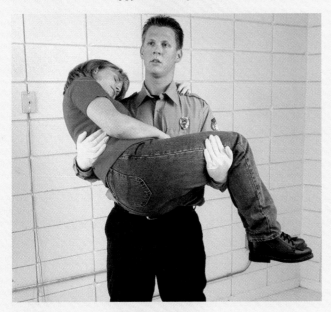

FIGURE 5-4G *Cradle carry.*

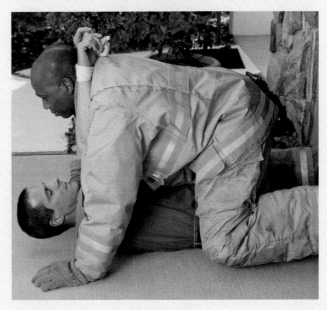

FIGURE 5-4H *Firefighter's drag.*

2. *Cradle the patient.* That is, have the first rescuer place one arm under the neck and shoulder to cradle the head. He must place his other arm under the patient's lower back. The second rescuer should then place one arm under the patient's knees, and one arm above the buttocks.

   If a third rescuer is available, he is to place both arms under the patient's waist. Then, the first rescuer should slide his arms up to the middle of the back. The second rescuer should slide his arms down to the buttocks.

3. *On signal, lift the patient as a unit.* First, lift to knee level. Then, with a gentle rocking motion, roll the patient as a unit toward your chests until she is cradled in the bends of your elbows. Tuck the patient's head in toward your chests.

4. *On signal, rise to a standing position.* Then carry the patient to the stretcher.

5. *To lower the patient onto the stretcher, reverse the steps.*

SKILL SUMMARY *Performing a Firefighter's Carry*

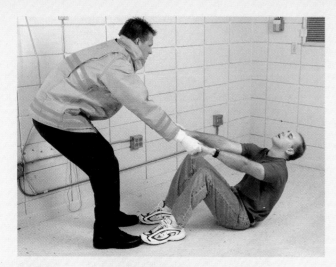

FIGURE 5-5A *Grasp the patient's wrists.*

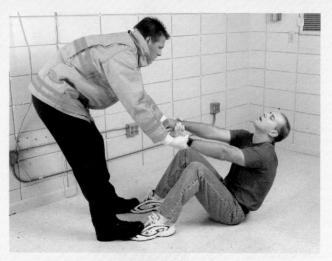

FIGURE 5-5B *Stand on the patient's toes and pull.*

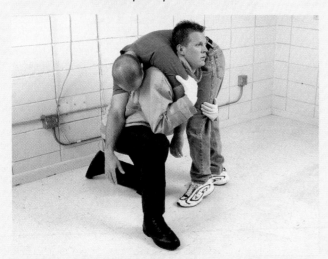

FIGURE 5-5C *Pull the patient over a shoulder.*

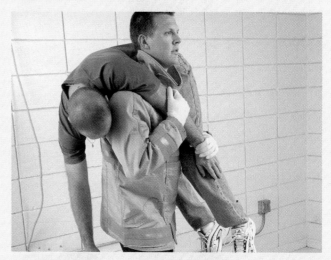

FIGURE 5-5D *Pass an arm between the legs and grasp the arm nearest you.*

Extremity Lift

The extremity lift requires two rescuers (Figure 5-7). Use it to move an unresponsive patient from a chair to the floor. Do not use it if the patient has injuries to his or her arms or legs. To perform an extremity lift, first get into position. One rescuer should move to the patient's head and place one hand under each shoulder, reaching through to grab the patient's wrists. The other rescuer should kneel at the patient's side by the knees and slip his hands under them. Then, on signal, move up to a crouch. Finally, on signal, rise to a standing position and move the patient to the desired location.

Positioning the Patient

Unless there is a life-threatening emergency, a First Responder should not move an injured patient. The EMTs will evaluate, stabilize, and move the patient as necessary. However, how you position the patient depends on the patient's condition. General guidelines include:

■ An unresponsive patient who is not injured should be placed in the *recovery position* (lateral recumbent position). This is done by rolling the patient onto his or her side, preferably the left side. (See Chapter 6 for more information.)

SKILL SUMMARY   *Performing a Direct Ground Lift*

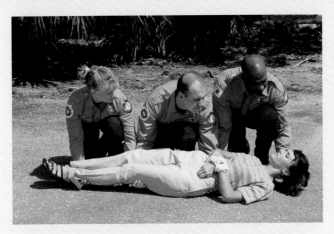

FIGURE 5-6A *Kneel on one knee, and then get into position to cradle the patient.*

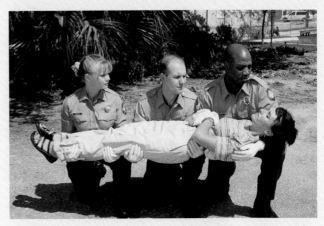

FIGURE 5-6B *In unison, lift the patient to knee level.*

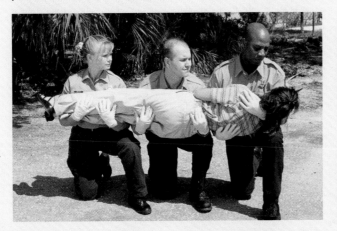

FIGURE 5-6C *Slowly turn the patient toward you.*

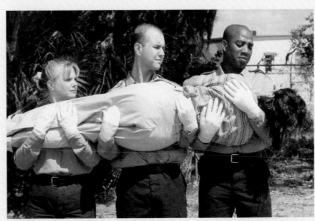

FIGURE 5-6D *In unison, rise to a standing position.*

- A patient who shows signs of shock may need to be positioned. If it will not aggravate injuries to the legs or spine, do this by elevating the supine patient's legs 8 to 12 inches. (See Chapter 18 for more information.)

- A patient who has pain or breathing problems may be in any position that makes him more comfortable, unless his injuries prevent it. Generally, a patient with abdominal pain will want to lie on his side with knees drawn up. A patient who has breathing difficulties will want to sit up.

- A responsive patient who is nauseated or vomiting should be allowed to remain in a position of comfort. However, always be positioned so you can manage the patient's airway if needed.

1. When may a First Responder make an emergency move?

2. What is the greatest danger to a patient during an emergency move?

3. How can you protect a patient from further injury during an emergency move?

Section 3 Equipment

Become completely familiar with the equipment used to move patients in your EMS system. Decide which piece of equipment to use based on the patient's condition, the

SKILL SUMMARY   *Performing an Extremity Lift*

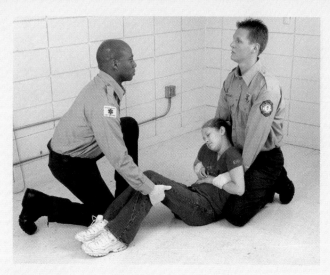

FIGURE 5-7A   *Get in position at the head and feet of the patient.*

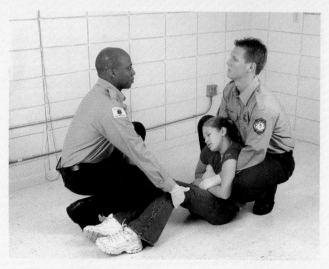

FIGURE 5-7B   *On signal, move up to a crouching position.*

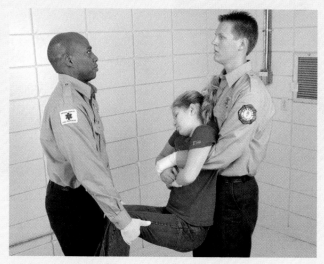

FIGURE 5-7C   *Then move to a standing position.*

environment in which he is found, and the resources available.

Generally, the best way to move a patient is the easiest way that will avoid injury or pain. Let your equipment do the work whenever possible. Drag or slide the patient (do not lift), whenever you can. If you must lift a patient, use a device designed for that purpose. As a rule, carry a patient only as far as absolutely necessary. Make sure you have adequate help. If you don't have it, get it. Never risk injuring yourself.

Typical equipment used in EMS includes various types of stretchers, the stair chair, and backboards.

Stretchers

There are a number of different kinds of stretchers (Figure 5-8). A **standard stretcher,** or cot, has wheeled legs. It also has a collapsible undercarriage so that it can be loaded into an ambulance.

A **portable stretcher** is lightweight, folds compactly, and is easy to clean. It has no undercarriage or wheels. It is comfortable to rest on, especially if the head is padded. It is valuable when there is not enough space for a standard stretcher or when there are multiple patients. It comes in a variety of styles. The most common has an aluminum frame with canvas fabric.

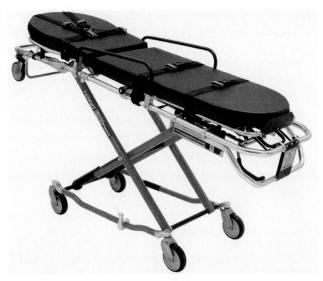

a. *Standard wheeled stretcher. (Ferno Corporation)*

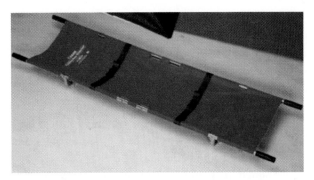

b. *Portable stretcher.*

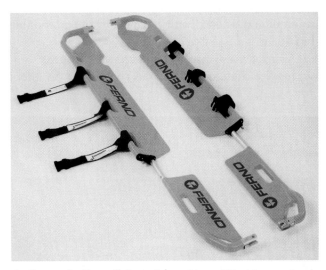

d. *Scoop (orthopedic) stretcher. (Ferno-Washington, Inc.)*

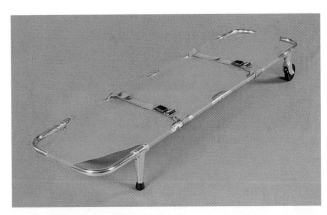

c. *Portable ambulance stretcher.*

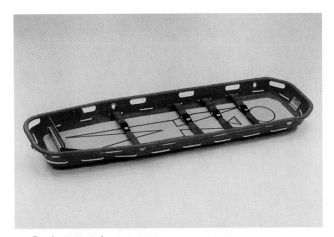

e. *Basket stretcher. (Ferno Corporation)*

FIGURE 5-8 Stretchers, or patient-carrying devices, are designed to help rescuers carry the patient to an ambulance or to the hospital.

A **scoop stretcher,** also called an *orthopedic stretcher,* splits into two or four sections. Each section can be fitted around a patient who is lying on a relatively flat surface. It is used in confined areas where larger stretchers will not fit. Once secure in a scoop stretcher, a patient can be lifted and moved to a standard one. To operate a scoop stretcher, split it apart lengthwise. Carefully slide it under the patient from both sides. Then lock the brackets at each end, and lift the patient.

Designed to surround and protect the patient, the **basket stretcher,** or Stokes stretcher, is used to move a patient from one level to another or over rough terrain. The basket should be lined with a blanket before positioning the patient.

A stretcher also can be improvised with a blanket, canvas, brattice cloth, or a strong sheet and two 7- to 8-foot poles. To improvise a stretcher with two poles and a blanket, follow these steps (Figure 5-9):

1. *Position the first pole.* Place it about one foot from the center of the unfolded blanket. Then, fold the short side of the blanket over it.

2. *Position the second pole.* Place it on top of the two folds of blanket. It should be about two feet from the first pole and parallel to it.

3. *Fold the remaining side of the blanket over the second pole.*

4. *Place the patient on the blanket.* The weight of the patient's body will secure the poles.

A stretcher can be made from cloth bags or sacks. (Make holes in the bottoms of bags or sacks so that the

---

SKILL SUMMARY *Improvising a Stretcher*

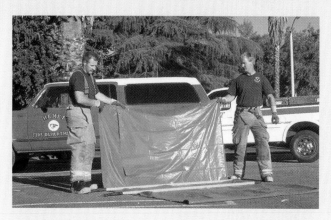

FIGURE 5-9A *Position the first pole. Then, fold the blanket over it.*

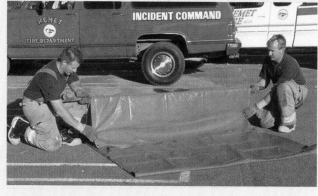

FIGURE 5-9B *Position the second pole.*

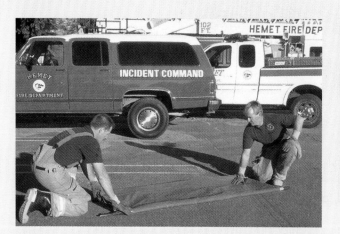

FIGURE 5-9C *Fold the remaining side of the blanket over the second pole.*

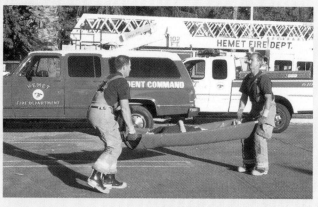

FIGURE 5-9D *When the patient is placed on the blanket, his or her weight will secure the poles.*

SKILL SUMMARY *Using a Stair Chair*

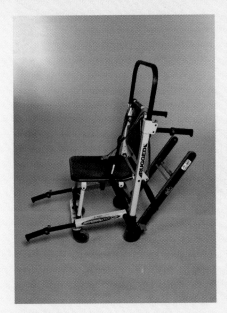

FIGURE 5-10A *Example of a stair chair.*

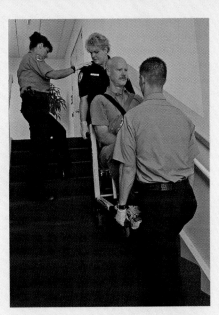

FIGURE 5-10B *Moving a patient up steps with a third rescuer as spotter.*

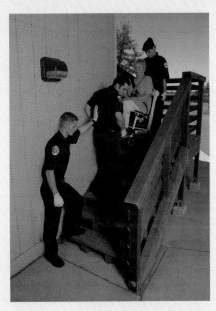

FIGURE 5-10C *Moving a patient down steps with a third rescuer as spotter.*

poles pass through them. Use enough bags to provide the required length.) A stretcher also can be made from three or four coats or jackets. (First turn the sleeves inside out. Then fasten the jackets with the sleeves inside. Place the poles through the sleeves.)

Stair Chair

Moving patients up or down stairs dramatically increases the potential for rescuers to be injured. The safest method is to use a stair chair. A **stair chair** is a lightweight folding device. It has straps to confine the patient, wheeled legs, a grab bar below the patient's feet, and handles that extend behind the patient's shoulders.

When you use a stair chair (Figure 5-10), make sure as many people as necessary are helping. Always use a "spotter" to help maneuver the stair chair down stairs. He should continually tell how many stairs are left and what conditions are ahead. A spotter also can place his hand on the back of the rescuer who is moving backward to help steady him.

Rescuers carrying a patient in a stair chair should keep their backs in a locked position. They should flex at the hips instead of at the waist, bend at the knees, and keep arms (and the weight of the chair) as close to their bodies as possible. Once off the stairs, the patient can be transferred to a more conventional stretcher.

Stair chairs work well for patients in respiratory distress who must be moved up or down stairs. The sitting position does not worsen the patient's breathing problems.

Backboards

There are both long and short backboards (Figure 5-11). A **long backboard** may be six to seven feet long, which means it can stabilize the patient's entire body. It is used for patients with suspected spine injury who are lying down. A **short backboard** is three to four feet long and can stabilize the patient down to the hips. It is used for a patient with suspected spine injuries who is in a sitting position. Both the long and short backboards feature handholds and straps. Most are made of synthetic material that will not absorb blood and is easy to clean.

Another type of device used much like the short backboard is the *vest-type immobilization device.* As the

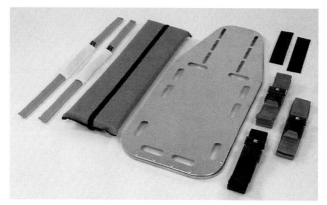

a. *Traditional short backboard.*

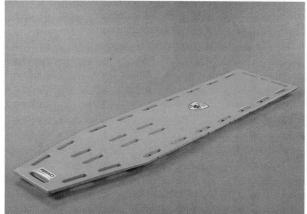

c. *Long backboard.*

b. *Vest-type immobilization device.*

FIGURE 5-11 **Backboards are used to help stabilize a patient's spine.**

name implies, it is designed to wrap around and stabilize the patient's head and torso.

Regardless of whether you use a long or short backboard, always maintain manual support of the patient's head and neck in the normal anatomical position. Maintain that support until the patient is *fully* secured and immobilized.

1. What are three common types of stretchers?

2. What is the safest way to move a patient up or down stairs?

3. What are two common types of backboards? When should each be used?

The Call Follow-up

At the beginning of this chapter, you read that the First Responders were at the scene of a collision. They were faced with a patient with unknown injuries and in serious danger from smoke and fire. To see how the First Responders handled this emergency, read the following. It describes how the call was completed.

Scene Size-up (continued) We glanced at each other quickly. We both knew the patient was in mortal danger and had to be moved immediately. Although we were concerned about her possible injuries, we knew it would do no good to leave her in the smoke-filled, flaming car. I grabbed her under her shoulders and began the move. I cradled her head in my arms to help minimize problems with her spine. My partner grabbed her legs. We moved her a safe distance from the car and set her down carefully.

Initial Assessment My partner stabilized her head as I assessed her mental status. She moaned when I spoke loudly. My partner kept an eye on her airway and saw she was breathing adequately and had no foreign material in her mouth. But that could change quickly. There also were no signs of external bleeding.

Our general impression was that this woman was about 50 years old and in potentially serious condition. She may have had injuries from the crash and from the smoke. We had oxygen available, so we applied a nonrebreather mask immediately.

We updated the incoming units of our suspicions so they could be prepared when they arrived on scene.

Physical Examination Based on our observations of the scene, we knew that any type of injury was possible. The patient was not alert and couldn't tell us what hurt. Palpation of her head and neck were negative for signs of injury. I palpated her chest and she groaned, indicating that she felt pain from an injury there. I listened to her chest and found unequal breathing sounds, diminished on the right. She had some abrasions on her lower legs and no other injuries that I could find. As I finished the exam, my partner told me that respirations were becoming inadequate. My partner began to assist them. I checked the patient's pulse, which was 112, regular, and weak. Her respirations were 36 and shallow.

Patient History We didn't notice any medical information tags on the patient. She couldn't tell us anything about her condition and no family members were present.

Ongoing Assessment We continued to assist her ventilations. They remained shallow and rapid. Her pulse increased slightly to 120 and remained weak. We concentrated on ventilating the patient until the EMTs arrived.

Patient Hand-off When the EMTs arrived, we described our initial observations of the scene. They agreed that the patient had to be moved fast. We then went on to report on the patient's condition (see below). It turned out the patient experienced a collapsed lung in the crash. The smoke from the fire really didn't help. The EMTs told us they corrected the lung problem right in the emergency department and the patient improved dramatically. She was expected to recover fully. We were pleased to hear that our actions at the scene were an important part of her doing so well.

 ## Hand-off Report

"This is a female, about 50 years of age, involved in a motor-vehicle crash. She responds only by moaning. We are currently stabilizing the spine and assisting ventilations because of inadequate breathing. We noted pain in her chest while we palpated. Breath sounds on the right are diminished compared to the left. Her pulse is weak and increased from 112 to 120. Her respirations are 36 and shallow. We have no information on history. We'll give you a hand with the backboarding so you can get off the scene quickly."

The Last Word *When to move a patient is determined by the patient's condition and the environment in which she is found. How to move a patient is determined by considering her condition, location, and resources. Remember, in general, a First Responder does not move a patient unless an emergency move must be made or the EMTs ask for assistance. When you do move a patient, be sure to follow the rules of good body mechanics.*

Chapter Review

Focus on the EMS Team

You will find that most patients are in safe locations. Others have problems that would be worsened by movement. So, in most cases, you will not move a patient until the EMTs arrive on scene. However, being first on scene means you will be the first to recognize any problems you and other EMS personnel need to solve, such as lifting an unusually heavy patient or making an especially difficult move. Recognizing these problems and reporting them to dispatch as soon as possible after you arrive on scene will go a long way in making sure the call runs safely and smoothly.

Remember that lifting and moving takes teamwork between you and your partner as well as with other rescuers who may be on scene. Don't risk injuring yourself. Don't risk causing additional injury to your patient. Ask for help when you need it, and practice the skills presented in this chapter. You will use them more than you think.

Summing Up

- Good body mechanics for lifting include placing, your feet on a firm, level surface; using your legs to lift, not your back; keeping the weight close to your body; aligning shoulders, hips, and feet; reducing the height or distance from you before moving the object.

- Good body mechanics for reaching, pushing, and pulling include not twisting while reaching; not reaching more than 15 to 20 inches in front of you; pushing rather than pulling when possible; when weight is below your waist, move the weight from a kneeling position; never push or pull items that are over your head.

- When possible, let equipment do the work for you.

- Ideally, when lifting and moving, partners should have adequate and equal strength and height. Good verbal coordination is also ideal.

- Use the power lift to help prevent injuries during a lift. Use a power grip to get the maximum force from your hands.

- Good posture is an important part of good body mechanics. While standing, your ears, shoulders, and hips should be in vertical alignment; knees should be slightly bent; and your pelvis slightly tucked forward. When sitting, your weight should be evenly distributed on both ischia; ears, shoulders, and hips should be in vertical alignment; feet should be flat on the floor or crossed at the ankles; lower back should be in contact with the support of the chair.

- Proper body mechanics cannot protect you if you are not physically fit. A proactive, wellbalanced physical fitness program should include flexibility training, cardiovascular conditioning, strength training, and nutrition.

- In general, do not move a patient. However, you may perform an emergency move when there is an immediate danger to the patient. Emergency moves include the shirt drag, blanket drag, shoulder or forearm drag, piggyback carry, one-rescuer crutch, one-rescuer cradle carry, and firefighter's drag.

- The greatest danger in an emergency move is the possibility of making a spine injury worse. To provide as much protection to the spine as possible, pull the patient in the direction of the long axis of the body.

- Non-emergency moves are generally performed with other rescuers. Do not use such a move with possible spine-injured patients, since it offers no spinal protection. Non-emergency moves include the direct ground lift and the extremity lift.

- In certain circumstances, a First Responder may position a patient to help keep the airway clear (recovery position) or as part of the emergency care of specific conditions. (This will be discussed further in subsequent chapters.)

- If you must lift a patient, use a device designed for that purpose. That includes various types of stretchers, the stair chair, and backboards.

Key Terms

basket stretcher designed to surround and protect the patient, this stretcher is used to move a patient from one level to another or over rough terrain. *Also called* Stokes stretcher.

body mechanics the safest and most efficient methods of using the body to gain a mechanical advantage.

emergency move a move made when there is an immediate danger to the patient.

long backboard a rigid device, about six to seven feet long, that can help stabilize a patient's entire body.

non-emergency move a move made by several rescuers usually after a patient has been stabilized. *Also called* non-urgent move.

portable stretcher commonly made of an aluminum frame and canvas, this cot has no wheels. It is valuable when there is not enough space for a standard stretcher or when there are multiple patients.

power grip a technique used to get maximum force from the rescuer's hands while lifting and moving.

power lift a technique used for lifting that helps prevent injury to rescuers and provides a stable move for the patient.

scoop stretcher this cot splits in two or four sections, so it can be used where larger stretchers cannot fit. *Also called* orthopedic stretcher.

short backboard three to four feet long, this device can help stabilize a patient down to the hips. It is used for patients with suspected spine injuries who are in a sitting position.

stair chair a lightweight folding device that is used to safely move patients up or down stairs.

standard stretcher a cot with wheels. It may also have a collapsible undercarriage that makes it possible to load it into an ambulance.

Knowledge Check

1. **Which one of the following steps is included in the power-lift technique?**
   a. Keep your knees locked.
   b. Use the balls of your feet when lifting.
   c. Place your feet about shoulder width apart.
   d. Bend at the waist to lift objects from the ground.

2. **In which one of the following situations would an emergency move be appropriate?**
   a. An injured patient is lying supine on the ground.
   b. A patient who has fallen has possible spine injuries.
   c. Two patients with spine injuries are in a crashed car.
   d. A patient is in a vehicle with fire in the engine compartment.

3. **Which one of the following statements about body mechanics is TRUE?**
   a. Use your back, not your legs, to lift objects.
   b. Before you lift an object, move it farther away from your body.
   c. When team members are lifting, their heights should be similar.
   d. Physical fitness and posture are *not* important to body mechanics.

4. **A patient who is unresponsive but breathing adequately should be placed in the ___ position.**
   a. recovery
   b. sitting
   c. supine
   d. prone

5. **The device most appropriate for a patient with a spine injury is the:**
   a. stair chair.
   b. long backboard.
   c. wheeled stretcher.
   d. improvised stretcher.

6. Because emergency moves do NOT protect the patient's spine, you should always perform them by pulling the patient:

   a. sideways, along the short axis of the body.
   b. feet first on any inclined or sloping surface.
   c. in the direction of the long axis of the body.
   d. in a stair chair or secured to a long backboard.

7. An emergency move of a patient who is lying supine on the ground may be performed by:

   a. rolling her like a log.
   b. securing her to a backboard.
   c. using one rescuer on each extremity.
   d. pulling her clothing at the shoulders.

8. When moving or lifting a patient using a non-emergency move, you should do all of the following EXCEPT:

   a. apply the principles of body mechanics.
   b. communicate clearly with your partner.
   c. twist from the hips while lifting her.
   d. consider your physical limitations.

Matching

Match the patient with the appropriate carrying device. Write the letter of the carrying device on the appropriate line.

PATIENT	CARRYING DEVICE
_____ A patient with respiratory distress in an upstairs back bedroom.	A. long backboard
_____ A patient with suspected spine injury. He fell about 15 feet from a tree in his backyard.	B. stair chair
_____ A patient who is one of 47 involved in a multiple-casualty incident.	C. scoop stretcher
_____ A patient with a possible hip injury who is on the floor in a confined area.	D. portable stretcher

Scenario

You come upon a motor-vehicle collision where a patient has been thrown from one of the vehicles. He is unconscious and lying in the road, in danger from oncoming rush-hour traffic. What type of move would you perform for this patient? Explain your choice.

_____

_____

_____

_____

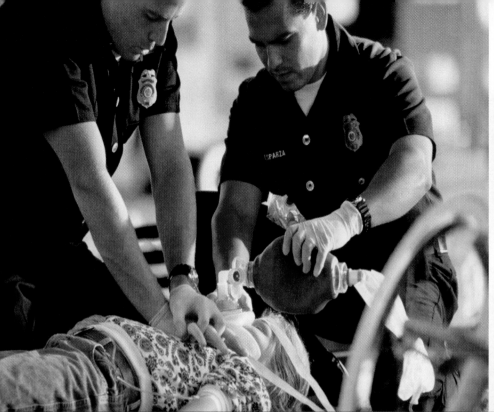
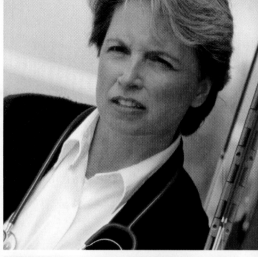
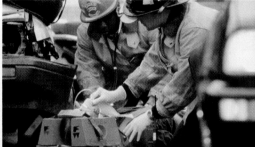

6 | Breathing and Ventilation

Objectives

From the U.S. Department of Transportation (DOT) 1995 "First Responder: National Standard Curriculum." Material supplemental to the DOT curriculum is listed under "Enrichment." DOT's airway objectives are covered in Chapters 6 and 7.

Cognitive

2-1.1 ▶ Name and label the major structures of the respiratory system on a diagram. (pp. 95–96)

2-1.2 ▶ List the signs of inadequate breathing. (pp. 102–103)

2-1.3 ▶ Describe the steps in the head-tilt chin-lift. (pp. 98–99)

2-1.4 ▶ Relate mechanism of injury to opening the airway. (p. 99)

2-1.5 ▶ Describe the steps in the jaw thrust. (p. 99)

2-1.8 ▶ Describe how to ventilate a patient with a resuscitation mask or barrier device. (pp. 103, 106–110)

2-1.9 ▶ Describe how ventilating an infant or child is different from an adult. (pp. 110–112)

2-1.10 ▶ List the steps in providing mouth-to-mouth and mouth-to-stoma ventilation. (pp. 109–110)

Affective

2-1.19 ▶ Explain why basic life support ventilation and airway protective skills take priority over most other basic life support skills. (pp. 95, 98, 116)

2-1.20 ▶ Demonstrate a caring attitude towards patients with airway problems who request emergency medical services. (pp. 97, 114)

2-1.21 ▶ Place the interests of the patient with airway problems as the foremost consideration when making any and all patient care decisions. (p. 102)

2-1.22 ▶ Communicate with empathy to patients with airway problems, as well as with family members and friends of the patient. (p. 97)

Psychomotor

2-1.23 ▶ Demonstrate the steps in the head-tilt chin-lift. (pp. 98–99)

Introduction

The most important part of your job as a First Responder involves a patient's airway and breathing. No matter what a patient's problem may be, you must determine if a patient has an open, clear airway and is breathing adequately. That can spell the difference between life and death—for a business executive having a heart attack, a child who falls into a swimming pool, or an unresponsive patient whose problem is unknown.

This chapter will help you focus on the anatomy of the respiratory system. It also provides information on airway techniques and procedures such as how to open an airway, how to assess breathing, and how to perform artificial ventilation in adults and children. Chapter 7 will continue discussion of the airway with topics related to airway care and maintenance.

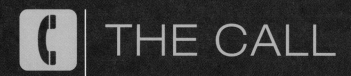

THE CALL

Dispatch Our first-response unit was dispatched to an "unresponsive person."

Scene Size-up We moved toward the house carefully, as we always do. A man came to the door. He looked very concerned as he explained that his wife slumped over in her chair minutes ago. "She looks bad," he told us. "She's not breathing right. Please help her." As we approached the patient, we asked her husband if she had sustained any falls or injuries. He assured us that she had not.

Initial Assessment We already had our gloves and eye-wear on by the time we reached the patient's side. We observed that she was unresponsive, with snoring respirations.

This patient requires immediate attention. No matter what the underlying reason for her condition, she will not survive without adequate respirations. Consider this patient as you read Chapter 6. What can the First Responders do for her?

Section 1 The Respiratory System

The body can store food for weeks and water for days, but it can store enough oxygen for only a few minutes. When oxygen is cut off, brain cells begin to die in about 4 to 6 minutes. The respiratory system supplies the body with the oxygen it needs. It also removes carbon dioxide.

Anatomy of the Respiratory System

The major components of the respiratory system are the nose and mouth, pharynx (throat), epiglottis, larynx (voice box), trachea (windpipe), and the bronchi, lungs, and diaphragm. (See the upper airway in Figure 6-1. You also may wish to review Chapter 4.)

- *Nose and mouth.* Air normally enters the body through the nose and mouth. There it is warmed, moistened, and filtered as it flows over the damp, sticky mucous membranes.

- *Pharynx.* At the back of the nose and mouth, the air enters the pharynx (throat), the passageway for both food and air. Air from the mouth enters through the oropharynx. Air from the nose enters through the nasopharynx. At its lower end, the pharynx divides in two. One division is the esophagus, which leads to the stomach. The other is the trachea (windpipe), which leads to the lungs.

- *Epiglottis.* The trachea is protected by a small, leaf-shaped flap called the epiglottis. Normally, this flap covers the entrance of the larynx during swallowing so that food and liquid cannot enter. However, with injury or illness, that reflex may not work properly. As a result, a patient could **aspirate** (inhale) liquid, blood, or vomit into the trachea and lungs, causing obstruction, infection, and death.

- *Trachea and larynx.* The trachea (windpipe) carries air from the nose and mouth to the lungs. Immediately above it is the larynx (voice box) or "Adam's apple." The larynx can be easily felt with your fingertips at the front of the throat.

- *Bronchi and lungs.* The lower end of the trachea divides into two tubes called bronchi. The bronchi lead to the lungs. Each bronchus divides into the smaller *bronchioles,* somewhat like the branches of a tree. At the ends of the bronchioles are millions of tiny air sacs called *alveoli.* Each alveolus is enclosed in a network of capillaries and is responsible for the exchange of oxygen and carbon dioxide.

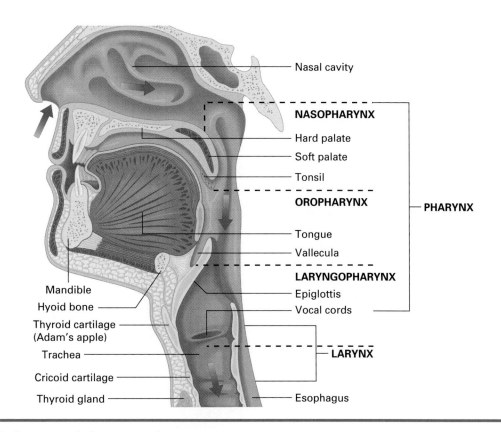

FIGURE 6-1 Anatomy of the upper airway.

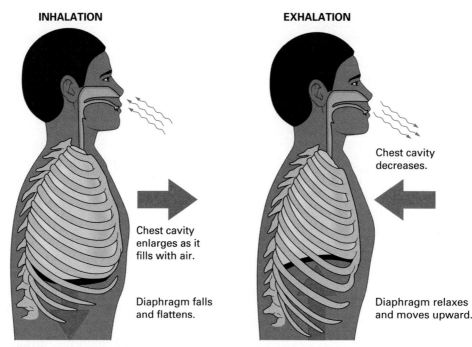

INHALATION

Chest cavity enlarges as it fills with air.

Diaphragm falls and flattens.

Air pressure inside the chest cavity is less than outside, so air rushes into lungs to balance the pressure.

EXHALATION

Chest cavity decreases.

Diaphragm relaxes and moves upward.

Air pressure inside the chest cavity is greater than outside, so air is pushed out of the lungs.

FIGURE 6-2 How respiration works.

The principal organs of respiration are the lungs. The lungs are two large, lobed organs that house millions of tiny alveoli.

- *Diaphragm.* The diaphragm is a powerful, dome-shaped muscle essential to breathing. It separates the thoracic cavity from the abdominal cavity. If it cannot contract effectively because of illness or injury, a patient will breathe inadequately and develop significant respiratory distress.

How Respiration Works

During inhalation, the diaphragm and the muscles between the ribs contract. This increases the size of the thoracic cavity, making it possible for the lungs to expand. The diaphragm moves down slightly, flaring the lower portion of the rib cage, which then moves upward and outward. This decreases pressure in the chest and causes air to flow into the lungs. (See Figure 6-2.)

In the lungs, gases pass through the thin walls of the alveoli and capillaries. Oxygen enters the alveoli during inhalation and passes through the capillary walls into the bloodstream. Carbon dioxide and other waste gases pass from the blood through the capillary walls into the alveoli so they can be exhaled.

During exhalation, the diaphragm and the muscles between the ribs relax. This decreases the size of the tho-

racic cavity. The diaphragm moves up, the ribs move down and in, and air flows out of the lungs.

With some respiratory diseases, a patient has a hard time moving air out of the lungs. He has to use muscles not only to draw air in but also to force air out. As a result, both inhalation and exhalation require energy. Such patients tend to get exhausted quickly and will deteriorate rapidly.

Adequate breathing occurs at a normal rate (Table 6-1). For adults, that is 12 to 20 breaths per minute. For children, it is 15 to 30 breaths per minute. For infants, it is 25 to 50 breaths per minute. Breathing is adequate when it is regular in rhythm and free of unusual sounds, such as wheezing or whistling and when chest expansion and depth of respirations are sufficient to support life without assistance.

TABLE 6-1 **Normal Breathing Rates**	
Infant	25–50 breaths per minute
Child	15–30 breaths per minute
Adult	12–20 breaths per minute

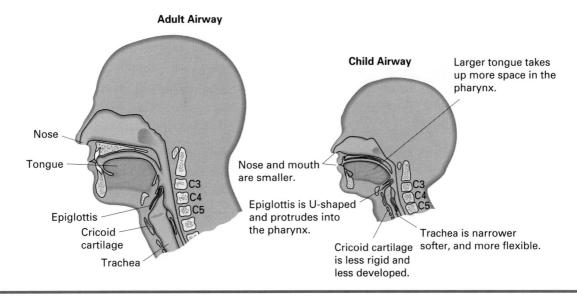

FIGURE 6-3 Comparison of the airways of an adult and an infant or child.

Breathing should be virtually effortless. It should be accomplished without the use of **accessory muscles** (additional muscles) in the neck, shoulders, and abdomen.

Infants and Children

When providing emergency care to infants and children, remember the anatomical differences in their respiratory systems (Figure 6-3). All structures, including the mouth and nose, are smaller than those of adults. They are more easily obstructed by even small objects, blood, or swelling. Take extra care to keep the airway of infants and children open.

The tongue of an infant or child takes up proportionally more space in the pharynx than the tongue of an adult. It can therefore block the airway more easily.

The trachea of an infant or child is narrower than an adult's. It also is softer and more flexible. So, tipping the head too far back or allowing it to fall forward can close the trachea. Because the head of an infant or young child is quite large relative to the body, a folded towel or similar item under the shoulders may be needed to keep the airway aligned and open.

Because the chest wall is softer, infants and children tend to rely on the diaphragm for breathing. Watch for excessive movement there. It can alert you to respiratory distress in an infant or child. Remember, the primary cause of cardiac arrest in infants and children is an uncorrected respiratory problem.

Whether your patient is an infant, child, or adult, remember that family members also need you. Be calm and caring as well as professional. Place the patient's interests first, but consider the family, too.

1. How does air move from the nose and mouth to the lungs? Describe the pathway it takes.

2. Where is the diaphragm located? What role does it play in respiration?

3. What are normal breathing rates for an infant, child, and adult?

Section 2 Airway Techniques

Opening the Airway

The tongue is the most common cause of airway obstruction in an unresponsive patient. A patient who loses consciousness will lose muscle tone. When that happens, the base of the tongue can fall back and **occlude** (block) the airway. The patient's effort to breathe then creates negative pressure, which pulls the tongue, epiglottis, or both into the throat. In some cases, the patient requires **artificial ventilation** (forcing air into the patient's lungs). But before a patient who is not breathing or is breathing inadequately can receive it, he must have an open airway.

Two maneuvers are commonly used to open an airway: the **head-tilt/chin-lift maneuver** and the **jaw-thrust maneuver.** Both techniques move the tongue from the back of the throat and allow air to pass into the lungs. (The tongue is attached to the lower jaw. So, moving the lower jaw forward will relieve the obstruction.)

Head-Tilt/Chin-Lift Maneuver

The head-tilt/chin-lift maneuver is the method of choice for opening the airway of an uninjured patient. The American Heart Association (AHA) recommends it for opening the airway of patients who do not have injuries to the head, neck, or spine. Use it first for unresponsive patients who are not injured. To perform the head-tilt/chin-lift maneuver (Figure 6-4):

1. *Position your hand* on the patient's forehead. Use the hand closest to the patient's head.

SKILL SUMMARY   *Performing a Head-Tilt/Chin-Lift Maneuver*

ADULT

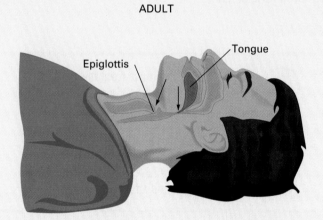

Figure 6-4a *An adult airway occluded by the tongue.*

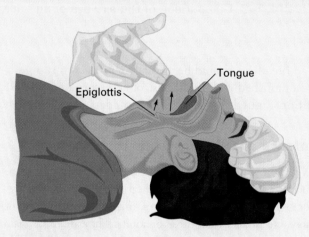

FIGURE 6-4B *Opening the airway by tilting the head back and lifting the chin.*

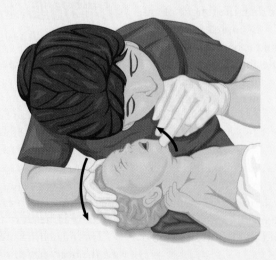

FIGURE 6-4C *Performing the head-tilt/chin-lift for an infant.*

2. *Tilt the head back* by applying firm backward pressure with the palm of your hand.

3. *Position the fingertips of your other hand* under the bony part of the patient's lower jaw. (If the patient is an infant or child, place only one finger under the jaw.)

4. *Lift the chin forward.* At the same time, support the jaw and tilt the head back as far as possible. The patient's teeth should be nearly together. (If the patient is an infant or child, tilt the head back only slightly, as if the child is "sniffing." Remember not to overextend the head.)

5. *Continue to press the other hand on the patient's forehead* in order to keep the head tilted back.

Remember the following important precautions when performing the head-tilt/chin-lift. One is never let your fingers press deeply into the soft tissues under the chin. Doing so could block the patient's airway. Also, if necessary, you may use your thumb to press in the patient's lower lip, keeping the patient's mouth slightly open. But never use your thumb to lift the patient's chin. A third precaution is to never let the patient's mouth close. And, finally, if the patient has dentures (false teeth), try to hold them in place. This will help prevent the patient's lips from interfering with breathing. If you are unable to manage the dentures, remove them.

Jaw-Thrust Maneuver

Use a jaw-thrust maneuver instead of the head-tilt/chin-lift when injuries to the spine are suspected. Note that this maneuver is tiring and technically difficult. However, it is the safest approach to opening the airway in a patient with suspected spine injury. With it, the patient's head and neck are brought into a neutral position. This means the head is not turned to the side, tilted forward, or tilted back.

To perform the jaw-thrust maneuver, follow these steps (Figure 6-5):

1. *Get in position.* Kneel above the patient's head. Place your elbows on the surface where the patient is lying. Place one hand on each side of the head.

2. *Grasp the angles of the patient's lower jaw on both sides.* (If the patient is an infant or child, place two or three fingers of each hand at the angle of the jaw.)

3. *Move the jaw forward with both hands,* using a lifting motion. This pulls the tongue away from the back of the throat.

4. *Keep the patient's mouth slightly open.* If necessary, pull back the lower lip with the thumb of your gloved hand.

First on Scene

The jaw-thrust maneuver is taught only to professional rescuers and health-care providers. It is no longer taught to laypeople. You may come upon a scene where a bystander has tilted back a spine-injured patient's neck. When you take over ventilations, stabilize the spine and use the jaw-thrust maneuver.

If the jaw-thrust maneuver does not open the patient's airway, try again. Reposition the jaw and determine whether or not the airway is open. If repositioning does not work, insert an airway adjunct (described later in this chapter).

Inspecting the Airway

Assess the airway of each and every one of your patients. A clear and open airway, or **patent airway**, is absolutely necessary for adequate breathing. You can determine that a patient's airway is patent if he is alert and talking to you in a normal voice. If you see that his mental status is altered, however, you have to look more closely. A patient who is drowsy, disoriented, confused, or unresponsive may have blood, vomit, or excess saliva in the airway.

To inspect the airway of an unresponsive patient, first open the patient's mouth with a gloved hand. If necessary, use a **cross-finger technique.** That is, kneel above the patient. Then cross the thumb and forefinger of one hand. Place the thumb on the patient's lower incisors and the forefinger on the upper incisors. Then use a scissors-like or finger-snapping motion to open the patient's mouth.

When the mouth is open, look inside for fluids and solids, including broken teeth or dentures that may be blocking the airway. Finally, listen for unusual sounds. Sounds that may indicate an airway obstruction include snoring, **crowing**, gurgling, and **stridor:**

- *Snoring* may indicate the upper airway is blocked by the tongue or by relaxed tissues in the throat.

- *Crowing,* like the cawing of a crow, may mean the muscles around the larynx are in spasm.

- *Gurgling* occurs when blood, vomit, mucus, or another liquid is in the airway.

- *Stridor,* which is a harsh, high-pitched sound during inhalation, may indicate the larynx is swollen and blocking the upper airway.

SKILL SUMMARY *Performing a Jaw-Thrust Maneuver*

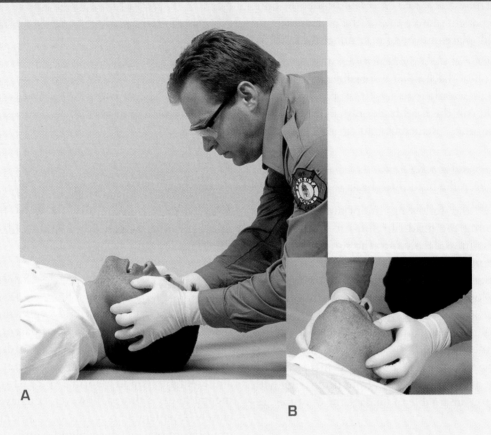

A

B

FIGURE 6-5 *Jaw-thrust maneuver. Inset shows view of First Responder's finger position at angle of the jaw just below the ears.*

Clearing the Airway

A First Responder can clear an airway of secretions in three ways—by using the **recovery position, finger sweeps,** or **suctioning.** These techniques are not performed sequentially. The technique you choose depends on the patient's condition. (NOTE: Suctioning will be discussed in detail in Chapter 7.)

Recovery Position

If the patient is breathing adequately and has a pulse, the American Heart Association (AHA) recommends that you place him in the recovery position. It is the first step in maintaining an open airway. This position uses gravity to keep the airway clear. It allows fluids to drain out of the mouth instead of into the airway, making it more likely for the patient's airway to remain open and airway obstructions not to occur. Note that even though the patient is in a recovery position, you should continue to monitor him until the EMTs arrive and take over care.

Do not move the patient into the recovery position if you suspect trauma or spinal injury. It should be used for an unresponsive, uninjured patient who is breathing adequately. He or she should stay in that position until the ambulance arrives. (If not breathing or breathing inadequately, the patient must be supine so you can provide artificial ventilation.)

To move a patient into the recovery position (Figure 6-6), first lift his left arm above his head. Then, cross the right leg over the left one. Support the patient's face as you grasp his right shoulder. Next, roll the patient toward you onto his side (the left side, preferably). Then, place his right hand under the side of his face. If possible, move the patient's head, shoulders, and torso simultaneously as a unit without twisting. The head should be in as close to a midline position as possible. Finally, flex the patient's top leg at the knee.

Finger Sweeps

A finger sweep is performed *only* on unresponsive patients and *only* when you see in the airway an object that needs to

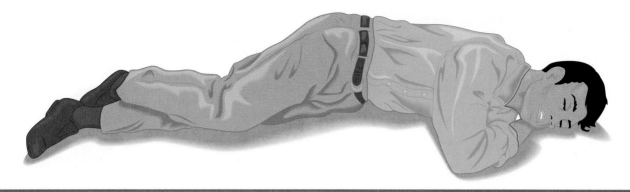

FIGURE 6-6 The recovery position.

be removed. In a finger sweep, you use your gloved finger to remove solid objects from the airway. Always wear protective gloves when performing a finger sweep. Foreign material or vomit in the mouth should be removed quickly. Never perform a "blind finger sweep." If you do not see an object in the mouth, do not perform a finger sweep.

To perform a finger sweep when an object is observed in the airway (Figure 6-7):

1. *Roll the patient,* if uninjured, onto his left side. This position allows material to drain out of the mouth. It also helps to keep the tongue away from the back of the throat.

2. *Open the patient's mouth.* If you see liquids or semi-liquids, cover your gloved index and middle fingers with a cloth.

3. *Wipe out the patient's mouth.* Insert your index finger, and pass it along the inside of the cheek and into the throat at the base of the tongue. (Use your little finger

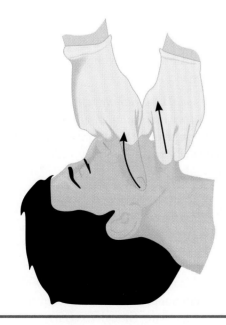

FIGURE 6-7 A finger sweep.

for an infant or child.) Hook your finger to dislodge and remove any foreign object. Take extreme care that you do not force an object deeper into the patient's throat.

Suctioning

Liquid materials such as saliva, blood, and vomitus can be removed by suctioning. It is vital to remove them to prevent **aspiration** (entry of such materials into the lungs). If they do enter the lungs, it can be fatal. (Suctioning is covered in detail in Chapter 7.)

Assessing Breathing

After you establish an open airway, determine if the patient is breathing and if that breathing is adequate.

Determining the Presence of Breathing

Breathing should be effortless. Watch to determine whether or not the chest rises and falls as the patient breathes. Also check to see if the patient is using accessory muscles to breathe. Look for excessive use of the neck muscles or pulling inward of the muscles between the patient's ribs.

Observe a responsive patient for the ability to speak. This ability means the air is moving past the vocal cords. If the patient can only make sounds or can speak just a few words, breathing may be inadequate. Patients who can speak full sentences without showing signs of distress or obstruction are breathing adequately.

In an unresponsive patient, use the cross-finger technique, if needed. Then, open the airway with the head-tilt/chin-lift or jaw-thrust maneuver. Place your ear close to the patient's mouth and nose for no more than 10 seconds and:

- *Look* for the rise and fall of the patient's chest.

- *Listen* for air coming out of the patient's mouth and nose.

- *Feel* for air coming out of the patient's nose and mouth.

If the airway is obstructed, the patient's chest may still rise and fall. However, air will not be moving in and out of the patient's nose or mouth. Note that **agonal respirations** (reflex gasping with no regular pattern or depth) may occur with cardiac arrest. They also may be a late sign of impending respiratory arrest. These reflex gasps should not be confused with breathing.

Pulse Oximetry

A **pulse oximeter** is a device that can be used to evaluate a patient's breathing. When attached to a patient's finger (Figure 6-8), it can measure *oxygen saturation,* or the amount of oxygen bound to hemoglobin. For example, if the pulse oximeter reads 96%, it means that 96% of the patient's hemoglobin molecules are saturated with oxygen. Normal pulse oximetry readings are in the 95% to 100% range. A reading of 90% to 95% indicates hypoxia. Readings below 90% indicate severe hypoxia.

If you use a pulse oximeter often, you will notice that some patients have low oxygen saturation readings but appear to have no significant difficulty breathing. In contrast, some patients who have good readings may describe serious breathing difficulties. So, when using a pulse oximeter, remember this: *Never withhold oxygen from a patient because of a normal reading. Never delay giving oxygen in order to obtain a pulse oximeter reading.* (Pulse oximetry will also be discussed in Chapter 11.)

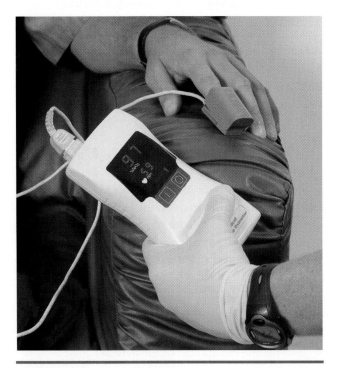

FIGURE 6-8 Pulse oximeter.

SIGNS OF INADEQUATE BREATHING

Breathing rates:
  less than 8 in adults
  less than 10 in children
  less than 20 in infants

Rapid, shallow breathing

Inadequate chest wall motion

Cyanosis

Mental status changes

Increased effort to breathe

Gasping and grunting

Slow or rapid heart rate accompanied by slow or irregular breathing rate

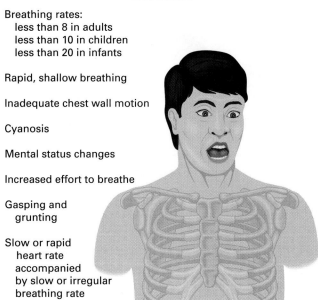

FIGURE 6-9 Inadequate breathing in a patient requires ventilatory assistance.

Signs of Inadequate Breathing

Breathing is not an all-or-nothing proposition. In between patients who are breathing normally and patients who are not breathing at all is a condition called **inadequate breathing.** It is very important for you to recognize it (Figure 6-9). Some signs are subtle and require careful evaluation. If you are not sure that a patient needs breathing assistance, it is better to err on the side of safety and provide ventilations.

Inadequate breathing is characterized by the signs listed below. Note, however, that not all of the signs will be present at the same time. Any one of them may be reason enough to ventilate a patient without delay. Signs of inadequate breathing include:

- *Too fast or too slow breathing rate.* Rates of less than 8 respirations per minute in an adult, less than 10 in a child, and less than 20 in an infant are ominous signs of inadequate breathing. Rapid breathing is often shallow and inadequate.

- *Inadequate chest wall motion.* Adequate breathing is normally accompanied by the rise and fall of the chest. This motion indicates the *depth of breathing.* If the chest wall is not rising and falling as it should, or if the sides of the chest rise and fall unequally, breathing is inadequate.

- *Cyanosis.* This is a bluish discoloration of the skin and mucous membranes. **Cyanosis** is a sign that body tissues are not receiving enough oxygen.

- *Mental status changes.* Mental status typically correlates with airway and breathing status. A patient who becomes drowsy, disoriented, confused, or unresponsive may not be breathing adequately.
- *Increased effort to breathe.* Normal breathing is effortless. When you see a pronounced use of abdominal muscles to breathe, the patient is pushing on the diaphragm to force air out of the lungs. An infant also may develop a "seesaw" motion in which the abdomen and chest move in opposite directions. You may note **retractions** (pulling inward) between the ribs, above the collarbone, around the muscles of the neck, and below the rib cage as the patient inhales. Flaring of the nostrils during inhalation is also seen in infants and children.
- *Gasping and grunting.* These sounds mean the patient is having a difficult time moving air through the respiratory tract. Be alert for other abnormal sounds, such as snoring, crowing, gurgling, or stridor.
- *Slow or rapid heart rate accompanied by slow or irregular breathing rate.* Abnormally slow heart rate in infants and children is always presumed to be the result of inadequate breathing.

Minute Volume

There are times when a patient appears to be moving air in and out of the lungs but the amount of air in each breath is simply not enough to sustain life. Two factors determine what is enough: rate and depth. To be adequate, breaths must be of a sufficient rate and deep enough to get the air to the alveoli for the exchange of gases to occur (Figure 6-10).

Both the rate and depth combined is called the **minute volume** (Table 6-2). For example, if a patient is breathing 12 times per minute and taking in 500 ml of air per breath, he is breathing in 6,000 ml of air per minute (the minute volume). Of that 6,000 ml of air, some will not reach the alveoli. About 150 ml per breath will remain in the **deadspace** located between the pharynx and the alveoli. This area must be filled before the air can reach the alveoli. So, instead of 6,000 ml of air, the patient is really only getting the oxygen from 4,200 ml. Look at the math:

> 12 breaths per minute × 500 ml per breath = 6,000 ml of air
>
> 12 breaths per minute × 150 ml deadspace per breath = 1,800 ml
>
> 6,000 ml − 1,800 ml = 4,200 ml
>
> 4,200 ml = adequate volume

Now imagine a patient who is breathing at a rate of 30 breaths per minute (twice as fast) at a volume of 250 ml per breath (half as much). You might think that because he is breathing faster, he is getting plenty of oxygen. Check the math:

> 30 breaths per minute × 250 ml per breath = 7,500 ml of air
>
> 30 breaths per minute × 150 ml deadspace per breath = 4,500 ml
>
> 7,500 ml − 4,500 ml = 3,000 ml
>
> 3,000 ml = inadequate volume

After subtracting the deadspace, the patient has a relatively small amount of air reaching the alveoli (3,000 ml). If this patient's breaths get faster and shallower, it could mean that almost no oxygen is reaching the alveoli. This is why patients can appear to be breathing but in reality require ventilatory assistance. Without it, they will die.

Note: Patients must have both an adequate rate and adequate depth of breathing to support life. If either one is not adequate, then breathing is inadequate.

:

1. What is the most common cause of airway obstruction in an unresponsive patient? How can you clear that obstruction?

2. What are two ways to clear a patient's airway of secretions, vomitus, and foreign materials?

3. How can you determine if a patient is breathing adequately or inadequately?

4. If a conscious patient is breathing inadequately, what should you do?

Section 3 Artificial Ventilation

If a patient is breathing inadequately or is not breathing at all, that patient needs your immediate assistance. Artificial ventilation is a way of breathing for these patients. The air we inhale contains about 21% oxygen. The body uses only 5%. The remaining 16% is exhaled. Since the air you breathe into a patient contains more than enough oxygen to keep him alive, artificial ventilation is sufficient

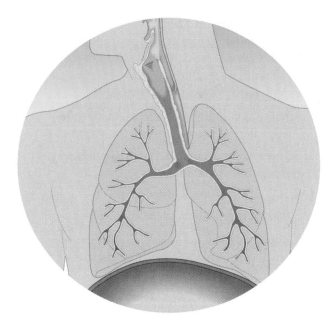

a. *No air in respiratory system.*

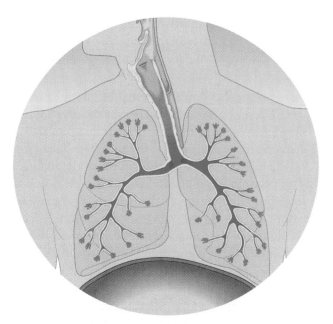

b. *Deadspace is filled with air, but it cannot reach the alveoli for gas exchange.*

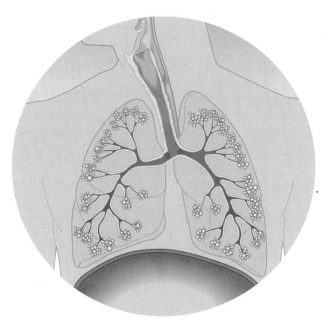

c. *Normal volume, with air filling the lungs including the alveolar sacs.*

FIGURE 6-10 Even when a patient's respiratory rate increases, ventilation may still be inadequate. If breathing is also shallow, the air may remain in the "deadspace," and never get to the alveoli.

TABLE 6-2 **Minute Volume**

Effects of Minute Volume and Deadspace on Respiration

Not all of the air breathed in reaches the alveoli for gas exchange with the blood. Some—an estimated 150 ml of the air taken in with each breath—remains trapped in deadspace (the bronchi and bronchioles). So how much air really does get to the alveoli?

Formula

The breathing rate per minute *multiplied by* the volume of air per breath *equals* the total volume of air breathed in per minute, or:

Rate × volume per breath = minute volume

The breathing rate per minute *multiplied by* 150 ml deadspace *equals* the amount of air breathed in per minute that never reaches the alveoli, or:

Rate × deadspace = volume lost per minute

The minute volume *minus* the amount of air per minute that never reaches the alveoli *equals* the actual amount of air that reaches the alveoli, or:

Minute volume − volume lost per minute = minute volume reaching alveoli

Examples

Example 1: Normal Breathing 12 breaths per minute × 500 ml per breath = 6,000 ml minute volume. 12 breaths per minute × 150 ml = 1,800 ml lost per minute. 6,000 ml minute volume − 1,800 ml lost per minute = 4,200 ml 4,200 ml = minute volume reaching alveoli, which is **adequate.**	**Adequate Breathing**
Example 2: Shallow Breathing at a Normal Rate 12 breaths per minute × 250 ml per breath = 3,000 ml minute volume. 12 breaths per minute × 150 ml = 1,800 ml lost per minute. 3,000 ml minute volume − 1,800 ml lost per minute = 1,200 ml 1,200 ml = minute volume reaching alveoli, which is **inadequate.**	**Inadequate Breathing**
Example 3: Shallow Breathing at a Faster Rate 24 breaths per minute × 250 ml per breath = 6,000 ml minute volume. 24 breaths per minute × 150 ml = 3,600 ml lost per minute. 6,000 ml minute volume − 3,600 ml lost per minute = 2,400 ml 2,400 ml = minute volume reaching alveoli, which is **inadequate.**	**Inadequate Breathing**
Example 4: Shallow Breathing at a Rapid Rate 36 breaths per minute × 200 ml per breath = 7,200 ml minute volume. 36 breaths per minute × 150 ml = 5,400 ml lost per minute. 7,200 ml minute volume − 5,400 ml lost per minute = 1,800 ml 1,800 ml = minute volume reaching alveoli, which is **inadequate.**	**Inadequate Breathing**

Adequate breathing requires adequate rate and adequate depth. If either is inadequate, breathing is inadequate. Note: Exact measurements are not important. Respiratory depth is best measured by observing the patient's respiratory effort.

to support life until high-concentration oxygen is available. (See Table 6-3.)

When performing artificial ventilation, monitor the patient continuously to make sure your breaths are adequate. Indications of *adequate* ventilations include:

- Rate of respiration is adequate–for infants and children, once every 3 to 5 seconds (12 to 20 breaths per minute) and for adults, once every 5 to 6 seconds (10 to 12 breaths per minute).
- The force of air is consistent. It also is sufficient to cause the chest to rise during each ventilation.

- Patient's heart rate decreases or returns to normal. However, underlying medical conditions may prevent this from happening even when ventilations are adequate.
- Patient's color improves.

Inadequate ventilation may occur because of problems with the patient's airway or because of improper use of a ventilation device. Indications of *inadequate* ventilations include:

- Chest does not rise and fall with each ventilation.
- Ventilation rate is too fast or too slow.
- Heart rate does not decrease or return to normal.

TABLE 6-3 Respiratory Status and First Responder Care

Respiratory Status	Signs	First Responder Care	
Breathing adequately.	• Rate and depth of breathing are normal. • No abnormal breath sounds. • Air moves freely in and out of the chest. • Skin color appears to be normal.	Monitor the patient's breathing for any changes. If allowed, also administer oxygen by nonrebreather or nasal cannula.	
Breathing inadequately. Patient is moving some air in and out but breathing is slow or shallow and not enough to sustain life.	• Rate and/or depth of breathing not within normal range. • Shallow breathing. • Diminished or absent breath sounds. • Noises with breathing such as crowing, stridor, snoring, gurgling, or gasping. • Blue or gray skin color (cyanosis). • Decreased minute volume.	Assist ventilations. If allowed, also administer supplemental oxygen during ventilation by way of a pocket face mask or bag-valve mask.	
No breathing at all.	• No chest rise. • No evidence of air being moved from the mouth or nose. • No breath sounds.	Provide ventilations. If allowed, also administer supplemental oxygen during ventilation by way of a pocket face mask or bag-valve mask.	

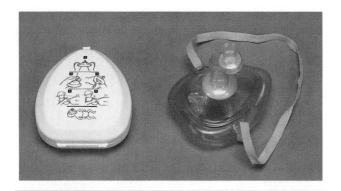

FIGURE 6-11 A pocket face mask with one-way valve and carrying case.

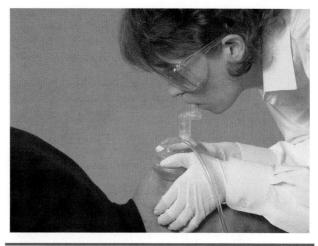

FIGURE 6-12 You must maintain a jaw-thrust during artificial ventilation of a patient with suspected spinal injury.

The risk of coming in contact with a patient's secretions, blood, or vomit while ventilating is high. Therefore, you must take BSI precautions. At a minimum, use gloves, eyewear, and a pocket face mask or other barrier device with a one way valve and filter. If large amounts of blood or secretions are present, use a face mask.

There are many techniques for artificial ventilation. A First Responder must be competent in three, listed here in order of preference: **mouth-to-mask, mouth-to-barrier device,** and **mouth-to-mouth.**

Mouth-to-Mask Ventilation

The most effective First Responder technique for ventilation is mouth-to-mask. A pocket face mask with a one-way valve is used to form a seal around the patient's nose and mouth (Figure 6-11). You blow into a port at the top of the mask to deliver a ventilation. The one-way valve diverts the patient's exhaled breath. Mouth-to-mask is the preferred technique because it eliminates direct contact with the patient's nose, mouth, and body fluids, and it prevents exposure to the patient's exhaled air. It also allows you to deliver ventilations of adequate force.

The mask you use should be transparent, so you can see vomit, blood, or other substances in the patient's mouth. It must fit snugly enough on the patient's face to form a good seal, so it should be available in an average adult size and in additional sizes for infants and children. The mask should have a one-way valve, or it must be able to connect to a one-way valve at the ventilation port. If you have oxygen available, the mask must have an oxygen inlet port.

Mouth-to-mask ventilation is very effective because both hands are used to create a seal around the mask. To perform mouth-to-mask ventilation (Figures 6-12 and 6-13):

1. *Get in position* at the patient's head and attach oxygen to the mask, if available.

2. *Position the mask on the patient.* The narrower top portion of the mask should be seated on the bridge of the nose. The broader portion should fit in the cleft of the chin. The position of the mask is critical. If it is wrong, the mask will leak and prevent you from delivering adequate ventilations.

3. *Seal the mask.* Place both thumbs on the top portion. Place the heels and palms of both hands along the sides. Compress the mask firmly around the edges to form a good seal.

4. *Open the patient's airway.* Place your index fingers on the part of the mask that covers the chin. Using your middle and ring fingers of both hands, grasp along the *mandible* (the bony part of the jaw). Pull upward to perform the maneuver. Use a jaw-thrust maneuver if trauma is suspected.

 First Responder Practice

When it comes to ventilation, more is *not* better. The American Heart Association (AHA) guidelines require ventilations to be given at about one second each and in an amount that makes the chest rise visibly. The reason is this: when ventilations are too forceful or have too much volume, air goes into the stomach. This causes gastric distention and vomiting in the patient. Vomiting causes airway problems and aspiration, which can kill the patient through infection and pneumonia.

SKILL SUMMARY   *Performing Artificial Ventilation*

Mouth-to-mask ventilation is the preferred technique because it eliminates direct contact with the patient's nose, mouth, and body fluids.

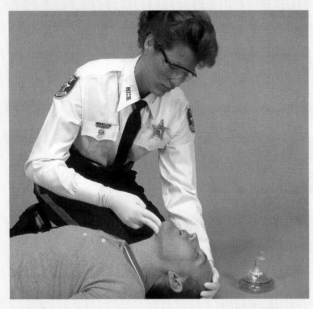

FIGURE 6-13A *Open the airway using the head-tilt/chin-lift maneuver.*

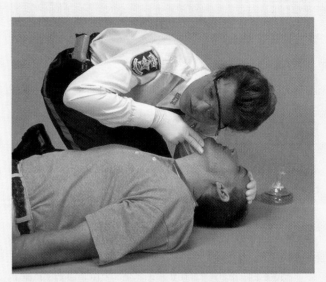

FIGURE 6-13B *Look, listen, and feel to establish breathlessness.*

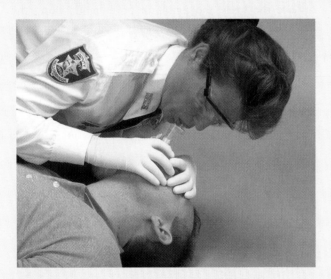

FIGURE 6-13C *Deliver two slow initial breaths.*

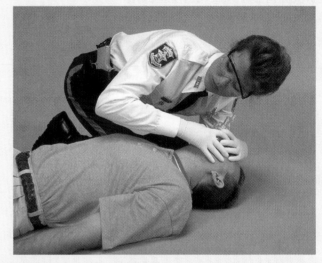

FIGURE 6-13D *If successful, you will see the chest fall and feel the exhaled air on your cheek after each breath. Continue ventilations at the proper rate.*

TABLE 6-4 **Artificial Ventilation Rates**	
Newborn	30–60 breaths per minute at approximately 1 second each
Infant	12–20 breaths per minute at 1 second each
Child	12–20 breaths per minute at 1 second each
Adult	10–12 breaths per minute at 1 second each

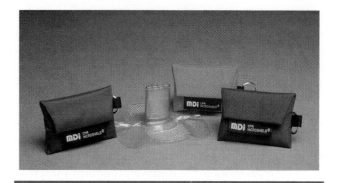

FIGURE 6-14 Example of a barrier device.

5. *Deliver two initial breaths.* Place your mouth around the one-way valve and blow into the ventilation port. Each breath should be delivered over one second. It also should be steady and of sufficient volume to make the chest rise without over-inflating and causing gastric distention.

6. *Determine if ventilations are adequate.* Watch the chest rise and fall. Listen and feel for air escaping when the patient exhales.

7. *Continue ventilations at the proper rate* (Table 6-4). For adults, deliver 10–12 breaths per minute with each breath lasting one second. For infants and children, deliver 12–20 breaths per minute with each breath lasting one second. For a newborn, deliver 30–60 breaths per minute with each breath lasting approximately one second.

If you cannot ventilate the patient or if the chest does not rise adequately, position the patient's head and try again. (Improper head position is the most common cause of difficulty with ventilation.) If subsequent tries also fail, assume the airway is blocked by a foreign object. Follow the guidelines for removing it. (Foreign body airway obstruction is described in detail in Chapter 7.)

Mouth-to-Barrier Device Ventilation

A barrier device, such as a face shield, can be used during artificial ventilation (Figure 6-14). It provides some of the same protection to the First Responder as a pocket face mask. A thin and flexible plastic face shield also can be folded and carried easily. Some are available in keyring and belt-storage containers. Barrier devices are thin enough to provide very low resistance to the ventilations you deliver to the patient. And they can provide some protection against contamination from body fluids. However, many do not have a one-way valve to divert the patient's exhaled air.

To perform mouth-to-barrier device ventilation:

1. *Get in position* at the patient's head.

2. *Position the device* on the patient.

3. *Open the patient's airway,* using a head-tilt/chin-lift or a jaw-thrust maneuver, as appropriate.

4. *Deliver two initial breaths.* Place your mouth over the barrier device and blow into it. Each breath should be delivered over one second. It also should be steady and of sufficient volume to make the chest rise. Make sure that you do not deliver too much air too fast, or you will force air into the patient's stomach.

5. *Determine if ventilations are adequate.* Watch the chest rise and fall. Listen and feel for air escaping when the patient exhales.

6. *Continue ventilations at the proper rate.* For adults, deliver 10–12 breaths per minute. For infants and children, deliver 12–20 breaths per minute. For a newborn, deliver 30–60 breaths per minute, each lasting approximately one second.

If you cannot ventilate the patient or if the chest does not rise adequately, position the patient's head and try again. If the second try also fails, assume the airway is blocked by a foreign object. Then follow the guidelines for removing a foreign body airway obstruction (Chapter 7).

Mouth-to-Mouth Ventilation

The risk of contracting infectious diseases makes mouth-to-mouth ventilation too dangerous for regular use by First Responders. As described earlier, barrier devices and face masks with one-way valves are available. You should always have a one on hand and use it as a BSI precaution. However, since you may find yourself in the position of caring for a loved one, your decision may be a personal one.

Mouth-to-mouth ventilation is a quick, effective method of delivering oxygen to a nonbreathing patient. It involves ventilating the patient with your exhaled breath while making mouth-to-mouth contact. Use the mouth-to-mouth technique only in emergency situations in which no protective devices are available. For example, you may find that you need to perform mouth-to-mouth on a family member at home where a barrier device is not available.

In mouth-to-mouth ventilation, you form a seal with your mouth around the patient's mouth. The obvious risk to you is exposure to body fluids and thus to infectious disease. To perform mouth-to-mouth ventilation:

1. *Get in position at the patient's head.*

2. *Open the patient's airway,* using a head-tilt/chin-lift or a jaw-thrust maneuver.

3. *Form an airtight seal.* Gently squeeze the patient's nostrils closed with the thumb and index finger of the hand that is holding the patient's head tilt. Take a deep breath and form an airtight seal with your lips around the patient's mouth. If you are ventilating an infant or small child, cover both the nose and mouth with your lips.

4. *Deliver two slow initial breaths* over one second for all patients. Each breath should be steady and of sufficient volume to make the chest rise. Make sure that you do not deliver too much air too fast, or you will force air into the patient's stomach.

5. *Determine if ventilations are adequate.* Watch the chest rise and fall. Listen and feel for air escaping when the patient exhales.

6. *Continue ventilations at the proper rate.* For adults, deliver 10–12 breaths per minute. For infants and children, deliver 12–20 breaths per minute (every three to five seconds). For a newborn, deliver 30–60 breaths per minute, each breath lasting approximately one second.

If you cannot ventilate the patient or if the chest does not rise adequately, position the patient's head and try again. If the subsequent tries also fail, assume the airway is blocked by a foreign object. Then follow the guidelines for removing a foreign body airway obstruction (Chapter 7).

Mouth-to-Stoma Ventilation

A patient who has had all or part of the larynx surgically removed has had a *laryngectomy* (Figure 6-15a). This patient will have a **stoma,** a permanent opening that connects the trachea directly to the front of the neck. These patients breathe only through the stoma.

To perform mouth-to-stoma ventilation (Figure 6-15b):

1. *Expose the stoma area.* Remove all coverings such as scarves or ties.

2. *Clear the stoma of any foreign matter.* Use a gauze pad or handkerchief. Do not use tissue, which can shred and cling.

3. *Form an airtight seal around the stoma.* Whenever possible, use a barrier device such as a pocket face mask or shield with one-way valve.

4. *Blow slowly through the stoma for one second.* Use just enough force to make the patient's chest rise.

5. *Determine if ventilations are adequate.* Allow time for exhalation. Watch for the patient's chest to fall. Feel to make sure air is escaping back through the stoma as the patient exhales.

6. *Continue ventilations at the proper rate.* For adults, deliver 10–12 breaths per minute. For infants and children, deliver 12–20 breaths per minute. For a newborn, deliver 30–60 breaths per minute.

If the chest does not rise, the patient may be a "partial neck breather." This patient has had only part of the larynx removed. He or she can breathe through both the stoma and the mouth and nose. Seal the patient's nose and mouth with one hand. Pinch off the nose between your third and fourth fingers. Seal the lips with the palm of the same gloved hand. Hook your thumb under the patient's chin, and press up and back. Then continue ventilations through the stoma.

Special Considerations

Infants and Children

Many of the steps involved in managing the airway of an infant or child are the same as those for an adult. However, remember there are important differences. You must position the head carefully when preparing for artificial ventilation. Keep an infant's head in a neutral ("sniffing") position. You can extend the head slightly beyond neutral if the patient is older than one year. But do not extend the patient's head too far. The airway is more flexible than an adult's and can be easily overextended, which can in itself block the airway.

Consider an oral airway for an infant or child. The primary cause of blocked airway in these patients is the tongue. Try positioning the head and pulling the jaw forward to move the tongue away from the back of the throat. If that is unsuccessful, use an oropharyngeal airway to keep the tongue away from the throat and the airway open (Chapter 7).

SKILL SUMMARY *Performing Mask-to-Stoma Ventilation*

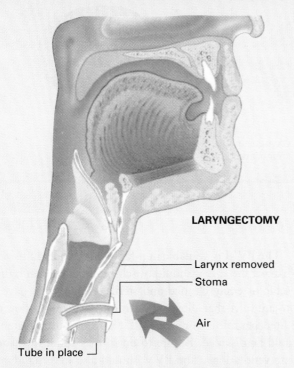

LARYNGECTOMY

Larynx removed

Stoma

Air

Tube in place

FIGURE 6-15A *The neck breather's airway has been changed by surgery.*

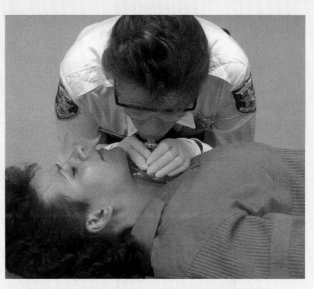

FIGURE 6-15B *Mask-to-stoma ventilation.*

Depending on the age and size of an infant, you may be able to form a seal with your mouth over the infant's mouth and nose. If you must use an adult pocket face mask, position the mask upside down (Figure 6-16).

Guard against **gastric distention** (inflation of the stomach). It is common in infants and children who are being ventilated. During artificial ventilation, air may get into the esophagus and stomach if ventilations are too forceful. Gastric distention may significantly impair your attempts at ventilation, because it forces the diaphragm up, limiting the amount of air that can enter the lungs. Monitor the infant or child carefully to make sure the chest is rising and falling with ventilations. Listen and feel for exhaled air. Watch carefully to make sure the abdomen does not start to extend.

The American Heart Association (AHA) recommends against pressing on the abdomen to relieve gastric distention. To help avoid gastric distention in infants and children, keep the following points in mind:

- Breathe slowly and with just enough force to make the chest rise. If you notice that the abdomen is starting to distend, reduce the force of your ventilations.

- Keep the infant or child's head in a neutral position.

- Allow the infant or child to exhale between ventilations.

- Monitor against vomiting. If it looks like the infant or child is about to vomit, stop ventilating immediately, and roll him onto his side. This position allows the

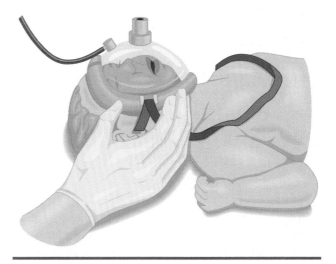

FIGURE 6-16 For an infant, the pocket face mask is reversed.

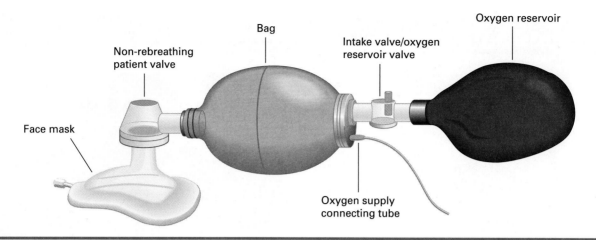

FIGURE 6-17 Bag-valve-mask unit.

vomit to flow from the mouth rather than into the lungs. If the infant or child vomits, suction or quickly wipe out the mouth with gauze pads. Wipe off the face, and return to ventilation.

Patients with Dental Appliances

If the patient has dentures that are secure in the mouth, leave them in place. It is much easier to create an airtight seal with them there. If the dentures are extremely loose, remove them so they do not block the airway. Partial dentures—plates and bridges—may become dislodged, too. If they are loose, remove them. Reassess the mouth frequently in patients who have dental appliances to make sure they have not come loose.

Bag-Valve-Mask Ventilation

The **bag-valve mask (BVM)** is a hand-operated device (Figure 6-17). It consists of a self-inflating bag, one-way valve, face mask, and oxygen reservoir. The BVM device has a volume of about 1,600 ml. When used with oxygen, it can deliver almost 100% oxygen to the patient.

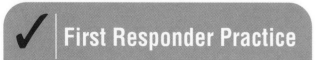

✔ First Responder Practice

It is highly recommended that two rescuers operate a BVM, because the task is too difficult and tiring for one rescuer. If you are alone, use a pocket face mask instead.

The BVM is available in infant, child, and adult sizes. Whatever the size, it should be self-refilling bag that is disposable or easily cleaned and sterilized. It should have a non-jam valve that allows a maximum oxygen inlet flow of 15 liters per minute or greater. If it has a pop-off valve, this should be disabled. Failure to do so may result in inadequate ventilations. The BVM should also have standardized 15/22 mm fittings, an oxygen inlet and reservoir that allows for a high concentration of oxygen, a true nonrebreather valve, and the ability to perform in all environments and temperature extremes. To perform bag-valve-mask ventilation (Figures 6-18 and 6-19):

1. *Open the patient's airway.* An oral or nasal airway may be necessary in conjunction with the BVM. NOTE: if you suspect injury to the head or spine, stabilize the patient's head between your knees or have an assistant manually stabilize it while performing a jaw-thrust maneuver.

2. *Select the correct size mask*—adult, child, or infant size. And position the mask. Place your thumbs over the top half of the mask. Index and middle fingers should be over the bottom half. Then, put the narrow end (apex) of the mask over the bridge of the patient's nose. Lower the mask over the mouth and upper chin. If the mask has a large, round cuff around a ventilation port, center the port over the patient's mouth. Use your ring and little fingers to bring the jaw up to the mask. Use the jaw-thrust maneuver, if you suspect head or spine injury. Be sure to avoid tilting the head or neck.

3. *Connect the mask to the bag,* if this has not already been done.

4. *Operate the bag.* Your partner should squeeze the bag with two hands until the patient's chest rises. For

SKILL SUMMARY *Bag-Valve-Mask Ventilation—Nonbreathing Patient*

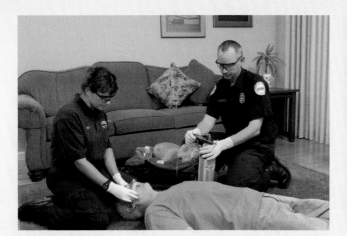

FIGURE 6-18A *Open the patient's airway. Then, select the correct mask size.*

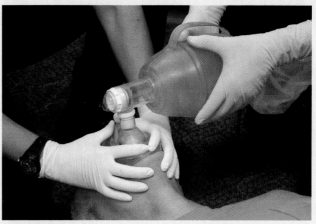

FIGURE 6-18B *Positioning of the mask and your hands (side view).*

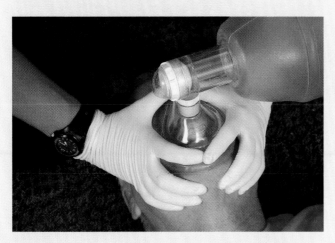

FIGURE 6-18C *Positioning of the mask and your hands (top view).*

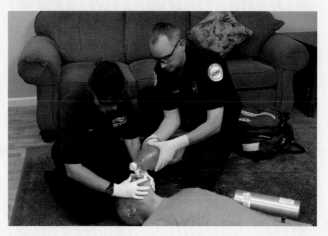

FIGURE 6-18D *After the mask is in position, connect the oxygen and begin to ventilate the patient.*

adults, deliver 10–12 breaths per minute. For infants and children, deliver 12–20 breaths per minute.

If you are alone, form a "C" around the ventilation port with your thumb and index fingers. Use your middle, ring, and little fingers under the jaw to maintain a chin lift and complete the seal. Squeeze the bag with your other hand while observing the chest rise and fall.

If the chest does not rise and fall with your ventilations, reposition the patient's head or jaw. Check again for an airway obstruction. If air is escaping from under the mask, reposition your fingers and check the position of the mask. If the patient's chest still does not rise, use an alternative method such as mouth-to-mask ventilation.

Assisting Inadequate Breathing

If your patient is breathing but breathing inadequately, you must assist (Figure 6-20). Provide ventilations while the patient is inhaling or trying to breathe on his or her own. Since inadequate breathing is often slower than usual, you will need to provide additional ventilations in between the patient's own attempts to breathe. If breathing is rapid and very shallow, and therefore inadequate, provide assisted ventilations when the patient begins a respiration. You will find that providing a ventilation while the patient is exhaling can create resistance or an unusual noise.

Simply continue to time your assisted ventilations as best you can with the patient's own respiratory effort. To

SKILL SUMMARY *Bag-Valve-Mask Ventilation—Breathing Patient*

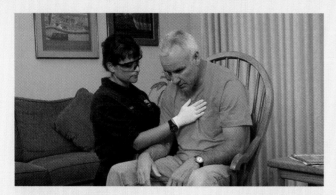

FIGURE 6-19A *Assess the patient's respiration.*

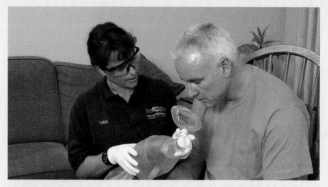

FIGURE 6-19B *If breathing is inadequate, calm the patient and explain what you are about to do.*

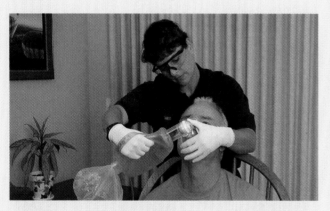

FIGURE 6-19C *Squeeze the BVM when the patient attempts to breathe and between the patient's own respirations.*

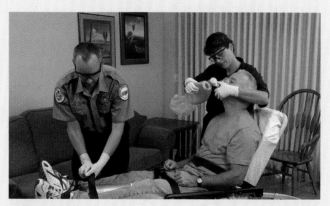

FIGURE 6-19D *Continue ventilating and transport promptly.*

 First Responder Practice

Does ventilating a conscious patient seem odd to you? It isn't. In fact, if you are providing emergency care to a patient who is breathing inadequately, it is something you must do. Note that when a patient is not breathing adequately, he or she can get anxious or panicky. During these times, oxygen is needed most. So, do your best to calm the patient. Coach him on how to accept the breaths you are giving.

recognize inadequate breathing and then to assist the patient with ventilations are among the best things you can do for your patient. Your intervention may prevent him or her from lapsing into complete respiratory and cardiac arrest.

:

1. What are the signs of inadequate artificial ventilation?

2. Why is mouth-to-mask ventilation preferred over other artificial ventilation techniques?

3. What are the artificial ventilation rates for newborns, infants, children, and adults?

PATIENT'S CONDITION   **WHEN AND HOW TO INTERVENE**

Adequate breathing:
Speaks full sentences;
alert and calm

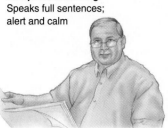

Nonrebreather mask or nasal cannula

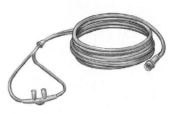

Increasing respiratory distress:
Visibly short of breath;
Speaking 3-4 word sentences;
Increasing anxiety

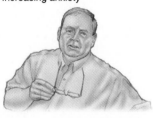

Nonrebreather mask

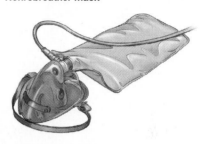

Key decision-making point:

Recognize inadequate breathing
before respiratory arrest
develops.

Assist ventilations
before they stop altogether!

Severe respiratory distress:
Speaking only 1-2 word sentences;
Very diaphoretic (sweaty);
Severe anxiety

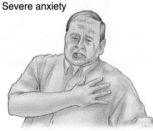

Assisted ventilations
Pocket face mask (PFM),
bag-valve mask (BVM), or
flow-restricted, oxygen-powered
ventilation device (FROPVD)

Assist the patient's own
ventilations, adjusting the
rate for rapid or slow
breathing

Continues to deteriorate:
Sleepy with head-bobbing;
Becomes unarousable

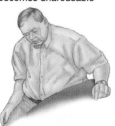

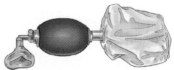

Respiratory arrest:
No breathing

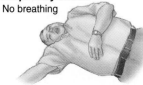

Artificial ventilation
Pocket face mask (PFM),
bag-valve mask (BVM), or
flow-restricted, oxygen-powered
ventilation device (FROPV)

Assisted ventilations at
12/minute for an adult or
20/minute for a child or infant

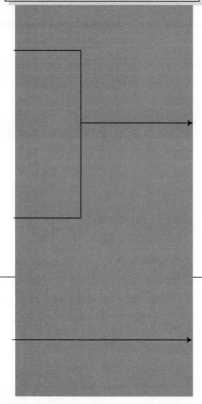

FIGURE 6-20 First Responder care includes recognizing the need for assisted ventilations, even before severe respiratory distress develops.

▶▶ The Call Follow-up

At the beginning of this chapter, you read that First Responders were called to help an unresponsive adult with snoring respirations. To see how they responded to this emergency, read the following. It describes how the call was completed.

Initial Assessment *(continued)* Since it was not possible to assess the patient's airway while she was slumped in a chair, we quickly but carefully moved her to the floor. My partner, Pete, immediately performed a head-tilt/chin-lift maneuver. It eliminated the snoring sounds.

Pete suctioned the airway to remove the built up secretions. Mrs. Constantino didn't have a gag reflex, so she accepted the oropharyngeal airway well.

Our assessment of her breathing revealed minimal chest movement and slow respirations. She also was beginning to show signs of blue coloring around her lips. Realizing that Mrs. Constantino was breathing inadequately and her pulse was rapid and weak, we ventilated her using a pocket face mask with one-way valve and supplemental oxygen.

Physical Examination We believed that Mrs. Constantino had a medical problem rather than a traumatic condition, but I wanted to be sure. So I did a quick physical examination while my partner continued to assist ventilations. There were no signs of injury on her head, neck, chest, abdomen, or extremities. Her pulse was 96 and bounding. The respiratory rate was 8 and shallow.

Patient History Mr. Constantino told us that his wife had a heart attack several years ago. She takes medications for her heart and high blood pressure. She had complained of a headache about an hour before she became unresponsive. She ate breakfast earlier. She has no allergies.

Ongoing Assessment Our primary focus was on making sure Mrs. Constantino was ventilated properly. We also checked her pulse frequently. Her pulse on our second check was 104, bounding and regular. Her respirations were about 6 and shallow, being assisted.

Patient Hand-off We had the airway under control when the paramedics arrived. The patient's color had improved. Her pulse also had slowed a bit. Pete gave them the hand-off report (see below).

I saw Mr. Constantino in the grocery store recently. He told me that his wife had had a severe stroke. She remained in the hospital for some time and was eventually moved to a rehabilitation center. I hope she will be able to go home soon.

Hand-off Report

"This is Mrs. Constantino. She is 74 years old. She had a headache about an hour ago. She was found by her husband slumped over in a chair. We moved her to the floor and found that she had inadequate ventilations. We began assisting with a pocket mask and oxygen. She groans with loud verbal stimulus. Her respiratory rate was about 6, pulse 104 and bounding. She has a history of heart attack and high blood pressure. She ate breakfast. She has no allergies."

The Last Word *It has been said that the priorities in patient care are the airway, the airway, and the airway. Without a clear and open airway plus adequate ventilations, no patient can survive. So even as you approach your patient's side, the first questions in your mind should be "Is she breathing? Is she breathing adequately?" Remember, without an airway, there is no chance of survival.*

Chapter Review

Focus on the EMS Team

If one person has one airway, why does it take a team to manage it? Consider the patient who has a spine injury and is not breathing. One rescuer will maintain stabilization of the head and use a jaw-thrust to open the airway. Another will administer ventilations. If the patient is vomiting, he will be rolled to his side by several rescuers, who protect his spine during the move. The patient's airway would then be suctioned. CPR may become necessary as well. Finally, someone else may be needed to get specialized equipment from the emergency vehicle or to ensure scene safety. All this is teamwork.

Summing Up

- The major components of the respiratory system are the nose and mouth, pharynx, epiglottis, trachea, larynx, and the bronchi, lungs, and diaphragm.

- Adequate breathing occurs in adults at 12 to 20 breaths per minute. For children, it is 15 to 30 breaths per minute. For infants, it is 25 to 50 breaths per minute.

- Breathing is adequate when it is regular in rhythm, free of unusual sounds, such as wheezing or whistling, and when chest expansion and depth of respirations are sufficient to support life without assistance.

- Breathing should be virtually effortless. It should be accomplished without the use of accessory muscles in the neck, shoulders, and abdomen.

- Two maneuvers are commonly used to open an airway in an unresponsive patient: the head-tilt/chin-lift maneuver and the jaw-thrust maneuver. The head-tilt/chin-lift is used for patients who are not injured. The jaw-thrust is used for patients who are injured, especially those who are suspected of having a spine injury.

- Clear an airway of secretions by using the recovery position, finger sweeps, or suctioning. Use the recovery position when the patient is *not* suspected of trauma or spinal injury, is breathing adequately, and has a pulse. Use finger sweeps (never "blind" ones) only on unresponsive patients.

- To assess breathing in an unresponsive patient, *look* for the rise and fall of the patient's chest, *listen* for air coming out of the patient's mouth and nose, and *feel* for air coming out of the patient's nose and mouth.

- Signs of inadequate breathing are too fast or too slow breathing rate, inadequate chest wall motion, cyanosis, mental status changes, increased effort to breathe, gasping and grunting, slow heart rate accompanied by slow breathing rate. When you observe these signs, perform artificial ventilation.

- To assess breathing properly, you have to consider both the rate and depth of a patient's breathing. That is, you have to know if breathing is both fast enough *and* deep enough to keep your patient alive. One way to do this is by calculating the minute volume that actually reaches the alveoli for gas exchange.

- Many First Responders now use pulse oximetry with their patients. This device indicates the amount of oxygen carried in the patient's blood. However, even if the device gives you a "normal" reading, never withhold oxygen from a patient with respiratory distress.

- There are many techniques for artificial ventilation. A First Responder must be competent in three (listed here in order of preference): mouth-to-mask, mouth-to-barrier device, and mouth-to-mouth. You should also know how to perform mouth-to-stoma ventilation and bag-valve-mask ventilation.

- Artificial ventilation is delivered at a rate of one ventilation every 3 to 5 seconds for infants and children and once every 5 to 6 seconds for adults. The force of air is consistent and sufficient to cause the chest to rise during each ventilation. In addition, if no underlying disease or injury prevents it, the patient's heart rate will decrease or return to normal and the patient's color will improve.

- During artificial ventilation, you can give to a patient a higher concentration of oxygen (higher than the oxygen in your breaths) by connecting supplemental oxygen to your pocket face mask.

- If a conscious patient is breathing inadequately, you must assist his efforts to breathe. If the patient is breathing too slowly, provide ventilations between the patient's own attempts to breathe. If breathing is rapid and very shallow, provide ventilations when the patient begins a respiration.

Key Terms

accessory muscles additional muscles; in regard to breathing, these are the muscles of the neck and the muscles between the ribs.

agonal respirations reflex gasping with no regular pattern or depth; related to death or dying.

artificial ventilation a technique used to help maintain lung function in a patient who is either breathing inadequately or not breathing at all. *Also called* pulmonary resuscitation *or* rescue breathing.

aspirate inhale material into the lungs.

bag-valve mask (BVM) an aid for artificial ventilation; consists of a self-inflating bag, one-way valve, face mask, and oxygen reservoir.

cross-finger technique a method of opening an unresponsive patient's clenched jaw.

crowing a breathing sound similar to the cawing of a crow; may indicate that muscles around the larynx are in spasm.

cyanosis bluish discoloration of the skin and mucous membranes; a sign that body tissues are not receiving enough oxygen.

deadspace the areas of the respiratory system that hold the portion of inhaled air that does not participate in gas exchange.

finger sweeps technique used to remove a foreign object from the mouth.

gastric distention inflation of the stomach.

head-tilt/chin-lift maneuver a manual technique used to open the airway of an ill (uninjured) patient.

jaw-thrust maneuver a manual technique used to open the airway of an unresponsive patient who is injured or any patient who has a suspected spine injury.

mouth-to-barrier device technique of artificial ventilation that involves the use of a barrier device such as a face shield to blow air into the mouth of a patient.

mouth-to-mask ventilation technique of artificial ventilation that involves the use of a pocket face mask with one-way valve to blow air into the mouth of a patient.

mouth-to-mouth ventilation technique of artificial ventilation that involves a rescuer using his mouth—with no protective barrier—to blow air into the mouth of a patient.

occlude block, close up, or obstruct.

patent airway an airway that is open and clear of obstructions.

pulse oximeter an electronic device for determining the amount of oxygen in the blood (oxygen saturation or SpO_2).

recovery position lateral recumbent position; used to allow fluids to drain from a patient's mouth instead of into the airway.

retraction a pulling inward; a shortening; the condition of being drawn back.

stoma a permanent, surgically created opening that connects the trachea directly to the front of the neck.

stridor a harsh, high-pitched sound made during inhalation, which may mean the larynx is swollen and blocking the upper airway.

Knowledge Check

1. The passage that takes air from the pharynx into the lungs is called the:
   a. trachea.
   b. alveolus.
   c. esophagus.
   d. epiglottis.

2. The correct rate for artificial ventilation in an adult patient is ____ breaths per minute, each breath lasting ____ second(s).
   a. 8–10, 2
   b. 10–12, 1
   c. 30–60, 2
   d. 20, 1 to 1.5

3. The correct rate for artificial ventilation in a child is ____ breaths per minute, each breath lasting ____ second(s).

   a. 8–10, 2

   b. 10–12, 2

   c. 30–60, 1

   d. 12–20, 1

4. In the average adult, approximately _____ ml of air taken in with each breath remains trapped in the "deadspace" of the respiratory system.

   a. 50

   b. 100

   c. 150

   d. 250

5. You may have to ventilate a patient who is conscious.

   a. True

   b. False

6. The two factors that determine whether or not a patient is breathing adequately are:

   a. respiratory rate and depth.

   b. heart rate and stroke volume.

   c. chest expansion and pulse.

   d. respiratory rate and pulse.

7. Which is more efficient, one-rescuer BVM ventilation or two-rescuer BVM ventilation? Explain your answer.

_____

_____

_____

8. Place the following methods of artificial ventilation in the preferred order.

   _____ Mouth-to-mouth ventilation

   _____ Mouth-to-mask ventilation

   _____ Mouth-to-barrier device ventilation

9. A respiratory status of a faster-than-normal breathing rate plus shallow breathing suggests that the patient may NOT be breathing adequately.

   a. True

   b. False

Scenario

For each of the following patients decide if breathing is likely to be adequate or inadequate. Then, describe the airway and breathing care you would provide.

a. A 16-year-old male patient fell and broke his leg. He is breathing at a rate of 22 breaths per minute. His skin is pink and warm. He has a normal mental status.

_____

_____

b. A 72-year-old male patient has had a respiratory infection for a week. Today, his wife noticed that he seemed "sleepy" and he was breathing faster than normal. You observe shallow respirations at 44/minute.

_____

_____

_____

c. A 56-year-old female patient is having trouble breathing and chest pain. She can speak only in four-to-five word sentences. She is pale and clammy. She appears slightly anxious.

_____

_____

_____

d. A 24-year-old female patient has crashed her motorcycle. She is found unresponsive with respirations of about 6 to 8 per minute and appears to be gasping.

_____

_____

_____

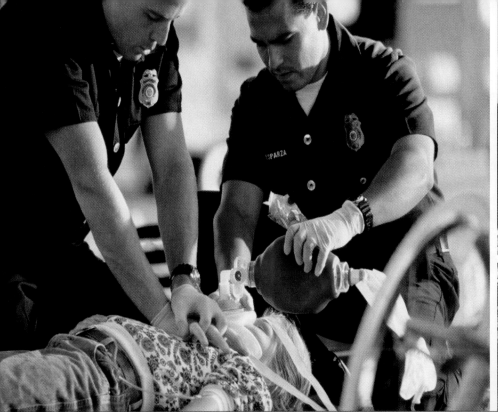
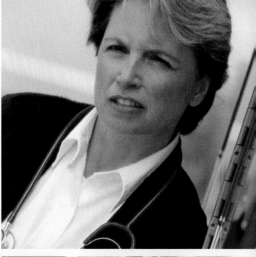
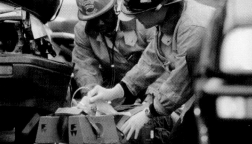

7 | Airway Care and Maintenance

Objectives

From the U.S. Department of Transportation (DOT) 1995 "First Responder: National Standard Curriculum." Material supplemental to the DOT curriculum is listed under "Enrichment."

Cognitive

2-1.6 ▶ State the importance of having a suction unit ready for immediate use when providing emergency medical care. (pp. 125–126)

2-1.7 ▶ Describe the techniques of suctioning. (pp. 126–127)

2-1.11 ▶ Describe how to measure and insert an oropharyngeal (oral) airway. (pp. 127–128)

2-1.12 ▶ Describe how to measure and insert a nasopharyngeal (nasal) airway. (pp. 128–129)

2-1.13 ▶ Describe how to clear a foreign body airway obstruction in a responsive adult. (pp. 137–138)

2-1.14 ▶ Describe how to clear a foreign body airway obstruction in a responsive child with complete obstruction or partial airway obstruction and poor air exchange. (p. 141)

2-1.15 ▶ Describe how to clear a foreign body airway obstruction in a responsive infant with complete obstruction or partial airway obstruction and poor air exchange. (pp. 139–140)

2-1.16 ▶ Describe how to clear a foreign body airway obstruction in an unresponsive adult. (p. 138)

2-1.17 ▶ Describe how to clear a foreign body airway obstruction in an unresponsive child. (p. 141)

2-1.18 ▶ Describe how to clear a foreign body airway obstruction in an unresponsive infant. (pp. 140–141)

Psychomotor

2-1.25 ▶ Demonstrate the techniques of suctioning. (pp. 126–127)

2-1.29 ▶ Demonstrate how to measure and insert an oropharyngeal (oral) airway. (pp. 127–128)

2-1.30 ▶ Demonstrate how to measure and insert a nasopharyngeal (nasal) airway. (pp. 128–129)

2-1.32 ▶ Demonstrate how to clear a foreign body airway obstruction in a responsive adult. (pp. 137–138)

2-1.33 ▶ Demonstrate how to clear a foreign body airway obstruction in a responsive child. (p. 141)

2-1.34 ▸ Demonstrate how to clear a foreign body airway obstruction in a responsive infant. (pp. 139–140)

2-1.35 ▸ Demonstrate how to clear a foreign body airway obstruction in an unresponsive adult. (p. 138)

2-1.36 ▸ Demonstrate how to clear a foreign body airway obstruction in an unresponsive child. (p. 141)

2-1.37 ▸ Demonstrate how to clear a foreign body airway obstruction in an unresponsive infant. (pp. 140–141)

Enrichment

▸ Describe oxygen cylinders, oxygen delivery equipment, and oxygen administration guidelines. (pp. 127–129)

▸ Describe the special considerations related to administering oxygen to patients with chronic obstructive pulmonary diseases (COPD). (p.129)

▸ Describe how a First Responder may be able to assist advanced EMS providers with a patient's airway care. (pp. 129, 132–133)

Introduction

After you open the airway and assess breathing, you will use the devices discussed in this chapter. Many First Responders have the ability to administer oxygen—a truly life-saving drug. It has been said already and is worth saying again: if you do anything for your patient, the airway care you provide—opening and maintaining an airway and ensuring adequate breathing—is the most important thing you will ever do.

Section 1 Ensuring an Open Airway

Airway Adjuncts

Once the airway is open, it may be necessary to insert an **airway adjunct** (an artificial airway) to keep it open. There are two kinds—the **oropharyngeal (oral) airway** and the **nasopharyngeal (nasal) airway**. Both extend down to, but do not pass through, the larynx. They often are used when patients are being artificially ventilated.

When using airway adjuncts, remember: they must be clean and clear of any obstructions. The proper size must be used to be effective and to prevent complications. And the patient with an airway adjunct can still aspirate (inhale) secretions, blood, vomit, or other foreign substances into the lungs.

The patient's mental status and gag reflex will tell you if an airway adjunct is appropriate. That is, in general, if the patient is unresponsive with no gag reflex, use the oropharyngeal airway. If the patient is responsive or has a gag reflex, use the nasopharyngeal airway. You must continually and carefully monitor the patient's mental status. If he becomes completely responsive or gags, you must remove the airway adjunct.

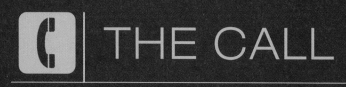

THE CALL

📡 **Dispatch** The tones came out for a snowmobile accident in a rural section of the county. We'd been having a bad year with snowmobile fatalities. I hoped we weren't about to respond to another.

◎ **Scene Size-up** When we arrived in our first-response truck we saw two deputies on scene. They motioned us over. The patient was about 50 feet from his machine, which had hit a tree. The deputy said, "He looks pretty bad." Even from a distance, I could see he hadn't worn a helmet and that he had blood on his face. That was all I needed to call for ALS.

✔️ **Initial Assessment** The patient was a 19-year-old male who was unresponsive and had blood flowing into his airway. He was gurgling pretty badly.

As you read Chapter 7, think about this patient and ask yourself these questions: What are the priorities for this patient? How do you expect the First Responders to proceed?

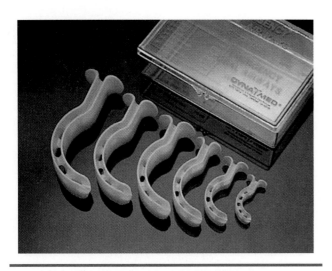

FIGURE 7-1 Oropharyngeal (oral) airways.

Oropharyngeal Airway

The oropharyngeal airway, or oral airway, is a semicircular device made of hard plastic or rubber (Figure 7-1). It is designed to hold the tongue away from the back of the throat at the level of the pharynx. It also allows secretions to drain in a patient without a gag reflex.

There are two common types. One is tubular, and the other has a channeled side. Both types are disposable and come in a variety of adult, child, and infant sizes.

The oral airway can be used to help maintain an open airway in an unresponsive patient who has no gag reflex. Do not use this device on a patient who is responsive or has a gag reflex. If you do, it may cause vomiting, which will further compromise the airway.

To insert an oropharyngeal airway (Figure 7-2):

1. *Select the proper size.* It should extend from the corner of the lip to the angle of the jaw or to the tip of the

SKILL SUMMARY *Inserting an Oropharyngeal Airway*

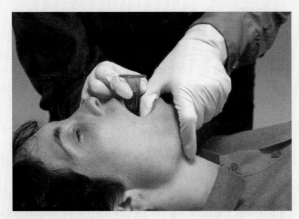

FIGURE 7-2A *Measure to ensure correct size.*

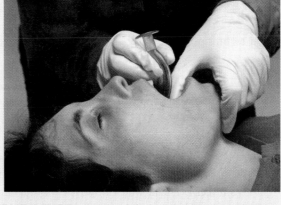

FIGURE 7-2B *In an adult, insert with top pointing up toward the roof of the mouth and then . . .*

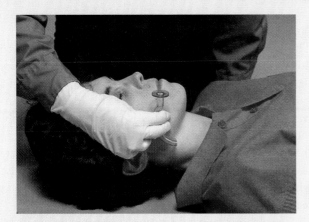

FIGURE 7-2C *. . . gently rotate it until it reaches the proper position.*

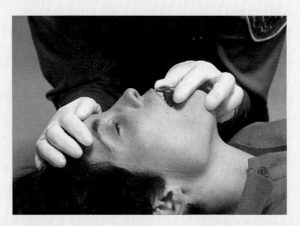

FIGURE 7-2D *Continue until the flange rests on the patient's teeth.*

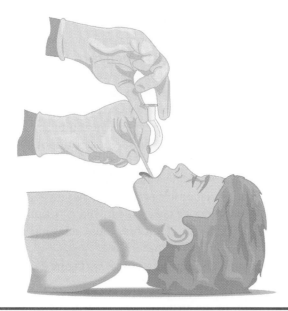

FIGURE 7-3 Inserting an oropharyngeal airway in an infant or child.

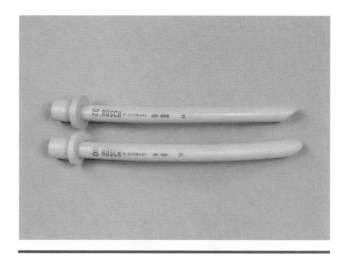

FIGURE 7-4 Nasopharyngeal (nasal) airways.

earlobe. Note that if the device is too long, it can push the epiglottis over the opening of the trachea, closing off the airway completely.

2. *Open the patient's mouth.* If necessary, use the cross-finger technique.

3. *Insert the adjunct upside down.* Be sure the tip is pointing toward the roof of the patient's mouth.

4. *Advance the adjunct gently.* Stop when you encounter resistance. Resistance occurs when the device comes in contact with the soft back of the roof of the mouth.

5. *Turn the airway 180°.* Do so while continuing to advance it until the flat flange at the top rests on the patient's front teeth. The airway follows the natural curve of the tongue and the oropharynx.

If the patient is an infant or child, the preferred alternative method is to use a tongue depressor (blade) to help insert the device (Figure 7-3). To do so, first select the proper size of airway. Open the patient's mouth, and insert the tongue depressor until its tip is at the base of the tongue. Then, press down on the tongue depressor, and therefore the tongue, toward the floor of the mouth and away from the opening of the throat. Next, insert the airway in its normal upright position. Stop when the flange is seated on the patient's teeth. (Do not insert it upside down as you would in an adult. If you do, it could cause bleeding in the airway.)

NOTE: If a patient gags when you suction the airway, he has a *gag reflex.* It is otherwise difficult to tell if an unresponsive patient has a gag reflex until you actually begin to insert an oral airway. If you observe gagging or retching during insertion, remove the device and be prepared for vomiting. If the unresponsive patient has a gag reflex, you will not be able to insert an oral airway, but it will still be important to monitor and suction the airway as needed.

Nasopharyngeal Airway

The nasopharyngeal airway, or nasal airway, is a curved hollow tube of soft plastic (Figure 7-4). It has a flange or flare at the top and a bevel at the bottom and comes in a variety of sizes. Nasal airways are less likely than oral airways to cause vomiting. This is because the soft tube moves and gives when the patient swallows. Use it to keep the tongue from blocking the airway in patients who are not fully responsive or who have a gag reflex. Use it also when the patient cannot take the oral airway or if his teeth are clenched tightly and will not open.

Even though a nasal airway is lubricated before insertion, it can be painful and may cause the lining of the nose to bleed into the airway.

To insert a nasopharyngeal airway (Figure 7-5):

1. *Select the proper size.* It should extend from the tip of the patient's nose to the tip of the earlobe. Also, the diameter should fit inside the nostril without **blanching** (losing color from) the skin of the nose. If it is too long, it could send air into the stomach instead of the lungs, causing massive **gastric distention** (inflation of the stomach) and inadequate ventilation.

2. *Use a sterile, water-soluble lubricant on the device.* It makes it easier to insert. It also reduces the chances of injuring the nasal lining. Do not use petroleum jelly, which can damage the lining of the nose and throat.

3. *Insert the airway posteriorly.* The bevel should point toward the **septum** when it is inserted into the right

SKILL SUMMARY   *Inserting a Nasopharyngeal Airway*

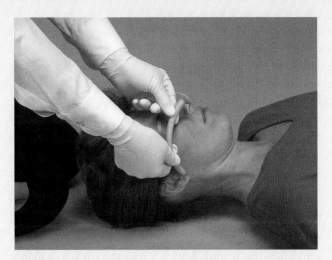

FIGURE 7-5A   *Measure the nasopharyngeal airway.*

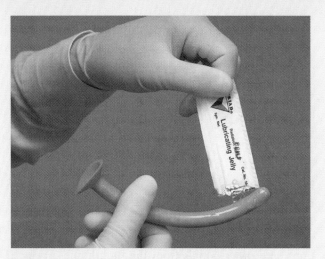

FIGURE 7-5B   *Lubricate it with a water-soluble lubricant.*

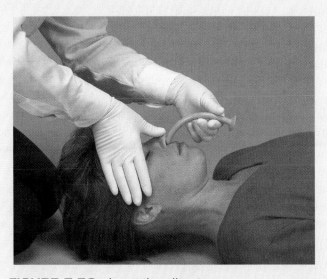

FIGURE 7-5C   *Insert the adjunct.*

nostril. (The *septum* is the wall dividing the two nostrils.) Insert the device close to the midline, along the floor of the nostril, and straight back into the nasopharynx. When the airway is properly inserted, the flange should lie against the flare of the nostril.

4. If the airway cannot be inserted in one nostril, try the other nostril. Do not force a nasal airway into place. If you meet resistance, gently rotate it from side to side. If you still feel resistance, remove the airway.

   After insertion, check to see that air is flowing through the airway as the patient breathes. If the patient is breathing spontaneously but you feel no air movement through the tube, remove it immediately and try inserting it in the other nostril. Note that it is still necessary to maintain a head-tilt/chin-lift or jaw-thrust once the device is inserted.

Suctioning

Every effort should be made to prevent vomitus and secretions from entering an unresponsive patient's lungs. A tiny amount can cause infection and even death. Remember,

✓ | First Responder Practice

It's good news when you have cared for a patient near death and your actions helped him to survive. It's bad news when you later find out he died in the hospital from pneumonia and a severe infection, the result of aspirated foreign materials. Remember, suctioning is important.

it is important to keep the patient's airway clear. Suction the airway when needed, early and often.

Suction devices use negative pressure to keep the airway clear (Figure 7-6). They remove blood, vomit, secretions, and other liquids from the mouth and airway. If you hear a gurgling sound during assessment or artificial ventilation, immediately suction the airway. Most suction units cannot remove solid objects like teeth, particles of food, and other foreign bodies. Some cannot remove very thick vomit. In such situations, you may need to use an alternative piece of suction equipment or a finger sweep.

Suctioning Equipment

Portable suction units can be manually or electrically powered. Some are oxygen- or air-powered. All produce a vacuum that can suction substances from the throat. Each should be inspected before a shift or on a regular basis.

Manual units require no energy source other than the person operating it. As a result, they lack some of the typical problems associated with electric- or oxygen-powered devices. They also can more effectively suction heavy substances, such as thick vomit.

Electric units must have fully charged batteries to function effectively. A low battery charge reduces the vacuum and the length of time the unit can be used. Some units allow for constant charging, so batteries remain full.

Any type of suction unit must have a wide-bore, thick-walled, non-kinking tubing that fits a standard suction catheter. It should have several sterile disposable suction catheters, including a "tonsil tip" (rigid plastic), which is used to suction unresponsive patients. An unbreakable collection bottle or container and a supply of water for rinsing and clearing tubes and catheters should be included. The unit also should have enough vacuum pressure and flow to suction substances from the throat effectively.

Principles of Suctioning

The procedure for suctioning varies, depending on the type of unit and catheter used. However, some general principles apply. One is to be sure to take body substance isolation (BSI) precautions. Suctioning involves removal of body fluids, and the potential for coughing and fluid

SKILL SUMMARY *Suctioning*

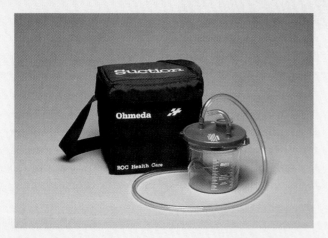

FIGURE 7-6A *Example of a portable suction unit.*

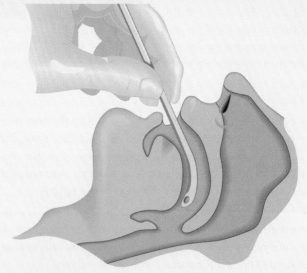

FIGURE 7-6B *Suctioning technique.*

spatter is high. So, wear protective eye wear, a mask, and gloves. If you suspect tuberculosis (TB), wear an N-95 or HEPA respirator the entire time you are in contact with the patient.

Another important principle is to use the correct type of catheter for your patient. Use a "tonsil tip" or "tonsil sucker" catheter to suction the mouth and throat of an unresponsive patient, or an infant or child. Then, insert the catheter, without suction, only to the base of tongue. Place the convex (bulging) side of the catheter against the roof of the patient's mouth. If the patient vomits copiously, or if the vomitus is thick, use the end of the suction tubing (without a catheter attached).

A third principle is to apply suction by moving the catheter (or tubing) from side to side as you withdraw it from the mouth. Stop after 15 seconds in an adult, 10 seconds in a child, and 5 seconds in an infant. Do not exceed the maximum times noted here. Air and oxygen are removed during suctioning, which can cause a quick drop in blood oxygen levels and changes in heart rate. In an adult, watch for rapid, slow, or irregular heart rates. In an infant, watch for a decreased heart rate. If a decrease is noted, stop suctioning and reapply oxygen or ventilate for at least 30 seconds before suctioning again.

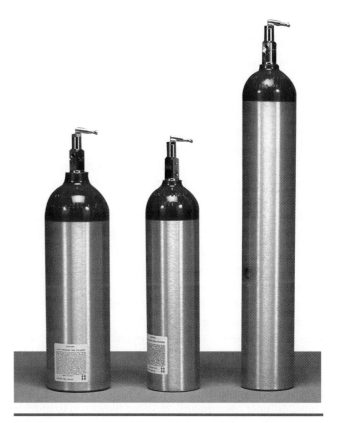

FIGURE 7-7 A basic portable oxygen cylinder.

 Q:

1. What is the difference between an oral airway and a nasal airway?

2. How long should you apply suction in an infant? A child? An adult?

Section 2 Oxygen Therapy

Oxygen equipment can be an excellent tool for a well-trained First Responder. It allows you to deliver oxygen to patients who desperately need it. However, if you are not allowed to administer oxygen in your EMS system, do not wait for it to arrive before providing emergency care.

Conditions that may require oxygen therapy include injury, heart or breathing problems, shock, and any other condition that prevents the efficient flow of oxygen throughout the body. Signs and symptoms that indicate the need for oxygen are:

- Poor skin color (blue, gray, or pale).
- Unresponsiveness.
- Cool, clammy skin.
- Difficulty breathing.
- Blood loss.

- Chest pain.
- Trauma (injury).

Note that when you provide artificial ventilation, you can give a higher concentration of oxygen to the patient by connecting supplemental oxygen to your pocket face mask.

Oxygen Cylinders

All oxygen cylinders are manufactured according to strict governmental (U.S. Department of Transportation) regulations. According to those regulations, cylinders must be checked for safety at least once in 5 years. New cylinders should be checked every 10 years. (See Figure 7-7 for an example of a portable oxygen cylinder.)

Different types of oxygen cylinders are available. They vary in size and volume. Even though the volume of oxygen may vary, all cylinders when full are at the same pressure, about 2,000 **psi**. Cylinder sizes are identified by letter. The following are sizes used in emergency medical care:

- D cylinder   —   350 liters.
- E cylinder   —   625 liters.
- M cylinder   —   3,000 liters.
- G cylinder   —   5,300 liters.
- H cylinder   —   6,900 liters.

Gas flow from an oxygen cylinder is controlled by regulators. These reduce pressure in the cylinder to a safe range of about 50 psi and control the flow from 1 to 25 liters per minute. Regulators are attached to the cylinder by a yoke. Each yoke fits only the cylinders made for one type of gas. In addition, all gas cylinders are color coded according to contents. Oxygen cylinders in the U.S. are generally steel green or aluminum gray.

Two types of regulators may be attached to oxygen cylinders: *high-pressure regulators and therapy regulators.* The high-pressure regulator can provide 50 psi to power a *demand-valve type resuscitator* (flow-restricted oxygen-powered ventilation device) or a suction device. It has a threaded outlet and one gauge, which registers cylinder contents. It cannot be used interchangeably with the therapy regulator. It has no mechanism to adjust flow rate, and it is designed specifically for use with other equipment. To use a high-pressure regulator, attach the equipment supply line to the threaded outlet and open the cylinder valve fully. Then back off one-half turn for safety.

The therapy regulator can administer a maximum of 15 to 25 liters of oxygen per minute. It has two gauges. One shows cylinder contents and the other allows you to provide a metered flow of oxygen to the patient. The cylinder is full when the pressure is 2,000 psi or greater. This pressure drops in direct proportion to the contents. For example, if the pressure is 1,000 psi, the cylinder is half full. Adjust the flow meter to provide oxygen appropriate to the device used and the condition of the patient. Follow local protocol.

Safety Precautions

Observe the following safety precautions when you handle oxygen cylinders:

- Never allow combustible materials such as oil or grease to touch the cylinder, regulator, fittings, valves, or hoses.

- Never smoke or allow others to smoke in any area where oxygen cylinders are in use or on standby.

- Always store the cylinders below 125°F.

- Never use an oxygen cylinder without a safe, properly fitting regulator valve.

- Never use a valve made for another gas, even if it has been modified.

- Always keep all valves closed when the oxygen cylinder is not in use, even when a tank is empty.

- Always keep oxygen cylinders secure to prevent them from toppling over. In transit, keep them in a carrier rack.

- Never place any part of your body over the cylinder valve. A loosely fitting regulator can be blown off with sufficient force to amputate a head.

- Never stand an oxygen tank upright near the patient. If the tank is not in a commercial pack, lay it on its side by the patient.

Using the Cylinders

Part of your daily routine should include checking the oxygen tank carried in your vehicle. To do so, you should open the main cylinder valve and check the pressure remaining on the cylinder. It is very discouraging, not to mention negligent, to arrive at the scene of a crash with lights, sirens, and other fanfare only to find that you have an empty oxygen cylinder. So, always replace a cylinder when the pressure is low. Have backup portable oxygen cylinders in your vehicle.

Prepare the tank, administer oxygen, and discontinue administration as described in Figure 7-8. Note that oxygen itself does not burn. It does, however, feed and support combustion, especially when the oxygen is pressurized. Make absolutely sure that there are no open flames in the area when you are using oxygen.

Oxygen Delivery Equipment

A variety of devices are available to deliver oxygen to the patient. Proper training in their use is essential. Follow all local protocols.

Oxygen equipment delivers either low- or high-flow oxygen. Use low-flow oxygen through a **nasal cannula.** Use high-flow oxygen through a **nonrebreather mask.** Note that the patient must be breathing in order for you to use either of these devices. If the patient is not breathing or is breathing inadequately, begin artificial ventilation with supplemental oxygen.

Nasal Cannula

One of the most common oxygen devices is the nasal cannula. Its two soft plastic tips are inserted a short distance into the nostrils. The tips are attached to the oxygen source with thin tubing. It is comfortable and convenient. Most patients tolerate it with ease.

The nasal cannula provides safe, comfortable, low-flow oxygen in concentrations of 24% to 44% with a one- to six-liter flow. It should be used at low rates of less than six liters per minute. Higher flows can cause headaches, drying of the membranes in the nose, and nosebleeds.

The nasal cannula is good for patients who are anxious about a mask, for patients who are nauseated or vomiting, and in situations in which you need to communicate with the patient.

To use a nasal cannula (Figure 7-9), first set liter flow to the desired rate. Make sure oxygen flows from the cannula tips. Then, insert the two tips into the nostrils with the tab facing out. Finally, position the tubing over and behind each ear and gently secure it by sliding the adjuster underneath the chin.

Do not adjust the tubing too tightly. If using an elastic strap, adjust it so that it is secure but comfortable. If the tubing causes irritation, pad the patient's cheeks and behind the ears with 2″ × 2″ gauze pads. Be sure to check placement often. The cannula can be dislodged easily.

Nonrebreather Mask

A nonrebreather mask has an oxygen reservoir bag and a one-way valve. The one-way valve allows the patient to inhale from the bag and exhale through the valve. Adjust the oxygen flow to prevent the bag from collapsing during inhalation, using about 10 to 15 liters per minute.

A nonrebreather mask requires a tight seal. If fitted properly to the face, it can deliver oxygen concentrations up to 90%. It is ideally suited for patients who are breathing adequately but have conditions such as difficulty breathing, chest pain, or trauma. Remember that flow rate must be adequate to keep the bag inflated as the patient breathes. If the bag collapses, the patient will not receive oxygen and may suffocate. Be ready to remove the mask if the patient vomits. Note also that you must exercise caution when using this device on patients with certain chronic lung diseases. (See "Special Considerations", which follows.)

To use the nonrebreather mask (Figure 7-10):

1. *Select a mask,* one with the oxygen supply tube preattached. The other end attaches to the oxygen source.

2. *Turn on the oxygen and set the flow.* Oxygen should be at 10 to 15 liters per minute to fill the bag. The flow should be set at the prescribed level. Make sure the bag is full before placing it on the patient's face.

3. *Position the mask.* Gently place it over the patient's face. Slip the loosened elastic strap over the head so that it is positioned below or above the ears. Then pull the ends of the elastic until the mask fits the patient's face. Note that you should not lift the head of a trauma patient. Such movement may worsen a spine injury. Instead, gently tape the mask to the patient's cheeks. Then, monitor the airway.

Some masks have a thin piece of metal where the mask covers the bridge of the patient's nose. To ensure a good seal, that metal should be pinched so that the mask conforms to the shape of the nose.

Patients who have trouble breathing or who are in shock may get anxious when you try to place a mask on them. To these patients, it feels as if they are being suffocated. Try to convince them to accept the mask. Explain to the patient what the mask is and why you are using it. You might tell them that the mask can feel confining, but that it also provides the high concentration of oxygen they need. As a last resort, use a nasal cannula to provide some oxygen.

Special Considerations

WARNING! The term *respiratory depression* refers to a slow breathing rate of less than 8 breaths per minute. It can occur—though rarely—when oxygen is applied to patients who have a chronic obstruction pulmonary disease (COPD) such as emphysema or chronic bronchitis. Beware of this rare complication.

Patients with COPD may, over time, lose the normal ability to use increased carbon dioxide levels in the blood as a stimulus to breathe. When this occurs, the COPD patient's body may use low blood oxygen as the factor that stimulates breathing. This is called "hypoxic drive."

Because of this *hypoxic drive,* EMS personnel have for years been trained to administer only low concentrations of oxygen to these patients. However, more harm is done by withholding high-concentration oxygen than could be done by administering it.

As a First Responder, you will probably never see adverse conditions resulting from oxygen administration. The time required for such conditions to develop is usually too long to cause any problem during emergency care in the field. The bottom line is this: Never withhold high-concentration oxygen from a patient who needs it.

Q:
1. What signs and symptoms indicate that a patient needs oxygen therapy?

2. What safety precautions should you keep in mind when handling oxygen cylinders?

3. What is the daily routine for checking an oxygen tank?

4. Among patients who need oxygen, which would benefit most from a nasal cannula? From a nonrebreather?

Section 3 Assisting with Advanced Airway Devices

As a First Responder, you will arrive on scene and provide emergency care for your patient's airway until the ambulance arrives. In many cases, ambulance personnel will have the ability to use advanced airway devices.

SKILL SUMMARY *Preparing the Oxygen Delivery System*

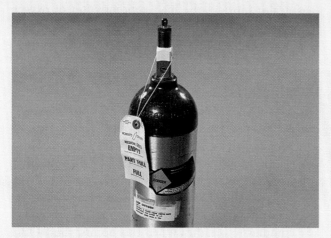

FIGURE 7-8A   *Select the desired cylinder. Check for the label, "Oxygen U.S.P."*

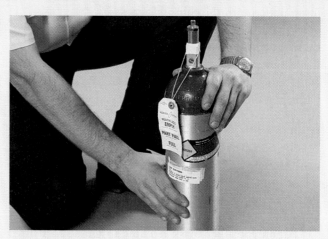

FIGURE 7-8B   *Place the cylinder in an upright position and stand to one side.*

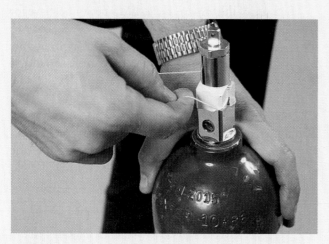

FIGURE 7-8C   *Remove the plastic wrapper or cap protecting the cylinder outlet.*

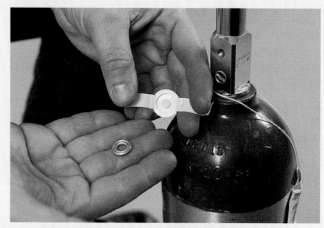

FIGURE 7-8D   *Keep the plastic washer (for some set-ups).*

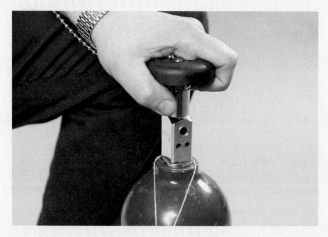

FIGURE 7-8E   *"Crack" the main valve for one second.*

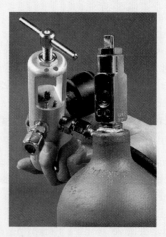

FIGURE 7-8F   *Select the correct pressure regulator and flowmeter.*

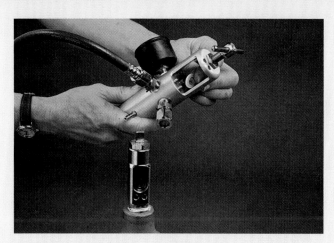

FIGURE 7-8G *Place the cylinder valve gasket on the regulator oxygen port.*

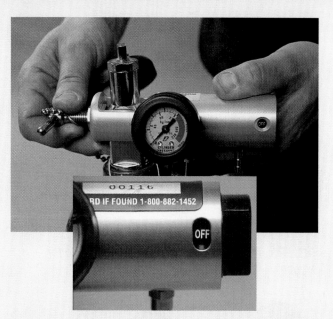

FIGURE 7-8H *Make certain that the pressure regulator is closed.*

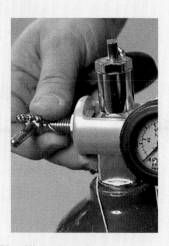

FIGURE 7-8I *Align pins.*

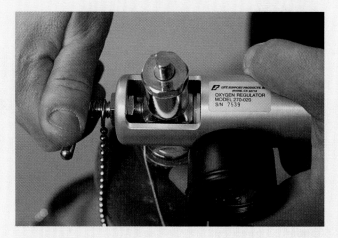

FIGURE 7-8J *Tighten T-screw for pin yoke.*

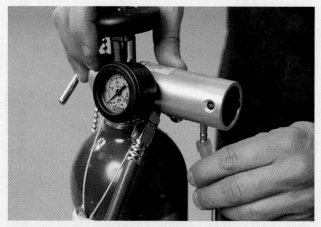

FIGURE 7-8K *Attach tubing and delivery device.*

SKILL SUMMARY *Administering Oxygen*

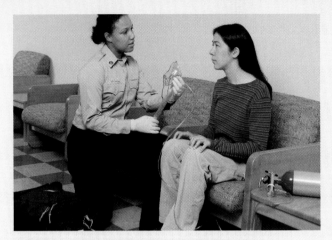

FIGURE 7-8L *Explain to the patient the need for oxygen.*

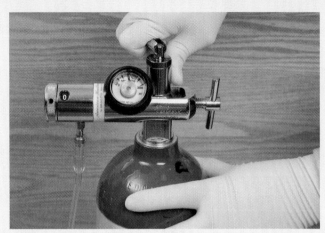

FIGURE 7-8M *Open the main valve and adjust the flowmeter.*

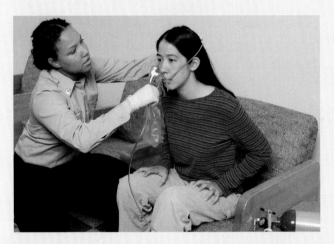

FIGURE 7-8N *Place the oxygen delivery device on the patient.*

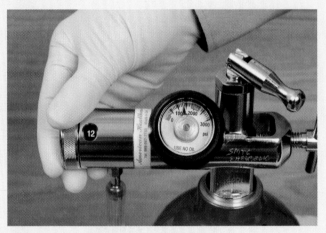

FIGURE 7-8O *Adjust the flowmeter.*

Sellick's Maneuver

One technique you may be asked to perform is *Sellick's maneuver* (Figure 7-11). Sellick's maneuver has two purposes: it compresses the esophagus so that vomiting is less likely, and it helps make the trachea more visible to the advanced provider who is attempting an *endotracheal intubation* (insertion of a tube into the trachea).

When requested to do so by an advanced provider, perform Sellick's maneuver as follows: On a supine patient, first locate the cricothyroid membrane. Use the finger and thumb of one hand to provide downward (posterior) pressure over it. Compress with a steady, gentle force, enough to compress the flexible esophagus but not enough to damage the trachea or cricothyroid

membrane. Maintain this pressure until instructed to stop by the advanced provider. Follow local protocols.

Ventilating Through an Advanced Airway

Several advanced airway devices are used in the field. The most common of these is the endotracheal tube. One major difference in ventilating a nonbreathing patient who has an advanced airway in place is that a mask seal is not necessary. The part of the BVM that fits into the mask will also attach to the end of the advanced airway device (also called the "tube") by way of the 15/22 mm standard connection.

To ventilate a patient through an advanced airway device, you must first attach the BVM to it. Then, squeeze

SKILL SUMMARY *Discontinuing Oxygen*

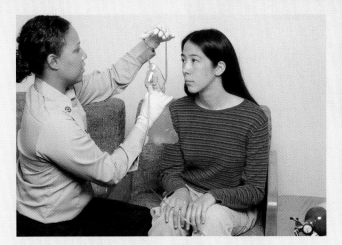

FIGURE 7-8P   *Remove the delivery device.*

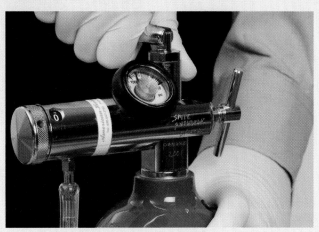

FIGURE 7-8Q   *Close the main valve.*

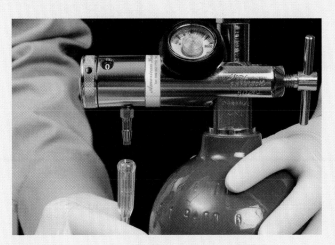

FIGURE 7-8R   *Remove the delivery tubing.*

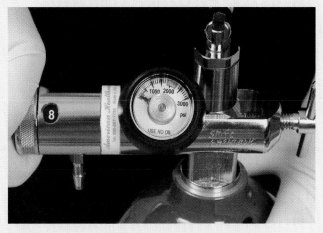

FIGURE 7-8S   *Bleed the flowmeter.*

the BVM so that full breaths enter the patient and cause the chest to rise. Do not squeeze too forcefully or rapidly. Ventilations may require slightly less volume and will be delivered more slowly than in a patient without the tube. The AHA recommends 8–10 breaths per minute (approximately every 7–8 seconds) for a patient who is being ventilated through an advanced airway.

Be very careful not to dislodge the tube. Although the advanced provider will secure the tube, never pull on the BVM or push directly down on the tube. This can cause the tube to dislodge or to go too deep into the airway.

If you are working a cardiac arrest or "code," always remove the BVM from the tube when you clear the patient during defibrillation. If you let go of the BVM, its

weight dangling from the tube may cause the tube to dislodge.

If you believe the tube has been dislodged or if the tube suddenly becomes much easier or more difficult to ventilate through, notify the advanced provider immediately.

Always follow all local protocols.

1. Why would you disconnect the BVM from the tube before defibrillation is performed?

2. What is Sellick's maneuver?

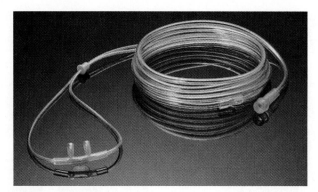

a. *Nasal cannula.*

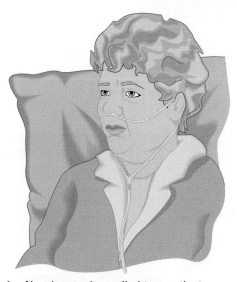

b. *Nasal cannula applied to a patient.*

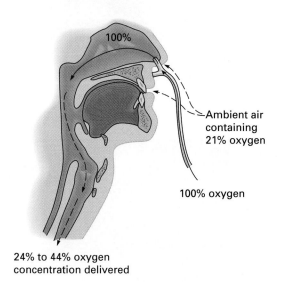

100%

Ambient air
containing
21% oxygen

100% oxygen

24% to 44% oxygen
concentration delivered

FIGURE 7-9 **The nasal cannula is used for patients who are anxious, nauseated, or vomiting, or when you need to communicate to the patient.**

Section 4 Foreign Body Airway Obstruction

An upper airway obstruction is anything that blocks the nasal passages, the back of the mouth, or the throat. A lower airway obstruction can be caused by breathing in a foreign body or by severe spasm of the bronchial passages. A **foreign body airway obstruction (FBAO)** is a *true emergency.* It must be cleared from the airway before the patient can breathe and before you can give artificial ventilation.

Airway obstruction in a responsive patient can be the cause of cardiac arrest. The most common FBAO is food. If your patient was eating before he collapsed, suspect that he choked on food. Elderly people are at risk for choking because they have a weaker gag reflex. As a result, they are more frequently misdiagnosed as having heart disease if they collapse. Other common causes of airway

obstruction in a responsive patient are bleeding into the airway and aspirated vomit.

In an unresponsive patient, an FBAO may be caused by vomiting, loose or broken dentures or bridges, or injury to the face or jaw. The most common source of

First on Scene

The first minute on scene is the one in which a tremendous difference can be made. Many times the actions you take during this time can correct the problem, such as expelling an FBAO. Be sure to update incoming EMS units with any changes in the patient's condition while are you are at the scene.

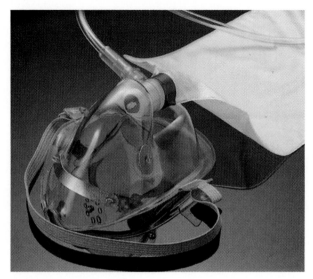

a. *Nonrebreather mask.*

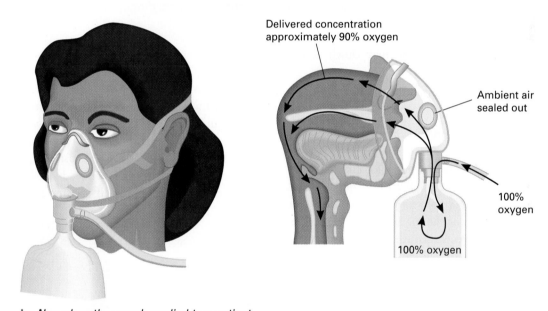

Delivered concentration
approximately 90% oxygen

Ambient air
sealed out

100%
oxygen

100% oxygen

b. *Nonrebreather mask applied to a patient.*

FIGURE 7-10 The nonrebreather mask is ideally suited for patients who have severe hypoxemia.

upper airway obstruction in an unresponsive patient is the tongue. Other causes of airway obstruction include secretions, blood clots, cancerous conditions of the mouth or throat, enlarged tonsils, and acute epiglottitis.

Types of FBAO

There are two types of foreign body airway obstruction (FBAO)—*mild* (also called *partial*) and *severe* (also called *complete*). A mild FBAO means an object is caught in the throat but does not totally occlude (block) breathing. Even if there is good air exchange, *never leave a patient with a mild airway obstruction.* The obstruction can shift and become severe.

A patient with a mild FBAO but with good air exchange may:

- Remain responsive.
- Be able to speak.
- Cough forcefully.
- Wheeze between coughs.

A patient with a severe FBAO may be either responsive or unresponsive, depending in part on how long the airway has been blocked. He may have some very limited ability to move air and have:

- Weak, ineffective cough.
- High-pitched noise when inhaling.

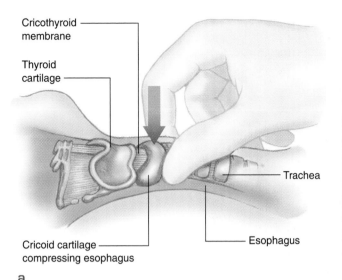

Cricothyroid membrane

Thyroid cartilage

Trachea

Cricoid cartilage compressing esophagus

Esophagus

a.

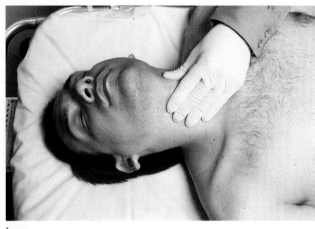

b.

FIGURE 7-11 In Sellick's maneuver, pressure is placed on the cricoid cartilage, pushing it posteriorly against the esophagus.

- Increased respiratory difficulty and may clutch at the throat.
- Cyanosis (bluish discoloration of the skin and mucous membranes).

A patient with a severe FBAO will soon be unable to breathe, cough, or speak. He may clutch at the neck with thumb and fingers (the universal signal for choking). All air exchange will stop because an object fully occludes the patient's airway. The amount of oxygen in the blood will decrease rapidly because air cannot enter the lungs. This will result in unresponsiveness. Death also will occur rapidly if the obstruction is not relieved.

The way you manage an obstructed airway depends on whether the obstruction is mild or severe.

FBAO in an Adult

Mild FBAO with Good Air Exchange

A patient with a mild obstruction and good air exchange is responsive and able to cough forcefully. In this case, do not interfere with the patient's own attempts to dislodge the obstruction by coughing. Instead, encourage him to "cough up" the foreign body. Do not make any other specific attempts to relieve the obstruction. If the patient cannot dislodge the object on his own, even if good air exchange continues, activate the EMS system. Place the patient in a position of comfort, where it is easiest for him or her to breathe. Finally, never leave the patient until you are certain the airway is clear and no other problems threaten the airway.

Severe Obstruction

The American Heart Association (AHA) recommends the **Heimlich maneuver** in cases of mild airway obstruc-

tion with poor air exchange and in cases of severe airway obstruction. Also called *abdominal thrusts,* the Heimlich maneuver pushes the diaphragm quickly upward (Figure 7-12). This action forces enough air from the lungs to dislodge and expel the foreign object. *The AHA recommends against the use of back slaps in an adult and a child.*

Each individual abdominal thrust must be delivered with enough force and pressure to dislodge the foreign object. You must keep trying if the first thrust is unsuc-

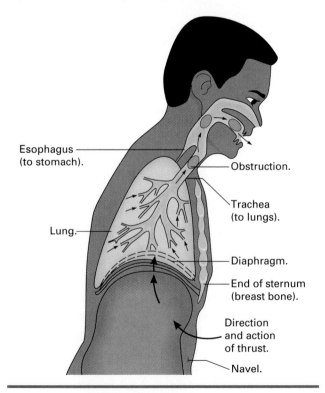

Esophagus (to stomach).

Obstruction.

Trachea (to lungs).

Lung.

Diaphragm.

End of sternum (breast bone).

Direction and action of thrust.

Navel.

FIGURE 7-12 Abdominal thrusts push the diaphragm up, forcing air to expel the foreign object.

cessful. Deliver each thrust with the intent of relieving the obstruction. It may take as many as five or more thrusts to succeed. Continue with thrusts until the item is dislodged or the patient becomes unconscious.

Responsive Adult.   If the patient is responsive, perform the Heimlich maneuver as follows (Figure 7-13):

1. *Get in position.* Stand behind the patient. Wrap your arms around his waist. Keep your elbows out, away from his ribs.

2. *Position your hands.* Make a fist with one hand. Place the thumb side of the fist on the middle of the abdomen slightly above the navel and well below the xiphoid process.

3. *Perform an abdominal thrust.* First, grasp your fist with your other hand, thumbs toward the patient. Then press your fist into the patient's abdomen with a quick inward and upward thrust.

4. If the first thrust does not dislodge the foreign body, make each new thrust separate and distinct. Continue

SKILL SUMMARY   *Foreign Body Airway Obstruction—Responsive Adult*

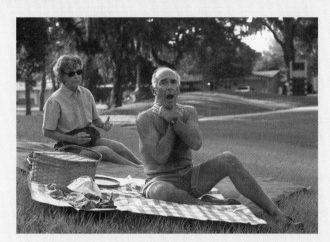

FIGURE 7-13A   *The universal sign of choking.*

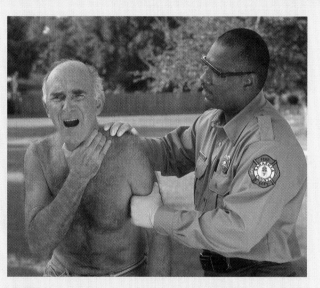

FIGURE 7-13B   *Determine if the patient can speak or cough by asking, "Are you choking?"*

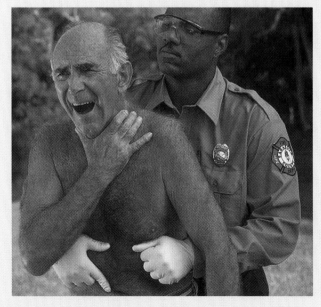

FIGURE 7-13C   *If so, perform the Heimlich maneuver to dislodge the object.*

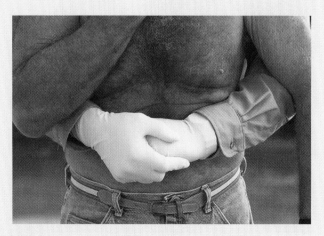

FIGURE 7-13D   *Hand position for Heimlich maneuver.*

until the object is expelled or the patient becomes unresponsive.

Beware of certain dangers. First, if you are improperly positioned or if you perform the thrusts too rapidly or too forcefully, you can lose your balance and fall into the patient. If your hands are positioned too high, you could cause internal injury. Finally, the Heimlich maneuver can cause vomiting. Correct hand placement and use of appropriate force minimizes this risk.

Pregnant or Obese Responsive Adult.   If the patient is in the advanced stages of pregnancy or is markedly obese, there may be no room between the rib cage and the abdomen to perform abdominal thrusts, or you may be unable to reach around the patient. In these cases, perform chest thrusts as follows (Figure 7-14):

1. *Get in position.* Stand behind the patient. Place your arms directly under the patient's armpits. Wrap your arms around the patient's chest.

2. *Position your hands.* Make a fist with one hand. Place the thumb of your fist on the middle of the patient's sternum. If you are near the margins of the rib cage, your hand is too low.

3. *Perform a chest thrust.* First, seize your fist firmly with your other hand. Then, thrust backward sharply.

4. If the first thrust does not dislodge the foreign body, repeat thrusts until the object is expelled or the patient becomes unresponsive.

Unresponsive Adult.   If your patient is unresponsive when you find him or becomes unresponsive, activate the EMS system if it had not been activated already. Then,

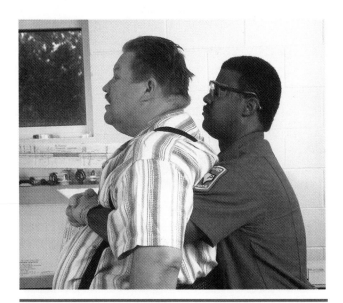

FIGURE 7-14 Chest thrusts on a standing obese patient with an FBAO.

place the patient in a supine position and proceed with the following (Figure 7-15):

1. *Attempt to ventilate the patient.* First, open the airway. Then, try to ventilate using the mouth-to-mask, mouth-to-barrier device, or mouth-to-mouth technique.

2. *If ventilation is unsuccessful,* reposition the patient's head and try again. If ventilation is still unsuccessful, proceed as follows:
   —*Begin CPR.* Perform 30 chest compressions.
   —*Look into the patient's airway.* If you see an object, reach in and remove it.
   —*Attempt to ventilate.*

3. *If the foreign body is not dislodged,* repeat the sequence. That is, in rapid succession attempt to ventilate, perform 30 chest compressions, and remove any objects you see. Continue until the foreign object is expelled and ventilation is successful or until you are relieved by other EMS personnel.

If a choking patient becomes unresponsive while you are attempting to dislodge an FBAO, activate the EMS system if it has not yet been activated. Then, look into the airway and remove any objects you see. If necessary, continue airway care as outlined above for an unresponsive adult.

Pregnant or Obese Unresponsive Adult.   Care for a severe airway obstruction in an unresponsive patient who is pregnant or obese is the same as for an unresponsive adult (see above).

FBAO in an Infant or Child

Manage a severe airway obstruction in children older than eight years the same way you would for adults. Care for infants (birth to one year) and children (one to eight years) is different.

More than 90% of childhood deaths from FBAO are in children younger than five years old. Nearly 65% of those who die are infants. The most common causes of FBAO in small children are toys, balloons, small objects such as plastic lids, and food such as hot dogs, round candies, nuts, and grapes.

Airway obstruction in an infant or small child also can be caused by swelling and infection. Both narrow the airway. Croup and epiglottitis can cause complete blockage of the airway.

Suspect that obstruction is caused by infection instead of by a foreign object if you detect gradual onset of the following:

- Fever, especially if accompanied by congestion.

- Hoarseness.

- Drooling.

SKILL SUMMARY *Foreign Body Airway Obstruction—Unresponsive Adult*

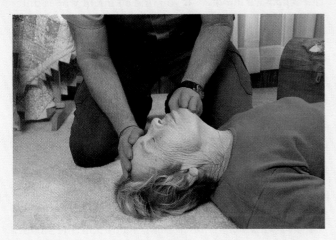

FIGURE 7-15A *If the patient is unresponsive, open the airway.*

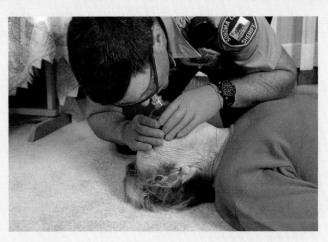

FIGURE 7-15B *Try to ventilate. If unsuccessful, reposition the head and try again.*

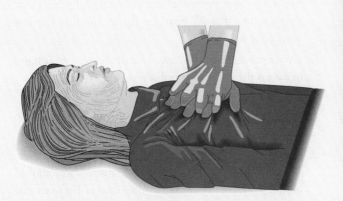

FIGURE 7-15C *If still unsuccessful, perform 30 chest compressions.*

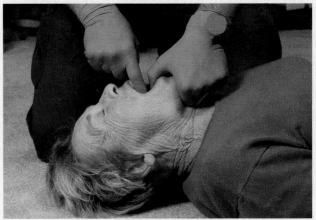

FIGURE 7-15D *Remove any visible object, or repeat until successful attempted ventilation, chest compressions, and removal of any visible objects.*

- Lethargy or limpness.
- Unexplained unresponsiveness in a normally healthy infant or small child.

If you suspect the obstruction is caused by infection, arrange for immediate transport to a medical facility.

Suspect an FBAO in an infant or child who has sudden onset of respiratory distress associated with coughing, gagging, stridor, or wheezing, especially when food or small items are found near the child. You should try to clear only a severe airway obstruction or a mild airway obstruction with poor air exchange.

Never perform a blind finger sweep on an infant or child. Look into the airway and use your finger to sweep the foreign body out *only* if you can actually see it.

Responsive Infant. If the infant has a mild airway obstruction but still has good air exchange, activate the EMS system. Let the infant try to expel the object by coughing. Place the patient in a position of comfort (in the parent's arms if possible) so that secretions and vomit will drain out of the mouth. The jaw will also fall forward, bringing the tongue and epiglottis away from the back of the throat.

If the infant is not breathing or has serious difficulty breathing, an ineffective cough, and no strong cry, he or she has a severe obstruction.

According to the AHA, you should perform the following procedure *only* if the infant has a severe obstruction with poor air exchange and *only* if the obstruction is due to a witnessed or strongly suspected foreign object.

Do not perform the following procedure if you suspect the obstruction is caused by infection. Instead, arrange for immediate transport to a medical facility.

If you cannot dislodge the FBAO in an infant within *one minute* using the following procedure, activate the EMS system.

To relieve an FBAO in a responsive infant:

1. *Get in position.* Straddle the infant over one of your arms, face down with his head lower than the rest of his body. Rest your arm on your thigh for support. Support the infant's head by firmly holding the jaw with your hand.

2. *Deliver up to five back slaps.* Use the heel of your hand between the shoulder blades (Figure 7-16).

3. *If the FBAO is not expelled,* turn the infant face up. Support him on your arm, with his head lower than the rest of his body.

4. *Position your hand.* Place your middle and ring fingers over the middle of the infant's sternum. They should be in the center of the chest just below an imaginary line drawn between the infant's nipples (Figure 7-17).

5. *Deliver up to five chest thrusts.* Use a quick downward motion.

6. *If the first set of thrusts does not dislodge the foreign body,* continue alternating sets of five back slaps and five chest thrusts until the FBAO is expelled or the infant becomes unresponsive.

When an FBAO is expelled, a responsive infant will usually start to cry and make noise. An unresponsive infant may not make noise or breathe spontaneously. You will need to try to ventilate the infant to determine if air is reaching the lungs.

Unresponsive Infant.   If you find an infant who is unresponsive:

1. *Call out "Help!"* When someone responds, have that person activate the EMS system. If you are alone, activate the EMS system within one minute, if you are unable to clear the airway.

2. *Position the patient.* Place the infant on his back on a firm, hard surface. Support his head and neck. Note that the infant's head should be in a neutral position. Overextension of the infant's neck can obstruct the airway.

3. *Attempt to ventilate.* First open the airway. Then seal your mouth over the infant's mouth and nose. Deliver breaths.

4. *If ventilation is unsuccessful,* reposition the infant's head and try again. If ventilation is still unsuccessful, proceed with the following steps.

5. *Get in position.* Straddle the infant over one of your arms, face down with his head lower than the rest of the body. Rest your arm on your thigh for support. Support the infant's head by firmly holding the jaw with your hand.

6. *Deliver up to five back slaps.* Use the heel of your hand between the infant's shoulder blades.

7. *If the FBAO is not expelled,* turn the infant face up. Support him on your arm, with his head lower than the rest of his body.

8. *Position your hand.* Place your middle and ring fingers over the middle of the infant's sternum. They should be just below an imaginary line drawn between the infant's nipples.

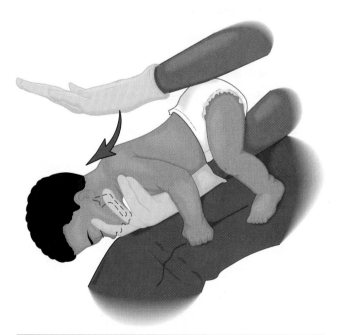

FIGURE 7-16 Back slaps for an infant with an FBAO.

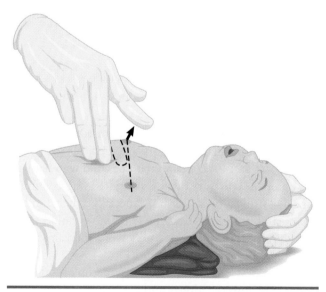

FIGURE 7-17 Locating the finger position for chest thrusts on an infant with an FBAO.

9. *Deliver up to five chest thrusts.* Use a quick downward motion.

10. *Look into the infant's mouth.* If you see the object, perform a finger sweep to remove it. (Never perform a blind finger sweep in an infant.)

11. *If the first set of ventilations, back slaps, and cchest thrusts do not dislodge the foreign body,* repeat the procedure. Continue with alternating sets of attempts to ventilate, five back slaps, five chest thrusts, looking into the airway and removing visible items until the FBAO is expelled or until you are relieved by other EMS personnel.

If a choking infant becomes unresponsive while you are attempting to dislodge an FBAO, have a second person activate EMS. If you can see the object, perform a finger sweep to remove it. If necessary, continue with airway care as described above for an unresponsive infant.

Once the foreign body is removed, check the infant for breathing and pulse. If there is no pulse, begin infant CPR as described in Chapter 8. If the infant is breathing and has a pulse, place him or her in a recovery position. Monitor breathing and pulse while you maintain an open airway.

Responsive Child. A patient one year old to the onset of puberty is considered a child. If a child has a mild obstruction with good air exchange, encourage him to expel it himself by coughing. If there is a severe obstruction, follow the steps outlined below (Figure 7-18):

1. *Get in position.* Stand behind the child. Wrap your arms around his waist. Keep your elbows out, away from his ribs.

2. *Position your hands.* Make a fist with one hand. Place the thumb side of the fist on the middle of the abdomen slightly above the navel and well below the xiphoid process. Never place your hands on the xiphoid process or on the lower edge of the ribs. Keep in mind a child's smaller size and proportions as you determine hand placement.

3. *Perform an abdominal thrust.* First, grasp your fist with your other hand, thumbs toward the patient. Then, press your fist into the patient's abdomen with a quick inward and upward thrust.

4. *If the first thrust does not dislodge the foreign body,* make each new thrust separate and distinct. Continue until the object is expelled or the patient becomes unresponsive.

Unresponsive Child. If you find an unresponsive child, have a second person activate the EMS system. Then:

1. *Position the patient.* Place the child in a supine position.

2. *Attempt to ventilate the patient.* First, open the airway. Then, try to give several rescue breaths using the

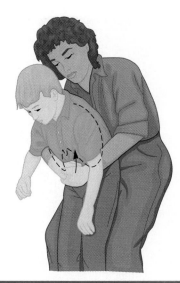

FIGURE 7-18 Performing the Heimlich maneuver on a standing or sitting responsive child with an FBAO.

mouth-to-mask, mouth-to-barrier device, or mouth-to-mouth technique.

3. *If ventilation is unsuccessful,* reposition the patient's head and try again. If ventilation is still unsuccessful, proceed with the following:
   —*Begin CPR.* Perform 30 chest compressions.
   —*Look into the patient's airway.* If you see an object, reach in and remove it.
   —*Attempt to ventilate.*

4. If the foreign body is not dislodged, repeat the sequence. That is, in rapid succession attempt to ventilate, perform 30 chest compressions, and remove any objects you see. Continue until the foreign object is expelled and ventilation is successful or until you are relieved by other EMS personnel.

If a choking child becomes unresponsive while you are attempting to dislodge an FBAO, have a second person activate EMS. If you can see the object, remove it with a finger sweep. Then, if necessary, continue with airway care as outlined above for an unresponsive child.

1. How can you tell the difference between good and poor air exchange in a patient who has a mild FBAO?

2. What is an abdominal thrust? How should it be performed?

3. What are the steps for clearing a severe FBAO in an unresponsive infant? An unresponsive adult?

▶▶ The Call Follow-up

At the beginning of this chapter, you read that First Responders were called to the scene of a snowmobile crash where a teenager was found unresponsive with blood flowing into his airway. To see how they responded to this emergency, read the following. It describes how the call was completed.

Initial Assessment *(continued)* My partner, Dave, put on gloves and a face shield and took stabilization of the head and neck. I donned the similar protective gear. Dave performed a jaw-thrust maneuver, and I began to suction. The patient's airway cleared pretty quickly. That and the jaw-thrust worked wonders.

I checked the rate and depth of breathing. His breathing was a bit rapid but adequate. Depth appeared to be adequate, too. His pulse was a little fast. We didn't get time to do much more than airway care. Nothing more important to do. The airway would get blood dripping into it, and I'd suction it out. I must've repeated that 10 or 15 times.

We put a nonrebreather mask on him and ran oxygen at 15 liters per minute.

I radioed the incoming units to bring equipment to get him boarded and to the ambulance. They also had to prepare for the cold temperature.

Patient Hand-off We gave our report to the ambulance crew (see below). They understood why it was so brief. I have to say that when we got the airway under control things certainly seemed more positive. It looked pretty bad, there, in the beginning. And it may have been over for him if someone hadn't called so quickly and if we hadn't been able to keep his airway open.

Hand-off Report

"This young man is 19 years old. He hit that tree with his snowmobile. No helmet. We have been suctioning his airway almost continuously. We stabilized his spine right away and gave oxygen by nonrebreather. No time for much more."

The Last Word *Airway, the airway, and the airway!*

Chapter Review

Focus on the EMS Team

After the first few minutes that a patient is without oxygen, his chance of survival drops dramatically. This explains the vital nature of the First Responder on the EMS team. The materials learned in this chapter—and the chapters before and after it—highlight what are perhaps your most important functions as an EMS team member: to open and maintain the airway, to support breathing, and to perform CPR and defibrillate.

Summing Up

- Airway adjuncts may be used to keep a patient's airway open, often during artificial ventilation. Use the oropharyngeal (oral) airway in an unresponsive patient who has no gag reflex. Use the nasopharyngeal (nasal) airway in patients who are not fully responsive, have a gag reflex, cannot take the oral airway, or have tightly clenched teeth that will not open.

- Clear an airway of secretions by suctioning whenever the patient cannot clear his own airway of blood, vomit, or other body fluids.

- If you are allowed to administer it to your patients, oxygen is indicated when you observe poor skin color, unresponsiveness, cool and clammy skin, difficulty breathing, blood loss, chest pain, or trauma.

- Whenever you handle oxygen cylinders, you must strictly observe safety precautions and be able to prepare the cylinder for use, properly shut it down after use, and routinely check the pressure and replace the tank as necessary.

- Oxygen delivery equipment includes the nonrebreather mask, which can deliver oxygen concentrations up to 90%. The nasal cannula can also deliver oxygen, but at a lower concentration (24% to 44%).

- Paramedics and EMT-Intermediates may ask First Responders to assist them with patient airway care. First Responders may also be asked to provide artificial ventilation to a patient who has already been intubated. Always follow your local protocols.

- *A foreign body airway obstruction (FBAO) is a true emergency.* The foreign body must be cleared from the airway before the patient can breathe and before artificial ventilation.

- Procedures involved in helping to clear the airway of an adult or child with an FBAO may include abdominal thrusts (responsive patient) or CPR compressions and removing visible objects (unresponsive patient). Procedures for an infant with an FBAO may include back slaps, CPR compressions, and removing visible foreign objects.

Key Terms

airway adjunct an artificial airway.

blanching losing color from.

FBAO foreign body airway obstruction.

gastric distention inflation of the stomach.

Heimlich maneuver a technique used to dislodge and expel a foreign body airway obstruction. *Also called* subdiaphragmatic abdominal thrusts *or* abdominal thrusts.

nasal cannula oxygen delivery device characterized by two soft plastic tips, which are inserted a short distance into the nostrils.

nasopharyngeal airway an artificial airway positioned in the nose and extending down to the larynx. *Also called* NPA *or* nasal airway.

nonrebreather mask oxygen delivery device characterized by an oxygen reservoir bag and a one-way valve.

oropharyngeal airway an artificial airway positioned in the mouth and extending down to the larynx. *Also called* OPA *or* oral airway.

psi pounds per square inch.

septum a wall that divides two cavities; an example is the wall dividing the two nostrils.

suctioning using negative pressure to keep a patient's airway clear.

Knowledge Check

1. Suctioning should be performed:

   a. as you pull the catheter out of the mouth.
   b. while you are ventilating a patient with oxygen.
   c. both on the way in and on the way out of the mouth.
   d. as you insert the catheter to the base of the tongue.

2. After identifying a severe FBAO in a responsive adult, you should deliver:

   a. back slaps.
   b. CPR.
   c. abdominal thrusts.
   d. blind finger sweeps.

3. Your patient is conscious with shallow breathing at a rate of 44 breaths per minute. Your emergency care for him is which one of the following?

   a. nasal cannula at 4 liters per minute
   b. nonrebreather at 10 liters per minute
   c. nonrebreather at 15 liters per minute
   d. artificial ventilation with supplemental oxygen

4. A "D" cylinder of oxygen contains 350 liters. If you were to administer oxygen to a patient via nonrebreather mask at 10 lpm, how many minutes would your tank last?

   a. 5
   b. 15
   c. 25
   d. 35

5. You are alone and your patient's breathing rate is 48 times per minute and shallow. Which one of the devices listed below would you use to care for this patient's airway?

   a. nasal cannula
   b. nonrebreather mask
   c. pocket face mask with supplemental oxygen
   d. bag-valve mask with supplemental oxygen

6. Chest thrusts should be used to clear a severe FBAO in a pregnant patient.

   a. True
   b. False

7. Never withhold oxygen from a patient because of a normal oxygen saturation level displayed on his pulse oximeter.

   a. True
   b. False

8. Fill in below the percentage of oxygen each device is capable of delivering to a patient.

   a. Nasal cannula at 4 liters per minute: _____
   b. Nonrebreather mask at 15 liters per minute: _____
   c. Pocket face mask: _____
   d. Bag-valve mask: _____

9. What is the difference between a mild airway obstruction and a severe one?

   _____

   _____

Scenario

You are called to a patient who is found unresponsive in an area frequented by drug dealers. The police have secured the scene. You enter to find a young man who has shallow breathing at just a few times per minute. You notice a frothy substance around the young man's lips.

a. What should you do first?

_____

_____

b. Your partner hands you a nonrebreather mask. Is this the correct device for this patient? Why or why not?

_____

_____

c. The patient stops breathing. What should you do?

_____

_____

d. The patient vomits while you are ventilating him. What should you do? What may be the cause of his vomiting?

_____

_____

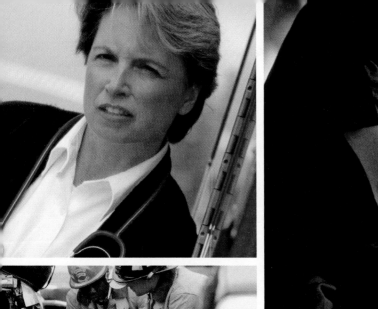
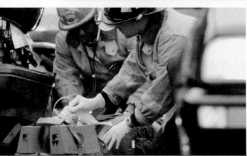
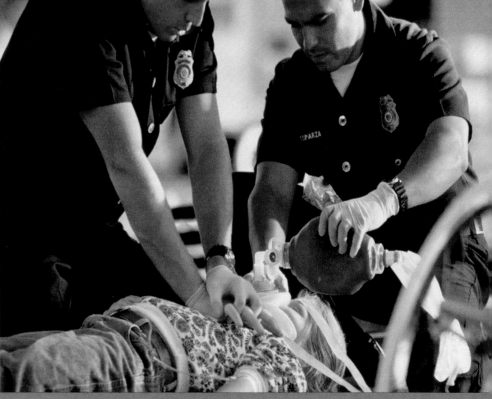

8 | Circulation

Objectives

From the U.S. Department of Transportation (DOT) 1995 "First Responder: National Standard Curriculum."

Cognitive

4-1.1 ▶ List the reasons for the heart to stop beating. (p. 148)

4-1.2 ▶ Define the components of cardiopulmonary resuscitation. (p. 149)

4-1.3 ▶ Describe each link in the chain of survival and how it relates to the EMS system. (pp. 148–149)

4-1.4 ▶ List the steps of one-rescuer adult CPR. (pp. 152–153)

4-1.5 ▶ Describe the technique of external chest compressions on an adult patient. (pp. 150–152)

4-1.6 ▶ Describe the technique of external chest compressions on an infant. (pp. 158–161)

4-1.7 ▶ Describe the technique of external chest compressions on a child. (pp. 158–161)

4-1.8 ▶ Explain when the First Responder is able to stop CPR. (p. 149)

4-1.9 ▶ List the steps of two-rescuer adult CPR. (p. 155)

4-1.10 ▶ List the steps of infant CPR. (pp. 158–161)

4-1.11 ▶ List the steps of child CPR. (pp. 158–161)

Affective

4-1.12 ▶ Respond to the feelings that the family of a patient may be having during a cardiac event. (p. 150)

4-1.13 ▶ Demonstrate a caring attitude towards patients with cardiac events who request emergency medical services. (p. 150)

4-1.14 ▶ Place the interests of the patient with a cardiac event as the foremost consideration when making any and all patient care decisions. (p. 147)

4-1.15 ▶ Communicate with empathy with family members and friends of the patient with a cardiac event. (p. 150)

Psychomotor

4-1.16 ▶ Demonstrate the proper technique of chest compressions on an adult. (pp. 150–152)

Introduction

In the U.S., heart disease takes the lives of about 350,000 people each year, many before they ever reach a hospital. The patients who can be saved need immediate CPR followed closely by defibrillation and advanced medical care within 8 to 10 minutes of collapse. But even with emergency care, many patients do not live. They may have been without a pulse or oxygen for too long or the attack may have caused irreversible damage to the heart. But don't let that discourage you. Emergency care in the field is critical to saving lives.

Section 1 The Circulatory System

The circulatory system is responsible for delivering oxygen and nutrients to and removing waste from the body's tissues. The basic components of the circulatory system are the heart, arteries, veins, capillaries, and blood. (See Chapter 4 for an illustration.)

The heart is a hollow, muscular organ about the size of a fist. It lies in the lower left central region of the chest between the lungs. It is protected in the front by the ribs and sternum (breastbone) and in the back by the spinal column. The heart contains four chambers. The two upper ones are the left and right **atria**. The two lower ones are the left and right **ventricles**. The *septum* (a wall) divides the right side of the heart from the left side. The heart also contains several one-way valves that keep blood flowing in the correct direction.

The circulatory system contains blood vessels. These vessels transport blood throughout the body. You will recall from Chapter 4 that the arteries transport blood away from the heart. Veins carry blood back to the heart. The tiny capillaries allow for the exchange of gases and nutrients between the blood and the cells of the body.

How the Heart Works

The heart is like a two-sided pump (Figure 8-1). The left side receives oxygenated blood from the lungs and pumps it to all parts of the body. The right side receives blood from the body and then pumps it to the lungs to pick up oxygen.

The blood is kept under pressure and in constant circulation by the heart's pumping action. Every time the heart contracts, a wave of blood is sent through the arteries. We feel that wave as a **pulse**. The pulse is a sign of the pressure exerted during each contraction of the heart. In a healthy adult at rest, the heart contracts between 60 and 80 times per minute.

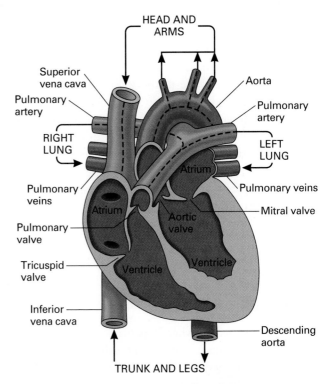

RIGHT HEART: Receives blood from the body and pumps it through the pulmonary artery to the lungs where it picks up fresh oxygen.

LEFT HEART: Receives oxygen-full blood from the lungs and pumps it through the aorta to the body.

FIGURE 8-1 The heart.

THE CALL

Dispatch Our engine company was dispatched for an EMS assist because the closest ambulance was unavailable. The call was for a cardiac patient. We knew that time would really count.

Scene Size-up There were three of us on the engine. I was the officer. I sized up the scene carefully from the cab before we got out. I reminded the others to put on their BSI equipment and to bring the AED.

Initial Assessment We observed a woman performing CPR on an older gentleman. The woman seemed to be doing pretty well, but she was getting tired. My crew approached, we told her who we were, and she turned over care to us. We applied the AED and got a "no shock advised" message. We continued CPR.

Though needed in only a small percent of calls, CPR, when used, is vitally important. In this scenario, the firefighters have taken over CPR. How long do you think they should continue? Could CPR injure the patient? Will the patient live? Consider these questions as you read Chapter 8.

The pulse can be **palpated** (felt) most easily where a large artery lies over a bone close to the skin. Sites include: the carotid pulse in the neck, the brachial pulse in the upper arm, the radial pulse in the wrist, and the femoral pulse in the upper thigh. The pulse is most easily felt over the carotid artery on either side of the neck and over the radial artery, which is on the thumb side of the inner surface of the wrist. The carotid artery should be palpated first when a patient is unresponsive. The radial artery should be palpated first when a patient is responsive.

The heart, lungs, and brain work together closely to sustain life. The smooth functioning of each is critical to the others. When one organ cannot perform properly, the other two are handicapped. If one fails, the other two soon will follow.

When the Heart Stops

Clinical death occurs when a patient is in **respiratory arrest** (not breathing) and **cardiac arrest** (the heart is not beating). Immediate **cardiopulmonary resuscitation (CPR)** may help sustain the patient's circulation enough to make other medical treatments such as defibrillation successful. However, if a patient is clinically dead for 4 to 6 minutes, brain cells begin to die. After 8 to 10 minutes without a pulse, irreversible damage occurs to the brain.

There are many reasons why a heart will stop. They include heart disease, stroke, allergic reactions, prolonged seizures, and other medical conditions. The heart also may stop because of a serious injury. In infants and children, respiratory problems are the most common cause of cardiac arrest. This is why airway care is so important in young patients.

The patient in respiratory and cardiac arrest has the best chance of surviving if all of the links in the **chain of survival** come together. This "chain," as identified by the American Heart Association (AHA), contains four links:

- *Early access.* Lay people must activate the EMS system immediately. Using a universal access number (9-1-1, for example) helps to speed system access.

First on Scene

As a First Responder, you have an important role. You can provide early CPR and, if permitted in your area, early defibrillation. The principle of CPR is to oxygenate and circulate the blood of the patient until defibrillation and advanced care can be given. Any delay increases the chances of nervous system damage and death. The faster the response, the better the patient's chances of survival. Survival rates improve when the time between arrest and the delivery of defibrillation and other advanced measures is short.

- *Early CPR.* Family members, citizens, and First Responders must be trained in CPR and begin administering it as soon as possible. CPR will help to sustain life until the next step.

- *Early defibrillation.* Defibrillation is the process by which an electrical current is sent to the heart to correct fatal heart rhythms. The earlier defibrillation can be performed, the better.

- *Early advanced care.* Advanced care, or administration of medications and other advanced therapies, must start as soon as possible. This may be done by paramedics at the scene or by prompt transportation to the hospital emergency department.

1. How does the heart create a "pulse"?

2. Where can a pulse be felt most easily?

3. What is the most common cause of cardiac arrest in children?

4. What are the four "links" in the chain of survival?

Section 2 Cardiopulmonary Resuscitation (CPR)

According to the American Heart Association (AHA), proper assessment of the patient's airway, breathing, and circulation is critical to successful CPR. The AHA also states that no patient should undergo the intrusive procedures of CPR until need is clearly established. You can establish the need for CPR by determining that the patient is *unresponsive, breathless,* and *pulseless.*

To provide CPR, you must maintain an open airway, provide artificial ventilation, and provide artificial circulation by means of chest compressions.

It was once thought that chest compressions work because they squeeze the heart between the sternum and spine to force blood out. Newer evidence indicates that they produce pressure changes inside the chest cavity. That pressure may be responsible for increased circulation to the body. So, pay as much attention to the duration of chest compressions as you do to the rate. Also be sure to stay current on all new CPR developments.

CPR must begin as soon as possible and continue until:

- Rescuer is exhausted and unable to continue.
- Patient is turned over to another trained rescuer or hospital staff.
- Patient is resuscitated.
- Patient has been declared dead by a proper authority.

A cardiac event is very serious. Without your intervention, the patient may not survive. Remember to always place the patient's interests first. Demonstrate a caring attitude. And, when possible, respond to the feelings of the patient's family and friends with empathy.

Steps Preceding CPR

Before providing CPR to a patient, you must first determine unresponsiveness, breathlessness, and pulselessness or the absence of any sign of circulation (Figure 8-2).

To determine unresponsiveness, tap or gently shake the patient and shout, "Are you okay?" If the patient does not respond, immediately activate the EMS system for an adult. (For an infant or child, activate EMS after two minutes of CPR.) This increases the patient's chances of early defibrillation and early advanced care. Then, continue with your assessment.

If, after opening the patient's airway, you determine breathlessness, provide artificial ventilation. Supplement your breaths with oxygen, if you are allowed, by attaching the oxygen supply to your pocket face mask. The oxygen should flow at 15 liters per minute.

To determine pulselessness, find the carotid artery pulse point (Figure 8-3). That is, first place two fingers on the larynx ("Adam's apple"). Then, slide your fingers to the side. Stop in the groove between the larynx and the large neck muscle. Finally, feel for the pulse. Press for at least 5 but no more than 10 seconds, gently enough to avoid compressing the artery. Do not use your thumb. Do not rest your hand across the patient's throat.

If the adult patient has a pulse—even a weak or irregular one, do *not* begin chest compressions. You could cause serious problems. If the patient has no pulse or any other sign of circulation including coughing or movement, assume that he or she is in cardiac arrest. Place the patient in a supine position on a firm, flat surface (such as the floor) and begin CPR immediately.

Note: As a First Responder, you will be trained as a professional rescuer in CPR. The training you receive will be more in depth than the training a lay rescuer, or bystander, would receive. The CPR course for people with no medical background differs from a First Responder course in the following ways:

- Lay rescuers are *not* trained to check for a pulse before beginning chest compressions. If the patient is not breathing and does not otherwise respond (cough or move), it is acceptable for the lay rescuer to begin compressions.

- As a First Responder, you will be taught additional techniques that are not taught to lay rescuers such as the two-thumbs/circling-hands technique for two-rescuer compressions in infants.

SKILL SUMMARY   *Steps Preceding CPR*

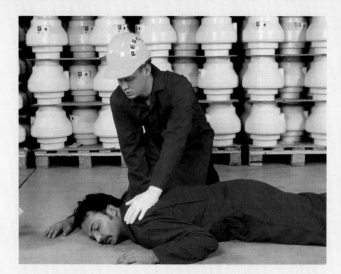

FIGURE 8-2A *Determine unresponsiveness.*

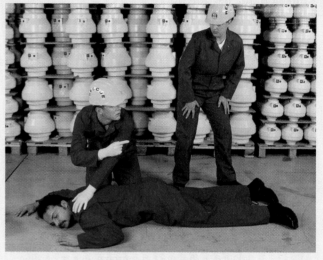

FIGURE 8-2B *Activate the EMS system.*

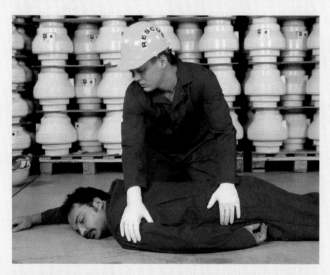

FIGURE 8-2C *Place the patient in a supine position on a firm, flat surface.*

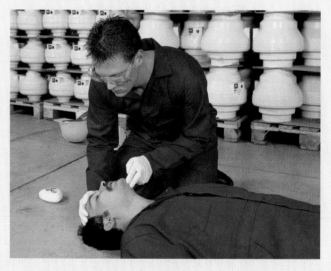

FIGURE 8-2D *Open the airway.*

You may come upon a bystander performing CPR and see some of the differences listed above. If you were to ask, for example, "Does the patient have a pulse?" he might not have checked nor was he required to do so. So, remember that performing CPR is quite stressful for the lay rescuer, who in many cases may be a member of the patient's family. It is important to be supportive and to use a nonjudgmental tone.

CPR for Adults

CPR involves a combination of skills. When a patient's heart has stopped, artificial ventilation alone cannot help

him. He also needs chest compressions to circulate the oxygen in the blood.

Chest compressions consist of rhythmic, repeated pressure over the lower half of the sternum. They cause blood to circulate as a result of the build-up of pressure in the chest cavity. When combined with artificial ventilation, they provide enough blood circulation to maintain life.

(*Note:* Remember that defibrillation, when available, is an important part of resuscitation. It will be discussed in detail in Chapter 9.)

To perform chest compressions, follow these steps (Figure 8-4):

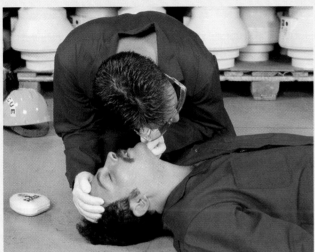

FIGURE 8-2E *Determine breathlessness.*

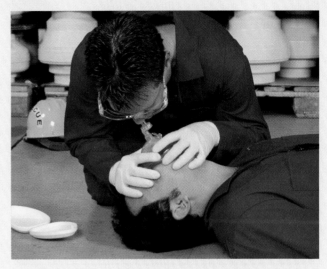

FIGURE 8-2F *Perform artificial ventilation.*

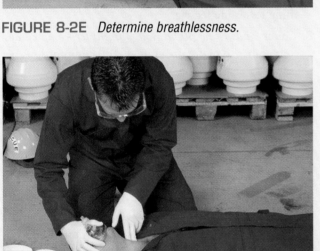

FIGURE 8-2G *Determine pulselessness or the absence of any sign of circulation.*

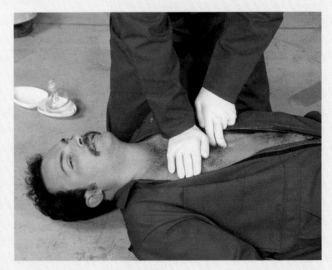

FIGURE 8-2H *Begin CPR.*

1. *Position the patient.* He or she must be supine on a firm, flat surface such as the floor.

2. *Uncover the chest.* Remove the patient's shirt or blouse. Do not waste time unbuttoning it. Rip it open or pull it up. Cut a woman's bra in two or slip it up to her neck.

3. *Get in position.* Kneel close to the patient's side. Have your knees about as wide as your shoulders.

4. *Locate the compression site.* Place the heel of one hand on the center of the patient's bare chest between the nipples.

5. *Position your hands.* Put your free hand on top of the hand on the sternum. Your hands should be parallel.

Extend or interlace your fingers to hold them off the chest wall. If your fingers rest against the chest wall during compressions, you increase the chance of separating and injuring the patient's ribs. (An alternative position for large hands and hands or wrists with arthritis is to use your free hand to grasp the wrist of the hand on the patient's sternum.)

6. *Position your shoulders.* Put them directly over your hands.

7. *Perform chest compressions.* Keeping your arms straight and your elbows locked, thrust from your shoulders. Apply firm, heavy pressure. Depress the sternum 1.5

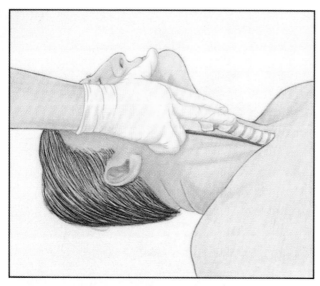

a. *Place two fingers on the larynx.*

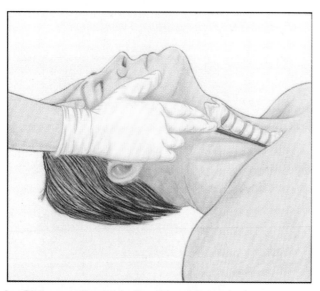

b. *Slide your fingers to the side and stop in the groove between the larynx and large neck muscle.*

FIGURE 8-3 Locating the carotid artery.

to 2 inches on an adult. Be sure the thrust is straight down into the sternum. If it is not, the torso will roll and part of the force of the thrust will be lost.

Use the weight of your body as you deliver the compressions. If necessary, add force to the thrusts with your shoulders. Never add force with your arms—the force is too great and could fracture the sternum. Compressions should be 50% of the cycle. That is, the compression and release time should be about equal.

8. *Completely release pressure after each compression.* Let the sternum return to its normal position and allow blood to flow back into the chest and heart. If you do not release all pressure, blood will not circulate

properly. Do not lift or move your hands in any way. You could lose proper positioning. Avoid sudden jerky movements. Effective compressions provide only one-fourth to one-third of normal blood circulation. Anything less is ineffective.

9. *Count quickly to 30 as you administer compressions.* Remember to maintain a rate of 100 compressions per minute.

This procedure should let you administer compressions to an adult at the rate of 100 per minute. Practice until you can perform 30 complete compressions in about 23 seconds.

CPR causes the circulation of some blood supply. Not as much as a healthy heart would circulate, but enough to provide some oxygen until defibrillation and other therapies can be administered. Recent research has shown that it is vital to perform compressions at an adequate rate and depth with minimal interruptions to maintain the flow of blood to vital organs.

One-Rescuer Adult CPR

To perform CPR alone, you must do the following: Determine unresponsiveness. Activate the EMS system. If a defibrillator is available to you, get it at this point. Open the airway and determine breathlessness. Perform artificial ventilation and remove FBAOs as needed. If breathing is restored and the patient has a pulse, place him or her in the recovery position. Do not begin CPR. If the pulse is absent, begin CPR as follows (Figure 8-5):

1. *Get in position.* Then, locate the proper hand position (described earlier).

2. *Perform 30 chest compressions* at a rate of 100 per minute. Either count out loud or use another way to keep track of the number of compressions you deliver.

3. *Open the airway and deliver two breaths,* each lasting one second. Be sure you inhale between breaths. Continue for about a minute.

SKILL SUMMARY *Correct Positioning for Adult CPR*

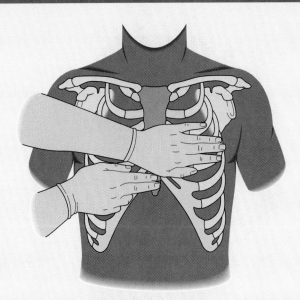

FIGURE 8-4A *Place the heel of your hand on the patient's sternum (center of the chest between the nipples).*

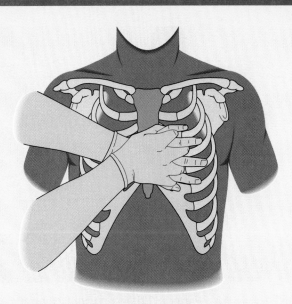

FIGURE 8-4B *Interlace your fingers.*

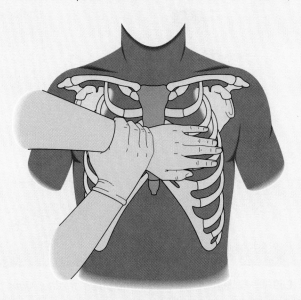

FIGURE 8-4C *Alternative hand placement for CPR.*

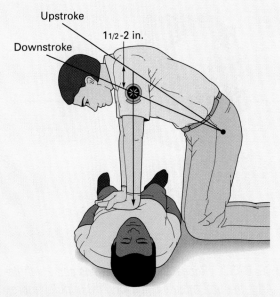

Upstroke

Downstroke

1 1/2 - 2 in.

FIGURE 8-4D *Position your shoulders and then perform chest compressions.*

4. *Check the patient's pulse.* Check for no more than 10 seconds at the carotid artery. Also look for other signs of circulation, such as breathing, coughing, or moving. If the pulse has returned, monitor it and breathing closely until the EMTs arrive. If the pulse has returned but the patient is not breathing, provide artificial ventilation at 10 to 12 breaths per minute. If there is still no pulse, resume CPR. Check again for pulse and breathing every two or three minutes.

If another rescuer trained in CPR arrives on scene, he should do two things: First, he should verify that the EMS system has been activated and is responding. Have him activate the EMS system, if necessary. Second, he should retrieve the AED, if one is available on scene. When both tasks are completed, he can join the first rescuer in performing CPR and defibrillation.

Studies have shown that a rescuer who performs compressions at the proper rate can tire quickly. So, rescuers

SKILL SUMMARY   *Performing One-Rescuer Adult CPR*

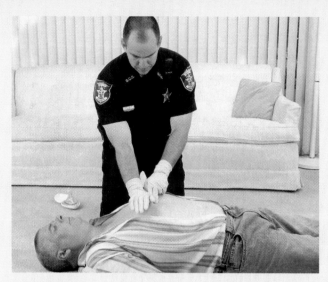

FIGURE 8-5A *Perform 30 chest compressions at a rate of 100 per minute.*

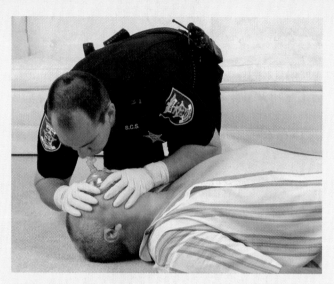

FIGURE 8-5B *After 30 compressions, open the airway and deliver two breaths.*

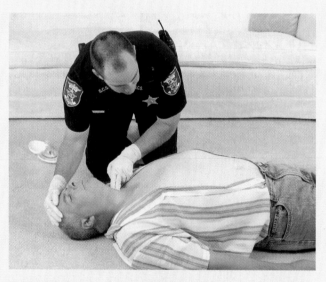

FIGURE 8-5C *Repeat 30 compressions and 2 ventilations. After the first minute and every few minutes thereafter, check for a pulse and other signs of circulation.*

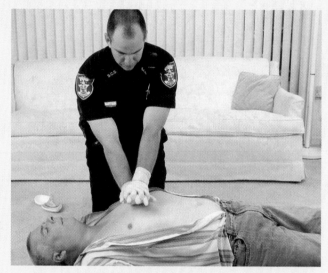

FIGURE 8-5D *If there is still no pulse or other signs of circulation, resume CPR.*

should switch after two minutes of CPR (five cycles of 30:2) to prevent fatigue and ensure quality compressions.

To relieve the first rescuer with as little interruption as possible, do one of the following:

■ If the first rescuer is currently performing chest compressions, take a position at the patient's head. Then check the pulse while the first rescuer compresses the chest. Adequate CPR will usually create a carotid pulse. When the first rescuer completes the compressions,

provide two ventilations and check the pulse. You can then resume CPR.

■ If the first rescuer is performing ventilations when you arrive, prepare to perform compressions. After the first rescuer completes two ventilations and checks the pulse, begin compressions.

No exact sequence covers all situations. The examples above are efficient ways for rescuers to take over CPR while it is being performed. The main goal is to minimize the amount of time the patient goes without CPR. It is usually convenient to incorporate pulse and breathing checks into the changes.

Any rescuers who are not currently performing CPR can help prepare the scene for the arrival of the ambulance. EMTs require space for stretchers, equipment, and additional personnel. Moving furniture away from the patient may help to create extra space. Directing the ambulance crew to the patient is also valuable. If time permits, find out from family the exact sequence of events leading to the cardiac arrest.

Two-Rescuer Adult CPR

All First Responders should learn both the one-rescuer and two-rescuer techniques. The two-rescuer coordinated technique is less tiring. Use an oral airway and a pocket face mask.

Before performing CPR, you and your partner must first determine that the patient is unresponsive, breathless, and pulseless. One rescuer may determine unresponsiveness, provide initial ventilations, and check the pulse. At the same time, the second rescuer can activate the EMS system and prepare to do compressions.

Note that in two-rescuer CPR, the ratio of compressions to ventilations is still 30:2 (30 compressions and two ventilations). The ventilations should be delivered during a pause after every 30 chest compressions.

If the patient remains unresponsive, breathless, and pulseless after your initial breaths, proceed as follows (Figure 8-6):

1. *Get in position.* The rescuers, if possible, should be on opposite sides of the patient. One rescuer kneels by the patient's side for compressions. The other kneels at the patient's head and provides ventilations.

2. *Perform chest compressions* at a rate of 100 per minute. The compression rescuer should count the sequence out loud up to 30.

3. *Deliver two breaths* when the compression rescuer pauses. Each breath should be sufficient to make the chest rise. The ventilations should be full, but not forceful. Breaths delivered too forcefully or with too much volume will cause air to enter the stomach and may cause vomiting. If you have the proper equipment and training, ventilate with 100% oxygen.

4. *After about two minutes or five cycles of 30:2, check the patient's pulse* at the carotid artery. Check for at least 5 but no more than 10 seconds. If the pulse has returned, monitor it and breathing closely until the EMTs arrive. If the pulse has returned but the patient is not breathing, provide artificial ventilation at 10 to 12 breaths per minute. If there is still no pulse, resume

CPR. Check again for pulse and breathing every two or three minutes.

When the compression rescuer gets tired, he should switch with the ventilation rescuer. This should occur about every two minutes to ensure the compressing rescuer is rested and performing appropriate chest compressions. Here is the seven-second method (Figure 8-7):

1. *Call for a switch.* The compression rescuer calls for a switch at the beginning of the compression cycle by substituting the word "change" for "one." The audible count remains the same for the remaining compressions. (Any memory aid that satisfactorily accomplishes the change is acceptable.)

2. *Both rescuers move simultaneously.*
   —After 30 compressions, the ventilation rescuer gives two breaths. Then, he moves to the patient's side, locates the correct hand position at the center of the chest between the nipples, and gets hands in place for compressions.
   —At the same time, the compression rescuer moves quickly to the patient's head. There, he checks the carotid pulse and breathing for a minimum of 5 and a maximum of 10 seconds. If no pulse is found, he gives a breath and announces, "No pulse. Continue CPR."

3. *When they are both in position,* the rescuer at the chest begins compression. If shortness of breath prevents him from giving a full count out loud, he says the numbers at the end of the count so that the ventilation rescuer will know when to breathe.

Note: You may be called to a scene with paramedics or other advanced providers. They practice *endotracheal intubation* (putting a tube directly into the patient's trachea). This is one of the best ways to secure the airway and provide 100% oxygen to the patient. When a patient is intubated, CPR is performed differently. For two-rescuer CPR, compressions and ventilations are performed asynchronously. That means there is no need to stop chest compressions while ventilations are delivered. As one rescuer performs compressions, the other provides a ventilation every six to eight seconds (8-10 per minute) in between compressions.

Monitoring the Patient

The patient's condition needs to be monitored throughout CPR. Monitoring will ensure that rescue efforts are effective. It also lets you know when spontaneous breathing and the pulse return.

In two-rescuer CPR, there is a ventilation rescuer and a compression rescuer. To monitor the effectiveness of chest compressions, the ventilation rescuer should feel for a pulse at the carotid artery during compressions. To determine if a spontaneous pulse has returned, the ventilation rescuer

SKILL SUMMARY   *Performing Two-Rescuer Adult CPR*

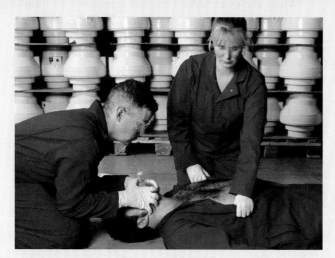

FIGURE 8-6A *Two rescuers get in position, one at the head and one at the patient's side.*

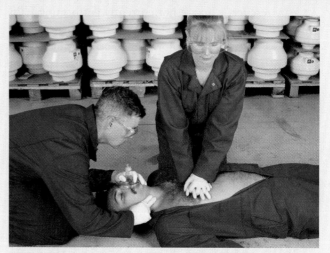

FIGURE 8-6B *The rescuer at the side performs 30 chest compressions at a rate of 100 per minute.*

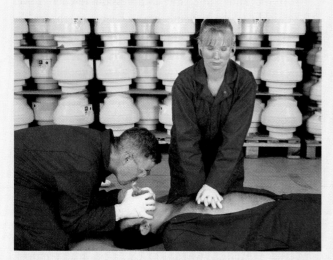

FIGURE 8-6C *After every 30 compressions, the rescuer at the head delivers two breaths.*

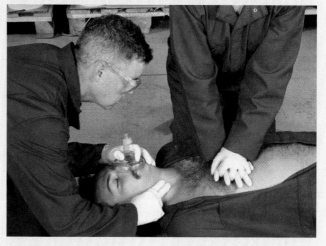

FIGURE 8-6D *After the first minute of CPR and every few minutes thereafter, the rescuer at the head checks the patient's pulse. If there is no pulse or no other sign of circulation, they resume CPR.*

should check the carotid artery for 5–10 seconds after two minutes of CPR and every few minutes thereafter. Note that the pulse must be checked when CPR is not in progress.

In general, CPR should be interrupted for no more than 10 seconds. One of the few exceptions to this rule applies to moving a patient. It may not be possible to perform CPR in a cramped bedroom or other small area. In that case, it is acceptable to move the patient so proper CPR can be performed. These actions must be kept as close to 10 seconds as possible.

Signs of Successful CPR

Signs of successful CPR include the following:

- Each time the sternum is compressed, you should feel a pulse in the carotid artery. It will feel like a flutter.
- Chest should rise and fall with each ventilation.
- Pupils may react or appear to be normal. (Pupils should constrict when exposed to light.)
- Heartbeat may return.
- Spontaneous gasp of breathing may occur.
- Skin color may improve or return to normal.

SKILL SUMMARY   *Changing Positions During CPR*

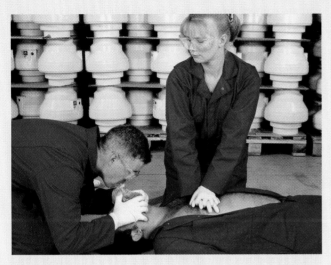

FIGURE 8-7A *The tired compression rescuer calls for a switch.*

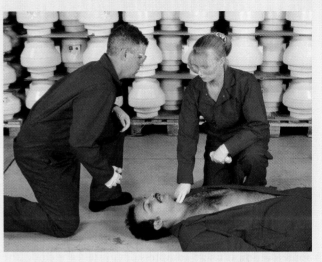

FIGURE 8-7B *The ventilation rescuer delivers a breath as usual, then moves to the patient's side. The second rescuer moves to the patient's head.*

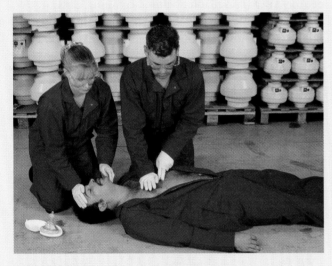

FIGURE 8-7C *The rescuer at the head opens the airway and checks respirations and pulse. The second rescuer prepares for compressions.*

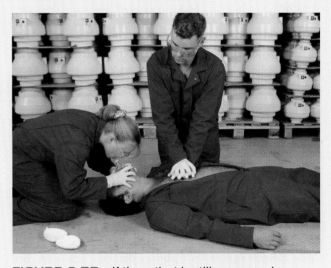

FIGURE 8-7D *If the patient is still unresponsive, breathless, and pulseless, they continue CPR.*

- Arms or legs may move.
- Patient may try to swallow.

Remember that "successful" CPR does not mean that the patient lives. "Successful" only means that you performed CPR correctly. Few patients will survive without defibrillation and/or **advanced cardiac life support (ACLS)**, such as that provided by paramedics and physicians. So, the goal of CPR is to prevent the death of cells and organs for a few crucial moments. Hopefully, advanced providers will arrive in time.

Mistakes in Performing CPR

The most common ventilation mistakes are as follows:

- Failing to maintain an adequate head tilt.
- Failing to maintain an adequate seal around the patient's mouth, nose, or both with a pocket face mask or face shield. The seal should be released when the patient exhales.
- Failing to watch and listen for exhalation.
- Providing breaths too rapidly or too forcefully.

First on Scene

CPR is a procedure that can help circulate blood and oxygen when a patient's heart has stopped. It helps keep the patient viable until defibrillation and advanced care becomes available. Alone, it will rarely start a stopped heart. Unfortunately, not all patients can be saved. If you perform CPR on a patient who ultimately dies, remember that it is not your fault. All you can do is perform CPR to the best of your ability. If you respond to a call where a patient dies—and that will happen—be sure to talk about it with someone you trust and, if needed, seek out stress counseling.

Some common chest compression mistakes include the following:

- Failing to keep your elbows straight. Instead, bending them.
- Failing to align your shoulders directly above the patient's sternum.
- Placing the heel of your bottom hand too low or not in line with the sternum (Figure 8-8).
- Failing to depress the sternum to the proper depth.
- Touching the patient's chest with your fingers instead of extending them.
- Pivoting at the knees instead of at your hips.
- Failing to perform compressions at the correct rate.
- Moving your hands from the compression site between compressions.
- Not releasing compressions fully between compressions.

Note: Several studies have shown that you can lose your CPR skills unless you have frequent practice and retraining. Retraining should occur often. Recertification should occur every one to two years.

Complications Caused by CPR

Even properly performed, CPR may cause rib fractures in some patients. Other complications that can occur with proper CPR include: fracture of the sternum, pneumothorax (collapse of the lungs caused by air in the chest), hemothorax (accumulation of blood in the chest), cuts and bruises to the lungs, and lacerations to the liver.

These complications are rare. However, you can help minimize the risk by giving careful attention to your performance. Remember that effective CPR is necessary, even if it results in complications. After all, the alternative is death.

In addition, note that the rib cartilage in elderly patients separates easily. You will hear it crunch as you compress. Be sure that your hand is positioned correctly and that you are compressing to the correct depth, but do not stop.

CPR for Infants and Children

Infants (up to one year old) and children (one year of age to the onset of puberty) need slightly different care. Cardiac arrest in them is rarely caused by heart problems. The heart nearly always stops beating because of too little oxygen due to injuries, suffocation, smoke inhalation, sudden infant death syndrome (SIDS), or infection.

See Chapters 6 and 7 for how to determine if your infant or child patient is unresponsive and breathless. Follow the directions there, too, for caring for an infant or child who is not breathing. Remember that according to AHA guidelines, you should resuscitate an infant or child for five cycles of compressions and ventilations (about two minutes) before you activate the EMS system. When children collapse suddenly, activate the EMS system and get the AED (if available) before beginning CPR.

Determining that your infant or child patient is pulseless is important. For an infant, check the brachial pulse on the inside of the upper arm between the elbow and shoulder. Press the artery gently with your index and middle fingers. Never use your thumb. In a child, check the pulse at the carotid artery. CPR guidelines also allow the use of the femoral artery for a pulse check.

It can be difficult to find a pulse in an infant or child. So, do not spend too much time trying to locate one. According to the AHA, if the infant or child is not breathing, heart rate is probably inadequate and chest compressions are usually necessary.

Note this important difference between adult CPR and CPR for infants and children: *The AHA recommends CPR for infants and children with a pulse below 60 beats per minute.* The reason is that these patients respond to a low oxygen level by exhibiting a slow pulse. This is a dire condition. CPR will benefit these patients because 60 beats per minute are not enough to sustain life.

Performing Infant or Child CPR

If the infant or child is breathless and pulseless or if the pulse is below 60 beats per minute, begin CPR. Follow these guidelines to perform chest compressions (Figures 8-9 and 8-10):

1. *Position the patient.* Make sure he is lying on a firm, flat surface. If the patient is an infant, put him in your lap with head tilted back slightly. Use your palm to support the baby's back. Make sure his head is not higher than the rest of the body.

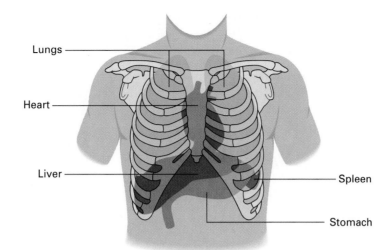

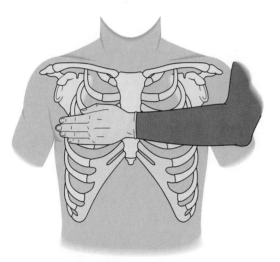

Too far right:
May fracture ribs and cause
lacerations to lung and liver.

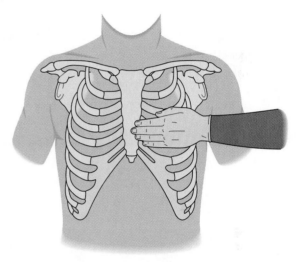

Too far left:
May fracture ribs and cause
lacerations to lung and heart.

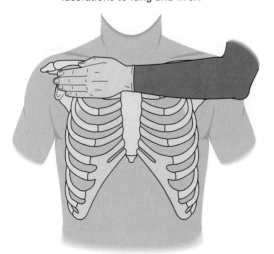

Too high:
May crack sternum.

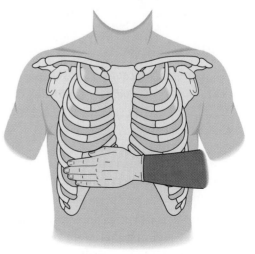

Too low:
May break off xiphoid process
and lacerate the liver.

FIGURE 8-8 Consequences of improper hand placement.

SKILL SUMMARY *Performing Infant and Child CPR*

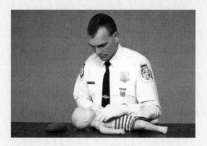

FIGURE 8-9A *Determine unresponsiveness with a "shake and shout" method.*

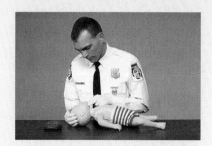

FIGURE 8-9B *Gently open the airway.*

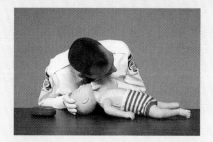

FIGURE 8-9C *Determine breathlessness.*

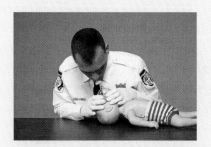

FIGURE 8-9D *Cover the infant's mouth and nose with a pocket mask. Ventilate until the chest rises.*

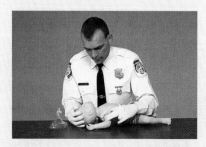

FIGURE 8-9E *Determine pulselessness at the brachial artery in an infant or carotid artery in a child.*

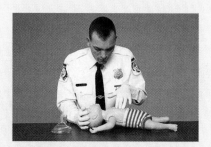

FIGURE 8-9F *Locate the correct hand position.*

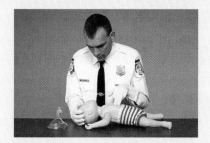

FIGURE 8-9G *Provide chest compressions at a rate of 100 per minute.*

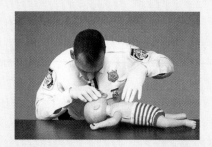

FIGURE 8-9H *Two breaths are given after every 30 compressions.*

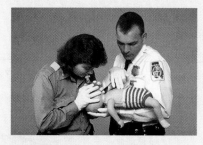

FIGURE 8-9I *VARIATION: Performing CPR while carrying the baby.*

2. *Locate the compression site.* For an infant or a child, the compression site is at the center of the chest just below the level of the nipples.

3. *Perform chest compressions.* For an infant, use the flat part of your middle and ring fingers to compress the infant's sternum one-third to one-half of the depth of the chest. The compression rate for an infant is 100 per minute.

For a child, you also will compress the sternum one-third to one-half of the depth of the chest, with the heel of one hand or, in larger children, two hands. The compression rate for a child is 100 compressions per minute.

The ratio of compressions to ventilations in both infants and children for one-rescuer CPR is 30:2 (30 compressions and two ventilations). The two-rescuer CPR ratio of compressions to ventilations is 15:2.

After five cycles of 30:2 (about two minutes), check for the return of a spontaneous pulse. If there is no pulse, activate the EMS system.

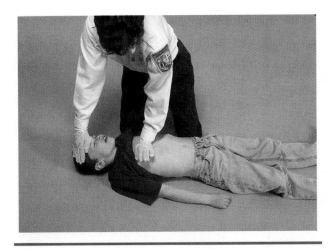

FIGURE 8-10 **Chest compressions on a larger child.**

Alternative Technique for Newborns

For a newborn, the AHA recommends two-rescuer CPR using the two-thumbs/circling-hands technique for compressions (Figure 8-11). This technique is preferred only for two rescuers because of the difficulty one rescuer would have switching between compressions and ventilations.

Locate the compression site just as you would for any infant. But instead of placing your fingers on the site, use two thumbs to perform the compressions. Place them side by side or, if the newborn is very small, one thumb on top of the other. Encircle the torso and support the back with the fingers of both hands.

Signs of Successful Infant or Child CPR

The methods of checking for successful CPR in infants and children are almost the same as for adults. That is, you should check the patient's pulse periodically. In the infant, check the brachial pulse. In the child, check the carotid pulse. Also check the pupils. CPR is successful if they are reacting normally or appear to be normal. Finally, watch for a spontaneous heartbeat, spontaneous breathing, and responsiveness.

Complications of Infant or Child CPR

One of the most common complications with injury and sudden illness in children is hypothermia (a below-normal body temperature). Keep the infant or child patient warm.

 :

1. How can you determine unresponsiveness in a patient?

2. After you determine unresponsiveness and breathlessness in your patient, what are your next steps?

3. What are the ratios of compressions to breaths for adult, child, and infant patients?

4. What are the rates of compressions for adult, child, and infant patients?

5. When is it appropriate to stop performing CPR on a patient?

SKILL SUMMARY *Performing Newborn CPR*

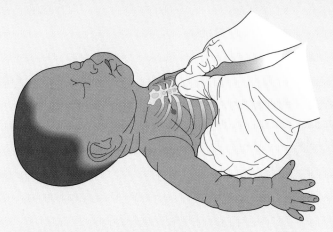

FIGURE 8-11A *For a newborn, perform compressions by placing two thumbs, side by side, at the center of the chest just below the level of the nipples.*

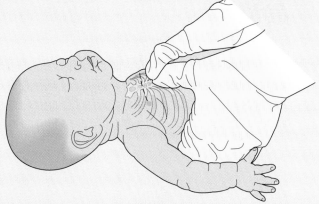

FIGURE 8-11B *If the newborn is very small, you may place one thumb on top of the other.*

The Call Follow-up

At the beginning of this chapter, you read that First Responders were performing CPR on a patient in cardiac arrest. To see how chapter skills apply to this emergency, read the following. It describes how the call was completed.

Physical Examination Our first concern was providing good CPR. Two men in my crew were doing that. A thorough physical exam would have to wait. The patient was on the grass and didn't appear to have any injuries from falling to the ground.

Patient History I talked to the bystander who had been performing CPR when we arrived. She told me that the patient had been mowing the lawn when he collapsed. She wasn't sure how long her neighbor had been down, but she thought it had been less than five minutes.

I went to the house to find the patient's wife. She told me that her husband was 71 and had bypass surgery two years ago after a heart attack. He was on medication for his heart and high blood pressure. She went to get it, as I radioed the incoming EMS units with an update.

Ongoing Assessment We monitored the patient. The AED reanalyzed the heart rhythm, but we still received a "no shock advised" message. All we could do at this point was perform CPR. We checked the carotid pulse during chest compressions, and the chest rise and fall during ventilations.

Patient Hand-off When the EMTs arrived, I gave them the hand-off report (see below). We helped the EMTs with CPR as they continued emergency care. They analyzed the heart rhythm once again and this time were advised to shock. The CPR and oxygen did some good. It took three shocks to get the patient's heart started again, but he still had no respirations. One of the EMTs continued to ventilate the patient while the others put him on a backboard. The backboard would give them a hard surface to compress against in case they had to start CPR again.

Later, the EMTs told me that the patient had improved slightly in the ambulance and was transferred to the cardiac unit at the hospital. Not all patients survive. I was happy we helped one who did.

Hand-off Report

"This is Sam Garfinkel, a 71-year-old male. He was found in cardiac arrest by a neighbor, who began CPR. The patient was unresponsive with no pulse or respirations when CPR was continued by our crew. Heart rhythm was analyzed with a "no shock advised" upon arrival and one subsequent assessment. I don't believe the patient has any injuries. He has a history of bypass surgery and high blood pressure, and took medication. Here are his medication vials."

The Last Word *Heart disease is still the number one killer in the U.S. Be prepared to provide CPR to any patient who needs it. Remember to* *take refresher courses frequently. And get recertified as per local protocol or every one or two years.*

Chapter Review

Focus on the EMS Team

Over the years, scientists have discovered that CPR has limitations. It is not nearly as effective as the patient's own heartbeat. This is why CPR procedure calls for you to activate EMS before beginning CPR on an adult. By doing so, you do two things: You give the ACLS rescuers as much time as possible to get to the scene. And you give your patient the best chance of getting the advanced care he needs in time to save his life.

Summing Up

- The basic components of the circulatory system are the heart, arteries, veins, capillaries, and blood.

- The heart, lungs, and brain work together closely to sustain life. When one cannot perform properly, the other two are handicapped. If one fails, the other two soon will follow.

- Reasons why a heart will stop include heart disease, stroke, allergic reaction, diabetes, prolonged seizures, and other medical conditions as well as serious injury. In infants and children, respiratory problems are the most common cause of cardiac arrest.

- The patient in respiratory and cardiac arrest has the best chance of surviving if all of the links in the chain of survival come together. Those links are early access, early CPR, early defibrillation, and early advanced care.

- Before providing CPR to a patient, you must first determine unresponsiveness, breathlessness, and pulselessness or the absence of any sign of circulation.

- To provide CPR, you must maintain an open airway, perform artificial ventilation, and provide artificial circulation by means of chest compressions.

- Chest compressions consist of rhythmic, repeated pressure over the lower half of the sternum. They cause blood to circulate as a result of the build-up of pressure in the chest cavity. When combined with artificial ventilation, they provide enough blood circulation to maintain life.

- CPR must begin as soon as possible and continue until the rescuer is exhausted and unable to continue, the patient is turned over to another trained rescuer or hospital staff, the patient is resuscitated, or the patient has been declared dead by a proper authority.

- The chart below summarizes the techniques of CPR.

CPR Summary

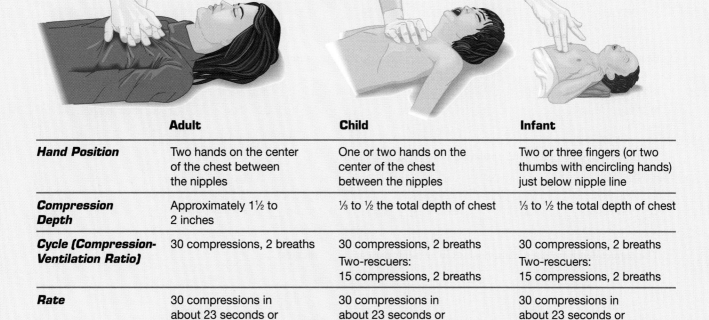

	Adult	**Child**	**Infant**
Hand Position	Two hands on the center of the chest between the nipples	One or two hands on the center of the chest between the nipples	Two or three fingers (or two thumbs with encircling hands) just below nipple line
Compression Depth	Approximately 1½ to 2 inches	⅓ to ½ the total depth of chest	⅓ to ½ the total depth of chest
Cycle (Compression-Ventilation Ratio)	30 compressions, 2 breaths	30 compressions, 2 breaths Two-rescuers: 15 compressions, 2 breaths	30 compressions, 2 breaths Two-rescuers: 15 compressions, 2 breaths
Rate	30 compressions in about 23 seconds or 100 per minute	30 compressions in about 23 seconds or 100 per minute	30 compressions in about 23 seconds or 100 per minute

Key Terms

advanced cardiac life support (ACLS) prehospital emergency care that involves the use of intravenous fluids, drug infusions, cardiac monitoring, manual defibrillation, intubations, and other advanced procedures.

atria the two upper chambers of the heart. Singular *atrium.*

cardiac arrest the cessation of circulation.

cardiopulmonary resuscitation (CPR) heart-lung resuscitation procedure; combined compression and ventilation techniques that maintain circulation and breathing in a patient.

chain of survival term used by the American Heart Association for a series of interventions that provide the best chance of survival for the cardiac-arrest patient.

palpate feel; sense by touch.

pulse the wave of blood propelled through the arteries as a result of the pumping action of the heart.

respiratory arrest the cessation of spontaneous breathing.

ventricles the two lower chambers of the heart.

Knowledge Check

1. To establish pulselessness in an unresponsive adult or child, palpate the ___ pulse first.
   a. carotid
   b. brachial
   c. radial
   d. tibial

2. To establish pulselessness in an unresponsive infant, palpate the ___ pulse.
   a. carotid
   b. brachial
   c. radial
   d. tibial

3. Compressions for an adult patient are performed at a rate of ___ per minute.
   a. 60
   b. 80
   c. 100
   d. 120

4. The one-rescuer compression/ventilation ratio for all patients is:
   a. 5:1
   b. 15:2
   c. 20:2
   d. 30:2

5. The correct depth for chest compressions in an adult patient is ___ inch(es).
   a. 1
   b. 1 to 1.5
   c. 1.5 to 2
   d. 2 to 2.5

6. Infants and children should be given CPR if their pulse is less than ___ beats per minute.
   a. 120
   b. 100
   c. 80
   d. 60

7. Most patients who receive CPR live.
   a. True
   b. False

8. During CPR, a chest compression may cause a pulse in the carotid artery.
   a. True
   b. False

9. For what reason must you hold your fingers off a patient's chest while performing compressions?

   _____

   _____

10. If you positioned your hands on the patient's chest incorrectly, what would be the likely result of the chest compressions? Write your answers beside each incorrect location.
    a. Too far to the right: _____
    b. Too far to the left: _____
    c. Too high: _____
    d. Too low: _____

Scenario

You are at your office. You are a volunteer First Responder in your community. You hear a commotion and look over to find an older coworker on the floor. Several employees are standing around. You approach, examine the patient, and find him unresponsive and pulseless. Your building has a defibrillator by the elevator about two minutes away.

a. As a First Responder, what are your initial tasks and decisions?

   _____

   _____

b. Which tasks would you delegate? Which would you perform yourself?

   _____

   _____

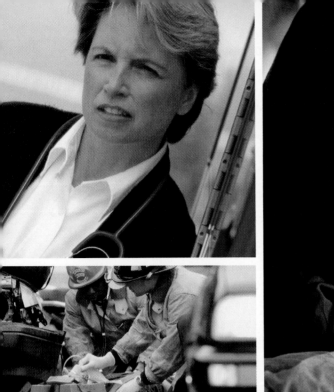
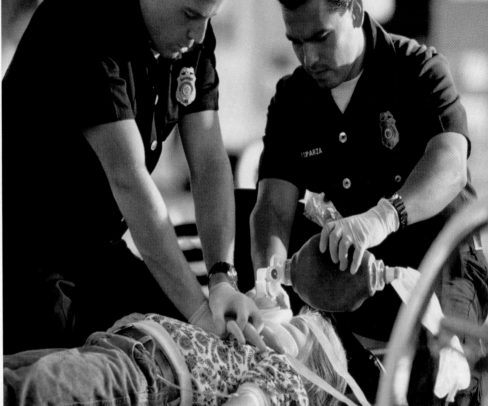

9 | Automated External Defibrillation

Objectives

From the U.S. Department of Transportation (DOT) 1995 "First Responder: National Standard Curriculum." Material supplemental to the DOT curriculum is listed under "Enrichment."

Cognitive

No objectives are identified by the DOT.

Affective

No objectives are identified by the DOT.

Psychomotor

No objectives are identified by the DOT.

Enrichment

- List the indications and contraindications for automated external defibrillation. (pp. 169–171)
- Differentiate between fully automated and the semi-automated external defibrillators. (pp. 167–168)

- List the steps in the operation of an automated external defibrillator. (pp. 171–173)
- Describe the care for a patient whose pulse has returned after automated external defibrillation. (p. 173)
- Discuss the need to complete the automated defibrillator operator's shift checklist. (p. 173)
- Explain the role medical direction plays in the use of automated external defibrillation. (p. 173)
- Describe the maintenance of an automated external defibrillator. (p. 173)

Introduction

As you will recall from Chapter 8, early defibrillation is part of the "chain of survival." To get defibrillation to patients early enough, as many trained people as possible—not just physicians and paramedics—must be able to perform this life-saving skill. Automated external defibrillators (AEDs) have made that possible. Now First Responders, EMT-Basics, and even members of the public can defibrillate a patient when it is needed.

Section 1 About Defibrillation

What Is an AED?

Defibrillation is the process by which an electric shock is applied to the chest of a patient who is in cardiac arrest—an unresponsive, nonbreathing, pulseless patient—in order to correct fatal heart rhythms. For many years, science has known that certain patients in cardiac arrest require prompt defibrillation if they are to survive. Each minute the heart is stopped significantly reduces a patient's chances of survival. Science is clear: cardiac-arrest patients cannot wait for a paramedic or physician to arrive on scene to interpret heart rhythms, decide if electric shocks are needed, and then manually defibrillate with "paddles." Something faster is needed.

Today, the concept of automated external defibrillation extends to First Responders, EMTs, and the public. With **public access defibrillation (PAD)**, you will now see defibrillators on airplanes, in shopping malls, in office buildings, and in other public places.

The **automated external defibrillator (AED)** has a microprocessor that actually interprets heart rhythms, just as a physician or paramedic would. When necessary, the AED delivers shocks directly to the patient by way of adhesive pads. These pads are connected to the AED through cables, which can transmit a shock to the chest powerful enough to correct a lethal heart rhythm. The pads make defibrillation safer, since no one needs to touch the patient at all during analysis or shocks.

EMS systems that allow First Responders to use AEDs should have all of the following in place:

- *All of the links in the "chain of survival."* Without early access, early CPR, and early advanced care, the patient will not have the best chance of survival (Figure 9-1).

- *Medical direction.* A physician must issue standing orders for First Responders to use an AED.

- *Quality improvement programs* to monitor the use of AEDs in the field.

- *Mandatory continuing education and practice* in defibrillation techniques.

Types of AEDs

There are two types of automated defibrillator. One is fully automated. The other is semi-automated. The operator of a fully automated machine attaches it to the patient and turns it on, and it does all the rest. The semi-automated external defibrillator is most common and performs the same tasks, but the operator must push a button to analyze the patient's heart rhythm

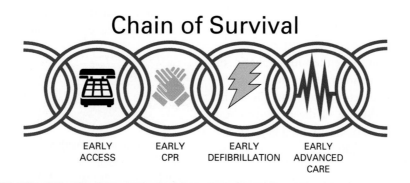

Chain of Survival

EARLY ACCESS   EARLY CPR   EARLY DEFIBRILLATION   EARLY ADVANCED CARE

FIGURE 9-1 All four links of the "chain of survival" should be in place.

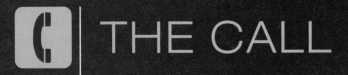

THE CALL

 Dispatch Our engine company was sent on a call to an unresponsive woman.

 Scene Size-up We approached the scene carefully and saw a man frantically waving to us. When we got to the house, the man said his neighbor, a nurse, was performing CPR. We saw her working on an elderly woman who was lying on the lawn. "My wife collapsed while she was carrying in the groceries," the man said. "Please help her. Please!"

We decided to call for the medics right away. After putting on our gloves and grabbing a pocket face mask, we joined the nurse at CPR. She was doing a good job.

Initial Assessment We checked the patient's pulse and respirations. There were none.

Cardiac arrest is literally a life-or-death situation. Consider this patient as you read Chapter 9. See if you can decide if she needs defibrillation or not.

and to deliver the shock. Many newer devices will analyze automatically, which usually takes about 5 to 15 seconds.

There are many brands of AED (Figure 9-2). Many of them include the following features: An on/off button, which controls power to the AED. A shock button that, when pressed, delivers an electric shock to the patient. At the appropriate time, a voice synthesizer will prompt the operator to perform specific actions, such as "analyze rhythm" or "push to shock." Some AEDs have an optional built-in digital data recorder, which documents the events of a cardiac arrest, including the time, cardiac rhythms, and shocks delivered, all data that can be used for training and quality improvement at a later date. Even though First Responders do not analyze heart rhythms, some AEDs also have a built-in screen or light that shows the electrical activity of the heart.

Defibrillators may also be either monophasic or biphasic. Monophasic defibrillators deliver shocks at 360 joules. In contrast, biphasic defibrillators can gauge the thickness and electrical resistance of the patient's chest and deliver a more exact dose of electricity. They can deliver shocks at 120 joules to 200 joules, depending on manufacturer and technology.

The number of joules, timing, and sequence of shocks delivered by an AED are preprogrammed into the device before you use it.

Q:
1. What is defibrillation?
2. What does an automated external defibrillator (AED) do?
3. What are some of the features of an AED?

Section 2 Operating a Defibrillator

AEDs are very safe and accurate. Even so, you must follow operation guidelines carefully. They will ensure safe and proper use of the defibrillator. Make time to become familiar with the AED you are to use. At the start of each shift, check your defibrillator. Many do self-checks and indicate when there is a problem.

 First Responder Practice

Never be in contact with a patient during AED analysis or when a shock is being delivered. And, if you are the First Responder responsible for delivering the shock, make sure everyone else is clear of the patient, too.

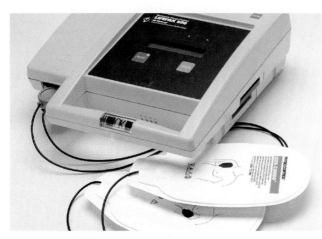

a. *An adult AED.* (Physio Control Corporation)

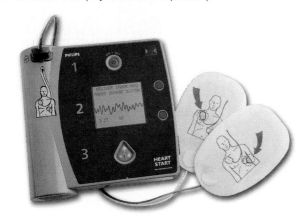

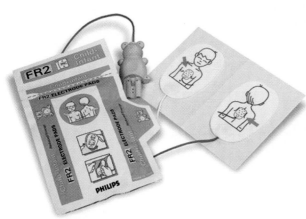

b. *An AED with dual connections: one for adults and one for pediatric patients.* (Philips)

FIGURE 9-2 Examples of automated external defibrillators.

On scene, carefully follow your local protocols on the use of an AED. Make sure no one touches the patient while the AED is analyzing a heart rhythm or while a shock is being delivered. If someone is in contact, the shock could be transferred to that person. Touching the patient or the cables also can cause interference with

the accuracy of the AED. Finally, do not apply the AED to a patient with a pulse. The shock could cause the patient's heart to stop.

According to AHA guidelines, AEDs should be used on any patient older than one year of age in cardiac arrest. To defibrillate patients between the ages of one and eight years of age, the preferred device has pediatric pads or settings. If a pediatric defibrillator is not available, the AHA recommends using an adult defibrillator and pads rather than not defibrillating at all.

Heart Rhythms

The normal electrical impulses of the heart occur in an orderly, rhythmic fashion. When you place an AED on a patient, it evaluates his heart rhythm (Figure 9-3). Heart rhythms that require a shock from the AED are:

- *Ventricular fibrillation.* This is a chaotic, unorganized heart rhythm. It cannot create a pulse or circulate blood to sustain life.

- *Ventricular tachycardia.* This rhythm is more organized but very rapid and inefficient. It is capable of producing a pulse. (Note that AED shocks must only be delivered to patients with no pulse.)

Heart rhythms that do not require an AED shock are:

- *Pulseless electrical activity (PEA).* If you were to look at an electrocardiogram (ECG) displaying this rhythm, you might think nothing was wrong. You would find electrical activity on the display, but you would not find a pulse.

- *Asystole.* Also known as "flatline," this is a condition where there are no electrical impulses present and, therefore, no pulse. The ECG shows a flat line.

If your AED displays a patient's heart rhythms on the screen, you must be careful not to base your decision to shock a patient solely on it. Remember that an AED does not check a pulse. It is the AED's rhythm analysis plus your pulse determination that makes for a safe and accurate decision to defibrillate or not. Always follow your local protocols when determining a candidate for defibrillation. If you have questions, contact medical direction. Also be sure to practice AED procedures frequently and attend continuing education sessions.

(See ideal positioning of responders and patient in Figure 9-4.)

Operation Guidelines

There are two different situations in which you will use an AED. The first is for a patient who has experienced a witnessed arrest and CPR is in progress or down time is

Chaotic electrical discharge as occurs
in heart muscle wall.

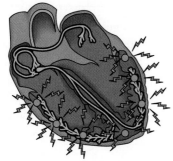

Ventricular tachycardia.

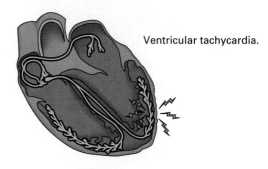

Chaotic electrical discharge as seen on an ECG tracing.

ECG tracing of ventricular tachycardia.

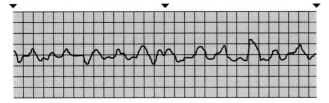

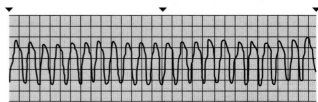

a. *Ventricular fibrillation.*

b. *Ventricular tachycardia.*

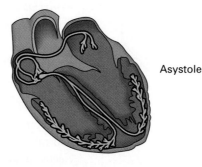

Asystole

ECG tracing of asystole, the absence of electrical activity

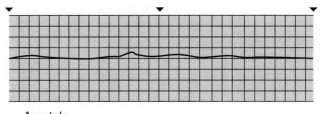

c. *Asystole.*

FIGURE 9-3 The electrical impulses of the heart, or heart rhythms, are monitored and analyzed by an AED.

less than four to five minutes. For that patient, apply the AED immediately. The second situation in which you will use an AED is for a patient who has been down longer than five minutes and CPR has not yet been performed. In this case, CPR should be performed for about five cycles of 30:2 before attaching the AED.

Using an AED is a definitive step toward returning a patient's heart to a normal rhythm and function. CPR is vital, but its main purpose is to prolong life until defibrillation can be performed.

Applying Adhesive Pads
The AED monitors heart rhythm and delivers shocks through the adhesive pads (Figure 9-5). So, the pads must be placed in very specific locations. Remember, all directions refer to the *patient's* right and left, not yours.

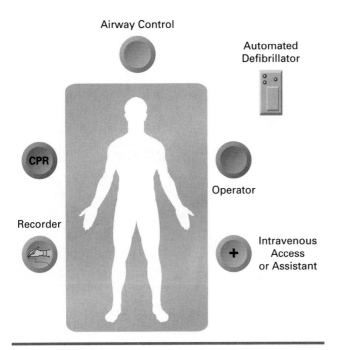

Airway Control

Automated Defibrillator

CPR

Operator

Recorder

Intravenous Access or Assistant

FIGURE 9-4 Ideal crew positioning. (Alternatives may be needed.)

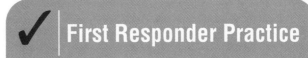

First Responder Practice

When you are called to the scene of a patient in cardiac arrest, you will feel considerable stress, especially if you have not been on many such calls. The old adage "practice makes perfect" applies here. If you practice with your AED frequently and if you know AED protocols well, you will be able to perform at your best.

Place one pad just below the patient's right clavicle and to the right of the sternum. Place the other pad over the patient's left lower ribs. The memory aid "white to right, red to ribs" may help you remember where the pads and cables are to be placed. Most pads also have a placement diagram on the pad itself.

Occasionally, you will find patients who have medication patches on their chests (nitroglycerin or nicotine patches, for example). Do not place pads on or near them. Arcing or burning of the patient's skin could occur. The patches also can prevent the effective transfer of electricity to the patient's chest. Instead, remove the patches and use a towel to wipe off any paste that remains.

Be sure the AED's adhesive pads are not positioned over a pacemaker. It is possible to observe or feel a pace-

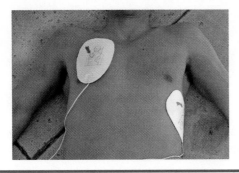

FIGURE 9-5 The AED monitors heart rhythms and delivers shocks through its adhesive pads.

maker once you bare the patient's chest. Or you may be told by a family member that the patient has one. Place the AED's adhesive pads so they are not touching the pacemaker.

Adhesive pads should be securely applied to the chest. This may not be possible if the patient is extremely hairy. Be sure to carry a razor with your AED. Use it to quickly but safely shave the areas where the pads are to adhere. If you do not have a razor, apply the pads. If they are not in contact with the chest, the AED will advise "check electrodes." In response, remove the pads. Much of the hair will come off with them. Place a new pair of pads on the patient and reanalyze.

Operating the AED

If CPR is in progress, stop it. Then check the patient's pulse and respirations (Figure 9-6). If the patient is pulseless, attach the AED. If there will be a delay in administering a shock, resume CPR. Then, turn on the AED power. Stop CPR and instruct everyone to clear the patient. When all are clear, press the "analyze" button.

If the AED does NOT advise a shock, then recheck the patient's pulse. If the pulse is not present, perform CPR for two minutes (five cycles of 30:2), and then reanalyze the heart rhythm. If a pulse is present, check respirations and assist with ventilations, if needed.

If the AED advises a shock, make sure everyone is clear and deliver the shock. After the shock, perform CPR for two minutes. Even if the patient has a pulse, it often takes a few minutes to restore circulation and respiration. Then check for a pulse. If there is no pulse, the AED will reanalyze the rhythm. Voice prompts should advise you to do this. The AED will then reanalyze the patient's heart rhythm and deliver a shock, if necessary.

If a pulse is present, check respirations. Remember, the patient most likely will have inadequate breathing at this point, if he or she is breathing at all. If there is no

SKILL SUMMARY   *Using an AED*

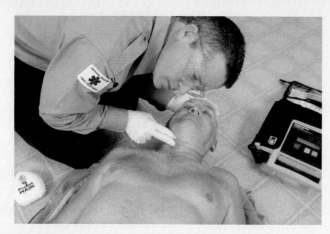

FIGURE 9-6A *Determine the patient is breathless and pulseless.*

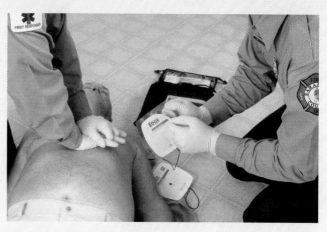

FIGURE 9-6B *Have your partner initiate CPR while you prepare the AED.*

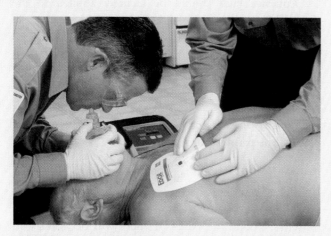

FIGURE 9-6C *Place electrodes on the patient's chest.*

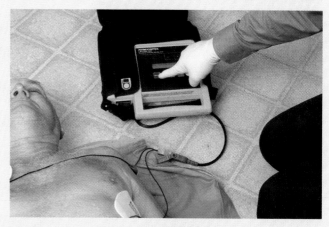

FIGURE 9-6D *Turn on the AED.*

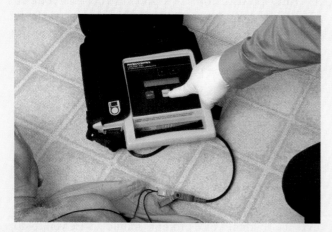

FIGURE 9-6E *Stop CPR and get clear of the patient as the AED analyzes heart rhythm.*

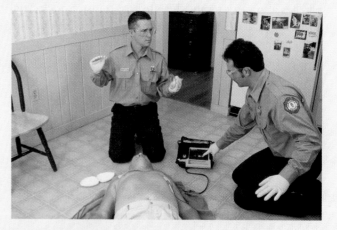

FIGURE 9-6F *If a shock is advised, clear all others from the patient and deliver the shock.*

pulse, begin CPR for two minutes (five cycles of 30:2). Then check the pulse again. If there is still no pulse, press the "analyze" button. Deliver one shock if advised by the AED. Repeat this sequence as allowed by local protocols. Transportation should occur after two shocks, when an ambulance is at the scene.

Note: Always follow your local protocols for defibrillation policies and protocols. Older defibrillators may not be programmed for the new standards. Their voice prompts and defibrillation sequence may be outdated. Find out if AEDs near you have been reprogrammed.

If you are alone and find an unresponsive patient, your actions depend on whether or not you witnessed the patient go into cardiac arrest or if down time is less than one or two minutes. Follow these guidelines:

■ *If you suspect a short down time (or see a witnessed arrest) and your AED is immediately available,* apply the AED and analyze the heart rhythm immediately. Do not begin CPR first. Defibrillation is more important at this point and more beneficial to the patient. Then follow the instructions outlined above in response to the AED's prompts.

■ *If the patient was down before your arrival* and may have been down longer than four or five minutes, perform CPR for two minutes. Then apply the AED and follow the instructions outlined above in response to the AED's prompts.

Post-Resuscitation Care

In some, but not all cases, your patient will regain a pulse. This is exciting, but there is much more to be done. Your patient is still in serious condition. Remember the following points when caring for a patient whose pulse has returned:

■ Monitor the pulse carefully. It may disappear.

■ Many patients will not breathe, even though a pulse has returned. This is common. Ventilate the patient as necessary.

■ If your patient has regained a pulse and adequate respirations—and has not been injured, place him or her in a recovery position.

■ Apply high-concentration oxygen, if you are trained and allowed by local protocol. If the patient is breathing adequately, use a nonrebreather mask. If the patient is breathing inadequately or not at all, ventilate with a BVM or pocket face mask.

■ Keep the AED attached to the patient. EMS personnel who take over care will want it attached during transport.

■ Your assessment of the patient should be ongoing until you turn over care.

It will help the patient if advanced care is available. Arrange for ACLS personnel to respond to the scene, if you have not done so already. Whether the advanced care is performed by them or by physicians, advanced care includes medications and other interventions that will help stabilize the patient and prevent another cardiac arrest. If the ACLS team cannot respond in a reasonable amount of time, an ambulance should transport the patient promptly to the nearest hospital emergency department.

Call Review

After using an AED, the call should be reviewed by a quality improvement committee to determine if protocols were followed. (Your medical director will be involved.) This review uses the run report and, if your AED was equipped, the recording of the call. While the call review looks for problem areas, it is not designed to get people into trouble. If needed, the committee may recommend further training for some or all rescuers who use AEDs. The goal of the review is to have trained First Responders providing quality care to patients.

AED Maintenance

The AED is a vital piece of equipment. It would be devastating to arrive at the side of a patient in cardiac arrest with a one that doesn't work. It may also be a cause of liability against you and your agency. So check your AED at the beginning of every shift. Many AEDs have a "self-check" feature and indicate by means of a light that the unit is charged and ready. Also make sure the leads are with the unit and there are several sets of adhesive pads available. Always treat the AED carefully. Do not expose it to unnecessary jarring or other rough moves. Finally, follow the manufacturer's guidelines for maintenance.

Q:

1. What are the two types of heart rhythm that require an AED shock?

2. How should you place AED adhesive pads on a chest that is very hairy?

3. If the AED advises not to administer a shock, what should you do next?

4. If you determine that your patient is unresponsive and you are alone but have an AED, what should you do?

▶▶ The Call Follow-up

At the beginning of this chapter, you read that First Responders were at the scene of a patient in respiratory and cardiac arrest. To see how chapter skills apply to this emergency, read the following. It describes how the call was completed.

Initial Assessment *(continued)* I had the AED. It took only a few seconds to hook up the electrodes and cables while CPR continued. I turned on the AED and instructed everyone to clear the patient while it analyzed the heart rhythm. The machine advised me to press the shock button.

After making sure everyone was clear, I shocked the patient. The AED advised me to perform CPR for two minutes. I did and then checked the pulse. I couldn't believe it. There it was. We immediately checked the patient's respirations. There were none. We hooked oxygen into the pocket face mask and ventilated her.

Patient History The patient's husband, Mr. Jones, told us that his wife was in good health. She hadn't been to a doctor in years. She took no medications. She had no complaints before she went down. They had sandwiches for dinner two hours

ago. She had no allergies. "She was always so healthy. I just don't understand," he said.

Physical Examination We checked quickly for any obvious signs of injury and found none.

Ongoing Assessment We never got to the ongoing assessment. The medics were already on scene.

Patient Hand-off We gave our hand-off report to the medics (see below) and they began advanced life support. They started intravenous lines (IVs), put in airway adjuncts, and gave medications. The patient went back into cardiac arrest once while they were caring for her. They used their manual defibrillator and got her pulse back with one shock. She made it to the hospital with a pulse, but the doctors said her heart and brain had suffered too much damage to survive.

After a day in the cardiac unit, Mrs. Jones passed away. We were sad to hear it and disappointed, but we realized that we had done the best we could. Many patients don't live. I know that. The next time maybe we'll get to shake the hand of the person we help when they walk out of the hospital.

Hand-off Report

"This is Georgia Jones. She is 66 and was carrying groceries into the house when she collapsed on the grass. A nurse who lives next door started CPR. She was doing a good job. We hooked up the AED and gave a shock, which caused the pulse to return, but no respirations. We ventilated the patient and monitored her pulse until you arrived. Mrs. Jones hasn't been to the doctor recently, has no meds, and no allergies. Her husband says she is in good health, and there were no problems before she collapsed. There are no obvious injuries from the fall. She had a sandwich two hours ago for dinner."

The Last Word *The AED has tremendous potential to save lives. But there are some patients who cannot be saved. Losing a patient is a difficult experience. Focus on the good you have done for prior patients and the good you will do* *for future ones. Also seek out experienced members of your agency. They undoubtedly felt the same at some point in their careers. If necessary, speak to your medical director about the call.*

Chapter Review

Focus on the EMS Team

Nothing represents teamwork more than the chain of survival. It means that for the best chance of survival, a patient will experience a true team effort from community resource personnel to First Responders, advanced cardiac life support (ACLS) personnel, and hospital staff. As a First Responder, you are a critical part of the chain of survival. By providing CPR, oxygenation, and defibrillation at the earliest possible moment, you bring the most critical elements of survival to your patients every day.

Yet, not all patients live. In fact, many don't. They have been down too long or damage is too severe. Here is another time when a team comes into play: When you may be sad or discouraged about a patient who did not live, talk it over with other members of your team. They will help you understand that it was not your fault. It is important that you remain a part of the team, ready to respond to the next emergency.

Summing Up

- EMS systems that allow First Responders to use AEDs should have all of the following in place: all of the links in the "chain of survival," medical direction, quality improvement programs to monitor AED use, and mandatory continuing education and practice in defibrillation techniques.

- AEDs may be used on any patient older than one year of age. AEDs that can deliver shocks at pediatric levels as well as adult levels are preferred.

- Indications for defibrillation include the AED's rhythm analysis plus determining that a patient is pulseless. Always follow your local protocols when determining a candidate for defibrillation.

- If you witness a patient go into cardiac arrest, the use of the defibrillator should be your first action. If you find the patient already down and you believe he may have been down for more than four or five minutes, perform CPR first and then use the defibrillator.

- The AED monitors heart rhythm and delivers shocks through the adhesive pads. Placement of the pads is "white to right, red to ribs" on the patient's dry bare chest.

- In general, operation of an AED is as follows: Determine breathlessness and pulselessness in your patient. Have your partner initiate CPR while you prepare the AED. Place the electrodes on the patient's chest. Turn on the AED. Stop CPR and get clear of the patient as the AED analyzes his heart rhythm. If a shock is advised, clear everyone from the patient and deliver the shock. *Always follow your local protocols on AED operation.*

- If you are alone and find an unresponsive patient, your actions depend on certain factors, such as whether or not you witnessed the cardiac arrest. *Follow all local protocols and policies related to defibrillation of a patient.*

- Even when the patient regains a pulse and is breathing adequately, keep the AED attached until more highly trained EMS personnel take over patient care.

- After an AED is used, the call should be reviewed by a quality improvement committee, including your system's medical director.

- Follow the manufacturer's guidelines for maintenance of your AED, and check it at the beginning of every shift.

Key Terms

automated external defibrillator (AED) an electrical apparatus that can detect fatal heart rhythms and deliver a shock through the patient's chest.

defibrillation the process by which an electric shock is applied to the chest of a patient who is in cardiac arrest in order to correct fatal heart rhythms.

public access defibrillation (PAD) the availability of fully automated external defibrillators in public and/or private places where large numbers of people gather or where people at high risk for heart attacks live.

Knowledge Check

1. Automated external defibrillators are able to check:

   a. pulse.
   b. respiration.
   c. electrical activity of the heart.
   d. all of the above.

2. A heart rhythm that should be shocked by an AED is:

   a. pulseless electrical activity.
   b. ventricular fibrillation.
   c. atrial fibrillation.
   d. asystole (flatline).

3. You are alone and respond to a patient in cardiac arrest at your workplace. You have an AED and arrive within two or three minutes of the collapse. After determining pulselessness, you should:

   a. perform one minute of CPR.
   b. contact medical direction for advice.
   c. apply the AED's adhesive pads and analyze the rhythm.
   d. perform CPR until another rescuer arrives to operate the AED.

4. An AED's adhesive pads are usually placed:

   a. on upper right chest and on upper left chest.
   b. on upper left chest and over lower right ribs.
   c. below the left clavicle and on the xiphoid process.
   d. below the right clavicle and over the left lower ribs.

5. You apply the AED to a pulseless patient and press the "analyze" button. The AED tells you to "check patient, no shock advised." You should:

   a. immediately begin CPR.
   b. press the "analyze" button again.
   c. deliver one shock.
   d. replace the defective electrodes.

6. While you are providing CPR, your partner is positioning the AED pads on the patient. Suddenly, your partner says, "Clear!" What should you do next?

   a. Deliver a shock to the patient.
   b. Check the patient's respirations and pulse.
   c. Stop CPR and move away from the patient.
   d. Press the AED's "analyze" button.

7. Touching the patient while the AED is analyzing the heart rhythm:

   a. is acceptable with the newest defibrillators.
   b. can cause the AED to misinterpret the rhythm.
   c. may be necessary to maintain cardiac function.
   d. requires specially made protective gloves.

8. While preparing the AED, what should you do for the cardiac-arrest patient who is wearing a nitroglycerin patch on her chest?

   a. Remove the patch.
   b. Place the AED pads far from it.
   c. Position an AED pad directly on it.
   d. Do not use the AED on this patient.

9. A patient who has been resuscitated from a cardiac arrest with an AED requires:

   a. periodic chest compressions.
   b. one more set of shocks.
   c. artificial ventilation.
   d. ongoing pulse checks.

10. One type of automated defibrillator requires a rescuer to do nothing but attach its pads to the patient and turn it on. The device will do all the rest, including delivering a shock.

    a. True
    b. False

11. Your patient has received two shocks and her pulse has returned. She also is breathing adequately. After you place her in a recovery position, you should remove the AED pads from her chest and turn off the AED.

    a. True
    b. False

12. Why is there a difference between defibrillation procedures for witnessed arrests and for patients who have been down prior to your arrival?

_____

_____

_____

13. Which has the greatest potential to restart a stopped heart, defibrillation or CPR? Why?

_____

_____

_____

Scenario

You have been called to the scene of an unresponsive patient. When you arrive, you take BSI precautions and determine the scene is safe to enter. You also note that someone is performing CPR on an elderly woman, who is lying on the ground.

a. What should you do first?

_____

_____

b. After you attach the AED and turn on the power, what should you do next?

_____

_____

c. When the AED does NOT advise a shock, you find the patient is still pulseless. You should:

_____

_____

d. The AED has advised you three times to shock the patient. After the third shock, the patient regains a pulse and begins to breathe. What is your post-resuscitation care?

_____

_____

_____

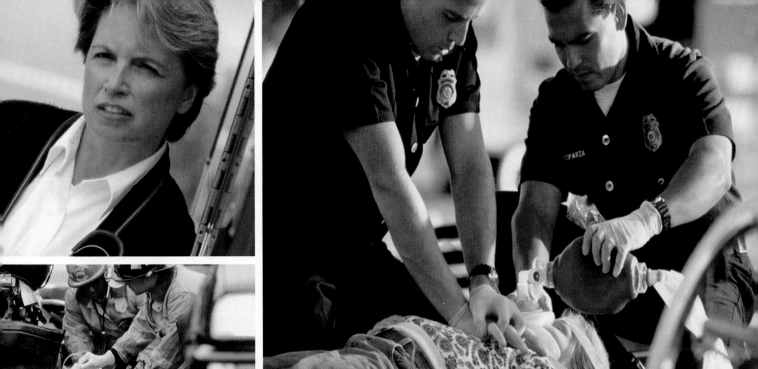

10 | Scene Size-up

Objectives

From the U.S. Department of Transportation (DOT) 1995 "First Responder:
National Standard Curriculum."

Cognitive

3-1.1 ▶ Discuss the components of scene size-up. (p. 179)

3-1.2 ▶ Describe common hazards found at the scene of a
trauma and a medical patient. (pp. 180–182)

3-1.3 ▶ Determine if the scene is safe to enter. (pp. 180–182)

3-1.4 ▶ Discuss common mechanisms of injury/nature of
illness. (pp. 182–190)

3-1.5 ▶ Discuss the reason for identifying the total number of
patients at the scene. (p. 191)

3-1.6 ▶ Explain the reason for identifying the need for additional
help or assistance. (p. 191)

Affective

3-1.22 ▶ Explain the rationale for crew members to evaluate
scene safety prior to entering. (pp. 180–182)

3-1.23 ▶ Serve as a model for others by explaining how patient
situations affect your evaluation of the mechanism of
injury or illness. (pp. 182–190)

Psychomotor

3-1.33 ▶ Demonstrate the ability to differentiate various scenarios and identify potential hazards. (pp. 179–182)

Introduction

Scene size-up is the first step a First Responder should take at the emergency scene. It includes three separate tasks: ensuring personal safety, identifying the mechanism of injury or nature of illness, and determining necessary resources. Never skipped or rushed, a good scene size-up will help you to ensure a safe and efficiently handled call.

Section 1 Overview of Scene Size-up

Scene size-up is an overall assessment of the emergency scene (Figure 10-1). It is the first step in the First Responder's patient assessment plan. It starts with taking the appropriate BSI precautions and assessing scene safety—before entering the scene. Next is identifying what caused an injury (mechanism of injury) or noting the signs of illness (nature of illness). Both the mechanism of injury and the nature of illness will help you focus on the type of care your patient will need.

The final component of scene size-up is determining and calling for the additional or specialized help you may need at the scene. This could include power company personnel for downed wires, multiple ambulances, fire or rescue personnel, or hazardous materials teams. Most likely, you will not have contact with your patient during scene size-up. Even so, your observations, decisions, and the actions you take at this time will set the foundation for the entire call.

1. What are the three major steps you should take in performing a scene size-up?

Section 2 Ensuring Personal Safety

The first step in scene size-up is to assess and ensure personal safety (Figure 10-2). That includes taking BSI precautions and determining if the scene is safe to enter.

BSI Precautions

BSI precautions must be taken on every call. First, observe the scene and the patient. If you see that the patient has been injured and has minor bleeding, put on protective gloves. If you observe serious bleeding or bleeding around the mouth that could spray you—or if you observe that the patient is vomiting or suspect a respiratory disease such as tuberculosis—protect yourself with eyewear and a mask or a face shield. (See Chapter 2 for a full discussion of BSI precautions.)

Personal protective equipment (PPE) used for BSI includes:

- *Gloves.* Wear them when there is any chance of coming in contact with a patient's blood or body fluids.

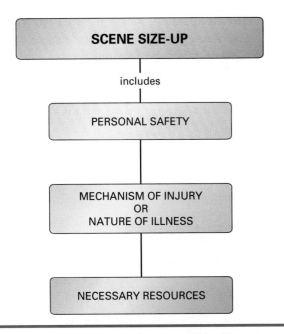

FIGURE 10-1 Scene size-up consists of ensuring personal safety, identifying the mechanism or nature of illness, and determining what resources are needed on scene.

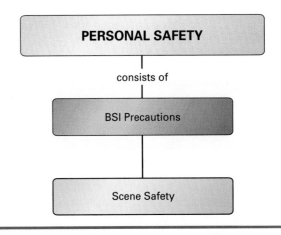

FIGURE 10-2 Before you enter an emergency scene, you must ensure your personal safety.

THE CALL

Dispatch I am a First Responder for the Fire Department. My partner and I were dispatched to a car crash at the corner of Central and Devine. The caller indicated that the crash involved one car only and that it seemed "pretty bad."

Scene Size-up When we approached the scene, we saw the caller was correct. It was a head-on into a telephone pole.

The scene size-up on this call will be very important, since car crashes can be dangerous. Not only might the crash vehicle be unstable, but other elements of the scene—such as the telephone pole and its lines as well as the oncoming traffic—can also pose hazards. How should these First Responders proceed? Consider what they should do as you read Chapter 10.

- *Face shield or protective eyewear and mask.* Wear them when there is any chance of blood or body fluids spraying or splashing into your eyes, nose, or mouth.

- *Gown.* Wear a disposable gown when there is any chance of clothing becoming soiled with blood or other body fluids.

Remember that you should always have personal protective equipment available. When you approach the scene, anticipate which items may be needed and then put them on. Waiting too long may cause you to become so involved in patient care that you forget to protect yourself.

Scene Safety

Nothing is more important at the emergency scene than your own safety. Hazards may be obvious, such as violence, downed power lines, or hazardous materials. But do not overlook the not so obvious dangers, such as those related

to car crashes, unstable vehicles, unstable surfaces (slopes, ice, and so on), and dangerous pets. Place your safety first. If you do not, you may become a patient yourself.

The vast majority of calls go by uneventfully. When there is danger, three words sum up the actions required to respond appropriately: *plan, observe,* and *react* (Figure 10-3).

Plan

Many First Responders work together to prevent danger and know what to do when danger strikes. However, scene safety begins long before the actual emergency. For example, as soon as you start your shift, you should:

- *Put on safe clothing.* Nonslip shoes and other practical clothing will help you respond to danger without restriction.

- *Prepare your equipment properly.* Make sure it is not cumbersome. Remember that you will be carrying it into emergencies. If your first-response kit is too heavy or large, it will distract your attention from where it should be—on observing the scene.

- *Carry a portable radio.* A radio allows you to call for help if you are separated from your vehicle.

- *Plan safety roles.* If there will be more than one rescuer on any call, tasks can be split. One rescuer can care for the patient, while the other observes for safety. The "observer" could look for nearby weapons or other threats, for example, and for clues to the patient's condition, such as prescription medications.

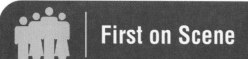

First on Scene

Your first concern at any scene must be your own safety. Resist the temptation to rush in. If you are injured, you'll not only become a patient yourself, you'll also be unable to provide proper care to the patient you came to help—and quite possibly prevent other rescuers from caring for the patient as well.

SKILL SUMMARY *Ensuring Scene Safety*

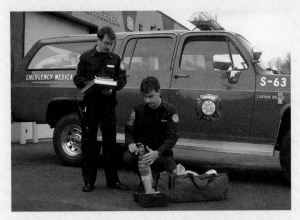

FIGURE 10-3A *Plan*—Wear safe clothing, make sure your equipment is ready, carry a portable radio, and determine safety roles.

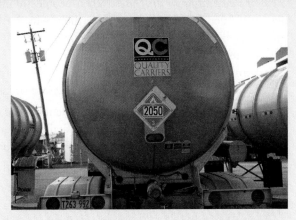

FIGURE 10-3B *Observe*—Look for signs of danger such as hazardous materials, violence, weapons, intoxication or drug use, or anything out of the ordinary.

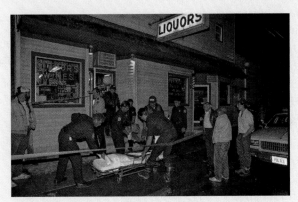

FIGURE 10-3C *React*—Retreat from danger. Radio dispatch to request assistance and to warn other rescuers. Finally, reevaluate the scene after it has been secured and then continuously while you are there. *(Craig Jackson/In the Dark Photography)*

Observe

It is always better to prevent danger than it is to deal with it. Observation and awareness are the best ways to accomplish this goal. Observation begins early in the call. Observe the neighborhood as you look for house or building numbers. If possible, do not park directly in front of the call. This provides two benefits. First, you may be able to approach the scene unnoticed, which allows you to size it up without distraction. Second, since many first response units do not transport, the area directly in front of the call is left open for the ambulance.

As you approach an emergency scene, look for the following signs of potential danger:

- *Violence.* Any indication that violence has or may take place is significant. These signs include arguing, threats, or other violent behavior. Also notice any broken glass, overturned furniture, or the like.

- *Weapons of any kind.* If a weapon is on scene, it is a serious potential danger.

- *Signs of intoxication or drug use.* When people are under the influence of alcohol or drugs, their behavior is unpredictable. In addition, even though you see yourself as there to help, other people may not. You may be mistaken for the police, because you are in uniform and you drove up in a vehicle that has lights and sirens.

- *Anything unusual.* Even an awkward silence should cause you to be wary. Emergencies are usually very active events. In situations where you observe an unusual silence, caution is advisable.

Note that nothing in this textbook is meant to create fear or unwarranted suspicion. Remember that the vast majority of EMS calls will go by uneventfully. Some calls, however, do pose a threat. Those calls usually provide subtle clues that may be picked up *before* the danger strikes. Use your observation skills on every call to determine important safety information. Remember, the general rule is: *If the scene is unsafe, make it safe if you are trained to do so. If not,* do not enter *and call for the appropriate teams to handle the situation.*

React

If you find danger at the scene, there are three "Rs" of reacting: *retreat, radio,* and *reevaluate.*

Retreat. With the exception of police who train with this textbook, it is not a First Responder's responsibility to subdue violent people or wrestle weapons away. A clear and justified course is to retreat from danger.

There are safer ways to retreat than others. When leaving the scene of danger, remember the following points:

- *Flee far enough away so that danger will not threaten you again.* Before you stop, make sure there are at least two major obstacles between you and the danger. If a threatening person moves in your direction and gets through one obstacle, the second obstacle will act as a buffer.

- *Take cover.* Find a position that hides your body and protects it from projectiles (get behind a brick wall, for example). This is preferred over concealment, which hides your body but offers no protection (like getting behind a shrub). When fleeing danger, moving a considerable distance from the scene and taking cover are usually the best options.

- *Discard your equipment.* Do not get bogged down. The equipment you carry can be thrown at the subject's feet to give you additional time to retreat.

Radio. The portable radio is an important piece of safety equipment. Its main function is to call for police assistance and to warn other rescuers of impending danger. When using the radio, speak clearly and slowly. Advise the dispatcher of the exact nature and location of the problem. Specify how many people are involved and whether or not weapons were observed. Remember that the information you have must be shared as soon as possible to prevent others from coming up against the same danger.

Reevaluate. Do not reenter the scene until the police have secured it. Even then, keep in mind that violence may begin again. Emergencies are situations packed with stress for families, victims, rescuers, and bystanders. Maintain a level of observation throughout the call. Occasionally, weapons or illegal drugs are found while you are assessing your patient. Notify the police immediately. After the call, document the situation on your run report.

Occasionally, on-scene danger can cause delays in reaching the patient. Courts have held this acceptable, provided that there has been a real and documented danger.

Q:
1. Why would you wear protective gloves as a BSI precaution?

2. Why would you wear a face shield or a gown?

3. What three words sum up the actions required to respond to danger appropriately? Give an example for each one.

Section 3 Identifying the Mechanism of Injury or Nature of Illness

During scene size-up, you must determine the nature of the patient's problem. Dispatch may already have given you some idea about whether your patient is a **medical patient** (ill) or a **trauma patient** (injured). So when you scan the emergency scene for safety factors, also try to determine if the patient is ill or injured.

A medical patient's condition is caused by some internal factor such as a heart or breathing problem. Nothing at the scene suggests injury. In this case, speak to the patient, family, or bystanders to determine why EMS was called and what the **nature of illness (NOI)** might be.

When you scan a trauma scene, note the **mechanism of injury (MOI)** (forces that caused the injury or injuries). For example, if your patient fell from a ladder, it would be important to note how far the patient fell. The greater the distance, the more serious and extensive the injuries may be.

First on Scene

Identify the mechanism of injury at every trauma call. Although it doesn't guarantee an injury will be present, it may help predict when serious hidden injuries exist. Knowing the mechanism of injury also will help you determine the need for additional resources on scene, such as paramedic advanced care, or special transportation needs such as multiple ambulances or a helicopter.

Occasionally, a patient may have a combination of illness and injury. Consider the patient who fell from a ladder, for instance. What if he passed out from a medical problem and then fell to the ground? As you approach the scene, the mechanism of injury may be obvious. The illness may not be. It will be your examination of the scene, as well as a patient history, that will make a difference. (See Chapter 11 for instructions on how to gather a patient history.)

Kinematics of Trauma

Trauma is the leading cause of death for people between the ages of 14 and 40. It also is the third leading cause of death overall—behind only heart disease and cancer.

Care of a trauma patient depends on the extent of the injuries. But beware, it is not quite that simple. Too often hidden injuries prove to be fatal. To understand how seriously a patient may be injured, you must determine the mechanism of injury. It will tell you what injuries or patterns of injury the patient may be suffering.

The science of analyzing the mechanism of injury is called the *kinematics of trauma*. The process is based on physical laws. For example, an object (mass) in motion contains energy, and energy is influenced by the interaction of velocity (speed) and mass. *Kinetic energy* is the total amount of energy contained by an object in motion. When the weight of that object is doubled, its energy also is doubled. In other words, it is twice as damaging to be hit by a two-pound baseball than by a one-pound baseball.

Velocity is the speed at which an object moves. According to physical laws, velocity is more important than weight in producing kinetic energy. The higher the speed of an object, the more energy it has. The rate at which an object changes speed (its acceleration and deceleration) is also significant. As you know, the faster a car travels, the longer it takes to stop.

The process of gaining and losing velocity occurs with each impact in a crash. The number of impacts varies, but there are three basic ones (Figure 10-4). First, the car impacts the object. Then, the occupant impacts the interior of the car. Finally, the occupant's organs impact the surfaces inside the body.

Each of the three impacts has the potential of causing harm. The amount of kinetic energy that is absorbed on impact, however, depends on how much energy is absorbed by other things first. For example, a person who falls on freshly plowed soil will not be injured as severely as the person who falls the same distance onto cement pavement.

Remember that the mechanism of injury is an important part of your assessment of a trauma patient. It can suggest which body parts are injured and how severe the injuries might be. Whenever you care for a trauma patient, maintain a high index of suspicion and take note of the part of the body impacted; the object that penetrated the body or the surface on which the body landed; and the distance involved, if any.

Common mechanisms of injury are falls, vehicular crashes, fire, explosions, and penetrating objects such as bullets and knives.

Car Crashes

There are five basic types of car crashes: *head-on impact, rear impact, side impact, rotational impact,* and *rollover.* Each one has its predictable pattern of injury, which may be affected by the type of restraint the occupant uses (seat belts, airbags, or a car seat).

Head-on Impact

A head-on impact occurs when a car hits an immovable object, such as a tree (Figure 10-5). The greater the car's speed, the greater the energy, and the greater the resulting damage. When the car stops, its occupants continue to travel forward. They take one of two possible pathways of motion—up-and-over or down-and-under (Figure 10-6). Each pathway has a distinctive pattern of injury, which can be affected by the use of a seat belt or the presence of air bags.

In the up-and-over pathway, the torso may be thrown over the steering wheel. The face, head, and neck strike the windshield. The chest and abdomen may then strike the steering wheel. The patterns of injury are as follows:

- *Face, head, and neck injuries.* Look for obvious clues like hair, tissue, or blood on the windshield or rearview mirror. The windshield also may bulge out in a classic bull's-eye or spider-web pattern.

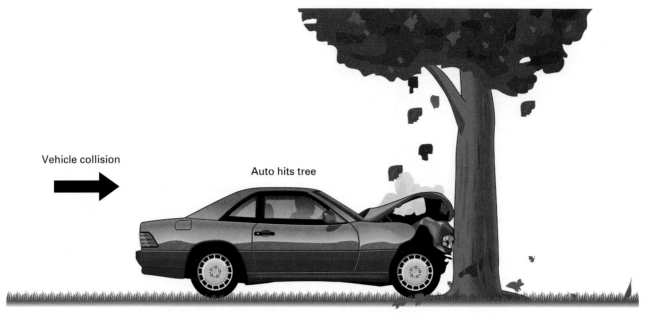

a. *First, the vehicle strikes an object.*

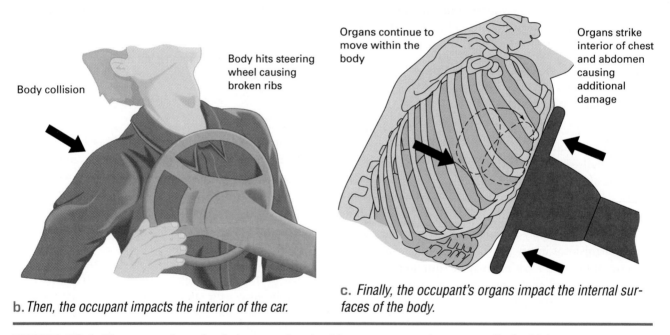

b. *Then, the occupant impacts the interior of the car.*

c. *Finally, the occupant's organs impact the internal surfaces of the body.*

FIGURE 10-4 **There are three basic impacts involved in any car crash, any or all of which can cause injury to the patient.**

The face can sustain extensive soft-tissue damage. However, bleeding from its rich supply of blood vessels may not be as serious as it looks. Watch for airway problems if there is bleeding from the mouth, nose, or face.

Skull fracture may occur. Almost all head injuries have the potential to cause damage to the brain. Brain tissue can compress, rebound against opposite sides of the skull, and bruise. Brain tissue also can be cut or bruised on the floor of the skull, which is very rough or jagged.

Energy can travel down the neck, causing the potential for cervical-spine injury. The neck may be flexed or extended too far, resulting in whiplash injuries or fractures. An impact at the top of the head can cause compression fractures of the cervical spine. The anterior neck also can be injured by hitting the steering wheel or

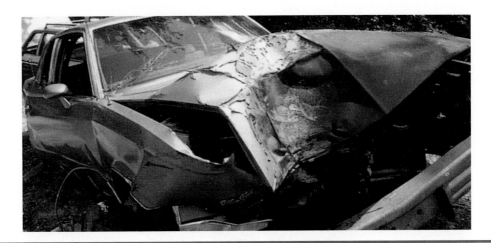

FIGURE 10-5 Head-on impact.

dashboard. Cartilage rings in the trachea (windpipe) can be separated, which would impair breathing.

■ *Chest injuries.* When the chest strikes the steering wheel, the ribs and sternum may break. The heart may

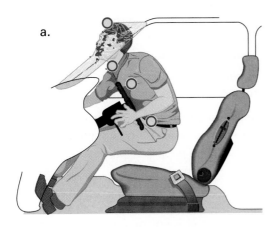

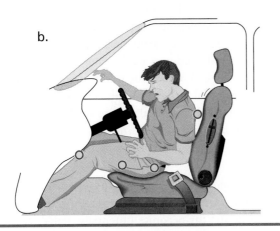

FIGURE 10-6 In a head-on crash, the patient is forced into either (a) an up-and-over pathway of motion or (b) a down-and-under pathway of motion.

be compressed and bruised, making it unable to pump blood effectively. The aorta may be torn, resulting in life-threatening bleeding. As the lungs are compressed, they can be bruised or ruptured. Remember that broken ribs can also injure the lungs and heart.

■ *Abdominal injuries.* When the abdomen strikes the steering wheel, the liver, spleen, and other organs are compressed. Sometimes they are cut. The liver may be cut in half as it is forced against the ligament that holds it in place. The spleen may be torn from its attachment, resulting in severe internal bleeding.

In the down-and-under pathway of motion, a body slides under the steering wheel. The knees strike the dashboard. Energy travels up the legs. The abdomen and then the chest strike the steering wheel. Classic injuries include dislocated hip and broken patella (knee cap), femur (thigh bone), and pelvis.

Rear Impact

Rear impact occurs when a car is struck from behind by another vehicle traveling at greater speed (Figure 10-7). The car that is hit accelerates suddenly, and the occupant's body is slammed backward and then forward (Figure 10-8). Suspect the same kinds of injuries as discussed for head-on collisions. If positioned properly, a headrest will prevent the head from whipping back. If the headrest is not in place, suspect soft-tissue injury to the neck, compression of the cervical spine, and cervical-spine fractures.

Side Impact

The side impact is often called a "broadside" or "T-bone" collision. The person closest to the impact absorbs more energy than a person on the opposite side. As the energy of the impact is absorbed, the body is pushed sideways

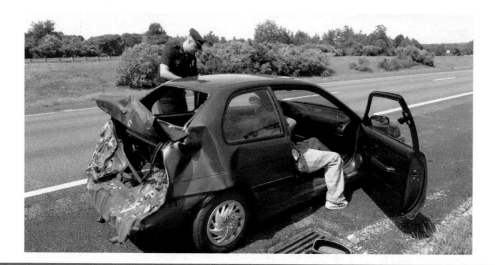

FIGURE 10-7 Rear impact. *(© Mark C. Ide)*

and the head moves in the opposite direction. The following injuries commonly occur:

■ *Head and neck injuries.* The head often impacts the door post. This can result in skull injury, brain injury, and tears in neck muscles and ligaments. Cervical-

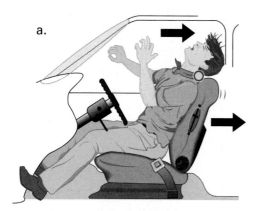

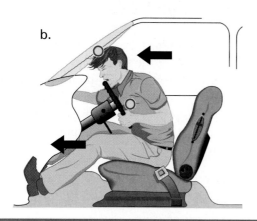

FIGURE 10-8 In a rear-end crash, the patient is forced (a) back and then (b) forward.

spine fractures are common, since the vertebrae are not designed for extreme lateral movement.

■ *Chest injuries.* If the door slams against the shoulder, the clavicle will probably break. If the arm is caught between the door and the chest, or if the door impacts against the chest directly, suspect broken ribs and possible breathing problems. Fractures low in the rib cage can injure the liver and spleen.

■ *Pelvis injuries.* Lateral impact to the pelvis often causes fractures of the pelvis and femur.

The person on the opposite side of the car is subject to similar kinds of head and neck injuries. In addition, if there is more than one person sitting on a seat, heads often collide.

Rotational Impact
A rotational impact is one that occurs off center. The car strikes an object and rotates around it until the car either loses speed or strikes another object. The sturdiest structures in the car (such as the steering wheel, dashboard, door posts, and windows) are the ones that cause the most serious injuries. A variety of injury patterns may occur due to the initial strike and subsequent striking of stationary objects. Look for the same kinds of injuries that occur with head-on and side impacts.

Rollover
During a rollover (Figure 10-9), car occupants change direction every time the car does (Figure 10-10). Every fixture inside the car becomes potentially lethal. A specific pattern of injury is impossible to predict, but rollovers almost always cause injuries to more than one body system. If car occupants are not wearing seat belts, they have a

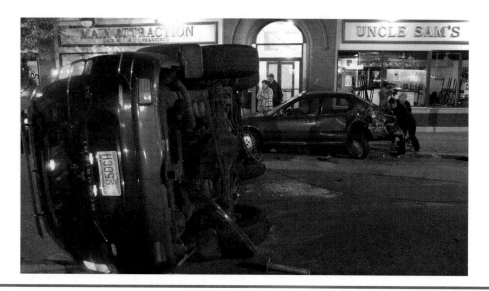

FIGURE 10-9 Rollover impact. *(© Mark C. Ide)*

much greater chance of being thrown from the car, either partially or fully. Common injuries include severe soft-tissue injuries, multiple broken bones, and crushing injuries resulting from the car rolling over the occupant.

Restraints

Restraints help to reduce the severity of injuries. However, occupants of a car can still be injured. Injury also can be caused when restraints are not used properly. Vehicle restraints include:

- *Lap belt.* When worn properly, a lap belt can prevent the occupant from being thrown out of the car. But it does not prevent the head, neck, and chest from striking the steering wheel or dashboard. When the torso is thrown forward, compression fractures of the lower back can occur. If the belt is worn across the upper abdomen instead of over the pelvis, the spleen, liver, intestines, or pancreas can be injured. There also may be enough pressure in the abdomen to injure the diaphragm and force abdominal contents into the chest cavity.

- *Lap-and-shoulder belt.* This type of restraint can prevent the occupant from striking the steering wheel or dashboard. A severe impact can cause the shoulder belt to break the clavicle. Even properly used, it does not prevent the head and neck from moving sideways or forward and back. If a headrest is not in place, suspect cervical-spine injury.

- *Air bag* (Figure 10-11). For air bags to deploy, a collision must have contact with a sensor in the bumper or the side of the vehicle at a specific speed or greater. Most vehicles have air bags in the steering wheel or dash. Some also offer air bags, or curtains, at the sides.

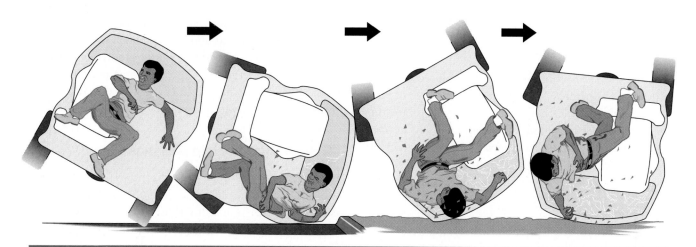

FIGURE 10-10 In a rollover, the unrestrained occupant changes direction every time the car does.

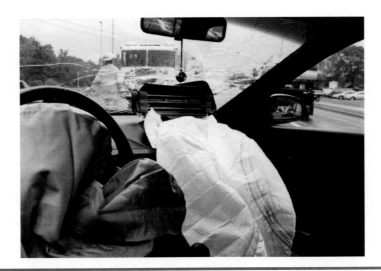

FIGURE 10-11 Airbag deployment in a car crash.

For maximum protection with air bags, vehicle occupants must also wear seat belts.

Air bags themselves may cause injury, including burns, contusions and, in some cases, more serious injury. Air bags deploy only once, so they will not offer protection for any impact after the initial collision.

- *Car seat.* An infant car seat that faces backwards in an upright position minimizes risk in a head-on collision. In such a crash, all unrestrained parts of an infant's body continue to move forward. The greatest danger is to the neck. An infant's head is large for its body, and it tends to snap forward with great force. Suspect injury to the neck any time the mechanism of injury indicates it may be possible, even if the patient appears to be uninjured.

It is possible for there to be more than one type of car seat in a vehicle, depending on the age, weight, and number of children involved. Note the type of seat and position as you assess the mechanisms of injury for each of these patients.

Motorcycle Crashes

Motorcycle crash injuries are greatly reduced when the rider wears a helmet. With no helmet, chances of severe head injury and death increase 340%. There are three types of impact in motorcycle collisions. They are *head-on, angular,* and *ejection. Laying the bike down,* an evasive action, often prevents serious injuries but can cause extensive scrapes, bruises, and burns.

Head-on Impact

In a head-on impact, the rider generally impacts the handlebars at the same speed the bike was traveling. A variety of injuries can be expected. For example, if the rider's feet get caught, the thighs or pelvis will strike the handlebars, resulting in fractures.

Angular Impact

In this type of impact, the rider strikes an object at an angle. The object then usually collapses on the rider. Common objects are the edges of signs, outside mirrors on cars, or fence posts. Severe amputations can result.

Ejection

If the rider clears the handlebars, ejection occurs. The body is thrown until it hits a stationary object or the ground. The body may hit several objects or strike the ground many times before stopping. Expect severe head and facial injuries if the rider is not wearing a helmet. Fractures and internal injuries are likely. Expect severe soft-tissue damage if the rider is not wearing boots and leather clothing.

Laying the Bike Down

A rider who anticipates a crash may try to "lay the bike down." That is, the rider may turn the motorcycle sideways and drag a leg on the ground to lose enough speed to get off. If successful, the rider slides along the ground, clearing the bike and the object it hits. Expect severe abrasions (scrapes) from contact with the pavement. Many victims are also burned by contact with the motorcycle's hot exhaust pipe.

Recreational Vehicle Crashes

One type of recreational vehicle is the ATV, or all-terrain vehicle. For ATV collisions, expect head, neck, and extremity injuries similar to those caused in motorcycle crashes. However, it may be more difficult and take longer to reach the patient, since ATVs often are used on fields and hilly terrain.

ATVs are prone to collisions. A simple turn in a three-wheel ATV can cause a rollover, resulting in head and crush injuries. Unfortunately, many of those who ride ATVs are children, whose lesser body weights make ATVs even more unstable.

Another type of recreational vehicle is the snow mobile. It is often driven at high speed. When there is a crash, riders sustain severe head and neck injuries. Rollovers also are common.

Falls

The most common mechanism of injury is a fall. Falls account for a significant number of trauma-related emergencies. The severity of injury depends on the following:

- Distance of the fall.
- Anything that interrupts the fall.
- Body part that impacts first.
- Surface on which the victim lands.

Some experts say that the surface on which a victim lands and the part of the body that impacts are more important than the height of the fall. For example, diving into deep water from a high diving board is a recreational activity. Diving the same distance onto a concrete sidewalk is not.

Generally, a fall of two to three times a patient's height onto an unyielding surface is considered severe. (The U.S. DOT suggests that any fall of 15 feet or greater onto an unyielding surface is severe.) In either case, you should have a high degree of suspicion about internal injuries no matter how the patient looks.

Feet-First Fall

A feet-first landing causes energy to travel up the skeleton (Figure 10-12). If the knees are flexed when the person lands, injury to the bones will be less severe. Common injuries include fractures of the spine, hip socket, femur, heel, and ankle. Head, back, and pelvis injuries are common if the victim falls backward. If the victim extends arms to break a forward fall, expect broken wrists. A broken shoulder and clavicle are common, too.

In falls of 15 feet or more, internal organs are likely to be severely injured from sudden deceleration. The liver may be sliced in two. The spleen or kidneys may be torn from their attachments. The heart may be torn from the aorta.

Head-First Fall

In head-first falls, the pattern of injury begins with the arms and extends to the shoulders. Head and spine injuries are very common. There is usually extensive dam-

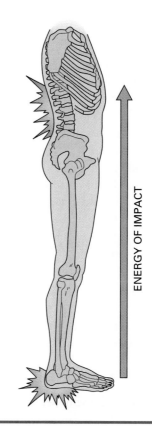

FIGURE 10-12 In feet-first falls, the energy of impact is transmitted up the skeletal system.

age to the neck. When the body is falling, the torso and legs are thrown either forward or backward, commonly causing chest, lower spine, and pelvis injuries.

Penetrating Trauma

Penetrating trauma occurs when an object is pushed through the surface and into the soft tissues of the body. Hand-powered weapons, such as knives or arrows, generally cause low-velocity injuries. These are limited to the immediate site of impact. Projectiles powered by another source, such as bullets from a handgun, cause medium-velocity or high-velocity injuries. These affect tissues far from the site of impact.

(Remember: When you encounter a scene of violence, do not enter it until it is safe to do so. It is absolutely essential that you make sure the scene is safe before you try to reach a patient. Follow local protocol.)

Low-Velocity Injuries

Among the factors that help determine the severity of a low-velocity injury are the location of the injury, the length of the object used to penetrate the body, and the gender of the person doing the stabbing.

The length of the weapon provides valuable clues. For example, a person stabbed in the chest with a three-inch paring knife would probably suffer a pneumothorax (collapse of the lungs due to air in the chest). The same stab wound inflicted by an eight-inch knife could cut the pulmonary veins, the aorta, and the heart muscle itself.

The gender of the offender also can give you important clues to the severity of the injury. Women generally have less upper-body strength, so they usually stab overhand, or downward. Men have more upper-body strength, so they usually stab up and out. For example, if a man stabbed the victim in the right side, the most likely injuries would be to the liver, kidney, and intestine. If a woman stabbed the victim in the right side, the most likely injury would be to the lungs.

Medium- and High-Velocity Injuries

A medium-velocity weapon is a shotgun or handgun. An example of a high-velocity weapon is a high-power rifle. Knowing a weapon's velocity helps to determine how severe an injury might be. Other factors include:

- Trajectory, or the path the bullet travels after it enters the body.

- Drag, or the factors that slow a bullet down.

- Impact point, or the bullet's point of entry into the body.

- Whether or not the bullet fragments (breaks apart).

- Pressure wave caused by the energy of the bullet as it travels through body tissue. A soft-nose, high-velocity bullet can cause a wave of energy through the body that is 30 times the diameter of the bullet (Figure 10-13).

- Complications such as clothing, gun powder, bacteria, and other foreign matter that can be pulled into the wound.

As you care for a gunshot victim, remember that tissue damage can be much more widespread than the surface wound indicates. A bullet wound that bleeds very little can be accompanied by a devastating internal injury. If all the energy of a bullet is absorbed by the body, the bullet will remain there. If all is not absorbed, the bullet will exit the body. You need to assess the victim carefully. Look for both an entry and an exit wound. Note that an exit wound can be much larger than the entrance wound.

Blast Injuries

The most common explosions involve natural gas, gasoline, fireworks, or grain elevators. They occur in three phases, each with a typical pattern of injury: primary phase, secondary phase, and tertiary phase.

In the primary phase, the pressure wave of an explosion affects gas-containing organs such as the lungs,

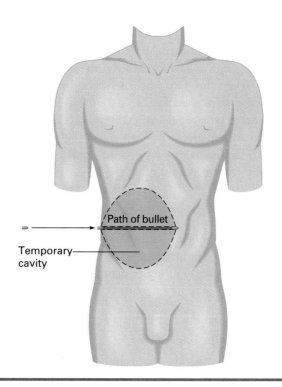

FIGURE 10-13 A gunshot can cause devastating damage, much more than a surface wound might suggest.

stomach, intestines, inner ears, and sinuses. Blood vessels and membranes of the organs can be ruptured. Death can occur without any obvious external injury. Common primary blast injuries include pneumothorax (collapse of the lungs due to air in the chest), pulmonary contusion (bruising of the lungs), and perforation of the stomach and intestines.

During the secondary phase, injuries result from flying debris created by the force of the blast. Unlike primary-blast injuries, these are obvious. They most commonly include open wounds, impaled objects, and broken bones.

Injuries in the tertiary phase occur when the victim is thrown away from the source of the explosion onto a hard surface. The injuries are basically the same as those of a victim who is ejected from a car during a collision.

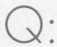

1. What are the five basic types of car crashes? Explain why it is important to recognize each one.

2. What happens to the patient during a head-on collision? Describe the two pathways of motion.

3. What is the most common mechanism of injury? When is it considered severe?

Section 4 Determining Necessary Resources

Once you have ensured personal safety and identified the patient's mechanism of injury or nature of illness, you must decide what additional resources are needed on scene (Figure 10-14). For example, if the scene involves hazardous materials, you need to call a specialized hazmat team. If you have two or more patients, you may need to call for extra EMS personnel and ambulances.

When special teams or extra units are needed, call dispatch to request them. Do this before you begin patient care. Experience has shown that getting immersed in patient care can cause any First Responder to forget to call for additional assistance. Call first. It will prevent inefficiency and confusion later. *Never be too proud to ask for help when you need it!*

Situations in which you may need help include the following:

■ *Number of patients.* When there are more patients than you can deal with in a multiple-casualty incident, call for additional personnel and ambulances. If there is a doubt about how many ambulances to request, call for

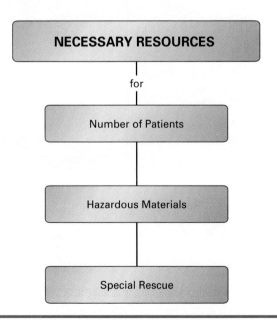

NECESSARY RESOURCES

for

Number of Patients

Hazardous Materials

Special Rescue

FIGURE 10-14 Once you have ensured personal safety and determined the patient's MOI or NOI, you must obtain the resources appropriate for the emergency.

First on Scene

Call for additional help before you become involved with patient care or other aspects of the emergency scene. Call early, because once you become involved, you may forget to call until it is too late. Remember that it will take time for EMS resources to get to you and your patient.

slightly more than you think you'll need. (It is always easier to cancel an ambulance than to wait for one.)

Until help arrives, you will need to make decisions about who must be treated first based on the severity of injuries. This is called "triage." (See Chapter 30 for details.)

■ *Hazardous materials.* They are everywhere. They are stored in homes and businesses. They are transported by ground, sea, and air. Hazmat incidents require specialized training to manage and decontaminate. Be alert and call for a hazmat team as soon as an incident is suspected. (See Chapter 30 for details.)

■ *Special rescue needs.* It may be necessary to call for law enforcement if violence or the potential for violence exists. Situations such as problems with traffic, bystanders and crowds, or violations of the law will also require the police. Other situations may require the fire service for fire or rescue, or the power company for downed wires. Confined-space rescue, high- and low-angle rescue, and helicopter rescue or evacuation also may be needed.

Call for the resources you need immediately. If later you find they are not needed, they may be canceled. Time is of the essence.

1. When is the best time to call dispatch to request the extra assistance you need on scene? Explain your reasoning.

2. Why should the number of patients be determined during scene size-up?

3. In what situations will you need to call for law enforcement?

At the beginning of this chapter, you read that fire service First Responders were at the scene of an auto vs. telephone pole. To see how chapter skills apply to this emergency, read the following. It describes how the call was completed.

Scene Size-Up *(continued)* At a safe distance from the car, we quickly but carefully sized up the scene. The pole seemed intact, and no wires were down. We didn't smell or see any gasoline leaks. I counted only one person in the car. He was responsive, so I told him not to move. The patient had blood on his face.

There was a lot of damage to the front of the car and a large star in the windshield where the patient's head must have hit. Considering the mechanism of injury, we knew he could have very serious internal injuries. So, I called the dispatcher to make sure the EMT-paramedics were on the way. We also called for an extrication team and truck.

Before we approached the patient, we put on turnout gear and eye protection. Over our latex gloves, we put on heavy duty gloves to protect ourselves from all the broken glass.

Initial Assessment Because of the severity of the MOI, we suspected the patient had serious internal injuries. The car was stable, so I climbed into the back seat and held the patient's head and neck in a neutral in-line position. I asked him some quick questions and saw that he was alert. His chief complaint was pain in the neck and chest.

The blood on the patient's face wasn't causing any airway problems, so we left it alone. He was breathing deeply at a good rate, and his pulse was good. My partner stayed at the window nearest the patient, where she talked to him to help keep him calm. We saw no severe bleeding.

My partner placed him on oxygen and then updated the incoming units.

Physical Examination What we found were cuts and bruises to his forehead, some of which were oozing blood. He admitted that he was not wearing a seat belt at the time of the crash. Upon palpation, we found that the back of his neck was tender. The left side of his chest was, too, but there were no signs of broken ribs or open wounds. My partner listened to the patient's lungs. Air was moving in and out of both, she said. The patient had no problems with his abdomen or hips. We could not get to his legs.

Patient History When the extrication team arrived, it got pretty noisy. We could not hear or do much when the tools were in operation, so we didn't try to ask the patient any more questions. It was more important to get him out of the car.

Ongoing Assessment We continued to monitor the patient's breathing and pulse during extrication. We also did our best to protect him from flying debris.

Patient Hand-off When the patient was extricated, the paramedics took over care. We told them what we had found so far (see below). We stuck around and helped with the backboarding. Later, we found out that the man got worse in the ambulance. He had a hemothorax, with blood accumulating in his left lung. Fortunately, the ambulance went to a trauma center, where he was rushed into surgery. He was in the hospital for a while and recovered fully.

 Hand-off Report

"This is a 30-year-old man. Name, Jim Kafa. He was the driver of the wrecked vehicle. He was not wearing a seat belt. Chief complaint is pain in his neck and chest. There are also cuts and bruises to his forehead. He is alert with adequate breathing and a rapid pulse. Upon examination, we found tenderness in his posterior neck and left lateral chest. We could not examine his legs, nor could we get a history during extrication. We kept his head and neck stabilized and administered oxygen."

The Last Word *As you can see, scene size-up is an important part of any call. It begins as you approach the scene, even before you see the patient. Do not rush in. Determine right away whether or not you will need help and what kind. Then call for it.*

Chapter Review

Focus on the EMS Team

You may notice that experienced First Responders seem to respond to every emergency calmly. This is because a calm, observant approach helps them perform an optimal scene size-up. Some experienced EMS personnel, when they feel as if they are rushing or not moving carefully enough, *will stop in their tracks and count to three. No one notices, not even crew members. But it can make all the difference. If you find yourself rushing, remember this pause. It could help return your focus to a proper scene size-up and quality patient care.*

Summing Up

- Scene size-up is an overall assessment of the emergency scene. It must be performed before you approach the patient. It includes taking the appropriate BSI precautions and assessing scene safety, identifying the mechanism of injury or nature of illness, and determining necessary additional resources.

- When you approach the scene, anticipate which BSI precautions may be needed and then take them. Waiting too long may cause you to become so involved in patient care that you forget to protect yourself.

- Ensuring scene safety involves the following:
  - Plan for safety before you go out on a call. Put on nonrestrictive clothing, which helps to ensure your safety, and carry equipment that has been properly stored and maintained, including a portable radio. Safety roles should also be planned ahead with your partner.
  - As you approach an emergency scene, look for signs of potential danger. If the scene is unsafe, do not enter it. Instead, call for the appropriate teams and equipment to make it safe.

  - If once on scene you find a potential threat or actual danger, retreat. Then, radio for police assistance. When the threat has been eliminated, return to the scene but stay alert for a possible recurrence.

- When nothing at the scene suggests injury, or the call is reported to be a medical emergency, identify the nature of the patient's illness. It will suggest how serious the patient's condition may be.

- Common mechanisms of injury include car crashes, motorcycle crashes, recreational vehicle collisions, falls, penetrating trauma, and explosions. Each one has its own predictable pattern of injury. Once you learn them, they will help you determine the best emergency care plan for your patient.

- The last step in scene size-up is deciding what additional resources are needed on scene. More than one patient, the presence of hazardous materials, or downed electrical wires are examples of emergencies in which extra resources are required. Be sure to call dispatch to request assistance *before* you begin patient care.

Key Terms

mechanism of injury (MOI) the force or forces that cause an injury.

medical patient a patient who is ill, not injured.

nature of illness (NOI) the type of medical condition or complaint a patient may be suffering.

scene size-up an overall assessment of the emergency scene, consisting of ensuring personal safety, identifying the mechanism of injury or nature of illness, and determining necessary resources.

trauma patient a patient who is injured, not ill.

Knowledge Check

1. **Which one of the following steps is part of a First Responder's scene size-up?**
   a. ensuring an open airway in a patient
   b. identifying a patient's mechanism of injury
   c. applying AED electrodes to a patient's chest
   d. determining if the patient's breathing is adequate

2. The term "nature of illness" refers to the patient's:

   a. mental status.
   b. mechanism of injury.
   c. past medical problems.
   d. current medical complaint.

3. Which one of the following observations should immediately cause you to suspect an injury to a patient's head?

   a. Steering wheel is bent.
   b. Right front tire of the car is flat.
   c. Windshield is cracked in a bull's-eye pattern.
   d. Rear bumper is twisted and hanging off the car.

4. Which one of the following collisions will most likely cause injuries to more than one body system?

   a. head-on
   b. rollover
   c. broadside
   d. rotational

5. As a result of the primary phase of an explosion, you can expect a patient's injuries to:

   a. be internal, with no obvious external injury.
   b. occur when he is thrown onto a hard surface.
   c. result from flying objects and other debris.
   d. be external only.

6. While at the scene of an emergency, all of the following can help to ensure personal safety EXCEPT:

   a. prepare your equipment properly.
   b. wear nonslip shoes and other practical clothing.
   c. keep your portable radio secured inside your vehicle.
   d. observe the scene while your partner provides patient care.

7. You respond to a scene where you observe an apparently unconscious patient lying on the floor. In the next room, you see someone who is unsteady on his feet, agitated, slurring words and swearing, and holding a broken bottle. You should:

   a. quietly remove the patient before the other person sees you.
   b. enter the room where the patient is and provide emergency care.
   c. notify the police and then enter the room where the patient is.
   d. retreat to a position of safety and then notify the police.

8. The police have secured the scene of an assault, where you find one patient has injuries around the mouth with minor bleeding. The appropriate BSI precautions to take with this patient are protective gloves plus:

   a. face shield.
   b. surgical mask.
   c. eye protection and a gown.
   d. eye protection, surgical mask, and gown.

9. When there is a significant mechanism of injury, you should suspect that your patient has serious injuries.

   a. True
   b. False

10. Front air bags will deploy in a vehicle that is struck in the rear.

   a. True
   b. False

Scenario

You pull up to an emergency scene where a car struck a pole. The pole is sheared in half and hanging by the power line wires. There is considerable damage to the vehicle. You observe two patients in the front seat of the car. Neither is moving. What additional resources would you call for? Why?

_____

_____

_____

_____

Scenario

You are called to an accident at a new home construction site. Scaffolding collapsed and sent two workers to the ground. One person on the ground was struck by falling pieces of scaffolding.

a. What hazards should you expect to be present?

_____

_____

_____

b. What resources and additional assistance should you request from dispatch?

_____

_____

_____

c. What factors would you consider when evaluating the mechanism of injury?

_____

_____

_____

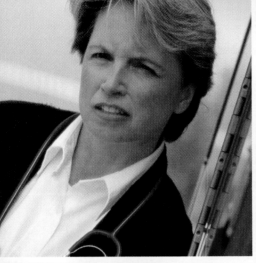
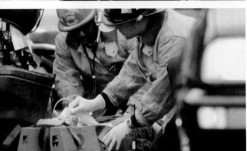
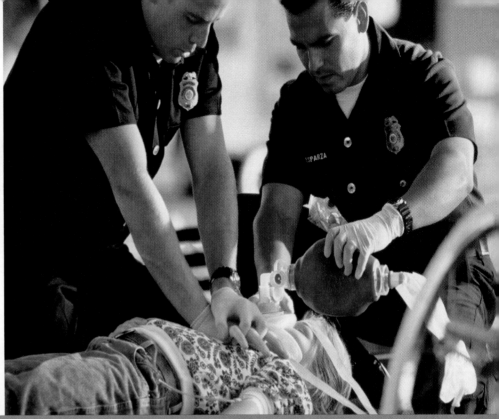

11 | Introduction to Patient Assessment and Vital Signs

Objectives

From the U.S. Department of Transportation (DOT) 1995 "First Responder: National Standard Curriculum." Material supplemental to the DOT curriculum is listed under "Enrichment."

Cognitive

No objectives are identified by the DOT.

Affective

No objectives are identified by the DOT.

Psychomotor

3-1.39 ▶ Demonstrate the techniques for assessing the patient's skin color, temperature, condition, and capillary refill (infants and children only). (pp. 202–203)

Enrichment

▶ Identify the components of an assessment of vital signs. (p. 200)

▶ Describe the methods used to obtain a breathing rate and a pulse rate. (pp. 201–202)

▶ Identify the terms that describe the quality of breathing and the quality of pulse. (pp. 201–202)

▶ Describe methods used to assess pupils. (pp. 203–204)

▶ Demonstrate application of the pulse oximeter. (p. 204)

▶ Describe the indications and interpretation of pulse oximetry. (p. 204)

▶ Describe methods used to assess blood pressure. (pp. 205–207)

▶ State the importance of accurately reporting and recording baseline vital signs. (p. 200)

Introduction

As a First Responder, you will assess every one of your patients. Some assessments will be relatively simple, such as for a patient with a twisted ankle. Others will be more challenging. This chapter will introduce you to a patient assessment plan. You will find it efficient, accurate, and adaptable to every patient. The chapter also will introduce you to vital signs, an important assessment skill many First Responders are required to use.

Section 1 Introduction to Patient Assessment

Patient assessment is a vitally important skill, one that will tell you what emergency medical care your patient needs. If you do not properly assess a patient, you cannot provide proper emergency medical care.

Patient assessment is a process performed in a variety of situations. Some patients have minor injuries, while others have serious ones. Some patients are in their homes, while others must be assessed and treated in automobiles, factories, or parks. You will learn to adapt your patient assessment skills to meet each of these situations.

Patient assessment involves the use of your senses. You will need to see, hear, touch, and occasionally use your sense of smell to obtain clues about your patient's condition. You will:

- *Observe.* As you are performing your scene size-up, you will also look at the patient to determine the level of distress, such as obvious difficulty breathing, external bleeding, deformities, and skin color.

- *Listen.* You will listen to your patients when they answer your questions and when they tell you what is wrong. You also will learn to listen to a patient's breathing to determine if it is adequate or problematic and, if you take blood pressure, you will listen for the sound of a pulse through a stethoscope.

- *Touch.* You will sometimes palpate (touch) a patient to see if something is wrong with a particular part of the body. Touching an area will allow you to feel for abnormalities or to elicit a response.

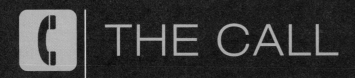

THE CALL

Dispatch I was off duty that day, so there was no initial call from Dispatch. I had been shopping. It was when I walked out of the mall that I saw the patient.

Scene Size-up An older woman was sitting on the curb, obviously in some distress. I quickly looked around and sized up the scene. It appeared to be safe. As I got closer, I saw that the woman's arm had a small abrasion with minor bleeding. Mall security arrived on scene and they called an ambulance.

Initial Assessment I introduced myself and told the woman that I am an EMS First Responder. She consented to my help. As she talked to me, I noticed that her breathing was adequate and her airway was clear. I saw no major bleeding, and the woman appeared to be alert and oriented.

To the untrained person, this patient's condition may not seem serious. But to an EMS-trained First Responder, it is too early in the patient assessment plan to draw any conclusions. As you read this chapter, consider what the First Responder should do next.

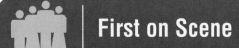

First on Scene

Often when you arrive at the scene of an emergency, you will find confusion and disorder. In the chaos, you may feel overwhelmed, wondering where to begin or what to do next. Those are the times when your patient assessment plan can be your best friend. Depend on it. It will work for all patient types and conditions.

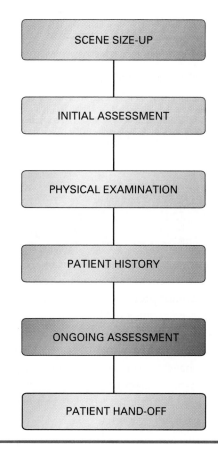

SCENE SIZE-UP

INITIAL ASSESSMENT

PHYSICAL EXAMINATION

PATIENT HISTORY

ONGOING ASSESSMENT

PATIENT HAND-OFF

FIGURE 11–1 The First Responder's patient assessment plan.

■ *Smell.* Sometimes the odor of a patient's breath will give you clues about his or her condition.

The final part of patient assessment is using your findings to make the appropriate decisions for your patient's care. For example, your assessment may reveal that the patient needs CPR or bleeding control. You may need to notify incoming EMS units that the patient's condition is serious or to request air medical (helicopter) transport. In any event, your patient assessment paves the way for appropriate patient care.

Patient Assessment Plan

The First Responder's patient assessment plan is a systematic evaluation of a patient. It is meant to help you determine the nature and extent of your patient's illness or injuries. It requires you to identify and treat life-threatening conditions, such as airway problems, early in the call. It makes no sense to evaluate a patient's legs for deformities, for instance, if the patient is not breathing.

The patient assessment plan can be broken down into six steps (Figure 11–1):

■ *Scene size-up.* You learned about this step in Chapter 10.

■ *Initial assessment.* As soon as you are at the patient's side, you must identify and care for any immediate threats to his airway, breathing, and circulation.

■ *Physical examination.* This is a head-to-toe examination of the patient. Vital signs may also be taken.

■ *Patient history.* Information about the events leading up to the emergency, as well as pertinent parts of the patient's past medical history are obtained.

■ *Ongoing assessment.* This step focuses on closely monitoring the patient until he or she is turned over to the EMTs or paramedics.

■ *Patient hand-off.* In this step, patient information is transferred to the EMS personnel who take over patient care.

Patient assessment findings allow you to make appropriate decisions for your patient's emergency care. For example, your initial assessment may reveal that the patient needs immediate CPR or bleeding control. Gathering your patient's history may suggest that an existing medical condition caused or is being affected by the current emergency. In any event, your assessment paves the way for appropriate patient care.

Medical vs. Trauma Patients

To help you remain consistent and accurate, the First Responder's patient assessment plan is always performed step by step for every patient. This is especially valuable when you encounter a seriously ill or seriously injured patient (Figure 11–2). When under the stress of a serious emergency, you will be using a procedure you know well and can depend on. However, that doesn't mean every call will be the same. Not every patient will need a full assessment in every area of his body. To illustrate this point, consider the following patients:

Patient #1 is a 24-year-old-male who twisted his ankle playing basketball. He did not fall to the ground, pass out, or injure himself in any other way.

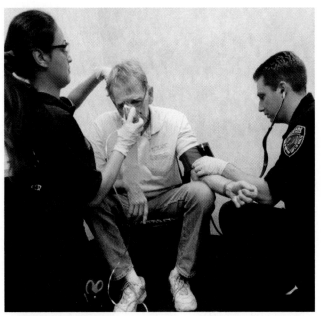

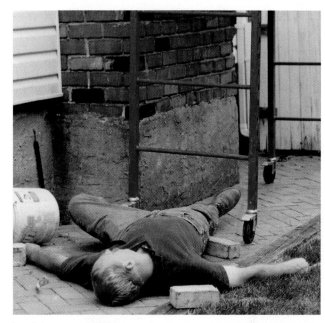

a. *A medical patient.*

b. *A trauma patient.*

FIGURE 11–2 The term "medical patient" refers to a patient who has an illness. The term "trauma patient" refers to one who has been injured.

Patient #2 is a 24-year-old male, who was involved in a serious motor-vehicle collision. He has been thrown from the vehicle, and you find him unresponsive on the ground.

Patient #1 is not critically injured. As you approach and he tells you emphatically, "My ankle hurts," you'll know his airway and breathing are fine. It makes no sense (and would aggravate the patient) if you were to use a jaw-thrust maneuver or attempt to suction his airway. If the patient did not fall to the ground or have any other mechanism of injury, it might not be necessary to palpate anything but his ankle and leg. Your approach to this patient—a patient with a non-serious injury—will not be the same as your approach to Patient #2.

Patient #2 is a critically injured patient. The mechanism of injury and the fact that he is unresponsive should cause you to be concerned about his airway, breathing, and circulation (ABCs). They would be your major focus of care until the EMTs arrive.

Now consider these patients:

Patient #3 is a 54-year-old woman who calls because she has chest pain. She is conscious and alert when you arrive on scene.

Patient #4 is a 54-year-old woman, who is found unconscious on the couch in her living room. Her husband could not awaken her.

Patients #3 and #4 are medical patients. One of the most significant differences between them is that you can ask Patient #3 questions. Patient #4 is unconscious and unable to answer your questions. She needs you to help maintain an open airway and adequate breathing. Her condition will also require you to obtain a history from her husband.

Note a difference between the first and second group of patients. Patients #1 and #2 are patients with injuries, or **trauma patients.** The most pertinent information you will gather about them will come from your physical examination.

In contrast, Patients #3 and #4 are **medical patients.** They probably have an illness. The histories of their current problem—including when the pain began and what they were doing when it started—plus their pertinent past medical histories will likely provide the most important information about their emergencies. It does not make sense to palpate the head and neck of a patient with a heart problem. A hands-on physical examination will not reveal significant information about these patients.

Of course, every rule has exceptions. Occasionally, patients have a heart attack and then crash the car, which results in both a medical and trauma emergency simultaneously. Other times, you will find a patient who has fallen. But was the fall caused by the patient tripping, or did the patient pass out from some medical condition and then fall?

One final but important word: *Follow your patient assessment plan.* If you are unsure about whether the patient has an illness or an injury—or if you are unsure of the extent of the injuries—complete a full head-to-toe exam and gather a complete patient history.

: 1. What are the six parts of a First Responder's patient assessment plan?

2. What is the difference between a medical patient and a trauma patient?

3. In what part of the patient assessment plan will you obtain the most important information about a medical patient? About a trauma patient?

Section 2 Vital Signs

Vital signs include the patient's respirations, pulse, skin, pupils, and blood pressure. (See Figure 11–3.) You can assess and monitor most vital signs by looking, listening, and feeling. However, it is best if you have the proper equipment. That includes a wristwatch to count seconds and a penlight to examine pupils. A **stethoscope** will help you listen to respirations and take blood pressure. You

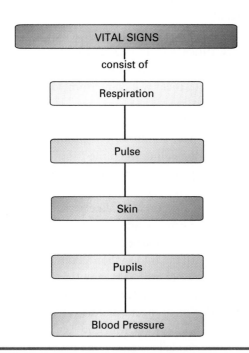

FIGURE 11–3 First Responders may be required to assess and document a patient's vital signs.

First on Scene

One set of vital signs is good. Two or more sets are better. Take multiple sets of vital signs if you are on the scene 5 or 10 minutes (or longer) before the EMTs arrive. Multiple sets of vital signs are called "trending." This is because more than one set shows changes (trends) over time. These trends, such as a rising pulse rate or a falling blood pressure, help identify or rule out serious medical conditions. Your measurements start the trending process.

will also need a **sphygmomanometer** (blood-pressure cuff). Finally, you must have a pen and notebook to record your findings. Many agencies also use pulse oximetry as an assessment tool.

More important than any one vital sign is change in vital signs over time. The vital signs taken by a First Responder are particularly important because they are taken early in the call. EMTs and hospital personnel will refer back to them to see if the patient has improved or gotten worse. For example, if you take a pulse and obtain a reading of 90 beats per minute, and later the pulse rises to 120, a serious condition may be developing. Without your early readings, this observation would not be possible.

Accuracy of vital signs is critical. The vital signs you take as a First Responder will be referenced as a *baseline* or starting point against which all future vital signs will be compared. If you have any difficulty taking accurate vital signs, say so. That is okay and better than placing something in a patient's record that may be incorrect. If you did not actually take vital signs, never say you did.

First Responder Practice

There is no "about" in vital signs measurement. All vital signs must be accurate, and they should be taken at regular intervals. If you are not sure about any reading, take it again. In most cases, you will take pulse and respirations for 30 seconds and multiply by 2. If you get an odd number, you've made a mistake. (You will never get an odd number when you multiply by 2.) Take the time to practice both the techniques and the math of vital signs.

TABLE 11–1 **Normal Respiratory Rates**	
Patient	**Respiratory Rate***
Infant	25–50 breaths per minute
Child	15–30 breaths per minute
Adult	12–20 breaths per minute
*Approximate per minute at rest	

Respiration

A **respiration** consists of one inhalation and one exhalation. The normal number of respirations per minute varies with gender and age. For an adult, that number is between 12 and 20 times per minute (Table 11–1). Count your patient's respirations by doing the following (Figure 11–4):

1. *Feel for breathing.* Place your hand on the patient's chest or abdomen.

2. *Count the number of breaths in one minute.* That is, count the number of times the chest (or abdomen) rises during a 30-second period. Then, multiply that number by 2.

3. *Record the breaths per minute.* Immediately write them down on your pad. Never rely on your memory.

The depth of respiration gives a clue to the amount of air that is inhaled. You can gauge depth by placing your hand on the patient's chest and feeling for chest movement. Feel the abdomen to see if it is moving instead of the chest. Normally, the work required by breathing is minimal. Some effort is required to inhale, but almost none is

required to exhale. For this reason, a normal inhalation takes slightly longer than a normal exhalation. When exhaling is prolonged, the patient may have a chronic obstructive pulmonary disorder (COPD) such as emphysema or may be in the midst of an asthma attack. Signs and symptoms of respiratory distress include:

- Shortness of breath, gasping for air.

- Breathing that is unusually fast, slow, deep, or shallow.

- Wheezing; gurgling; high-pitched, shrill sounds; or other unusual noises.

- Unusually moist, **flushed** skin. Later, may appear pale or bluish as the oxygen level in the blood falls.

- Difficulty speaking. Patient can say only a few words without catching his breath.

- Dizziness, anxiety.

- Chest pain and tingling in hands and feet.

If the patient is aware that you are assessing respiration, he may not breathe naturally. This can give a false reading. To get around this, take a pulse with the patient's arm draped over his chest or abdomen. Count the pulse for 15 seconds. Then, without moving the patient's arm, count respirations for the next 30 seconds. Readings are easily obtained by observing the chest rise and fall. You also can feel the motion with your hand, which is already on the patient's torso.

Pulse

Each time the heart beats, the arteries expand and contract with the blood that rushes into them. The pulse is the pressure wave generated by the heartbeat. It directly reflects the rate, relative strength, and rhythm of the contractions of the heart.

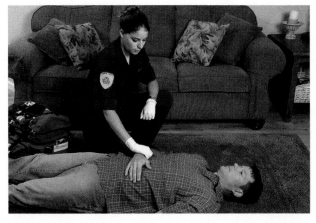

a.

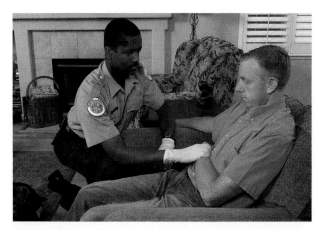

b.

FIGURE 11–4 Assessing respirations in a supine and a sitting patient.

TABLE 11-2 Normal Pulse Rates

Patient	Pulse Rate*
Infant	120–150 beats per minute
Child	80–150 beats per minute
Adult	60–80 beats per minute

*Approximate per minute at rest

When you take a pulse, note its *rate, strength,* and *regularity.* For rate, find out if the pulse is slow or fast. (See Table 11–2 for normal pulse rates.) For strength, find out if it is a **normal pulse** (full and strong), **thready** (weak and rapid), or **bounding** (unusually strong). For regularity, note the rhythm of the pulse. A normal pulse has regular spaces between each beat. An irregular one is spaced irregularly.

The rate, strength, and regularity of a pulse tell what the heart is doing at any given time. You can describe the pulse of a patient, for instance, as "72, strong, and regular."

The pulse can be felt at any point where an artery crosses over a bone or lies near the skin. First Responders often take a pulse at the wrist. This is where the radial artery crosses over the end of the forearm bone, the radius. To take the radial pulse (Figure 11–5):

1. *Position the patient.* Have him lie down or sit.

2. *Gently touch the pulse point* with the tips of two or three fingers. (Avoid using your thumb. It has a prominent pulse of its own, which can be counted by mistake.)

3. *Count the number of beats* you feel for 15 seconds. Then multiply that number by 4. This will give you the number of beats per minute. If a pulse is irregular,

slow, or difficult to obtain, count the beats for 30 seconds and multiply by 2 for a more accurate reading.

4. *Record the beats per minute.* Immediately write them down on your pad. Never rely on your memory.

Other points where a pulse may be taken include the brachial artery in the upper arm, the carotid artery in the neck, the femoral artery in the groin, the dorsalis pedis on the top of the foot, the posterior tibial artery on the medial surface of the ankle, and the **apical pulse** under the patient's left breast (requires a stethoscope).

Checking pulses in several areas will help to determine how well the patient's entire circulatory system is working. The absence of a pulse in a single extremity may indicate a blocked artery, for example. If left untreated, numbness, weakness, and tingling will follow the pain. The skin also gradually turns mottled, blue, and cold.

Skin

Assessment of skin temperature, color, and condition can tell you more about the patient's circulatory system.

Skin Temperature

Normal body temperature is 98.6°F (37°C). The most common way First Responders take temperature is by touching a patient's skin with the back of the hand. This is called **relative skin temperature.** It does not measure exact temperature, but you can tell if it is very high or low.

Changes in skin temperature can alert you to certain injuries and illnesses. A patient whose skin temperature is cool, for example, may be suffering from shock, heat exhaustion, or exposure to cold. A high temperature may be the result of fever or heat stroke. Body temperature can change over time, and it can be different in various parts of the body. A cold arm or leg, for example, may indicate circulatory problems. An isolated hot area could indicate a localized infection. Be alert to changes, and record them.

Skin Color

Skin color can tell you a lot about the condition of a patient's heart, lungs, and other areas as well. Assess visible areas of the skin, such as the face, neck, and arms. The nailbeds and lips may also show color changes. For example:

- *Paleness* may be caused by shock or heart attack. It also may be caused by fright, faintness, or emotional distress, as well as impaired blood flow.

- *Redness* (flushing) may be caused by high blood pressure, alcohol abuse, sunburn, heat stroke, fever, or an infectious disease.

- *Blueness* (cyanosis) is always a serious problem. It appears first in the fingertips and around the mouth.

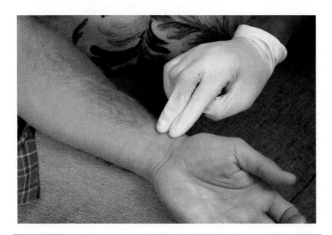

FIGURE 11-5 Assessing the radial pulse.

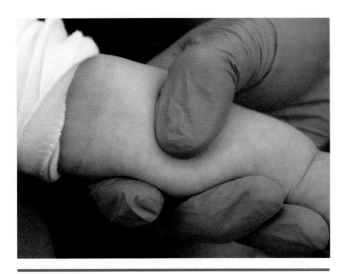

FIGURE 11–6 Assess capillary refill in children under 6 years of age.

Generally, it is caused by reduced levels of oxygen as in shock, heart attack, or poisoning.

- *Yellowish* color may be caused by a liver disease.
- *Black-and-blue mottling* is the result of blood seeping under the skin. It is usually caused by a blow or severe infection.

If your patient has dark skin, be sure to check for color changes on the lips, nail beds, palms, earlobes, whites of the eyes, inner surface of the lower eyelid, gums, and tongue.

Capillary Refill

Capillary refill (Figure 11–6) is one way of checking your patient for shock. It is recommended only for children under six years of age. Research has proven that it is not always accurate in adults.

This procedure is performed by squeezing one of the child's fingernails or toenails. In infants, squeeze the forearm or the area over the kneecap. When squeezed, the tissue turns white. When you let go, color returns. Measure the time it takes for the color to return (count "one one-thousand, two two-thousand," and so on). Two seconds or less is normal. If refill time is greater than two seconds, suspect shock or decreased blood flow to that extremity.

Note that when you recheck capillary refill, be sure to do it at the same place each time. Different parts of the body may have different refill times.

Skin Condition

Normally, a person's skin is dry to the touch. When a patient's skin is wet or moist, it may indicate shock, a heat-related emergency, or a diabetic emergency.

Abnormally dry skin may be a sign of spine injury or severe dehydration.

Pupils

Normally, pupils **constrict** (get smaller) when exposed to light and **dilate** (enlarge) when the level of light is reduced. In general, both pupils should be the same size unless a prior injury or condition changes this. (See Figure 11–7.)

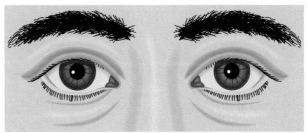

a. *Normal pupils*

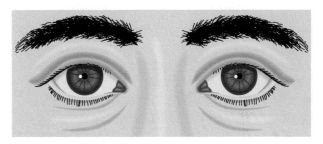

b. *Constricted pupils*

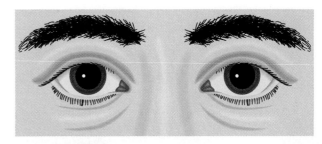

c. *Dilated pupils*

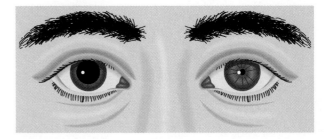

d. *Unequal pupils*

FIGURE 11–7 Check pupils for size, reactivity, and equality.

With these normal responses in mind, assess a patient's pupils. Shine your penlight into one of the patient's eyes and watch for the pupil to constrict in response to the light. If you are outdoors in bright light, cover the patient's eyes and observe for dilation of the pupils. Do not expose the patient's eyes to light for more than a few seconds. It can be very uncomfortable to the patient.

Abnormal findings for pupils include pupils that do not react to light. Pupils that remain constricted may be an indication of a drug overdose. Pupils that are unequal may indicate a serious head injury or stroke. Note that in a small percent of the population unequal pupils are normal.

Pulse Oximetry

The oxygen in the blood is carried by **hemoglobin.** A **pulse oximeter** is a device that measures the percentage of hemoglobin bound with oxygen (Figure 11–8). This finding provides one representation of how much oxygen the patient has in his or her blood. For example, if the pulse oximeter reads 99%, it is indicating that 99% of the patient's hemoglobin is saturated with oxygen.

Any numerical score displayed on the pulse oximeter displays a percentage of oxygen-saturated hemoglobin. Normal readings are 95%–100%. A reading of 90%–95% indicates **hypoxia** (an insufficiency of oxygen in the patient's tissues). Readings below 90% indicate severe hypoxia.

A significant limitation of the pulse oximeter is that it measures only oxygen in the blood, not oxygen levels in any other body tissue. Therefore, a patient in severe respiratory

distress could have a reading of 97%, while a patient who has only a minimum of distress has a 91% reading. This is why you will frequently hear "Never withhold oxygen from a patient based on a 'normal' pulse oximetry reading." All patients with trauma, breathing difficulty, chest pain, or other serious pain should receive oxygen regardless of the pulse oximetry reading.

So, why use a pulse oximeter? The best use of the pulse oximeter is to identify changes (improvements or decline) in the patient's condition. Keep your pulse oximeter readily available in your kit and place it on the patient before you administer oxygen. (NEVER delay administration of oxygen because pulse oximetry is not immediately available.) Observe an initial reading and then another after the patient has been receiving oxygen for a few minutes. If the patient reports feeling better or worse, this may correlate with changes on the pulse oximeter.

To use a pulse oximeter, follow these guidelines:

1. *Turn on the device.*

2. *Check the patient.* Make sure he or she is not wearing nail polish. Remove the nail polish, if necessary. (Commercially prepared polish removing wipes are available. Keep some with your oximeter.)

3. *Attach the device.* Place it over the patient's fingernail.

4. *Observe for a light or numerical reading indicating capture of a pulse.* If it matches the patient's pulse, which you have taken manually, this is a sign of proper functioning.

5. *Observe and record the oxygen saturation reading.* Remember: NEVER withhold supplementary oxygen from a patient based on normal pulse oximeter readings.

6. *Be alert to changes in subsequent readings.* Be sure to verify each reading. Never take pulse oximetry readings repeatedly without verifying each one with the radial or carotid pulse.

Note that some circumstances make pulse oximetry readings not valuable or not accurate. These include:

- *Carbon monoxide poisoning.* Falsely high readings will occur because the hemoglobin is saturated, but not with oxygen. Carbon monoxide can easily take the place of oxygen on the hemoglobin molecule. (Note that some newer oximeters can differentiate between oxygen and carbon dioxide.)

- *Hypothermia.* In this case, reduced circulation to the extremities will cause inaccurate oximetry readings.

- *Shock.* Shock is inadequate perfusion (blood supply to the body's tissues), so readings will be inaccurate in the extremities where perfusion is minimal. In some cases of shock, blood volume may be low due to internal or external bleeding. A pulse oximetry reading does not

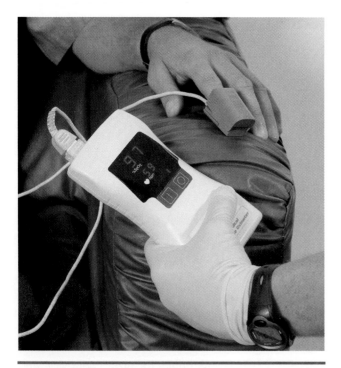

FIGURE 11–8 Using a pulse oximeter.

matter when there isn't enough blood to supply the body anyway.

- *Cardiac arrest.* In cardiac arrest, perfusion to the fingers is essentially absent, making readings unreliable. In fact, there usually is no time to consider pulse oximetry for these emergencies. CPR and defibrillation are more important considerations.

Blood Pressure

Blood pressure is the amount of pressure surging blood exerts against arterial walls. It is an important index of the efficiency of the whole circulatory system. In part, it tells how well the organs and tissues are getting the oxygen they need.

The blood-pressure cuff is the instrument used to measure blood pressure. The result of a contraction of the heart, which forces blood through the arteries, is called **systolic pressure.** The result of the relaxation of the heart between contractions is called **diastolic pressure.** With most diseases or injuries, these two pressures rise or fall together.

Blood pressure normally varies with the age, gender, and medical history of the patient. (See normal ranges in Table 11–3.) The usual guide for systolic pressure in the adult male is 100 plus the individual's age, up to 150 mmHg. Normal diastolic pressure in the male is 65 mmHg to 90 mmHg. Both the systolic and diastolic pressures are about 10 mmHg lower in the female than in the male.

Blood pressure is reported as systolic over diastolic (for example, 120/80).

Measuring Blood Pressure

There are two methods of obtaining blood pressure with a blood pressure cuff. One is by **auscultation,** or by listening for the systolic and diastolic sounds through a stethoscope. The second method is by **palpation,** or by feeling for the return of the pulse as the cuff is deflated.

To assess blood pressure by *auscultation,* follow the steps described below (Figure 11–9):

1. *Apply the blood pressure cuff.* First, choose the proper size cuff. It must be able to encircle the arm so that the

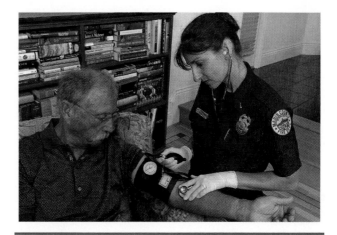

FIGURE 11–9 Taking a patient's blood pressure by auscultation.

Velcro on opposite ends meet and fasten securely. The cuff's bladder should cover half the circumference of the arm. If it covers less, it will not compress the blood vessels properly. If it covers more, it will suppress the pulse too quickly. The cuff should fit snugly with the lower edge at least an inch above the *antecubital space* (the hollow, or front, of the elbow) and the bladder centered over the brachial artery. It should not be too tight. You should be able to place one finger easily under its bottom edge. Some cuffs have markers for overlap placement, but they are not always in the correct location.

2. *Inflate the cuff rapidly with the rubber bulb.* At the same time, palpate the radial pulse until it can no longer be felt. Make a mental note of the reading. Without stopping, continue to inflate the cuff to 30 mm above the level where the pulse disappeared.

3. *Apply the stethoscope.* Place the diaphragm of the stethoscope over the brachial artery just above the hollow of the elbow. The diaphragm may be held with the thumb.

4. *Deflate the cuff* at approximately 2 mm per second (faster if skill permits). Watch the mercury column or needle indicator drop.

5. *Record the systolic pressure.* That is, as soon as you hear two or more consecutive beats (clear tapping sounds of increasing intensity), record the pressure reading. This is the systolic pressure.

6. *Record the diastolic pressure.* First, continue releasing air from the bulb. At the point where you hear the last sound, record the pressure reading. This is the diastolic pressure. Continue to deflate slowly for at least 10 mm. Remember that slow pulses require slower-than-normal rates of deflation. With children and some adults, you may hear sounds all the way to zero.

TABLE 11–3	**Normal Blood Pressure Ranges**	
Patient	**Systolic**	**Diastolic**
Child	80 + (2 × patient's age)	50–80 mmHg
Adult	100 + patient's age (up to 150 mmHg)	65–90 mmHg

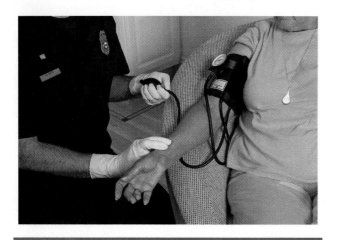

FIGURE 11–10 Taking a patient's blood pressure by palpation.

In such cases, record the pressure when the sound changes from clear tapping to soft, muffled tapping.

7. *Record where and how BP was taken.* Record the limb on which the blood pressure was taken. Record the position of the person when the blood pressure was taken, if other than supine. Record the size of the cuff if other than standard.

When it is too noisy for you to hear well enough to measure by auscultation, *palpate* the blood pressure (Figure 11–10). To palpate blood pressure, first rapidly inflate the cuff. As you do so, palpate the patient's radial pulse. Make a mental note of the level at which you can no longer feel the pulse. Without stopping, continue to inflate the cuff another 30 mmHg. Then, slowly deflate it. Note the pressure at which the radial pulse returns. This is the systolic pressure. Record it as a palpated systolic pressure (for example, 120/P).

Whether you auscultate or palpate the blood pressure, take several readings during the time the patient is in your care. Watch for changes, as this may indicate changes in the patient's condition. Carefully record the blood pressure when you measure it, including the time it was taken.

It is not unusual for a patient's blood pressure to vary between the first reading on scene and the reading at the hospital emergency department. Record the pressure accurately so that the receiving physician can tell how much it has changed.

Blood pressure may be normal even if the patient is seriously injured. You will learn in Chapter 18 that by the time the blood pressure drops, the patient already is in serious condition.

Standards for Adults

Blood pressures from person to person vary greatly. In general, systolic blood pressures above 180 and below 90 usually indicate problems. Diastolic blood pressures above 90 and below 60 also indicate problems. The most common blood pressure problem observed in the field is low blood pressure. However, if blood pressure increases dramatically, the patient may suffer a stroke.

In general, blood pressure changes occur late in an emergency. A person who has a blood pressure of 132/82 could actually be developing severe shock. On the other hand, an uninjured person may normally have a blood pressure of 92/62 and be perfectly healthy. Always consider the blood pressure reading as only one element of the patient's picture. Be sure to look at other vital signs, too.

Standards for Children

It is often difficult to take a child's blood pressure. Carrying a variety of cuff sizes is not always possible. But you must have a correctly fitting cuff if you are to get an accurate reading. Always try to get a complete set of vital signs. However, do not waste time attempting multiple blood pressure readings on a critical child if your first tries were unsuccessful. Note that a blood pressure reading is not recommended on children under three years of age.

Average blood pressures in children may be determined by the formula: 80 + (2 × age in years). This formula works until the child is about 12 years of age. From that point on, adult blood pressure values apply.

In children, adequate airway management is vital. Do *not* place blood pressure determination over assessment and care of life-threats. A child's blood pressure may not begin to drop until well over 40% of blood volume is lost. If the mechanism of injury suggests it, treat for shock regardless of vital signs.

Variable Factors

Trauma and most types of shock can *decrease* blood pressure. Factors that can *increase* blood pressure include conditions and substances that constrict blood vessels such as:

- Cold environment.
- High altitude.
- Physical and emotional stress.
- Pain.
- Full bladder.
- Upper arm lower than heart level.
- Cigarette smoke.
- Caffeine (coffee, tea, cola, and some analgesic medications).
- Decongestants.

With the many possible variables that affect blood pressure, it is essential that you recognize the mistakes that can occur in taking a reading. The most critical of these possible errors are:

■ Rescuer does not hear accurately due to noise, head cold, or distractions.

■ Stethoscope ear pieces are improperly placed.

■ Improper conditions exist, such as a cuff not at heart level or a patient not sitting or lying down.

■ Systolic pressure is not palpated at the highest level.

■ Cuff is the wrong size, either too wide or too narrow.

■ Bladder is too wide.

■ Cuff is deflated too quickly.

 Q:

1. What equipment should you have in order to take a patient's vital signs?

2. What are normal respiratory and pulse rates for the infant, child, and adult?

3. What is the most common way for a First Responder to take a patient's temperature?

4. For what conditions may pulse oximetry be inaccurate?

5. What should a First Responder look for during assessment of a patient's pupils?

6. What are the normal blood pressure ranges for children and adults?

The Call Follow-up

At the beginning of this chapter, you read that an off-duty First Responder happened upon an older woman who was sitting on a sidewalk curb. She has a small abrasion on her arm with minor bleeding. To see how chapter skills apply to this incident, read the following. It describes how the call was completed.

Physical Examination I knew the patient was injured, because I saw her arm. I also knew that she could be hurt somewhere else, so I quickly checked her from head to toe. Her pulse was a bit fast at 102, strong and slightly irregular. Respirations were 22 and adequate. Her forearm and wrist on the arm with the abrasion was painful. I thought she could have a broken bone in addition to the abrasion.

Patient History As I conducted the physical exam, the patient told me that she fell on the sidewalk. "Nothing serious," she said. "I just scraped my arm a bit. It happens when you get older." I asked her where she was coming from when she

fell. She said she couldn't remember. I asked her how she felt just before she fell, and she said she was a bit dizzy. She sometimes seems to "space out," she said. I was concerned and wondered if she had a medical problem that could have caused her fall. She told me she had a history of high blood pressure.

Ongoing Assessment The fire department ambulance pulled up before I could perform an ongoing assessment.

Patient Hand-off As one of the firefighter paramedics questioned the woman, I noticed that she was still a bit confused. I gave his partner my report (see below). The firefighter paramedics took over and moved Mrs. Hazelton into the ambulance. They agreed that she could have a medical problem. Maybe that problem caused her fall, maybe it didn't. I was happy that I recognized the fact that there could be more than one problem. I watched for a few minutes. They splinted her arm and put on a heart monitor. She was in good hands.

Hand-off Report

"This is Marge Hazelton. She is 74, and she told me that she took a fall. I saw the abrasion on her forearm. Palpation reveals some tenderness to that arm and wrist, as well. I did not find any other injury. I was concerned because she seemed a bit confused about what happened. She doesn't remember the fall, but said she was dizzy just before. You might want to check that out. She has a history of high blood pressure. Her baseline pulse and respirations are a bit high: pulse 102, strong and slightly irregular; respirations 22 and adequate."

The Last Word *It isn't always easy to tell the difference between a medical and trauma patient. Follow your patient assessment plan. It will help* *you avoid getting confused and prevent you from overlooking a problem.*

Chapter Review

Focus on the EMS Team

Vital signs are very important. As a First Responder, you will be on scene nearest to the time of the onset of illness or injury. The first set of vital signs you take show the condition of the patient early in the course of the emergency. These baseline signs will allow those who take over patient care—EMTs and hospital personnel—to monitor the progress of the patient's condition over time. Remember: Your patient depends on you. Be sure to obtain vitals accurately. Record your findings as soon as you have them.

Summing Up

- Patient assessment is a systematic evaluation of a patient, meant to help determine the nature and extent of a patient's illness or injuries. Findings from the assessment allow the appropriate decisions to be made for emergency care.
- The First Responder's patient assessment plan consists of scene size-up, initial assessment, physical examination, patient history, ongoing assessment, and hand-off report.
- The most pertinent information about a trauma patient will come from the physical examination. The most pertinent information about a medical patient will most likely come from the current and relevant past histories.
- If you are unsure about whether a patient has an illness or injury—or if you are unsure of the extent of the injuries—complete a full head-to-toe exam and gather a complete patient history.
- Vital signs include the patient's respiration, pulse, skin, pupils, and blood pressure.
- Respiratory rate is calculated by counting the number of times the chest rises during a 30-second period and then multiplying that number by 2. Respiratory quality is assessed by observing chest rise and fall and looking for extra effort to breathe, prolonged exhalations, or unusual breath sounds.
- Pulse rate is assessed by palpating an arterial pulse point, counting the number of beats for 15 seconds, and then multiplying that number by 4. For pulse strength, feel for a normal, thready, or bounding pulse. For regularity, notice the spaces between each beat.
- Skin temperature is assessed by feeling the patient's skin with the back of your hand. Inspect the skin for paleness or if it is somewhat red, blue, yellow, or mottled. Check capillary refill in children under six years of age. Finally, check skin condition to see if it is dry, wet, or moist.
- Pupil are assessed for size, reactivity, and equality.
- To measure the amount of oxygen in the patient's blood, use a pulse oximeter.
- Blood pressure may be assessed by either auscultation or palpation.
- Average or normal vital sign rates are summarized in the chart below:

Patient	Normal Respiratory Rate	
Infant	25–50 breaths per minute	
Child	15–30 breaths per minute	
Adult	12–20 breaths per minute	
Patient	**Normal Pulse Rate**	
Infant	120–150 beats per minute	
Child	80–150 beats per minute	
Adult	60–80 beats per minute	
Patient	**Normal Pulse Oximetry**	
All ages	95%–100%	
Patient	**Normal Blood Pressure**	
	Systolic	*Diastolic*
Child	80 + (2 × age in years)	50–80 mmHg
Adult	100 + patient's age (up to 150 mmHg)	65–90 mmHg

Key Terms

apical pulse an arterial pulse point located under the patient's left breast.

auscultation a method of examination that involves listening for signs of illness or injury. Taking a blood pressure by auscultation refers to listening for the systolic and diastolic sounds through a stethoscope.

blood pressure the amount of pressure surging blood exerts against arterial walls.

bounding a term used to characterize a pulse that is unusually strong.

capillary refill the time it takes for capillaries that have been compressed to refill with blood.

constrict get smaller.

diastolic pressure the result of the relaxation of the heart between contractions.

dilate enlarge.

flushed redness of the skin.

hemoglobin the iron-containing pigment of red blood cells that carries oxygen from the lungs to the tissues.

hypoxia an insufficiency of oxygen in the patient's tissues.

medical patient a patient who is ill, not injured.

normal pulse See *pulse*.

palpation a method of examination that involves feeling for signs of injury or illness. Taking a blood pressure by palpation refers to feeling for the patient's pulse as a blood pressure cuff is deflated.

patient assessment the gathering of information to determine a possible illness or injury. A First Responder's patient assessment plan includes scene size-up, initial assessment, physical examination, patient history, ongoing assessment, and patient hand-off.

pulse the wave of blood propelled through the arteries as a result of the pumping action of the heart. Characterized as full and strong (normal), bounding (unusually strong), thready (weak and rapid), regular (equal spaces between beats), irregular (unequal spaces between beats).

pulse oximeter an electronic device that measures the percentage of hemoglobin bound with oxygen.

relative skin temperature an assessment of the skin temperature obtained by touching the patient's skin.

respiration passage of air into and out of the lungs. When counting respirations, consider one inhalation plus one exhalation equal to one respiration.

sphygmomanometer an instrument used to determine arterial blood pressure.

stethoscope an instrument used to listen to sounds within the body.

systolic pressure the result of a contraction of the heart, which forces blood through the arteries.

thready a term used to characterize a pulse that is weak and rapid.

trauma patient a patient who is injured, not ill.

vital signs signs of life; assessments related to breathing, pulse, skin, pupils, and blood pressure.

Knowledge Check

1. **The pulse is:**
    a. the pressure wave generated by the heartbeat.
    b. arteries compressing and relaxing against bones.
    c. the blood in veins being compressed by arteries.
    d. blood vessels contracting and dilating.

2. The top number in a blood pressure reading is the ___ pressure.

   a. pulse
   b. systolic
   c. diastolic
   d. contracted

3. Bluish skin can be caused by:

   a. high blood pressure.
   b. sunburn.
   c. alcohol.
   d. shock.

4. Capillary refill is an assessment recommended for:

   a. adults.
   b. all patients.
   c. children younger than 6.
   d. children younger than 18.

5. Count the number of times the chest rises during a ___ period. Then multiply that number by ___ for the patient's respiration rate.

   a. 30-second, 2
   b. 12-second, 6
   c. 10-minute, 6
   d. 5-minute, 12

6. Which one of the following factors will decrease blood pressure?

   a. pain
   b. cigarette smoking
   c. decongestants
   d. shock

7. Which one of the following is NOT noted when assessing and documenting a pulse?

   a. rate
   b. rhythm
   c. strength
   d. pressure

8. Which one of the following statements about pulse oximetry is TRUE?

   a. Pulse oximetry approximates blood pressure.
   b. Pulse oximeters display the patient's pulse.
   c. Patients who have a saturation reading of 95% or above do NOT require oxygen.
   d. Pulse oximeters will display an accurate reading in hypothermia because the oxygen level does NOT change.

9. Palpation of blood pressure provides the patient's systolic blood pressure level.

   a. True
   b. False

10. Normally, when a light is shone into a patient's eye, the pupil will constrict.

    a. True
    b. False

11. The need for oxygen should be based on a pulse oximetry reading.

    a. True
    b. False

12. List the components of a First Responder's patient assessment plan.

_____   _____

_____   _____

_____   _____

13. List four ways in which your senses are used for patient assessment.

_____

_____

_____

_____

14. Describe the main difference between a medical patient and a trauma patient.

_____

_____

_____

Scenario

You are called to the scene of an unresponsive man in his backyard. As you begin scene size-up, you see the patient lying on the dirt just outside of his tool shed. It looks as if he was working on an old, freshly stripped door, which is flat on top of two sawhorses. On the ground beside the patient is a power sander, not running.

a. What should you do first?

_____

_____

_____

b. You and the patient's wife are at the patient's side. Your initial assessment found him to be unresponsive, with adequate respirations, a rapid weak pulse, and skin that is very dry and somewhat flushed. There are no signs of injury. While you wait for the EMTs to arrive with an ambulance, you follow local protocol and administer oxygen to the patient. What else should you do—gather the patient's history from his wife or conduct a thorough physical exam? Explain your answer.

_____

_____

_____

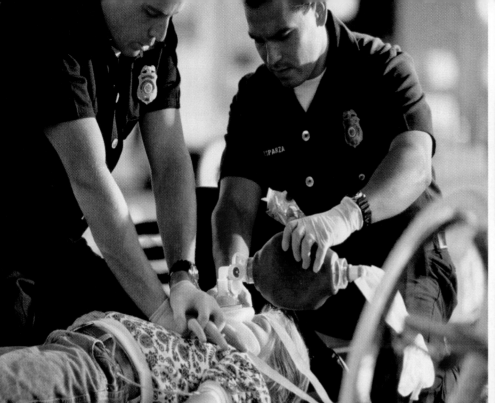
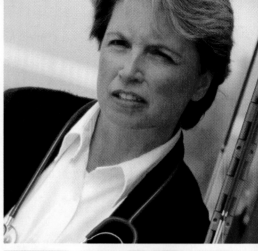
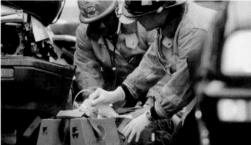

12 | Patient Assessment

Objectives

From the U.S. Department of Transportation (DOT) 1995 "First Responder: National Standard Curriculum." Material supplemental to the DOT curriculum is listed under "Enrichment."

Cognitive

3-1.7 ▸ Summarize the reasons for forming a general impression of the patient. (pp. 214–215)

3-1.8 ▸ Discuss methods of assessing mental status. (pp. 216–217)

3-1.9 ▸ Differentiate between assessing mental status in the adult, child, and infant patient. (p. 217)

3-1.10 ▸ Describe methods used for assessing if a patient is breathing. (pp. 217–219)

3-1.11 ▸ Differentiate between a patient with adequate and inadequate breathing. (pp. 218–219)

3-1.12 ▸ Describe the methods used to assess circulation. (pp. 219–220)

3-1.13 ▸ Differentiate between obtaining a pulse in an adult, child, and infant patient. (pp. 219–220)

3-1.14 ▸ Discuss the need for assessing the patient for external bleeding. (p. 220)

3-1.15 ▸ Explain the reason for prioritizing a patient for care and transport. (pp. 220–221)

3-1.16 ▸ Discuss the components of the physical exam. (pp. 221–222)

3-1.17 ▸ State the areas of the body that are evaluated during the physical exam. (pp. 223–226)

3-1.18 ▸ Explain what additional questioning may be asked during the physical exam. (pp. 223–226)

3-1.19 ▸ Explain the components of the SAMPLE history. (pp. 227–229)

3-1.20 ▸ Discuss the components of the ongoing assessment. (pp. 229–230)

3-1.21 ▸ Describe the information included in the First Responder "hand-off" report. (p. 230)

Affective

3-1.24 ▸ Explain the importance of forming a general impression of the patient. (pp. 214–215)

3-1.25 ▸ Explain the value of an initial assessment. (pp. 214–221)

3-1.26 ▸ Explain the value of questioning the patient and family. (pp. 227–229)

3-1.27 ▸ Explain the value of the physical exam. (pp. 223–226)

3-1.28 ▸ Explain the value of an ongoing assessment. (pp. 229–230)

3-1.29 ▸ Explain the rationale for the feelings that these patients might be experiencing. (pp. 212, 223, 228, 229–230)

3-1.30 ▸ Demonstrate a caring attitude when performing patient assessments. (pp. 212, 223, 228, 229–230)

3-1.31 ▸ Place the interests of the patient as the foremost consideration when making any and all patient care decisions during patient assessment. (pp. 212, 223, 228, 229–230)

3-1.32 ▸ Communicate with empathy during patient assessment to patients as well as with family members and friends of the patient. (pp. 212, 223, 228, 229–230)

Psychomotor

3-1.34 ▸ Demonstrate the techniques for assessing mental status. (pp. 216–217)

3-1.35 ▸ Demonstrate the techniques for assessing the airway. (pp. 217–219)

3-1.36 ▸ Demonstrate the techniques for assessing if the patient is breathing. (pp. 217–219)

3-1.37 ▸ Demonstrate the techniques for assessing if the patient has a pulse. (pp. 219–220)

3-1.38 ▸ Demonstrate the techniques for assessing the patient for external bleeding. (p. 220)

3-1.40 ▸ Demonstrate questioning a patient to obtain a SAMPLE history. (pp. 227–229)

3-1.41 ▸ Demonstrate the skills involved in performing the physical exam. (pp. 223–226)

3-1.42 ▸ Demonstrate the ongoing assessment. (pp. 229–230)

Enrichment

▸ Describe when and how to manually stabilize a patient's head and neck. (pp. 215, 224)

▸ Differentiate between a sign and a symptom. (p. 227)

Introduction

First Responders must be able to assess a patient's condition quickly and accurately. This chapter will help you learn how. It presents the step-by-step routine used by many experienced emergency care providers. The routine includes scene size-up, which you studied in Chapter 10. It goes on to include initial assessment, physical examination, patient history, ongoing assessment, and patient hand-off—all of which are described in this chapter.

Section 1 Initial Assessment

The **initial assessment** includes getting a general impression of the patient; assessing responsiveness; assessing the **ABCs** (airway, breathing, and circulation); and updating incoming EMS units about the patient's condition. (See Figure 12-1.) It may be the most important part of the patient assessment process. In it you must identify and treat conditions that cause an immediate threat to the patient's life. Life-threats usually involve airway obstruction, breathing problems, or severe bleeding.

General Impression

Form a general impression as you approach the patient (Figure 12-2). It should include the patient's *chief*

First Responder Practice

All components of patient assessment are important, but none is more important to your patient than the initial assessment. Never stop the initial assessment until it is complete. That means for some patients you will be able to do only an initial assessment. For example, if you find your patient is breathing inadequately, even with someone there to help, you won't be able to move on to the physical exam. Maintaining an open airway and assisting ventilations properly are much more important.

THE CALL

Dispatch My partner and I were dispatched to a call for an "unresponsive man." We were told the caller said she was unable to wake her husband after his nap.

Scene Size-up We approached the scene carefully. This call was in a quiet section of town but you never can tell. We realized that an unresponsive person could mean anything from a drunk to a cardiac arrest. A woman met us at the door, quite upset. She was about 60. We heard a dog in the yard, but the woman assured us that it couldn't get in the house. There was only one patient. The woman said her husband didn't fall or anything. We felt sure we had a medical problem on our hands.

Patient assessment is an important process for all levels of EMS responders. Here the First Responders performed a scene size-up. Put yourself in their place. What do you think should be done next? Consider this patient as you read Chapter 12.

complaint, the patient's age and sex, and a brief immediate assessment of the environment in which the emergency has taken place.

The **chief complaint** is the reason that EMS was called. It is generally the response to the question "Can you tell me why you called EMS today?" Record the response on your forms in the patient's own words. "I fell down the stairs" or "My chest hurts" are examples of chief complaints. If the patient is unresponsive, get the information from the person who called EMS.

The general impression is not designed to be the final word in the assessment of the patient's condition. Rather, it lets you get started on the right track with patient care. During this phase of the initial assessment, you are to determine if the situation is a trauma (injury) complaint or a medical (illness) complaint. Do this by listening to what the patient or bystanders tell you. Also make sure that you have looked around the scene to identify the forces involved in an injury.

If those forces suggest a possible head or spine injury, take **spinal precautions** at this time. This means you should hold the patient's head and neck stable and in a neutral position (Figure 12-3). To do so, first place your hands on either side of the patient's head. Then, spread your fingers apart. The object is to prevent movement until the patient can be fully immobilized. If the patient is conscious, explain what you are doing so he or she is not alarmed. Your hand position may reduce the patient's hearing. Be aware of the anxiety this may cause. (Spine injuries are covered in depth in Chapter 24.)

Once you have formed your general impression, you may find that you are facing a patient with a potentially serious injury or illness. If so, you may wish to ask EMS dispatch for advanced life support personnel or additional units to assist. (You may have already done this in the scene size-up.)

Consider the following examples of general impressions:

- A 12-year-old male patient, who was riding his bicycle, was struck by a dump truck. Your observation of the scene reveals that the boy's bicycle has been mangled by the truck. The boy appears unconscious.

- A 58-year-old woman is complaining of abdominal pain. She seems to be speaking normally, without a sign of strain. However, she is protecting her abdomen with one hand.

- A 26-year-old man is found on the floor of his bathroom, unconscious. No one is quite sure of what happened.

In the first case, the general impression leads you to believe the boy could be seriously injured. The second case appears to be a medical patient who is not in severe distress. The third case gives you little additional information on how to proceed. However, the mere fact that the man is unconscious can tell you that certain precautions must be taken.

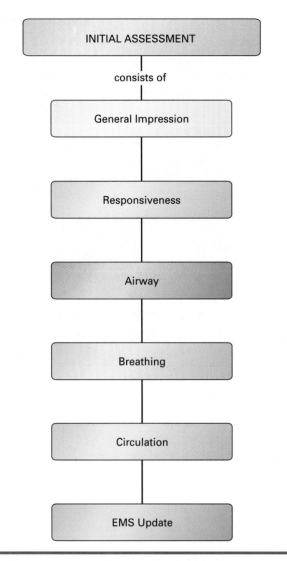

FIGURE 12-1 The initial assessment of your patient should take about one minute.

Responsiveness

The next part of the initial assessment is determining the patient's **level of responsiveness.** This is important for many reasons. One of the most important is the patient who has an **altered mental status** (a change in his or her normal mental state). That patient may need airway care as well as other life-saving aid.

Begin when you get to the patient's side. Introduce yourself. State your name. Then explain that you are an EMS First Responder who is there to help. Make sure your identity is clear. This interaction will help you begin your assessment of the patient's mental status.

Four levels of responsiveness are commonly used to classify patients. They are *alert, verbal, painful,* and *unresponsive.* Together, these terms make up the memory aid **AVPU.** The classifications, when applied to patients, are as follows (Figure 12-4):

A—*Alert.* A patient who is alert is responsive and oriented. That is, the patient is aware of his surroundings, the approximate time and date, and his name. This is commonly referred to as being "responsive to person, place, and date" (or "oriented × 3). Each distinction is important. Some patients may appear wide awake but in fact are not aware of their surroundings. A patient's mental status is important to determine because it can indicate injury or illness.

V—*Verbal.* This patient is disoriented but responds when spoken to. We say that he or she "responds to verbal stimulus." A patient who answers questions about place and date incorrectly is another example. He or she may be suffering from a medical condition such as seizures or diabetes or a traumatic condition such as shock.

P—*Painful.* The patient who responds only to a painful stimulus does not answer questions or open his eyes or respond to verbal commands. He or she only stirs or

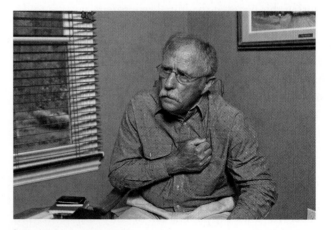

a.   b.

FIGURE 12-2 Form a general impression as you approach the patient.

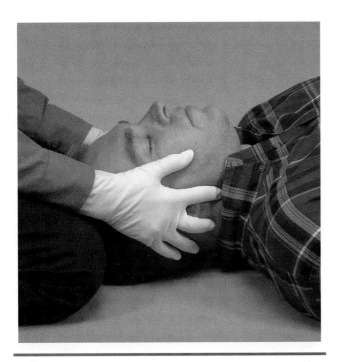

FIGURE 12-3 If there is a possible spine or head injury, immediately stabilize the patient's head and neck.

flinches. The stimulus may be a pinch or a careful but firm rub on the sternum in the absence of chest injuries. (Remember that you first check responsiveness by observation. If the patient is alert or verbal, there is no need to apply a painful stimulus.)

U—*Unresponsive.* This patient does not respond to any stimulus. He does not open his eyes, respond verbally, or even flinch when pain is applied. This patient is deeply

unconscious, most likely in a critical condition, and in definite need of airway and other supportive care.

Determining the level of responsiveness in infants and children and elderly patients is different. For infants and young children, assess their response to the environment. They should recognize their parents, and they usually wish to go to them. Expect your assessment to cause tears, too. Children who do not recognize their parents or who are indifferent to your assessment and treatment may be very sick.

In the elderly, common diseases and conditions such as Alzheimer's cause changes in responsiveness. In cases such as these, try to find out from the family if there has been a change. That is, the patient may normally be somewhat confused, but has it worsened with this episode?

Some elderly patients live alone and have neither the means nor reason to keep track of the date and current events. If an elderly patient does not know the date, try other questions to determine orientation. You might ask about the immediate surroundings, for example, or about what you are doing there. If the patient is responsive and oriented, obtain consent to continue care.

Airway

The patient's airway status is a foundation of patient care. No patient can survive without an adequate airway. Make sure the patient's airway is open and clear (Figure 12-5). The way you assess the patient's airway depends on whether the patient is responsive or not.

- *Responsive patient.* Notice if the responsive patient can speak clearly. Gurgling or other sounds may indicate

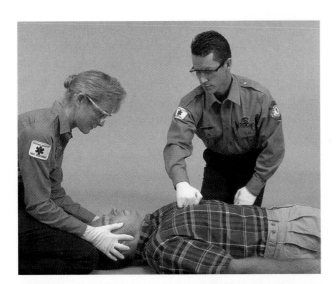

FIGURE 12-4 Use the AVPU scale—alert, verbal, painful, unresponsive—to assess the patient's level of responsiveness.

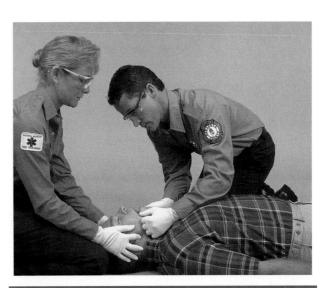

FIGURE 12-5 Open the patient's airway and make sure it is clear. Suction and insert an oral airway if necessary.

teeth, blood, or other matter in the airway. Also make sure the patient can speak full sentences.

■ *Unresponsive patient.* This patient needs aggressive airway maintenance. Immediately make sure the airway is open. If the patient is ill with no sign of trauma, use the head-tilt/chin-lift maneuver to open the airway. If trauma is suspected, use the jaw-thrust maneuver with great care to avoid tilting the head. Inspect the airway for blood, vomit, and secretions. Also look for loose teeth or other foreign matter that could cause an obstruction. Clear the airway using suction or a gloved finger. If there is no gag reflex, insert an oral airway.

Remember that an airway check is not a one-time event. Some patients with serious trauma, or unresponsive medical patients who are vomiting, will need almost constant suctioning and airway maintenance.

Breathing

After securing an open airway, *look, listen,* and *feel* for breathing (Figure 12-6). If there is breathing, determine if respirations are adequate. Remember, breathing is not an all-or-nothing proposition. There will be times when a patient is breathing but not at a sufficient depth or rate to sustain life.

Adequate breathing is characterized by three factors: adequate rise and fall of the chest, ease of breathing (breathing should appear to be effortless), and adequate respiratory rate.

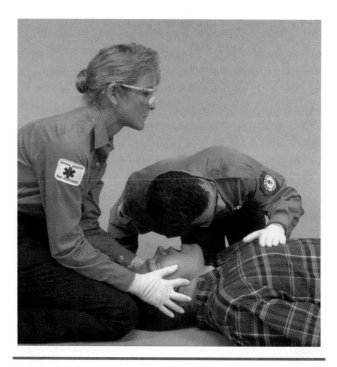

FIGURE 12-6 **Look, listen, and feel for breathing.**

Inadequate breathing may be identified by (Figure 12-7):

■ Inadequate rise and fall of the chest.

■ Increased effort to breathe.

■ Cyanosis (blue or gray color to the skin, lips, or nail beds).

SIGNS OF INADEQUATE BREATHING

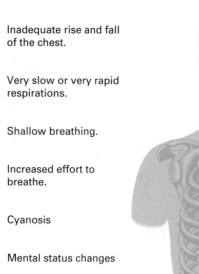

Inadequate rise and fall of the chest.

Very slow or very rapid respirations.

Shallow breathing.

Increased effort to breathe.

Cyanosis

Mental status changes

FIGURE 12-7 **Inadequate breathing in your patient requires ventilatory assistance.**

TABLE 12-1 **Oxygen Therapy**

Conditions that may require oxygen therapy include:
- Injury.
- Heart or breathing problems.
- Shock.
- Any other condition that prevents the efficient flow of oxygen throughout the body.

Signs and symptoms that indicate the need for oxygen are:
- Poor skin color (blue, gray, or pale).
- Altered mental status, including unresponsiveness.
- Cool, clammy skin.
- Difficulty breathing.
- Blood loss.
- Chest pain.
- Trauma (injury).
- Restlessness.

- Mental status changes.
- Inadequate respiratory rate (less than 8 per minute in adults, less than 10 in children, and less than 20 in infants).

If the patient is breathing adequately, there may be no need to assist respiration in any way. However, during your assessment, you may determine that your patient would benefit from oxygen therapy (Table 12-1). If you are trained and allowed, administer oxygen to these patients (Figure 12-8).

If you determine that the patient's respirations are inadequate or absent, you must begin ventilating immediately. Do not stop until you are relieved by another trained rescuer or until the patient regains adequate respirations. In most cases, you will continue ventilations until the EMTs arrive.

Circulation

When you assess circulation, you are checking to see that the heart is pumping blood to all parts of the body. You also must be sure that the heart is pumping adequately and that there is no life-threatening external bleeding.

To assess a patient's circulation, you must check the pulse (Figure 12-9):

- *Responsive patient.* In an adult, use the radial pulse point to assess circulation. Checking the carotid pulse may cause this patient undue anxiety. Use either the radial or brachial pulse point for the responsive child. For an infant, always use the brachial pulse point.

- *Unresponsive patient.* In an adult, check the carotid artery. In an unresponsive child, check the carotid or femoral arteries. For the unresponsive infant, check the brachial artery. If the pulse is absent, begin CPR.

When checking the pulse, note the approximate rate and rhythm. If the pulse is very irregular or feels extremely slow or fast, be on the lookout for serious conditions. Also note the patient's skin at this time. Check the

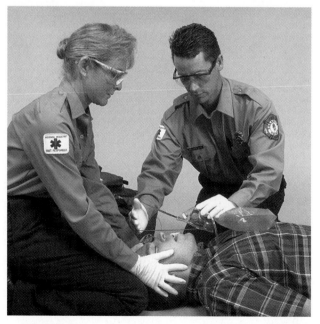

a. *If ventilations are adequate and the patient's condition warrants it, administer oxygen.*

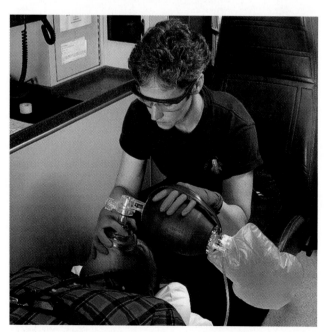

b. *Assist the patient's ventilations if breathing is inadequate or absent.*

FIGURE 12-8 Determine if ventilations are adequate.

SKILL SUMMARY   *Assessing the Pulse*

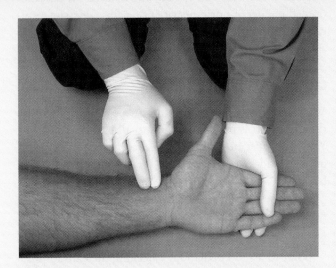

FIGURE 12-9A   *Assessing the radial pulse.*

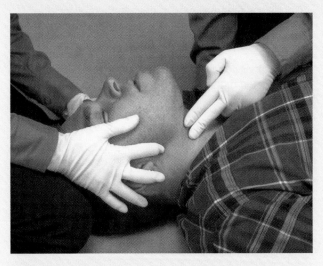

FIGURE 12-9B   *Assessing the carotid pulse.*

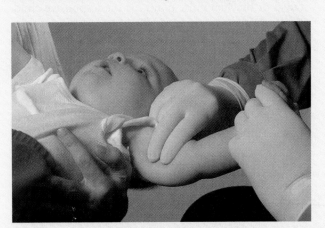

FIGURE 12-9C   *Assessing the brachial pulse.*

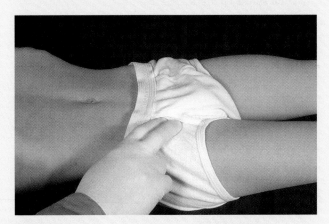

FIGURE 12-9D   *Assessing the femoral pulse.*

color, temperature, and condition (Figure 12-10). Skin that is pale, cool, and moist may indicate shock.

After checking the patient's pulse, check for serious external bleeding (Figure 12-11). Remember that the initial assessment is designed to identify and treat life-threatening problems. Be alert. Do not let minor wounds sidetrack you or keep you from caring for more serious injuries first.

Scan the patient for serious bleeding. Use your gloved hands to check areas that are hard to see, such as the small of the back and the buttocks. Remember that heavy clothes can absorb large quantities of blood. If you find serious bleeding, use the methods discussed in Chapter 18 to control it.

EMS Update

At this point, you will know if your patient is barely breathing and requires ventilation (a high priority) or if

your patient is stable with a minor complaint. In either case, the EMS units currently en route to the scene will be interested in an update. The information you provide will allow them to prepare for the patient and provide more efficient care.

If you have a phone or radio available, update EMS (Figure 12-12). Report the patient's age and sex, chief complaint, level of responsiveness, airway and breathing status, and circulation status. Also ask the incoming EMS units to give you their **ETA** (estimated time of arrival), so you can continue patient care and prepare for their arrival.

The following is an example of a radio report. It might have been given by the First Responders in "The Call," the scenario that opened this chapter:

"Dispatcher, we have an approximately 60-year-old male who was found responsive only to painful stimulus.

First on Scene

There are a number of findings that indicate a high priority for transport. These are conditions for which usually little or no treatment can be given in the field. They include:

- Poor general impression.
- Unresponsiveness.
- Responsive, but not following commands.
- Difficulty breathing.
- Shock.
- Complicated childbirth.
- Chest pain with systolic blood pressure less than 100.
- Uncontrolled bleeding.
- Severe pain anywhere.

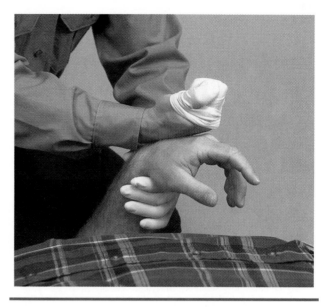

FIGURE 12-10 Assessing the patient's skin.

His airway required suctioning, and we are assisting ventilations. The patient's pulse is rapid and weak."

After your update report, the dispatcher will acknowledge your transmission and advise you of the ambulance's ETA (estimated time of arrival).

:

1. What should you do before you perform an initial assessment?

2. What does the term "chief complaint" mean?

3. What spinal precautions should you take in the initial assessment? For what reason should you take them?

4. What are the four levels of responsiveness commonly used to classify patients?

5. What are the signs of inadequate breathing?

6. During the initial assessment, what pulse point should be checked first in an infant? A child? An adult?

7. What patient information should be included in the EMS update?

Section 2 First Responder Physical Exam

The initial assessment is designed to help you identify and treat life-threats. However, not all problems will be life-threatening. The First Responder physical examination is a survey of the patient's entire body. It is meant to reveal any signs of illness or injury. (See Figure 12-13.)

The physical exam is designed to be thorough. In some cases, you will have time to perform it. In others, you will only have time for an initial assessment before the EMTs arrive. When you have time and the patient does not need continued life-saving care, begin the physical exam.

The physical exam proceeds in a logical order, usually from head to toe. It will be slightly different for each patient. A patient who falls a considerable height from a ladder, for instance, could have injuries anywhere on his body. This patient would require a full assessment. In the case of an isolated cut to a finger, a complete hands-on head-to-toe examination would not be necessary.

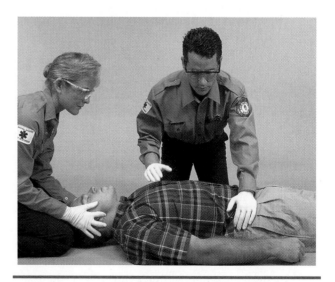

FIGURE 12-11 Assessing for major bleeding.

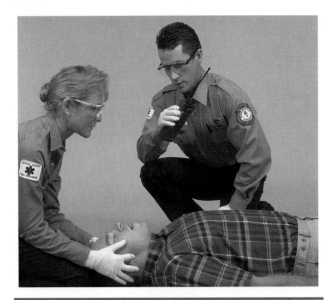

FIGURE 12-12 The last step in the initial assessment is to update incoming EMS units.

Patient assessment is a skill. Like other skills, the more you practice it, the better you will be. If you do not practice regularly, the result could be poor performance and missed injuries.

Principles of Assessment

The patient assessment process involves the use of your senses. There are three methods you will use during your patient assessment: **inspection** (looking), **auscultation** (listening), and palpation (feeling).

- *Inspection.* The first method is the easiest. Simply make an overall observation of the patient. Then, observe the various parts of the body. What you see is very important throughout a call. As you approach a patient, even before you talk to him, you may observe that he is clutching his fist to his chest and appears uncomfortable. This could be your first indication of a heart problem.

- *Auscultation.* The most important listening you will do is for the sound of air entering and leaving the lungs. It will help you to determine the status of the patient's breathing. If your EMS system requires you to perform this skill with a stethoscope, practice on your classmates. Become familiar with the sound of normal breathing.

- *Palpation.* Because it can cause pain, palpating, or feeling, with your fingertips is usually done last in the exam. The actual pressure you apply depends on the area you are palpating and the type of problem you suspect. For example, if you observe a swollen lower leg where the bone is normally near the surface, you would only gently palpate the area to determine if tenderness

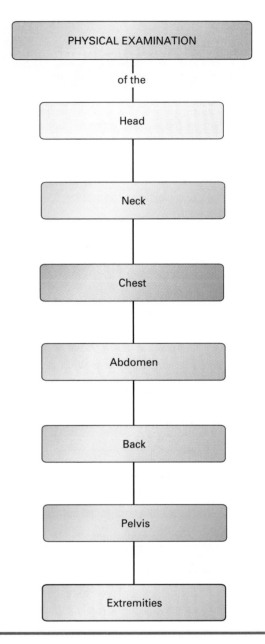

FIGURE 12-13 Components of the physical exam. Note that some EMS systems require assessment of vital signs as well.

is present. Assessing the abdomen of an obese patient would require more pressure. Palpation will also identify areas where bones are rubbing together, abnormally rigid areas, skin temperature, and sweating.

Inspect and palpate each part of the body before you move on to the next area. Also auscultate the chest. For example, observe the chest for rise and fall with breathing. Then, auscultate for adequacy of breathing and palpate for tenderness or other sensations. After examining the chest, you would move to the abdomen where you would inspect and palpate as appropriate.

When conducting the exam, you will be looking for the signs of injury. The first letters of the words *deformities, open injuries, tenderness,* and *swelling* form the memory aid **DOTS**. Use it to help you remember the signs you are looking for. Some signs will be obvious, such as a cut in the skin (open injury). Others, such as abdominal tenderness, will be less obvious but are certainly serious.

As you proceed through the physical exam, be sure to listen to what your patient tells you. This may seem too simple to even mention, but you could be distracted by other activities at a busy emergency scene. Listening shows that you care, and it gives you important information necessary to the proper emergency care of the patient.

Finally, remember that your patient will be anxious or scared. Reassure him or her throughout the call. When the EMTs arrive, introduce your patient to them and relay special concerns or fears the patient may have discussed with you.

The Physical Examination

The following text details the examination of specific areas of the body. Use the DOTS memory aid to guide your examination.

Examination of the Head

Assess all areas of the head, including the skull, face, and jaw (Figure 12-14). Also check pupils for size, equality, and reactivity. Note that injuries to the head may be serious. Bleeding can be severe. Many areas are covered by hair and can hide injuries. Use DOTS to guide you:

D—*Deformities.* Examine the skull, face bones, and jaw for signs of deformity (depressions or indentations, for example). Also look for deformities that can create airway problems, such as loose teeth.

O—*Open injuries.* Open head injuries can bleed profusely. So, they may have been treated in the initial assessment. Any injury that bleeds into the airway is of particular concern. Also look in the hair for hidden injuries.

T—*Tenderness.* When you are palpating the head, the patient may complain of pain or tenderness where there is no obvious injury. Make a note of the locations of tenderness.

S—*Swelling.* Swelling frequently accompanies injuries to the head. It may be noted around injuries to the skull and to facial structures such as areas around the eyes, nose, and mouth.

Examination of the Neck

The neck contains large blood vessels and major airway structures. Injuries there can be quite serious. To examine the neck (Figure 12-15):

D—*Deformities.* Look to see that the trachea is not deformed or shifted. Either can indicate a critical condition such as excessive pressure in the chest cavity. Palpate the vertebrae in the posterior (back) of the neck.

O—*Open injuries.* Open injuries to the neck can result in serious blood loss. Bandage them immediately. Use an occlusive (airtight) dressing, which prevents air from entering the neck.

T—*Tenderness.* Palpate the soft tissues, trachea, and vertebrae for tenderness.

S—*Swelling.* Examine for swelling. The neck may accumulate blood. Also, air may escape from the trachea or other airway structure and cause a popping or crackling sound under the skin.

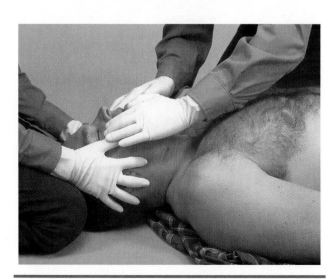

FIGURE 12-14 Assess all areas of the head, including the skull, face, and jaw.

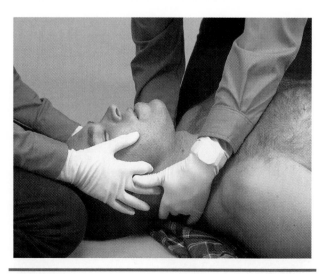

FIGURE 12-15 Examine both the front and back of the neck.

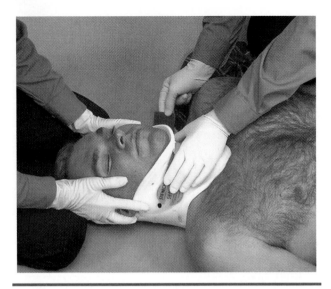

FIGURE 12-16 Apply a rigid cervical collar, if the patient needs one and if you are permitted to do so.

Whenever there is a possibility of spine injury, maintain manual stabilization of the head and neck until the patient can be completely immobilized. If you are equipped, trained, and allowed, apply a rigid cervical collar at this time (Figure 12-16). See Chapter 24 for a detailed discussion of the topic.

Examination of the Chest

Any injury to the chest may involve injury to the vital organs or to major blood vessels. If you are trained to do so, listen to the chest with a stethoscope. Determine if an adequate amount of air is entering the lungs. Compare both sides. The sounds you hear should be equal.

D—*Deformities.* Feel the rib cage for signs of deformity (Figure 12-17). Remember the ribs extend all the way back to the spine. Injuries to the back pose the same grave dangers as those to the front of the chest. Do not move the patient in order to examine the back until appropriate spinal precautions have been taken. Palpate the sternum. If the patient is responsive, ask him or her to take a deep breath. Determine if it causes pain.

O—*Open injuries.* Open injuries are of particular concern when they occur in the chest. If a wound extends into the chest cavity, air may enter the area around the lungs and cause a serious condition. Bandage open wounds to the chest immediately. Use an occlusive (airtight) dressing.

T—*Tenderness.* While palpating the chest, ask the patient if he or she feels any pain. Even when there is no obvious injury, internal injuries may be present.

S—*Swelling.* Observe the chest for swelling. If there is swelling or any other sign of possible injury, assess for underlying breathing problems.

Examination of the Abdomen

As you will recall from Chapter 4, the abdominal cavity contains many organs that can be injured. (Though the spine lies to the rear of the abdomen, it is not palpated in this location.) To examine the abdomen (Figure 12-18):

D—*Deformities.* Deformity of the abdomen usually refers to rigidity (hardness) or distention.

O—*Open injuries.* Open injuries to the abdomen include cuts and scrapes (lacerations and abrasions), penetrating wounds (from a knife or gunshot), or protruding organs (eviscerations). These wounds are severe because of the potential for bleeding and infection.

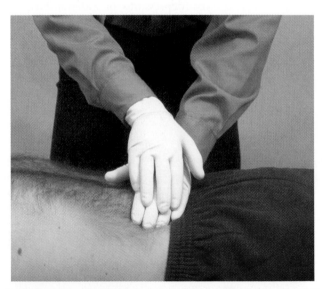

FIGURE 12-18 Palpating each quadrant of the abdomen.

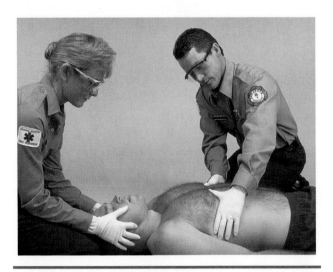

FIGURE 12-17 Examining the chest.

T—*Tenderness.* Tenderness is an important symptom because it may indicate an underlying injury. Recall the abdominal quadrants from Chapter 4. Palpate the quadrant where the patient complains of pain last. If you examine this area first, you could cause severe pain, making the examination of the other quadrants impossible or inaccurate.

S—*Swelling.* Skin swelling or discoloration is another indication of abdominal injury. Check the flanks (the lateral sides of the hips and buttocks) for pooling of blood.

Examination of the Back (Posterior)

Although it is important to check the patient's back, you must also realize that moving a patient could make a neck or spine injury worse. If enough rescuers are present and trained in moving or rolling the patient, you may wish to check the back. If you suspect spine injury and a long backboard is available, you may wish to move the backboard under the patient while he is being rolled. But do so only if you are trained and have enough help to do it safely. (See how to perform in "log roll" in Chapter 24.)

Check the patient's posterior as follows (Figure 12-19):

D—*Deformities.* Check for chest wall deformity, which may indicate broken ribs. Look for obvious deformity along the length of the spine.

O—*Open injuries.* Injuries to the posterior chest can cause the same serious conditions that occur in the anterior chest. Look for open or "sucking" chest wounds (open chest wounds sometimes make a sucking sound with respiration). Observe for scrapes, cuts, and other open injuries. Look for both entry and exit gunshot wounds.

T—*Tenderness.* Tenderness may indicate a broken rib or an abdominal injury. Tenderness along the spine may indicate serious injury to the spinal cord.

S—*Swelling.* Look for blood accumulation in the flanks, which could indicate bleeding in the abdomen. Swelling anywhere indicates some type of injury.

Examination of the Pelvis

The pelvis is a large, bony structure. As you may recall, it is composed of a left and a right *ilium, ischium,* and *pubis bone.* Palpate each of these areas for injury. The pelvis, or hips, may be fractured, which could result in life-threatening blood loss of two liters or more. Be sure to identify any possibility of pelvic injury.

D—*Deformities.* Unlike the bones of the arms and legs, deformities of the pelvis are not always obvious. Palpate the bones to feel for deformity (Figure 12-20).

O—*Open injuries.* There may be open injuries to the pelvis, although this is not as common as in other areas of the body. Open pelvic injuries can result in bleeding from the vagina or rectum.

T—*Tenderness.* Assess for tenderness. Palpate with less force if the bones of the pelvis are close to the skin. Palpate with more force if the patient is obese, with bones under a considerable amount of tissue. Though you may feel awkward assessing the pubis (groin) bone, be sure to check it.

S—*Swelling.* Look for swelling and discoloration around the hips.

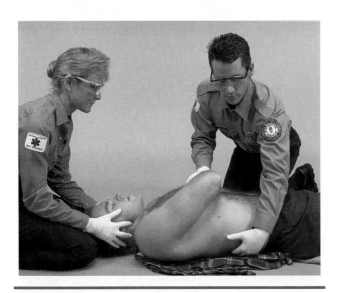

FIGURE 12-19 Examine the patient's back, keeping the head and neck in alignment at all times.

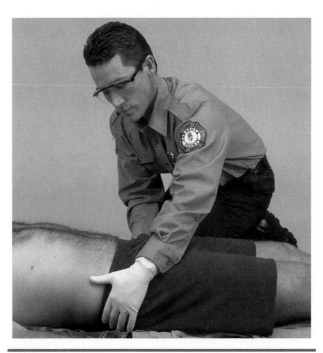

FIGURE 12-20 Examine the pelvis by applying gentle pressure.

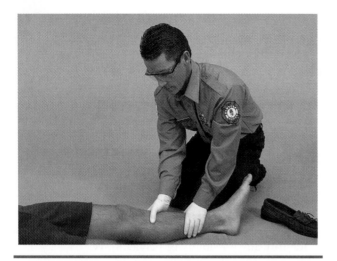

FIGURE 12-21 Inspect and palpate each extremity.

Examination of the Extremities

The extremities are common sites of injury. Be sure to inspect and palpate each one (Figure 12-21).

D—*Deformities.* Because bones are close to the surface, deformities may be seen easily in the extremities. Check the entire length of each bone and all joints for deformity.

O—*Open injuries.* Look for open injuries, which are quite common in the extremities.

T—*Tenderness.* Just like in other areas of the body, there may be underlying injury without obvious deformity. Palpate each extremity for tenderness.

S—*Swelling.* Since injuries to the extremities are often close to the skin, swelling and discoloration may be evident. Any extremity that is painful, swollen, or deformed may be broken and should be manually stabilized until it can be splinted.

The extremities may also be checked by feeling for the presence of a pulse in each extremity (Figure 12-22). The radial pulse in each wrist will tell you if circulation in the entire arm is adequate. There are two pulses in the feet, either of which may be palpated to see if circulation is adequate in the lower extremities. They are the *dorsalis pedis pulse* and the *posterior tibial pulse.* (Refer to Chapter 4, Figure 4-12, for the locations of the dorsalis pedis and posterior tibial arteries.)

The ability to move an extremity, such as wiggling fingers or toes, is also an important sign (Figure 12-23). Movement means that impulses from the nervous system can reach these points. If there is no movement, there may be a problem with a nerve. No movement on one side of the body or below a certain point could indicate problems with the central nervous system.

For the same reason, check to see that the patient has sensation in his limbs. Gently squeeze one extremity and

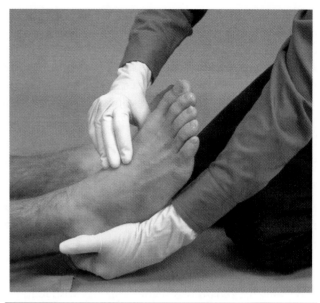

FIGURE 12-22 Also check the pulse in each extremity.

then the other. As you do, ask questions such as: Can you feel me touching your fingers? Can you feel me touching your toes?

1. What are the components of the physical exam?

2. When conducting a physical exam, what general signs should you be looking for?

3. During the physical exam, what senses are you using when you inspect a patient? Auscultate the chest? Palpate a limb?

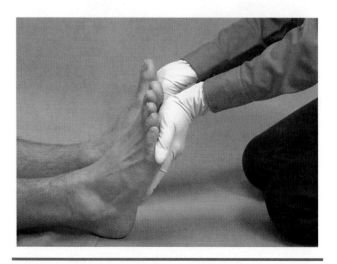

FIGURE 12-23 Check for sensation and the ability to move fingers and toes.

Section 3 Patient History

The **patient history** is an important part of a thorough patient assessment. It involves gathering facts that you would not be able to gather otherwise. For example, the answer to a simple question such as "What happened?" can provide a good amount of information on the patient's condition and the events leading up to it. If the patient is unresponsive, however, you would gather facts by observing the scene, looking for medical identification tags, and by questioning family members and bystanders (Figure 12-24).

One way to remember what you need to ask is by using the memory aid **SAMPLE.** Each letter identifies an important area of questioning (Figure 12-25):

S—Signs and symptoms.

A—Allergies.

M—Medications.

P—Pertinent past history.

L—Last oral intake.

E—Events.

Note: In trauma patients, you will most likely perform a physical exam first. For a medical patient, you most likely will gather a history first.

Signs and Symptoms

The term *sign* and the term *symptom* have quite different meanings (Figure 12-26). A **sign** is something you can observe directly. That is, you can see, feel, or hear signs.

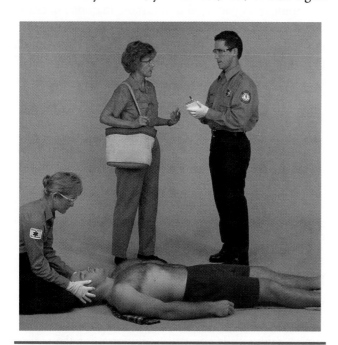

FIGURE 12-24 Gather facts from the patient or from family or bystanders.

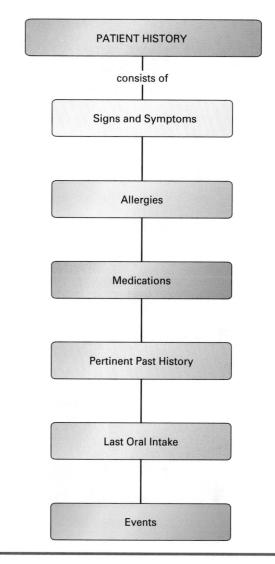

FIGURE 12-25 Components of a patient history.

Examples include deformities (see), skin temperature (feel), and wheezing (hear). A **symptom** cannot be observed by anyone but the patient. For you to be aware of symptoms, the patient must describe them. Examples of symptoms include pain, tenderness, or difficulty breathing.

A good starting point for determining signs and symptoms is to ask the patient an open-ended question such as "Why did you call today?" or "Describe how you feel." This technique allows patients to answer without restriction. They may even give you important information you may not have thought to ask about.

Responses to questions such as "Do you have chest pain?" are restricted to yes-or-no answers. They can cause you to miss important information. Such questions might be better phrased as "What do you feel in your chest?" or "Tell me what you feel in your chest."

You will find signs and symptoms of specific conditions in later chapters. Remember that you are not required to diagnose any medical condition. First Responder care of a patient is based on your assessment findings only.

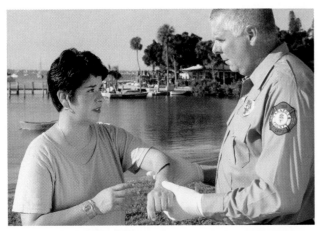

a. *A sign is something one can observe—a deformed wrist, for example.*

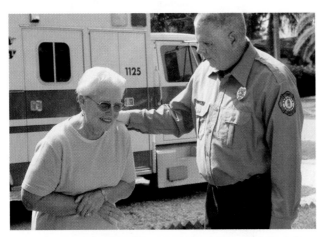

b. *A symptom is something the patient feels and describes, such as a stomach ache.*

FIGURE 12-26 Use the terms "signs" and "symptoms" correctly.

Allergies

Determine if your patient is allergic to anything, including medications, foods, and substances in the environment. Being aware of an allergy can help determine possible causes of the patient's condition. Identifying any allergies to medications also can help health-care personnel choose the proper treatment plans. Remember, an allergic reaction can be very serious. In fact, it can be life-threatening.

Medications

Identify all medications the patient is currently or has recently taken. This information may help identify a medical condition. For example, a patient who takes insulin has diabetes. Other specific medications are used for

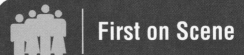

First on Scene

It's not only important for you to know what a patient might be allergic to, it's also important information for everyone who treats your patient. For example, finding out that a patient is allergic to a certain medication will help prevent other medical personnel—in the field and in the hospital—from administering it.

seizures, cardiac conditions, and respiratory problems. Many EMS rescuers carry a pocket guide that lists common prescription medications and their uses.

Pertinent Past History

Most patients have had some type of medical condition in their lifetimes. Some of these may be pertinent to the emergency care you provide to the patient. What is pertinent depends on the type of emergency.

For example, if a patient has shortness of breath, his history of heart problems is pertinent. The fact that he had foot surgery many years ago is not. However, if the patient's present emergency involves dropping a bowling ball on a foot that once was operated on, then the surgery is pertinent.

Patients and family members in the middle of a medical crisis may not know what to tell you. Some people say very little. Others are willing to tell you everything there is to know. It is your job to guide them.

Sometimes you need to ask more than one question to guide a patient to an answer. For example, you may begin by asking a patient to tell you about any medical problems he may have. Your patient may answer "None," even though he has diabetes. This is because he may have understood his physician to say that he has "a little sugar problem," which is controlled by diet or pills.

So your next question might be, "Do you see a doctor for anything?" or "Have you ever been admitted to the hospital?" It may cause the patient to disclose the information you need.

Most patients do not withhold answers or answer incorrectly on purpose. Remember, they may be scared, confused, or both.

Last Oral Intake

You must find out the time of your patient's last oral intake. It may be pertinent to the patient who is unresponsive or confused. It also will be important if the patient needs immediate surgery.

Do not ask "When was your last meal?" People may not consider a snack or several drinks a "meal." Instead ask, "When was the last time you had anything to eat or drink?" This may include anything from a glass of water to a large meal.

Events

Questions such as "What were you doing when this happened?" help to determine the events leading up to the emergency. However, this information might not be as clear-cut as it seems.

Say a patient falls from a ladder. You arrive to find her complaining of a possible broken arm. The patient is obviously a trauma patient, right? The answer is "yes," if the patient slipped on a broken rung of the ladder, for example. However, if she fell as a result of getting dizzy or losing consciousness, then she may also be a medical patient.

If a person is driving, has a heart attack, and passes out behind the wheel, he will surely crash. Upon your arrival at the scene, you could assume that the patient has suffered serious trauma and is unresponsive from that trauma. Your assessment of the events would help you determine what really happened. A passenger might tell you that he saw the driver clutch his chest before the crash, or a medical information tag may alert you to the heart condition.

As you can see, the patient history is an important part of the patient assessment process where information vital to patient care is obtained.

1. What is a patient history?

2. What do the letters in the memory aid SAMPLE stand for?

3. How can you gather a history if your patient is unresponsive?

Section 4 Ongoing Assessment

Some patients are stable, others are not. So your patient assessment process must be ongoing (Figure 12-27). Continually reassess your patient until he or she is turned over to the EMTs. To perform ongoing assessment, follow these steps:

- Reassess level of responsiveness (AVPU).

- Reassess and correct any airway problems.

- Reassess breathing for rate and quality. Ventilate if necessary.

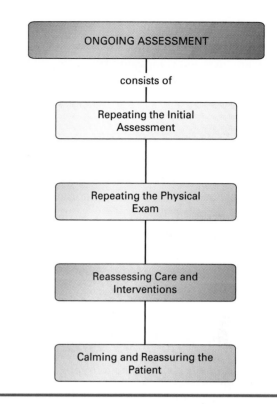

FIGURE 12-27 Components of the ongoing assessment. Note that some EMS systems require reassessment of vital signs as well.

- Reassess pulse for rate and quality.

- Reassess skin temperature, color, and condition.

- Repeat any portions of the physical exam that might be necessary.

- Reassess your **interventions** (treatment) to see if they are effective.

- Continue to calm and reassure the patient.

The more serious your patient's condition, the more often you should repeat ongoing assessment. The recommended intervals are as follows:

- *Every 15 minutes for a stable patient,* such as a patient who is alert, has vital signs in the normal range, and has no serious injury.

- *Every 5 minutes for an unstable patient,* such as a patient who has an altered mental status or difficulty with airway, breathing, and circulation, including severe blood loss or a significant mechanism of injury.

Remember that the patients you come across as a First Responder are in crisis. They may be uncomfortable, confused, and possibly afraid that they will die. It is important for you to have a professional, calm, and caring attitude. Try to address the patient's concerns. For example, if you can protect the patient's modesty, do so. Do not leave the patient alone. If the patient feels cold, even if you are not, turn up the heat or provide another blanket.

The kindness and compassion you show will help to calm the patient. It also will be remembered for a long time to come.

1. What are the components of an ongoing assessment?

2. How often should you perform an ongoing assessment?

Section 5 Patient Hand-off

When the EMTs arrive, you must be prepared to tell them appropriate information about your patient and the care you have given. This is called your **hand-off report**. The hand-off report contains the following information (Figure 12-28):

- Age and sex of the patient.
- Chief complaint.
- Level of responsiveness (AVPU).
- Airway and breathing status.
- Circulation status.
- Physical exam findings.
- Patient history.
- Interventions and the patient's response to them.

The hand-off report is designed to give the transporting EMTs an oral up-to-the-minute account of the condition of the patient, what care has been given, and other information that you feel is important, including any changes you have observed. Many agencies require First Responders to provide a written report to the EMTs. Do so before you leave the scene.

1. What are the components of a hand-off report?

2. To whom do you give a hand-off report?

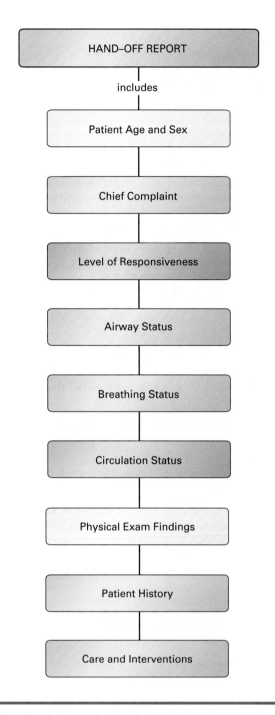

FIGURE 12-28 Information included in the hand-off report.

The Call Follow-up

At the beginning of this chapter, you read that First Responders were on scene with an unresponsive patient, a man whose wife could not wake him from a nap. To see how chapter skills apply to this emergency, read the following. It describes how the call was completed.

Initial Assessment We identified ourselves to the man, but received no response. As my partner assessed the patient's level of responsiveness, I took the pillows out from under his head and assessed his airway. I found some gurgling, so I suctioned him out, which helped. His respirations were slow and shallow. My partner found a pulse, which was rapid. There was no external bleeding visible. Our general impression was of a male unresponsive from unknown causes who required ventilation assistance.

Patient History We asked his wife if he had any problems before he went to sleep. She didn't know of any. In response to further questioning, she told us that he had no allergies and that he took insulin for his diabetes. He had taken his insulin in the morning but had been working in the yard all morning after a small breakfast. His wife added that he had a similar episode last year.

Physical Examination Although it seemed like we had a medical problem, you never can be too sure, especially with a patient who cannot talk. I continued to assist ventilations and monitored the airway while my partner did a quick head-to-toe exam to check for injuries that may have been hidden. There were none. My partner then took a set of vital signs.

Ongoing Assessment The patient required ventilation the entire time we were at the scene. I suctioned him one more time when I felt his secretions were building up. We continued to monitor the patient's mental status, and spoke to him by name just in case he could hear. His wife was quite upset, so we tried to reassure her and keep her calm.

Patient Hand-off When the EMTs arrived, one of them performed an initial assessment. "Good job," he said after assessing the patient's airway. Pretty quickly after my partner gave them the hand-off report (see below), we were dispatched to another run. A few days later I saw one of the EMTs. He told me that the hospital gave Mr. Jeffers glucose through an IV and he began to come around. By the time they left the hospital, he was sitting up and talking.

 Hand-off Report

"This is George Jeffers. He is 62, and his wife could not wake him up from a nap. He responds only to painful stimulus. We had to suction him and assist ventilations. The physical exam did not turn up anything, but his wife says he has diabetes. He took his insulin, had a small meal, and then worked all morning in the yard. His wife says this has happened before. His vitals were pulse 120 and weak, respirations 10 and shallow, blood pressure 110/68. Pupils were equal and reactive, skin cool and moist."

The Last Word *Patient assessment is performed on all patients you come in contact with. The procedure may vary depending on whether your patient is suffering from a medical problem or trauma and whether the patient has minor injuries or serious ones. It is important to be thorough and work in a logical order. Practice your patient assessment skills frequently to become proficient.*

Chapter Review

Focus on the EMS Team

If you are alone, perform patient assessment in order, one step at a time. But if another First Responder is present, work together so that more can be done for the patient. For example, while one First Responder takes a patient history, the other can take a blood pressure. While one holds manual stabilization, the other can perform a head-to-toe exam. The same kind of teamwork may be required when the EMTs arrive to take over patient care. Be prepared to assist, if requested.

Summing Up

- The initial assessment may be the most important part of patient assessment. It is meant to help you identify life threats and treat them immediately. Its components are forming a general impression, assessing the patient's level of responsiveness and ABCs, and updating incoming EMS units about the patient's condition.

- The physical examination involves the inspection, auscultation, and palpation of a patient. For a patient with a significant mechanism of injury or illness, it includes a thorough head-to-toe examination of the patient's body. For such an exam, use the memory aid DOTS (deformities, open injury, tenderness, swelling) to help you remember what to look for. In contrast, a patient who has an isolated minor injury needs only an exam focused on the injured part of the body.

- The patient history is composed of the facts that you would not be able to find out in any other way. Use the memory aid

  SAMPLE to remind you what questions to ask the patient (or the patient's family, friends, or bystanders, if the patient cannot respond). It stands for signs and symptoms, allergies, medications, pertinent past history, last oral intake, and the events leading up to the emergency.

- To perform an ongoing assessment, reassess the patient's level of responsiveness, reassess and correct any problems with the patient's ABCs, repeat any portions of the physical exam as needed, and reassess all interventions. Do so every 15 minutes for a stable patient and every 5 minutes for an unstable one.

- When the EMTs arrive to take over patient care, you must give them an oral hand-off report. It should include age and sex of the patient, chief complaint, level of responsiveness (AVPU), status of each of the ABCs, physical exam findings, patient history, and all interventions and the patient's response to them.

Key Terms

ABCs airway, breathing, and circulation.

altered mental status a change in a patient's normal level of responsiveness.

auscultation a method of examination that involves listening for signs of illness or injury.

AVPU memory aid for the four categories, or levels, of responsiveness: alert, verbal, painful, unresponsive.

chief complaint the reason that EMS was called, stated in the patient's (or the caller's) own words.

DOTS memory aid used to recall what signs to look for during a physical examination: deformities, open injuries, tenderness, and swelling.

ETA estimated time of arrival.

hand-off report a verbal report of the patient's condition and the care given, made to the EMS personnel who take over patient care.

initial assessment a component of patient assessment, conducted directly after the scene size-up, in which the rescuer identifies and treats life-threatening conditions.

inspection a method of examination that involves looking for signs of injury or illness.

interventions actions taken to correct a patient's problems.

level of responsiveness mental status; usually categorized as alert, verbal, painful, or unresponsive. See *AVPU*.

patient history facts about the patient's medical history that are relevant to the patient's condition. See *SAMPLE*.

SAMPLE memory aid for gathering a patient history; the letters stand for signs and symptoms, allergies, medications, pertinent past history, last oral intake, and events that led up to the emergency.

sign any injury or medical condition that can be observed in a patient.

spinal precautions methods used to protect the spine from further injury. For First Responders, this usually refers to manual stabilization of the head and neck until the patient is fully immobilized.

symptom any injury or medical condition that can be described only by the patient.

Knowledge Check

1. **Which one of the following lists the steps of initial assessment in the correct order?**
   a. general impression, responsiveness, ABCs, EMS update
   b. BSI, AVPU, mechanism of injury, and needed resources
   c. BSI, safety, needed resources, number of patients
   d. ABCs, AVPU, general impression, and EMS update

2. **If the mechanism of injury suggests a possible head or spine injury, you should immediately:**
   a. take a patient history before doing anything else.
   b. manually stabilize the patient's head and neck.
   c. determine the patient's level of responsiveness.
   d. conduct a thorough head-to-toe examination.

3. **For a trauma patient, what component of patient assessment is usually performed before the initial assessment?**
   a. scene size-up
   b. patient history
   c. ongoing assessment
   d. physical examination

4. **The memory aid DOTS stands for ___, open injuries, tenderness, and swelling.**
   a. disability
   b. deformity
   c. decapitation
   d. dorsalis pedis

5. **The "P" in the memory aid SAMPLE stands for:**
   a. palpation
   b. presentation
   c. pertinent past
   d. percussion problem

6. **An ongoing assessment for an UNSTABLE patient should be performed at least once every ___ minutes.**
   a. 3
   b. 5
   c. 10
   d. 15

7. Adequate breathing is characterized by all of the following EXCEPT:

    a. normal respiratory rate.
    b. easy, effortless breathing.
    c. verbal level of responsiveness.
    d. adequate rise and fall of the chest.

8. During the initial assessment, you determine that your patient's breathing is inadequate. What should you do?

    a. Begin ventilating immediately.
    b. Apply oxygen by nonrebreather.
    c. Reassess all vital signs every 5 minutes.
    d. Assess the pulse and check for external bleeding.

9. Generally, it is best to question a patient by asking open-ended questions. All of the questions below are open-ended EXCEPT:

    a. For what reason did you call EMS today?
    b. Why are you holding your abdomen?
    c. Do you have any pain?
    d. Can you tell me about your pain?

10. Which one of the following is a symptom, NOT a sign?

    a. nausea
    b. wheezing
    c. cyanosis
    d. rapid pulse

11. During your initial assessment, you should clean and dress all open, bleeding wounds.

    a. True
    b. False

12. Whenever there is a possibility of spine injury, maintain manual stabilization of the head and neck until the patient can be completely immobilized.

    a. True
    b. False

13. For an initial assessment, which arterial pulse point should you check for each patient?

    a. Responsive adult male: _____
    b. Responsive child: _____
    c. Responsive infant: _____
    d. Unresponsive adult female: _____
    e. Unresponsive child: _____
    f. Unresponsive infant: _____

14. Read the report below. It was given as an EMS update after the First Responder's initial assessment. Write what important information is missing.

    "Dispatcher, we have an obese patient who was found lying on the sidewalk. We are attempting to ventilate at this time. What is the ETA of the ambulance?"

    _____   _____

    _____   _____

    _____   _____

Scenario

You and your partner have been called to the scene of "two elderly women down." When you arrive, one of the policemen who found the women meets you. As he walks you to the patients, he assures you that the scene is safe to enter.

a. What step in your initial assessment should you perform first? Describe it.

_____

_____

_____

_____

b. Your partner takes responsibility for the unconscious patient. He finds her unresponsive. What should he do to assess her airway and breathing?

_____

_____

_____

_____

c. You take responsibility for the conscious patient, whom you find confused but able to follow directions. What should you do to assess her airway and breathing?

_____

_____

_____

_____

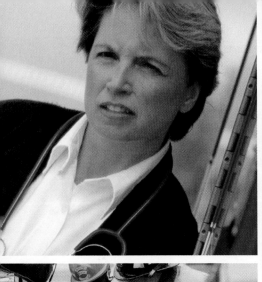
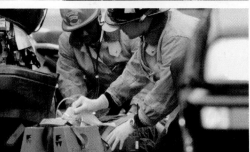
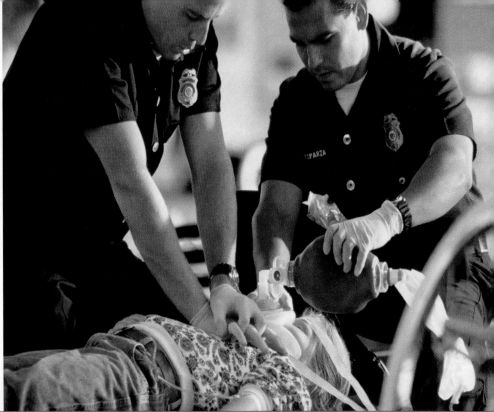

13 | Communication and Documentation

Objectives

From the U.S. Department of Transportation (DOT) 1995 "First Responder: National Standard Curriculum." Material supplemental to the DOT curriculum is listed under "Enrichment."

Cognitive

No objectives are identified by the DOT.

Affective

No objectives are identified by the DOT.

Psychomotor

No objectives are identified by the DOT.

Enrichment

▶ Explain the importance of effective verbal communication of patient information. (p. 237)

▶ Identify typical components of an EMS radio system. (pp. 237–238)

▶ List correct radio procedures. (pp. 237–238)

▶ Identify the essential components of a call to medical direction. (pp. 238–239)

▶ Discuss the communication skills that should be used to interact with the patient. (pp. 239–240)

▶ List the components of the written report. (pp. 240–243)

▶ Describe the legal implications associated with the written report. (pp. 240–243)

▶ Review the special considerations concerning patient refusal. (p. 243)

▶ List special EMS reporting situations. (p. 243)

Introduction

Communication is not limited to one-to-one conversations. It includes using a radio and writing reports as well. When the stress and confusion of an emergency arise, a First Responder must be able to communicate effectively and precisely—with the patient, family, bystanders, and other EMS personnel.

Section 1 Communication

Communication occurs throughout every First Responder call. For example, you must be able to determine a chief complaint, obtain a medical history, and properly reassure and comfort the patient. You also must be able to update incoming EMS units on your patient's status, request help from dispatch, ask medical direction for advice, and provide a hand-off report to the EMTs who take over patient care. All these tasks take skill.

Radio Communication

Radios operate on frequencies that are regulated and licensed by the Federal Communication Commission (FCC). The FCC makes sure that unauthorized persons do not disrupt emergency radio traffic.

There are many components to a radio system. They usually include a **base station, repeaters,** and mobile and portable radios:

- *Base station* (Figure 13-1) is a stationary radio located in a dispatch center, station, or hospital.
- *Mobile radios* (Figure 13-2) are radios mounted in vehicles.

- *Portable radios* (Figure 13-3), or hand-held radios, may be carried on your belt or elsewhere on your person.
- *Repeaters* are devices that receive a low-power radio transmission and rebroadcast it with increased power.

If your EMS system has a dispatch center and radios, you will need to advise the dispatcher of your activities. You must report when you are en route to a call, arrive at the scene, require additional assistance or specialized personnel, and return to service or are available for the next call. You also will use the radio when you update incoming EMS units or need to speak with medical direction. In each of these situations, you must communicate well—clearly, accurately, and briefly.

Using a radio can cause some anxiety, especially the first few times. It is important to remember to speak slowly and pronounce each word you use (don't slur them). Push the "push to talk" button one second before you begin to speak, and talk with your mouth two to three inches away from the microphone. It is best to keep your transmission brief in order to allow others to use the frequency. Listen before you transmit, so you do not disrupt another conversation.

Remember that people with scanners can hear what you say over the radio. Never use a patient's name or say

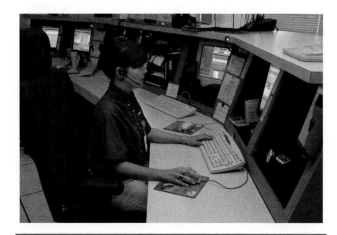

FIGURE 13-1 Example of an EMS communications center.

First on Scene

Radio communication, when available, is an important tool for First Responders. It will allow you to easily call for assistance, update incoming units, contact medical direction, and more. To obtain these benefits, you must use your radio properly. Remember to:

- Speak slowly and clearly.
- Push the "push to talk" button one second before speaking.
- Listen before you transmit.
- Avoid broadcasting personal information about a patient.
- Bring your portable radio with you. It will do you no good if it is left in your vehicle or at your base.

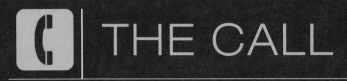

THE CALL

Dispatch Our first response unit was sent to the Bishop McGinn Senior Housing Center for an 80-year-old female patient who was "disoriented and behaving strangely."

Scene Size-up The outside of the complex was quiet. We were met at the door by the resident aide, who told us that Mrs. Gherson was acting "in a most peculiar manner." The aide took us up to the apartment. We remained cautious.

Initial Assessment Mrs. Gherson was sitting at her kitchen table, asking what all the fuss was about. Two neighbors stood beside her. They told us that just a short time ago Mrs. Gherson was wandering the halls, babbling incoherently. They were amazed that she had now suddenly improved.

We found the patient to be alert. She had no problems with her airway and could speak in full sentences. Her respirations seemed normal. She had no bleeding. Her friends had not witnessed or heard of a fall. And she refused permission for emergency care.

Patient refusals are challenging calls for any EMS provider. You must make sure you have tried your best to convince the patient to accept your care and that of the EMTs. Consider this patient as you read Chapter 13. Can communication and documentation affect this situation?

anything over the radio of a personal or confidential nature. Of course, never use profanities or speak in a less than professional tone of voice.

Note that cellular phones (Figure 13-4) may be used to contact medical direction or the dispatcher as well. They are often used where radio coverage is not available.

Communicating with Medical Direction

Consulting with a physician while you are on scene can help you and your patient. If possible, consult medical direction whenever you have questions about a patient that

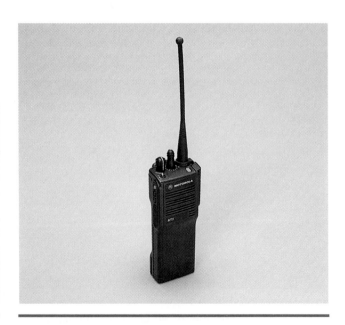

FIGURE 13-2 A mobile two-way radio.

FIGURE 13-3 A portable hand-held radio.

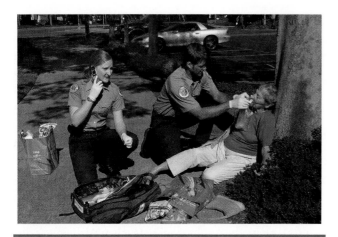

FIGURE 13-4 Cellular phones are commonly used in EMS.

First Responder Practice

In an emergency, the patient is under significant stress and is often in pain. How you communicate can help relax and reassure him, which often helps his condition. Make the patient as emotionally comfortable as possible. In short, treat the patient the way you would want to be treated. Using that as a guide, you won't go wrong.

cannot be resolved by protocols. Since the physician may be many miles away, it is up to you to present information clearly and concisely. Be prepared to give a report that includes:

- Unit identifier and the fact that you are a First Responder.
- Patient's age, sex, and chief complaint.
- Brief, pertinent history of the events leading to the injury or illness.
- Results of the patient's physical exam, including vital signs.
- Care given to the patient and the patient's response to that care.
- Reason why you are calling.

If the physician gives you orders, repeat the orders back to verify them. Be sure all orders and advice given to you by the physician are clear. If you have any questions, ask the physician for clarification.

Interpersonal Communication

Medical emergencies can be frightening to patients. Be sure to speak clearly and use language they and their families understand. Avoid medical terms that will confuse them.

When speaking to patients, make eye contact and, if possible, get down to their level to avoid appearing threatening (Figure 13-5). Also, address patients by name whenever possible. However, if your patient is elderly, do not use his or her first name unless you are invited to do so.

Listen carefully to what patients tell you. If a patient appears reluctant to speak about a topic, you may need to

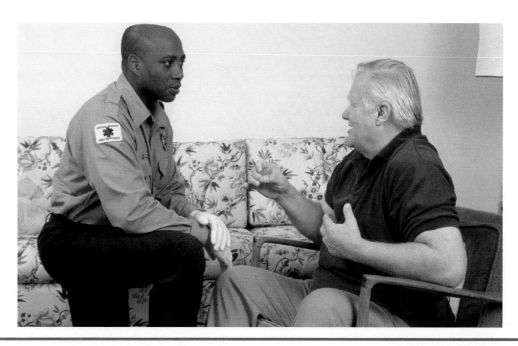

FIGURE 13-5 Use body language that shows you are open and interested in what your patient has to say.

reassure him. Tell him that any information he may have about the problem is important, even if it is upsetting to talk about.

Also observe patients while they are talking to you. It can help you to identify physical problems. For example, if a patient can speak only a few words before catching a breath, he may be in respiratory distress. Or if you observe the patient holding his stomach or clutching his chest, find out why. He may not even know he is doing it. A patient who winces with pain should be questioned about that pain.

Nothing is more annoying than not being listened to. Recall the last time you had to repeat information to someone several times. It is not a pleasant feeling. When you listen to a patient, you let him know that you believe he is important. If you ask a patient a question, wait for an answer. Make notes, if necessary, so you do not forget it. If you do forget the patient's answers, he will soon stop responding to your questions altogether.

If you are called to a patient who does not speak a language you understand, call for someone who can translate. A family member or a neighbor, for example, may be able to speak both your language and the patient's.

Remember that all patients deserve equal care. Each patient should be treated with the same respect and dignity afforded to any other.

Special Communication Situations

As a First Responder, you will encounter patients who have disabilities. Disabilities may affect how the patient perceives or communicates. This does not change the fact that disabled patients have the feelings and needs any other patient would have.

The way you communicate with patients is an important part of First Responder care. Always speak slowly and clearly, but do not speak to a disabled patient so slowly that it would be insulting. Do not use a patronizing tone or shout. Finally, do not assume that disabled patients who have trouble communicating also have trouble understanding. When possible, communicate with the patient directly, rather than with a family member.

Special communication situations and strategies include the following:

- *Blindness.* Blind patients are usually quite capable of getting around and functioning. However, an emergency can put the patient with visual impairment in a situation where assistance is needed. If your patient is blind, ask what help he or she needs. You may be asked to guide the patient and to explain any changes in the immediate surroundings.

- *Deafness.* Patients who have impaired hearing or deafness may need to see your mouth to read your lips. Speak normally. Do not exaggerate your speech or shout. A friend or family member may know sign language and be able to relay your questions to the patient. You also might write down questions the patient can answer verbally or in writing. Patients with a hearing impairment may not speak clearly. This does not mean they have reduced intelligence.

- *Mental impairment.* You will encounter many patients who have mental impairments that were present from birth, developed during their lives (such as a head injury), or are the result of aging (such as Alzheimer's disease). There are many points to consider. First, many patients have a level of function that will allow them to communicate with you and explain their condition. But some will not. You will need to rely on family members and other health-care providers to tell you about the patient.

Another consideration is determining how much of the patient's impairment is from an existing condition and how much is new or due to the present emergency. A patient with Alzheimer's disease could normally exhibit confused speech, but a stroke could make this worse. Family members may be able to report sudden or gradual changes in the patient that you would not be able to identify.

All patients deserve the best possible care delivered with compassion. Your efforts to communicate clearly will result in quality patient care and provide you with a sense of satisfaction that comes only with helping another.

Q:
1. In radio communications, what is a "base station"?

2. What are some of the "do's and don'ts" of radio communications?

3. When your patient is hearing or seeing impaired, how can you communicate with him?

Section 2 Documentation

Documentation should be considered an art. It can "paint a picture" of the patient and his or her condition. A properly completed written report not only provides all the pertinent facts, it also provides them in logical order.

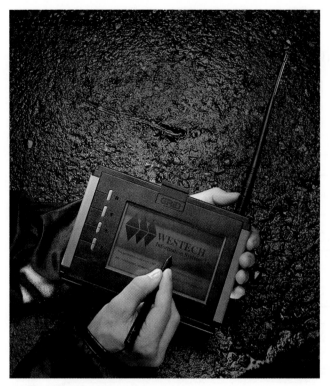

a. *Pen-based computer* (Westech, Inc.)

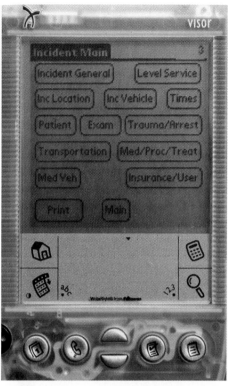

b. *Personal digital assistant (PDA).* (Carl Leet/ Youngstown State University)

FIGURE 13–6 **Direct data devices.**

Prehospital Care Report

A **prehospital care report (PCR)** is used for all of the following reasons:

- *To transfer patient information from one person to another.* Your report is turned over to the EMS personnel who transport your patient. They may turn it over to the hospital staff who use it to learn the patient's history, including the condition in which he was found, what emergency care was provided, and how the patient responded to that care.

- *To provide legal documentation.* A report prepared at the scene of an emergency is a legal record. If you provide care at the scene of an injury or act of violence, for example, your report may become evidence in court proceedings.

- *To document the care you provided.* This is important for legal reasons, too. Unfortunately, First Responders and other EMS professionals may be sued by patients and their families. As you will recall from Chapter 3, accurate documentation is one of your best defenses against lawsuits.

- *To improve your EMS system.* Research is performed in many different areas of your EMS system. It is used to improve such factors as response time and the effectiveness of certain procedures. Your accurate reports are vital to that research.

With the availability of notebook computers, pen-based computers, and other devices, more prehospital care reports are being made electronically (Figure 13-6).

Description

A prehospital care report (PCR) includes **run data**, patient information, and a narrative (Figure 13-7). For the run data you must fill in the date, time, unit involved, location of the call, and the names of the crew members.

The patient information you provide is extensive. It includes the patient's name, address, date of birth, gender, chief complaint, physical exam including vital signs, patient history, changes in the patient's condition, and the care you gave. Some of it can be written in specially designated areas of the form. Some can be recorded by way of check boxes. Some can be in narrative form.

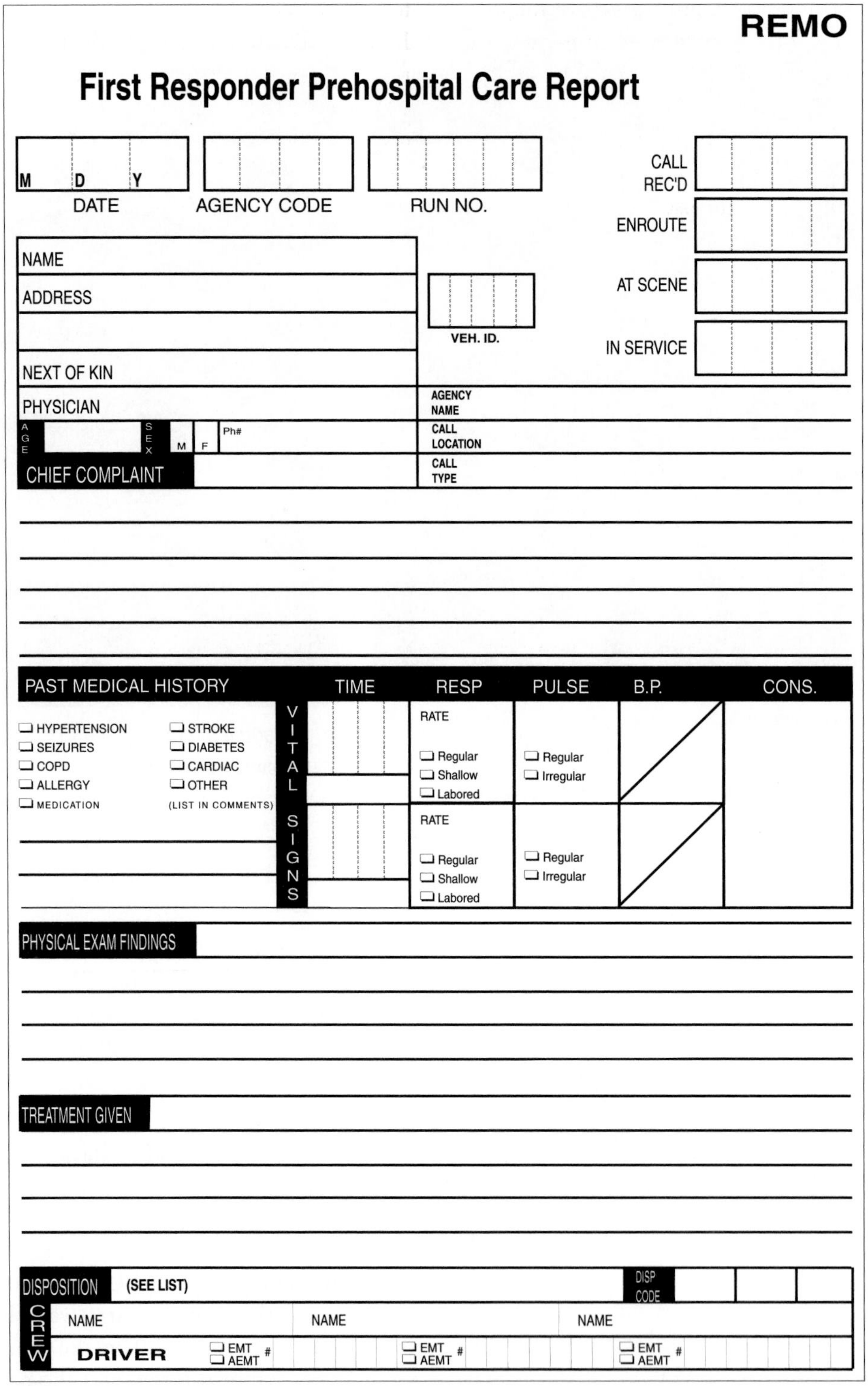

REMO

First Responder Prehospital Care Report

M	D	Y		AGENCY CODE		RUN NO.		CALL REC'D	

DATE   AGENCY CODE   RUN NO.

ENROUTE

NAME

ADDRESS

VEH. ID.

AT SCENE

IN SERVICE

NEXT OF KIN

PHYSICIAN

AGENCY NAME

AGE		SEX	M	F	Ph#

CALL LOCATION

CHIEF COMPLAINT

CALL TYPE

PAST MEDICAL HISTORY		TIME	RESP	PULSE	B.P.	CONS.

☐ HYPERTENSION ☐ STROKE
☐ SEIZURES ☐ DIABETES
☐ COPD ☐ CARDIAC
☐ ALLERGY ☐ OTHER
☐ MEDICATION (LIST IN COMMENTS)

VITAL SIGNS

RATE
☐ Regular ☐ Regular
☐ Shallow ☐ Irregular
☐ Labored

RATE
☐ Regular ☐ Regular
☐ Shallow ☐ Irregular
☐ Labored

PHYSICAL EXAM FINDINGS

TREATMENT GIVEN

DISPOSITION	(SEE LIST)			DISP CODE	

CREW

NAME	NAME	NAME

DRIVER	☐ EMT ☐ AEMT #	☐ EMT ☐ AEMT #	☐ EMT ☐ AEMT #

FIGURE 13-7 Example of a First Responder prehospital care report form. *(Courtesy of the Regional Emergency Medical Organization, Albany, New York)*

Also be sure to record your observations of the scene. Noting the mechanism of injury, for example, will help hospital personnel identify the extent of the patient's injuries.

It is important to fill out the report neatly and spell correctly. Do not draw conclusions or offer opinions. Simply state the facts. Avoid the use of radio codes or abbreviations that others might not understand. If you must correct an error while you are filling out the report, draw a single horizontal line through the error. Then, write the correct information beside it. If you try to totally cross out or otherwise deface a report, it will appear that you are trying to hide something.

If, after submitting a report, you realize that you made an error or omitted information, you may still be able to correct it. In general, you may cross out an error as described above. Write the correct information. Then, mark your initials and date by the new information. You may be required to send an amended copy of the report to any agency that received the original.

Confidentiality

In an emergency, you will observe the way a patient lives, the condition of the home, and his or her relationships with others. You also will be given a personal medical history. Whether the patient is a celebrity or private individual, you must respect his or her privacy. Everything you see, hear, and document at the scene is confidential. It may not be disclosed to anyone except in very specific circumstances. (See Chapter 3.)

Patient Refusal

Patient refusal is a major cause of lawsuits against EMS providers. Remember, a competent adult has the right to refuse care and transportation. However, it is your responsibility to advise the patient of the risks associated with that refusal.

As described in detail in Chapter 3, before allowing a patient to refuse care, take the following steps: Make sure the patient is competent and can make a rational, informed decision. Then try to persuade him to accept EMS care and transportation. Be sure to advise him of the risks associated with refusing care. Consult medical direction as required by local protocol. Finally, document each of these points thoroughly.

In addition, document the patient assessment you performed, that you offered care and transportation, and that you told the patient that you were willing to respond again at any time the patient desired.

Some systems may expect you to have the patient sign a refusal or "release from liability" form. Other EMS systems prefer to have EMTs respond and speak to the patient. Follow all local protocols.

Special Reporting Situations

Special incident reports may be required for infectious disease exposure, injury to EMS personnel, conflicts between agencies, multiple-casualty incidents, and other reasons (Figure 13-8). Since these situations can be very stressful, be sure to stick to the facts. They must be accurate and objective accounts in order to serve their purposes well.

One such special situation is the multiple-casualty incident. When many patients are involved in an emergency, there may not be time to provide full documentation on each one. This does not mean that records can be ignored or prepared poorly. Most EMS systems use special tags to record patient information. (See Chapter 31.) One copy of the tag remains with the patient, while another is kept for EMS records. Your local EMS plan for multiple-casualty incidents should explain the procedure for documentation.

Q: 1. What is a "prehospital care report"? How is it used?

2. How should you correct an error on a prehospital care report?

Special Incident Report

Town of Colonie
Department of Emergency Medical Services

EMERGENCY MEDICAL SERVICES
TOWN OF COLONIE

Date of Incident: _____ **Time:** _____ **REMO #:** _____

Town Run #: _____ **Reported by:** _____ **Zone:** _____

Type of Incident: ☐ MCI ☐ Rescue ☐ Personnel Matter ☐ Injury ☐ Accident with an EMS vehicle
☐ Infectious Disease Exposure ☐ Scene Conflict ☐ Other _____

Total # of Patients: ☐ #P-1: ____ ☐ #P-2: ____ ☐ #P-3: ____ ☐ #P-0: ____
Elapsed Scene Time: *(First unit arrival to last unit to hospital)* _____
Total Time of Incident: _____

Describe the Incident Below:
Attach any additional documentation such as news clipppings and the pre-hospital care report.
Attach additional sheets if necessary.

_____
_____
_____
_____
_____

Signature: _____ **Date:** _____

- -
Office Use Only
This incident relates to: ☐ Day Operation: TOT ☐ Night Operations: TOT: ☐ Administration: TOT:
_____ _____ _____

Disposition: _____
_____
Date: _____

Notifications/Copies: ☐ Director ☐ Deputy Director ☐ Supervisors
☐ Deputy Supervisors ☐ Senior Medics ☐ Zone Coordinator(s)
☐ Other _____ Zone: ☐ 2 ☐ 3 ☐ 4

FIGURE 13-8 **Example of a special incident report.** *(Courtesy of Town of Colonie EMS, New York)*

▶▶ The Call Follow-up

At the beginning of this chapter, you read that First Responders were on scene with an elderly patient who refused emergency care. To see how chapter skills apply, read the following to see how the call was completed.

Patient History We continued to question Mrs. Gherson. She had no idea why EMS was called. She didn't remember being out of her apartment. She denied having allergies. She took insulin for diabetes and a "heart pill" since her heart attack eight years ago. She had eaten dinner and taken her medications.

Physical Examination Mrs. Gherson had no complaints. We again asked for permission to perform a physical exam, but she refused. She said that she really didn't want our help. She felt she was fine. We convinced her to let us take her pulse and respiration. She told us that she would not go to the hospital.

Ongoing Assessment We observed Mrs. Gherson as we continued to try to get her to accept care. We were concerned that she had a serious condition. We felt she really needed to go to the hospital. Before we could change her mind, the ambulance arrived.

Patient Hand-off When the EMTs came on scene, we gave them our hand-off report (see below). I then called Mrs. Gherson's friends away. This let the EMTs get close and allowed me to enlist their help in convincing Mrs. Gherson to accept transport. After a while, one of the women, Mrs. Porter, went back in and explained how worried she was. "If you could have seen yourself, Ingrid," she began. She must have been very convincing, because after a few minutes of discussion, Mrs. Gherson finally agreed to go to the hospital.

We helped the EMTs and then carefully documented our actions. A few weeks later, we went back for a call. We saw Mrs. Porter, who told us that Mrs. Gherson had had a "mini-stroke." She also said that the doctors were watching her more closely now.

 ## Hand-off Report

"This is Mrs. Gherson, who is 80 years old. The resident aide told us that Mrs. Gherson was found wandering the halls, babbling incoherently. When questioned, Mrs. Gherson told us she had no memory of leaving her apartment and denies the incident occurred. Her pulse is 66, respiration 16. She refused all other attempts at assessment and care. She told us she had a heart attack eight years ago. She has no allergies. Medications include insulin for diabetes and a heart pill, which she refuses to or cannot identify."

The Last Word *Communication and documentation are key elements in every call you make. Your communication with patients is what they will likely remember most. Your documentation is all that is left behind after the call is done.*

Chapter Review

Focus on the EMS Team

Though communication and documentation may seem the least important aspects of a call, they are not. As a First Responder, you will have many opportunities to communicate with other EMS personnel on the radio, phone, and in person. In every one of those situations, it is important for you to be accurate and to speak slowly and clearly. Providing inaccurate information, omitting key information, or speaking in any way other than clearly could result in harm to your patient.

In addition, your documentation follows your patient, first to the EMTs who take over emergency care and transport and then to hospital personnel who provide ongoing medical care. So it must be accurate, to the point, and legible. And remember: "If you didn't write it, it didn't happen." That old saying means if you forget to document the care you gave to a patient, it will seem as if you never gave it—and that could be used against you if you are ever called to court.

The way you communicate, both orally and in writing, puts forth an image. Make it one you and EMS can be proud of.

Summing Up

- Radios operate on frequencies that are regulated and licensed by the Federal Communication Commission (FCC).

- A radio system includes a base station, repeaters, mobile radios, and portable or hand-held radios.

- When communicating over a radio, it is important to speak slowly, clearly, and briefly. You also must ensure confidentiality by never using a patient's name or providing information that could identify a patient.

- A consultation with medical direction over the radio or by way of a cell phone must include: unit identifier and the fact that you are a First Responder; patient's age, sex, and chief complaint; brief, pertinent history of the events leading to the injury or illness; results of the patient's physical exam, including vital signs; care given to the patient and the patient's response to that care; and the reason why you are calling. If the physician gives you orders, repeat them back to verify them. If you have any questions, ask the physician for clarification.

- Good interpersonal communication skills include how to speak, listen, and hold yourself when you are with a patient.

They will help reassure your patients and their families and allow you to elicit information you may not get otherwise. Use those skills with all patients so that each receives your best and equal care.

- A prehospital care report (PCR) is a legal document. It is used to transfer patient information from one health-care provider to another, to document the care you provided, and to improve your EMS system. It includes run data, patient information, and a narrative, all of which are confidential.

- Patient refusal is a major cause of lawsuits against EMS providers. Follow local protocols for documenting such situations. Generally, you should document your assessment findings and your attempts at persuading the patient to accept care and transport, including advising him of the risks associated with refusal.

- Special incident reports and documentation may be required for infectious disease exposure, injury to EMS personnel, conflicts between agencies, multiple-casualty incidents, and other reasons. Follow local protocols.

Key Terms

base station a stationary radio located in a dispatch center, station, or hospital.

prehospital care report (PCR) documentation of an emergency call; usually includes run data, patient information, and a narrative.

repeaters devices that receive a low-power radio transmission and rebroadcast it with increased power.

run data bare facts of an EMS response; include the date, time, unit involved, location of the call, and the names of the crew members.

Knowledge Check

1. The radio installed in a vehicle is called the ___ radio.

   a. portable
   b. mobile
   c. base station
   d. mobile repeater

2. When you call the medical director for advice, he or she will need to know all of the following information EXCEPT:

   a. patient's age.
   b. pertinent events leading to the emergency.
   c. patient's complete medical history.
   d. reason you are calling.

3. The prehospital care report should contain all of the following EXCEPT:

   a. history of family diseases.
   b. patient information.
   c. narrative.
   d. run data.

4. A prehospital care report is NOT used to:

   a. improve the EMS system.
   b. document the care provided.
   c. provide legal documentation.
   d. relay information to the press.

5. Which one of the following statements is TRUE?

   a. Using proper medical terminology to explain what you are doing will calm most patients.
   b. Regardless of native language, most patients can understand English in a crisis.
   c. If you speak loudly enough, most deaf patients will understand your questions.
   d. Getting down to their eye level can help you gain the trust of most patients.

6. People who have radio scanners can hear what you say on an emergency radio frequency.

   a. True
   b. False

7. When the emergency department physician gives you orders over a radio or phone, you must repeat the orders back to verify them.

   a. True
   b. False

8. List three rules to follow when using a mobile or portable radio.

   _____

   _____

   _____

9. List three examples of emergencies that may require a special incident report.

   _____

   _____

   _____

Scenario

You are the First Responder on scene. You find the patient has an altered mental status and appears to be injured. Apparently, he fell about 12 feet from a tree he was trimming. His family will not allow you to assess or provide care to him, and they are insisting they need to move him into the main house. You call medical direction for assistance in convincing them not to move the patient until the paramedics arrive on scene.

a. What information will the physician need before she can help you?

_____

_____

_____

_____

_____

_____

b. Why doesn't the First Responder want the family to move the patient?

_____

_____

_____

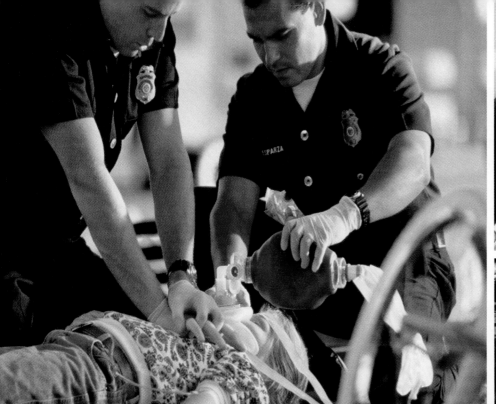
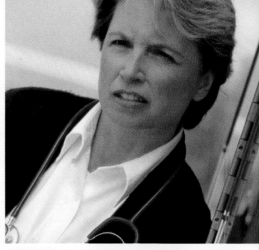
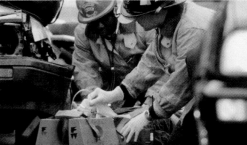

14 | Cardiac and Respiratory Emergencies

Objectives

From the U.S. Department of Transportation (DOT) 1995 "First Responder: National Standard Curriculum." Material supplemental to the DOT curriculum is listed under "Enrichment."

Cognitive

No objectives are identified by the DOT.

Affective

5-1.16 ▶ Attend to the feelings of the patient and/or family when dealing with the patient with a specific medical complaint. (pp. 252, 258, 261, 262)

5-1.21 ▶ Demonstrate a caring attitude toward patients with a specific medical complaint who request emergency medical services. (pp. 252, 258, 261, 262)

5-1.22 ▶ Place the interests of the patient with a specific medical complaint as the foremost consideration when making any and all patient care decisions. (pp. 258–261)

5-1.23 ▶ Communicate with empathy to patients with a specific medical complaint, as well as with family members and friends of the patient. (pp. 252, 258, 261, 262)

Psychomotor

No objectives are identified by the DOT.

Enrichment

▶ State the signs and symptoms of a cardiac emergency. (p. 252)

▶ Describe the emergency care of the patient experiencing chest pain or discomfort. (p. 252)

▶ Discuss common causes of chest pain or discomfort, including angina pectoris and acute myocardial infarction. (pp. 252, 254–256)

▶ List the signs of adequate breathing. (p. 257)

▶ State the signs and symptoms of a patient in respiratory distress. (p. 257)

▶ Describe the emergency care of the patient in respiratory distress. (p. 258)

▶ Discuss common causes of breathing difficulty, including chronic obstructive pulmonary disease, asthma, pneumonia, acute pulmonary edema, and hyperventilation. (pp. 258–261)

Introduction

In the U.S.A. each year almost a half-million people die of heart disease, almost 29 million more suffer from some form of it, and about 1.5 million have heart attacks. Respiratory illnesses also are common. Emphysema and chronic bronchitis alone affect more than 23 million people in the U.S. Asthma affects nearly 10 million. Both types of problems—respiratory and cardiac—can be life-threatening. When such emergencies occur, patients can benefit from the immediate care an emergency medical responder can provide.

Section 1 Cardiac Emergencies

Cardiac emergencies can occur from abnormal heart rhythm patterns. They also occur when there is an interruption of oxygen to some part of the heart muscle. The reduction of oxygen causes chest pain or discomfort, one of the most common symptoms of a cardiac emergency.

Coronary artery disease affects the inner lining of the arteries that supply the heart with blood. People who have it usually suffer from **arteriosclerosis**, a condition that causes the walls of the arteries to become thick and hard.

In coronary artery disease, the opening of the coronary artery is narrowed (Figure 14-1). This restricts the amount of blood that can reach and nourish the heart. The rough artery surfaces then cause a buildup of debris, further narrowing the artery. The more the artery narrows, the less oxygen gets to the heart. At some point, the patient may have chest pain. Finally, when the artery becomes blocked, the patient may suffer a heart attack that results in the death of heart muscle.

Researchers have identified a number of cardiac risk factors that predispose a person to heart attack. Obviously, some factors cannot be controlled. With awareness and determination, however, a person can change other factors and decrease his or her own risk (Figure 14-2). The major risk factors are physical inactivity, cigarette smoking, obesity, high serum cholesterol and triglycerides, diabetes, age (incidence increases over 30 years of age), hypertension (blood pressure above 140/90), and a family history of coronary artery disease occurring under age 60.

There are many reasons a patient may develop a condition that leads to a cardiac emergency. However, you do not have to identify them. A First Responder's assessment

 First Responder Practice

You will see many types of cardiac and respiratory conditions mentioned throughout this chapter. Remember that it is not necessary to diagnose or determine exactly which one your patient has. In fact, First Responder care for all cardiac and respiratory conditions is the same.

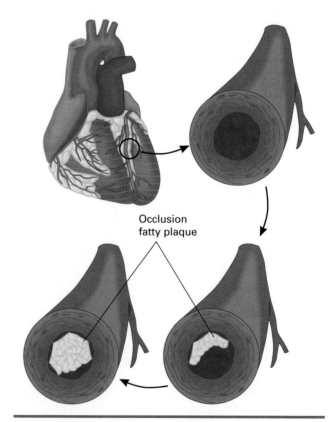

Occlusion
fatty plaque

FIGURE 14-1 Fatty deposits build up in arteries, depriving the heart muscle of blood and oxygen.

THE CALL

Dispatch I was working at the plant during my regular 4–12 shift. At about 6:30 p.m., my emergency response team was paged. A man was having chest pain.

Scene Size-up Other than a few concerned coworkers, everything was quiet. I recognized the man, Harry Nowack, because I used to work with him.

Initial Assessment Harry was alert. His airway was clear. He could speak in full sentences, but his breathing was labored.

Harry told me that he didn't fall or have any injuries. "My chest just hurts." I couldn't help but notice Harry's color. He looked ashen. It was definitely not normal. I radioed my findings to the plant office, and told them to notify the 9-1-1 ambulance. They told me the ETA of the ambulance was 10 minutes.

What do you think this patient's problem may be? Is it a cardiac problem or a respiratory one? Do you need to know? Consider this patient as you read Chapter 14. What should be done to assess and care for him?

CARDIAC RISK FACTORS

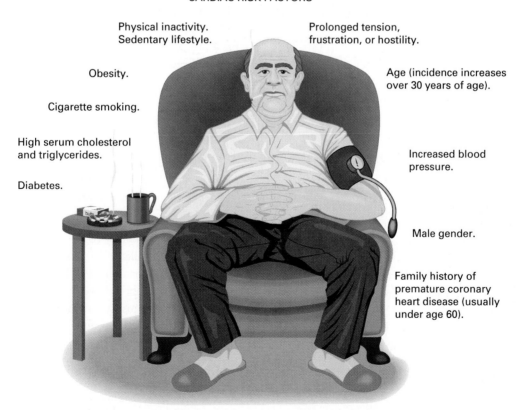

Physical inactivity. Sedentary lifestyle.

Prolonged tension, frustration, or hostility.

Obesity.

Age (incidence increases over 30 years of age).

Cigarette smoking.

High serum cholesterol and triglycerides.

Increased blood pressure.

Diabetes.

Male gender.

Family history of premature coronary heart disease (usually under age 60).

FIGURE 14-2 High cholesterol, high blood pressure, and heavy smoking increase risk 10 times.

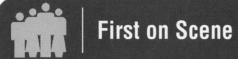

First on Scene

Sudden cardiac death is a death that occurs within two hours of the onset of symptoms. Unfortunately, the average time for a person to recognize symptoms and seek some sort of care is four to six hours. This means that lives could be saved by simply recognizing the problem and seeking help immediately.

and care of a patient with chest pain will be the same, no matter what the actual cause.

Patient Assessment

The general signs and symptoms of a cardiac emergency are as follows (Figure 14-3):

- Chest pain or discomfort described as heaviness or squeezing. The sensation also may radiate to the arms, shoulder, neck, or jaw.
- Difficulty breathing, shortness of breath.
- Unusual pulse (rapid, weak, slow, or irregular).
- Palpitations.
- Indigestion, nausea, vomiting.
- Sweating.
- Skin color, including mucous membranes, may be pale, gray, or cyanotic.
- Feeling of impending doom.
- History of heart problems or a previous similar experience.

Note that many patients experience a "silent" heart attack. This means that these patients do not experience the classic pain patterns. Patients who have diabetes, those who are elderly, and women may not experience pain. Instead, difficulty breathing and a feeling of weakness are the most common presenting symptoms.

As soon as you recognize a possible cardiac emergency, update the incoming EMS unit. Request advanced care if it is available in your area. Remember that a patient with chest pain will be very anxious. He may feel as if he is going to die. This requires compassion and reassurance. Make sure he understands that everything that can possibly be done is being done. Advise him and his family that further help is on the way and that he will be transported promptly to a medical facility.

Later, when you take the patient's history, use **OPQRRRST** as a memory aid to help you get a good

description of the pain. Each letter identifies an important area of questioning:

O—*Onset.* When did the pain begin?

P—*Provocation.* Did anything cause or start the pain (exercise, an activity)?

Q—*Quality.* What is the pain like (crushing, stabbing, etc.)?

R—*Region.* Where is the pain?

R—*Radiation.* Does the pain begin in one place and then seem to travel somewhere else?

R—*Relief.* Does anything relieve the pain?

S—*Severity.* On a scale of 1–10, with 10 the worst, how bad is the pain?

T—*Time.* How long have you had the pain?

When you perform a physical exam, palpate the chest for DOTS (deformities, open injuries, tenderness, swelling). Make a note if your touch causes pain. If you are trained to do so, listen to the lungs to determine if air is moving in and out of both sides equally. ■

First Responder Care

To provide care to a patient with chest pain or discomfort, follow these steps:

1. *Place the patient in a position of comfort.* This is usually a semi-reclining or sitting position. Also have him cease all movement.

2. *Ensure adequate breathing.* See that the airway is open. If breathing is adequate, administer high-flow oxygen with a nonrebreather mask. If breathing is not adequate, assist ventilations with a BVM and supplemental oxygen.

3. *Loosen tight clothing.*

4. *Maintain body temperature* as close to normal as possible.

5. *Continually monitor the patient.* He may become unstable rapidly. Be alert for changes in the patient's mental status and be prepared to perform CPR with supplementary oxygen, if possible, and to use an AED. ■

Your patient may tell you that he has had heart surgery or that he has a **pacemaker** or an implanted defibrillator. (An implanted defibrillator delivers shocks to a patient but at much less power than an AED.) Treat these patients in the same way as described above. Note that a malfunctioning pacemaker may cause a slow heart rhythm. If this occurs, monitor the patient carefully. Provide oxygen and be prepared to administer CPR if necessary.

Specific Cardiac Conditions

Two problems are commonly caused by coronary artery disease. They are *angina pectoris,* sometimes called *angina,* and *myocardial infarction,* the medical term for heart attack.

SIGNS AND SYMPTOMS OF A CARDIAC EMERGENCY

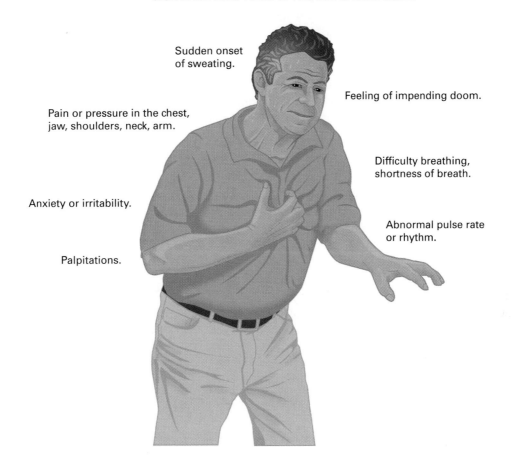

Sudden onset of sweating.

Feeling of impending doom.

Pain or pressure in the chest, jaw, shoulders, neck, arm.

Difficulty breathing, shortness of breath.

Anxiety or irritability.

Abnormal pulse rate or rhythm.

Palpitations.

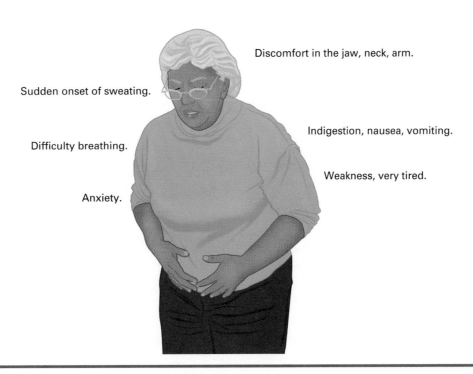

Discomfort in the jaw, neck, arm.

Sudden onset of sweating.

Indigestion, nausea, vomiting.

Difficulty breathing.

Weakness, very tired.

Anxiety.

FIGURE 14-3 In a cardiac emergency, men may be more likely to have the classic symptom—chest pain. Women, elderly people, and diabetics may not have chest pain at all.

First Responder care of patients with angina and myocardial infarction is the same. It is not necessary to differentiate between the two. Taking time to do so might even be harmful. Chest-pain patients need prompt care and constant monitoring. Early access to the EMS system and rapid transportation to a hospital can literally make the difference between life and death.

Angina Pectoris

The term **angina pectoris** literally means "pain in the chest." As you know, the heart relies on a constant supply of oxygen. If it does not get enough because of diseased or narrowed arteries, the patient experiences chest pain or discomfort. Most often the pain of angina occurs as a result of physical activity beyond the patient's limit, emotional stress, or extreme hot or cold weather. Sometimes, though rarely, it has no apparent cause.

The pain of angina can change from a mild ache to a severe crushing pain. It can appear suddenly, but usually it is associated with physical exertion. It usually is in the chest, but it can radiate to the jaw, neck, left shoulder, left arm, or left hand. It often is mistaken for indigestion. Note that angina does not always manifest itself as pain. It may be a feeling of tightness, gripping, heaviness, squeezing, burning, or a dull constriction. Other signs and symptoms include:

- Shortness of breath.
- Profuse sweating.
- Lightheadedness.
- **Palpitations** (a sensation of throbbing or fluttering of the heart).
- Nausea, vomiting.
- Pale, cool, moist skin.

Angina is reversible. It does not cause permanent damage to the heart muscle. Generally, the pain is relieved by rest, usually within a few minutes after the patient stops the activity, calms down, moves indoors, or takes nitroglycerin as prescribed by a physician.

Patients who have a history of angina are commonly prescribed *nitroglycerin* (Figure 14-4). This medication reduces the workload of the heart. It also dilates the arteries. Because you may come upon patients who have taken nitroglycerin or who are about to take it as you arrive, note the following:

- Nitroglycerin can lower blood pressure. Patients with systolic blood pressure below 100 mmHg should not take this medication. Carefully monitor the blood pressure of any patient who does.

- Before taking nitroglycerin, a patient's blood pressure should be at least 100 mmHg, but many systems use higher systolic pressures (110 mmHg or 120 mmHg). Always follow local protocol carefully.

- Nitroglycerin does not have a long shelf life. It can lose its potency quickly. It should taste bitter and may sometimes cause a headache in the patient. If these things do not happen, the medication may be old and thus may not be working properly.

- Generally, nitroglycerin is taken at the onset of chest pain. It may be repeated once or twice at five-minute intervals, if the pain is still present.

- *Do not administer this or any other medication without the approval of medical direction.*

Note that it is impossible for you to tell the difference between the pain of angina and the pain of a heart attack. While angina usually leaves the heart undamaged, if it is left untreated, it may eventually cause a heart attack.

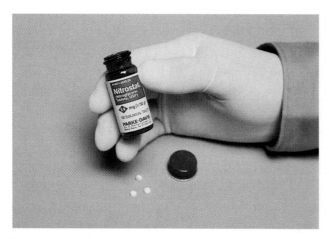

a.

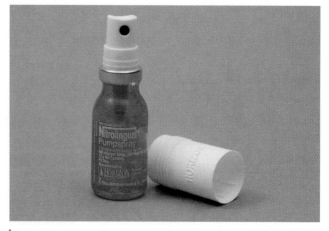

b.

FIGURE 14-4 Nitroglycerin in tablet or spray form is often prescribed to patients with a history of angina.

Acute Myocardial Infarction

Myocardial infarction means "death of heart muscle." When blood to part of the heart is blocked off or greatly reduced, that part dies. Myocardial infarction, or heart attack, is most commonly caused by blockage, the result of coronary artery disease. It has four serious consequences: sudden death, shock, **congestive heart failure**, and **cardiac dysrhythmias**:

- *Sudden death.* Of heart attack patients who die before reaching a hospital, most die within two hours of the first signs and symptoms.

- *Shock.* If 40% or more of the left ventricle is damaged after an attack, the heart cannot pump the proper amount of blood to the body. Shock usually occurs within 24 hours, with a mortality rate of about 80%.

- *Congestive heart failure.* This condition may develop after a heart attack. It causes pulmonary edema (a buildup of fluid in the lungs) and in other parts of the body. This is sometimes observed as swelling in the ankles. (See Figure 14-5.)

- *Cardiac dysrhythmias.* These are the abnormal heart rhythms that follow a heart attack. They are generally caused by injury to the electrical conduction system of the heart.

The most common symptom of heart attack is a sudden onset of chest pain. About 80% of all heart attack victims experience it. Many also have abnormal heart rhythms and may suffer nausea and vomiting. Note that 20% of all heart attack patients have no chest pain at all. (This is more likely to occur in women, the elderly, or patients with diabetes.) A heart attack without pain is called a **silent myocardial infarction.**

Chest pain associated with heart attack ranges from mild discomfort to severe pain. The sensation felt by the patient may be described as pain, crushing, tightness, or numbness. It usually lasts longer than 30 minutes. Though the pain can be experienced in a number of ways, the common location is substernal, radiating to the neck, jaw, left shoulder, and left arm (Figure 14-6). It often includes the burning and bloating sensations of indigestion. It can be continuous. It might subside, but do not ignore it if it does. Any adult with pain or discomfort to the chest, neck, shoulder, arm, or jaw should be suspected of heart attack. Treat the patient accordingly.

Other signs and symptoms include:

- Sudden onset of weakness, nausea and vomiting, and profuse sweating without a clear cause.

- Pain not related to physical exertion and not relieved by rest.

- Abnormal pulse, which may be rapid (over 100), slow (below 60), or irregular.

- Difficulty breathing or rapid, shallow respirations.

- Cool, pale, moist skin, and possible cyanosis.

- Lightheadedness, loss of consciousness.

- Anxiety, feelings of impending doom.

Note that patients may have been told by their physicians to take aspirin. Aspirin has been used for

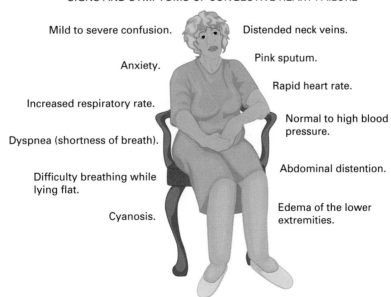

SIGNS AND SYMPTOMS OF CONGESTIVE HEART FAILURE

Mild to severe confusion.

Anxiety.

Increased respiratory rate.

Dyspnea (shortness of breath).

Difficulty breathing while lying flat.

Cyanosis.

Distended neck veins.

Pink sputum.

Rapid heart rate.

Normal to high blood pressure.

Abdominal distention.

Edema of the lower extremities.

FIGURE 14-5 Congestive heart failure may develop after a heart attack.

EARLY SIGNS OF HEART ATTACK

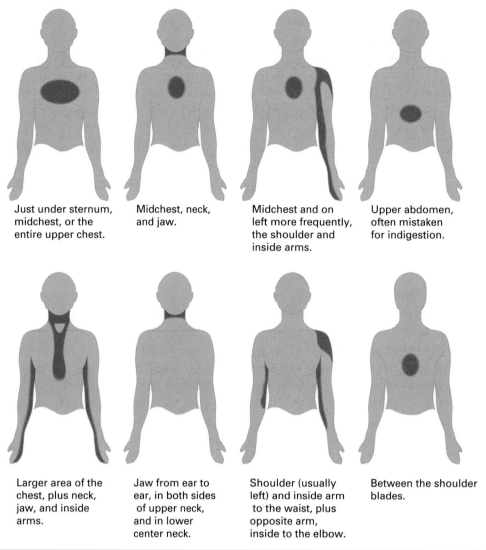

Just under sternum, midchest, or the entire upper chest.

Midchest, neck, and jaw.

Midchest and on left more frequently, the shoulder and inside arms.

Upper abdomen, often mistaken for indigestion.

Larger area of the chest, plus neck, jaw, and inside arms.

Jaw from ear to ear, in both sides of upper neck, and in lower center neck.

Shoulder (usually left) and inside arm to the waist, plus opposite arm, inside to the elbow.

Between the shoulder blades.

FIGURE 14-6 Pain or discomfort can occur in any one location or any combination of locations.

years to relieve pain and reduce fever. Now it has another role. It also is used in heart attack prevention and in helping to minimize damage if a heart attack occurs. As an EMS provider, you may be allowed to carry and administer aspirin or you may be allowed to help patients take their own. If either is the case, remember these points:

- Administering any medication is a serious responsibility. Be sure to follow your local protocols.

- An aspirin dose is usually two to four chewable baby aspirin (81 milligrams each).

- Some people have allergies to aspirin. Be sure to check for allergies before administering any medication.

- Although patients who are on blood-thinning medications, such as coumarin or warfarin, should not receive

aspirin routinely, local protocols may allow aspirin in the case of acute chest pain.

- Only patients who are conscious and have a gag reflex should receive oral medications.

1. Does the cause of chest pain affect First Responder care? Explain your answer.

2. How are the letters OPQRRRST used to gather a patient history? Explain what each letter stands for.

3. What is First Responder care for a patient with chest pain?

Section 2 Respiratory Emergencies

A variety of diseases and injuries can affect the body's ability to get enough oxygen. Without oxygen, cells such as those in the brain and heart can die within minutes, so rapid treatment is essential.

Remember, adequate breathing occurs at a normal rate. For adults, that is 12 to 20 breaths per minute. For children, it is 15 to 30 breaths per minute. For infants, it is 25 to 50 breaths per minute. Adequate breathing is regular in rhythm and free of unusual sounds, such as wheezing or whistling. The chest should expand adequately and equally with each breath. The depth of the breaths should be adequate, as well. In addition, breathing should be effortless. That is, it should be accomplished without the use of accessory muscles in the neck, shoulders, or abdomen.

Respiratory distress is shortness of breath or a feeling of air hunger with labored breathing. It is one of the most common medical complaints. Two circumstances may cause respiratory distress. Either air cannot pass easily into the lungs or air cannot pass easily out of them.

Patient Assessment

Signs and symptoms of respiratory distress include (Figure 14-7):

- Inability to speak in full sentences without pausing to breathe.

First on Scene

Respiratory distress in infants and children can be quite serious. It can rapidly lead to respiratory failure and death—much faster than in an adult. Recognize the signs of respiratory distress in infants and children, and notify incoming EMS units immediately.

- Noisy breathing.
- Use of accessory muscles to breathe. That includes neck muscles, muscles between the ribs, and abdominal muscles.
- **Tripod position.** In this position, the patient is sitting upright, leaning forward, fighting to breathe (Figure 14-8).
- Abnormal breathing rate and rhythm.
- Increased pulse rate.
- Skin color changes (pale, flushed, or cyanotic).
- Altered mental status.

Generally, breathing will be rapid and shallow. Patients may feel short of breath whether they are breathing rapidly or slowly. Remember, a certain amount of shortness of breath is normal following exercise, fatigue, coughing, or with the production of excess sputum. ■

SIGNS AND SYMPTOMS OF RESPIRATORY DISTRESS

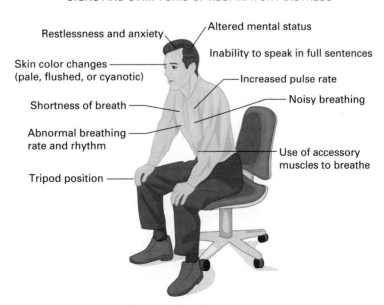

Restlessness and anxiety

Skin color changes (pale, flushed, or cyanotic)

Shortness of breath

Abnormal breathing rate and rhythm

Tripod position

Altered mental status

Inability to speak in full sentences

Increased pulse rate

Noisy breathing

Use of accessory muscles to breathe

FIGURE 14-7 Respiratory distress is one of the most common medical emergencies.

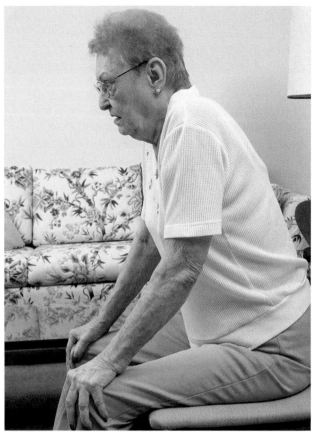

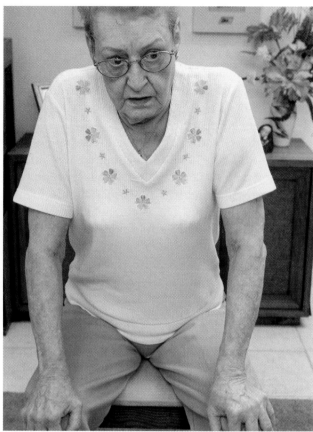

a.   b.

FIGURE 14-8 The tripod position is a sign of respiratory distress.

First Responder Care

To provide care to a patient in respiratory distress, follow these steps:

1. *Ensure adequate breathing.* Monitor it throughout the call. If breathing is adequate, administer oxygen at 10–15 liters per minute via nonrebreather. If breathing is inadequate, assist ventilation with a BVM and supplemental oxygen.

2. *Place the responsive patient with adequate breathing in a position of comfort.* This is usually a sitting position.

3. *Comfort and reassure the patient.* There are few feelings as terrifying as not being able to breathe. Because of this fear, the patient may become agitated or even angry. Do not take it personally.

4. *Activate the EMS system,* if not already done. Continue to monitor the patient's respiratory efforts. ■

Specific Respiratory Conditions

The following conditions are among the breathing problems you will commonly see in the field. They include chronic obstructive pulmonary disease (**COPD**),

asthma, pneumonia, **acute** pulmonary edema, and hyperventilation syndrome. Remember, although respiratory distress has a variety of causes, First Responder care is always the same.

Chronic Obstructive Pulmonary Disease (COPD)

Emphysema and **chronic bronchitis** are the most common chronic obstructive pulmonary diseases. Together they affect more than 23 million people in the U.S.

In *emphysema* the alveoli lose elasticity, become distended with trapped air, and stop working. As the total number of alveoli decreases, breathing becomes more and more difficult.

Chronic bronchitis is characterized by inflammation, **edema,** and excessive mucus in the bronchial tree. It features a productive cough that has persisted for at least three months per year over two consecutive years. Patients who get medical help early can lead fairly normal lives with proper medication and a good exercise program.

The most important known factor to cause COPD is cigarette smoking. It also is more common among city dwellers than among rural populations. Urban air pollution also plays a role.

Victims of COPD usually get colds or flu often. They also become winded under conditions that do not tax most healthy people (such as walking on a level surface). Other signs and symptoms include:

- Shortness of breath, gasping for air.
- Tripod position (sitting upright, leaning forward, fighting to breathe).
- Bulging neck veins.
- Coarse rattling sounds in the lungs.
- Cyanosis.
- Prolonged exhaling through pursed lips.
- Barrel-shaped chest.
- Presence of home-oxygen systems, breathing treatments, medications, and inhalers (puffers).

Both emphysema and chronic bronchitis patients may develop a hypoxic drive to breathe. Healthy people get their drive to breathe from the amount of carbon dioxide in the blood. Patients who have emphysema or chronic bronchitis build up consistently high levels of carbon dioxide. Because of this, the body looks to the levels of oxygen, rather than carbon dioxide, to determine the need to breathe. If oxygen levels are low, the body breathes faster to get more oxygen.

Giving oxygen to a patient with hypoxic drive can be a problem. After oxygen is administered, its level in the blood increases. In the patient with a true hypoxic drive, increased levels of oxygen may signal the body to slow down or even stop breathing. However, this occurs rarely in the field.

The general rule is to administer oxygen to all patients who need it. All patients with difficulty breathing, cyanosis, altered mental status, shock, or other signs of a serious condition should be given high-concentration oxygen by nonrebreather mask. If breathing is inadequate, assist ventilation with a BVM and supplemental oxygen. All patients in respiratory or cardiac arrest should receive high concentrations of supplemental oxygen by pocket face mask or BVM.

Asthma

Asthma affects approximately 3% of the people in the U.S., or about 10 million people. About 5,000 of those die from it every year. It is most common among children and middle-aged women. Often, it is present in more than one member of the same family.

Typically, people with asthma are free of symptoms between attacks. Some often do not know what causes an attack. Others have specific triggers such as exercise or animal dander.

The acute asthma attack varies in duration, intensity, and frequency. It reflects airway obstruction due to bronchospasm, swelling of mucous membranes in the bronchial walls, or plugging of the bronchi by thick mucus.

Signs and symptoms of an asthma attack include:

- Tripod position.
- Spasmodic, apparently unproductive cough.
- High-pitched wheezing during exhalation, which may also occur upon inhalation.
- Very little movement of air during breathing.
- Overinflated chest with air trapped in the lungs.
- Rapid, shallow respirations.
- Rapid pulse, often exceeding 120.
- Fatigue, confusion, agitation, lethargy.
- Inability to speak in full sentences without catching the breath.

Status asthmaticus is a severe, life-threatening, prolonged asthma attack. It is a dire medical emergency (Figure 14-9). The patient may begin shallow breathing or may stop breathing altogether. In these cases, the wheezing may stop, and it may appear that the patient has improved, but this is not true. Watch all asthma patients carefully for reduced respirations. Be prepared to provide artificial ventilation. Signs and symptoms of status asthmaticus include:

- Anxiety, exhaustion.
- Breathing through pursed lips.
- Wheezing at first, then inaudible breath sounds.
- Overinflated chest.
- Rapid heart rate.
- Tripod position.
- Extremely labored breathing.
- Cyanosis.
- Walking and talking only with great effort.

CAUTION: All that wheezes is not asthma. Many other diseases can cause wheezing, such as acute congestive heart failure, smoke inhalation, chronic bronchitis, anaphylaxis (an acute allergic reaction), and acute pulmonary **embolism**. If the patient is wheezing and breathing is adequate, administer high-flow oxygen with a nonrebreather mask. If breathing is not adequate, assist ventilations with a BVM and supplemental oxygen.

Note that patients with asthma and COPD often have constricted bronchioles. One common treatment for this is a *prescribed inhaler* (Figure 14-10). The medication in this device can dilate air passages and reduce difficulty breathing. In some areas, First Responders may assist patients in using a prescribed inhaler. To do so, follow all

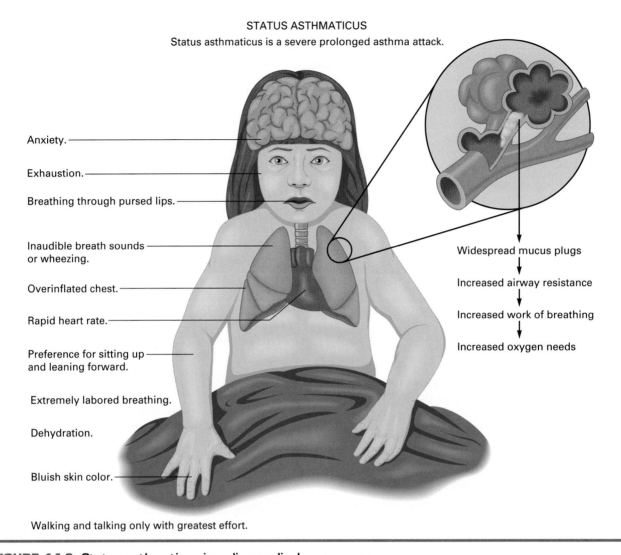

STATUS ASTHMATICUS
Status asthmaticus is a severe prolonged asthma attack.

Anxiety.

Exhaustion.

Breathing through pursed lips.

Inaudible breath sounds
or wheezing.

Overinflated chest.

Rapid heart rate.

Preference for sitting up
and leaning forward.

Extremely labored breathing.

Dehydration.

Bluish skin color.

Walking and talking only with greatest effort.

Widespread mucus plugs

Increased airway resistance

Increased work of breathing

Increased oxygen needs

FIGURE 14-9 Status asthmaticus is a dire medical emergency.

local protocols. In general, to assist a patient, keep the following points in mind:

- Be sure the medication is indicated. Contact medical direction prior to assisting with any medication.
- The patient must be able to inhale the medication properly. It is a fine powder, not a gas. It must be inhaled deeply into the lungs.
- Coach the patient to take a deep breath. As the patient begins to breathe, the inhaler should be activated. If it is activated before the breath, the medication will deposit in the mouth and not in the lungs.
- Instruct the patient to hold his breath to keep the medication in the lungs and then to exhale.
- Reassess the patient's vital signs and breathing.

Pneumonia

Pneumonia is a term used to describe a group of illnesses characterized by lung infection and fluid- or pus-filled

alveoli. Pneumonia can lead to inadequately oxygenated blood. Pneumonia is most frequently caused by bacteria

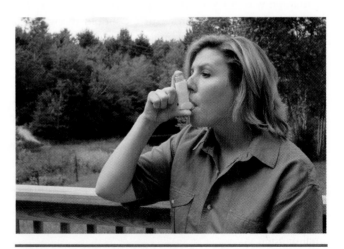

FIGURE 14-10 A prescribed inhaler delivers medication that can help a patient with asthma or COPD.

or a virus. It also may be caused by inhaled irritants such as vomit.

Pneumonia patients generally appear to be ill. Most complain of fever and chills "that shake the bed." Signs and symptoms may be influenced by the area of the lung that is affected. For example, pneumonia of the lower lobes of the lungs may not produce a cough but may cause abdominal pain. In general, look for the following:

- Chest pain, usually made worse with breathing.
- Rapid breathing.
- Respiratory distress.
- Productive cough with pus in the sputum or mucus.
- Fever, usually exceeding 101°F.
- Chills.
- Hot, dry skin.

Acute Pulmonary Edema

Acute pulmonary edema can be caused by damage to the heart or lungs. It occurs when extra fluids build up in the tissues around the spaces of the lungs. If you know your patient has acute pulmonary edema and he is responsive and in a sitting position, let his legs dangle to encourage blood to pool in the legs. You also can support the back and shoulders with pillows.

Signs and symptoms of acute pulmonary edema include:

- Shortness of breath.
- Rapid, labored breathing.
- Cyanosis.
- Frothy pink, blood-tinged sputum (a late sign).
- Bulging neck veins.
- Rapid pulse.
- Cool, clammy skin.
- Swelling or edema of the ankles.
- Restlessness.
- Anxiety.
- Exhaustion.

Note that oxygen therapy may be critical to this patient. So be sure to administer oxygen, if you are trained and allowed to do so. Also, monitor breathing and other vital signs carefully until help arrives.

Hyperventilation

Hyperventilation is a condition characterized by breathing too fast. Breathing too fast happens to most people occasionally, such as when they are surprised. That is normal, as long as the breathing quickly returns to a normal rate.

Hyperventilation syndrome is an abnormal state in which rapid breathing persists. It is a common disorder usually associated with anxiety. As the patient becomes more anxious, he or she breathes more rapidly, which in turn makes the patient more anxious, and so on.

The syndrome is characterized by rapid, deep breathing. The lungs overinflate, and the patient blows off too much carbon dioxide. In prolonged cases, the patient may pass out. It typically occurs in young, anxious patients, most of whom are not aware that they are breathing too fast. Signs and symptoms include:

- Air hunger, or "gulping" air.
- Deep, sighing, rapid breathing with rapid pulse.
- Sensation of choking.
- Dryness or bitterness of the mouth.
- Tightness or a "lump" in the throat.
- Marked anxiety escalating to panic and a feeling of impending doom.
- Dizziness, lightheadedness, fainting.
- Giddiness or unusual behavior.
- Drawing up the hands at the wrist and knuckles with the fingers flexed.
- Blurring of vision.
- Numbness or tingling of the hands and feet or around the mouth.
- Pounding of the heart with stabbing pains in the chest.
- Fatigue, great tiredness, or weakness.
- A feeling of being in a dream.

Note that most patients who are breathing rapidly or deeply are *not* hyperventilating. Any of several serious conditions may be the cause, including diabetes, asthma, or trauma. Rapid breathing also may have a medical origin, such as in aspirin overdose. If you are certain that no life-threatening condition exists, try to calm your patient. Be reassuring and listen carefully to his or her concerns. Try to talk the patient into breathing slowly. If the patient does not respond immediately to your efforts, administer oxygen. It will not make hyperventilation worse.

You may have heard that putting a paper bag over a patient's mouth is a cure for hyperventilation. This treatment is dangerous, especially if an underlying medical condition exists. As noted above, calming is a powerful benefit to the hyperventilating patient. Follow local protocol.

Q. 1. What is respiratory distress?

2. What is First Responder care for a patient in respiratory distress?

▶▶ The Call Follow-up

At the beginning of this chapter, you read that a First Responder was caring for a patient with chest pain, labored breathing, and poor skin color. To see how chapter skills apply to this emergency, read the following. It describes how the call was completed.

Physical Examination Two other members of the ERT arrived to help. They performed a head-to-toe exam, while I talked to Harry about his history.

Patient History Harry told me that he was working at his bench when he started getting severe pain in his chest. He had never felt anything like it before, and I had never seen Harry that scared. I reassured him and asked a few questions, using the OPQRRRST memory aid.

Harry was working when the pain came on. He told me it was crushing, like someone sitting right on the center of his chest. He held his fist there to show me. It didn't radiate, and nothing helped to relieve the pain. On a 1-to-10 scale, he said the pain was an "8." It started about 10 minutes before I arrived.

Harry hadn't seen a doctor in years. He took no medications and had no medical problems or allergies. He ate a big spaghetti dinner during his break.

When I heard Harry's vital signs—pulse 92 and irregular, respirations 18 and adequate, blood pressure 146/96, with skin that was cool, gray, and moist—I swore to myself that I'd do everything I could to make sure our plant gets an AED before this happens again.

Ongoing Assessment After helping to make Harry comfortable, I continued to talk and reassure him. We rechecked his ABCs, which remained okay. The chest pain did not diminish. A second assessment of vital signs revealed a pulse of 96 and irregular, and respirations 20 and still labored. Unfortunately, we didn't have oxygen to give him.

Patient Hand-off The paramedics arrived a short time later. We immediately called their attention to Harry's poor color, labored breathing, and chest pain to let them know how serious I thought it was. They agreed. Then we filled them in on the rest (see the hand-off report below).

The paramedics thanked us, and I helped them put the oxygen on Harry. He wanted me to come with him, and the paramedics didn't mind some help. I made sure that someone called Harry's wife.

Well, it turned out that Harry had a major heart attack. The word spread around the plant the next day. The way he looked was just like they described in the books. I always take chest pain seriously. I'm glad we did with Harry.

 ## Hand-off Report

"This is Harry Nowack, 55 years old. His chest pain started while he was working. It is in the center of his chest and is crushing. It is an 8 out of 10 on the scale, and it doesn't radiate. He has no medical problems that he knows of, but he hasn't been to a doctor in years. He has no meds or allergies. He ate a big spaghetti dinner a short time ago. His pulse is 96 and irregular, respirations 20 and slightly labored, blood pressure 146/96."

The Last Word *Few things are more frightening than chest pain or not being able to breathe. A patient with either problem will probably be anxious and may even become argumentative. Do your best to be calming and reassuring. If the patient yells or snaps at you, realize that he or she is reacting to the situation and not to you personally. Keep in mind that these emergencies require compassionate emotional care, as well as management of the patient's physical condition.*

Chapter Review

Focus on the EMS Team

Problems with cardiac and respiratory systems are frequently the reasons why First Responders are summoned. Quickly recognizing these problems as potentially life-threatening—and just as quickly making sure the proper medical help is on the way—can save your patient's life.

Summing Up

- Chest pain or discomfort is one of the most common symptoms of a cardiac emergency. As a First Responder, you do not have to identify the cause of that pain. Whatever the cause, your assessment and care of the patient will be the same.

- Assessment of a patient with a chief complaint of chest pain or discomfort is the same as assessment of any patient. That is, follow your patient assessment plan (initial assessment, patient history, physical exam, ongoing assessment). As soon as you recognize a possible cardiac emergency, update the incoming EMS unit or call dispatch to request advanced care. If possible, when you gather a patient history, attempt to get a good description of the pain.

- Emergency care of a patient with chest pain or discomfort includes ensuring adequate breathing and helping him get as comfortable and calm as possible. Continually monitor this patient, who could become unstable rapidly. Be prepared to assist ventilations, perform CPR, and use an AED if required.

- Two specific cardiac conditions are angina pectoris and myocardial infarction. Note that patients who have a history of angina are commonly prescribed a medication called *nitroglycerin*. Do not administer this or any other medication without the approval of medical direction.

- Note that 20% of all heart attack patients—usually the elderly or patients with diabetes—have no chest pain at all. A heart attack without pain is called a silent myocardial infarction.

- Respiratory distress, which is shortness of breath or a feeling of air hunger with labored breathing, may be a symptom of an injury or illness. Whatever the cause, First Responder assessment and care is the same.

- Emergency care of a patient in respiratory distress includes ensuring adequate breathing and keeping the patient as comfortable and as calm as possible.

- Specific respiratory conditions include chronic obstructive pulmonary disease (COPD), asthma, pneumonia, acute pulmonary edema, and hyperventilation syndrome.

- Administer oxygen to all patients who need it. All patients with difficulty breathing, cyanosis, altered mental status, shock, or other signs of a serious condition should be given high-concentration oxygen by nonrebreather mask. If breathing is inadequate, assist ventilation with a BVM and supplemental oxygen. All patients in respiratory or cardiac arrest should receive high concentrations of supplemental oxygen by pocket face mask or BVM.

Key Terms

acute having a sudden onset; severe.

angina pectoris pain in the chest, occurring when blood supply to the heart is reduced and a portion of the heart muscle is not receiving enough oxygen.

arteriosclerosis a condition that causes the walls of the arteries to become thick and hard.

asthma a condition in which the bronchioles constrict, causing a reduction of airflow and creating congestion.

cardiac dysrhythmias abnormal heart rhythms that follow a heart attack; generally caused by injury to the heart's electrical conduction system.

chronic bronchitis a condition characterized by inflammation, edema, and excessive mucus in the bronchial tree; one of the most common chronic obstructive pulmonary diseases.

congestive heart failure the failure of the heart to pump efficiently, leading to excessive blood or fluids in the lungs, body, or both.

COPD chronic obstructive pulmonary disease.

coronary artery disease the narrowing of one or more places in the arteries of the heart.

edema swelling resulting from a buildup of fluid in the tissues.

embolism a thrombus, or clot of blood and plaque, that has broken loose from the wall of an artery.

emphysema a condition in which the lungs suffer a progressive loss of elasticity; one of the most common chronic obstructive pulmonary diseases.

hyperventilation a condition characterized by rapid breathing.

myocardial infarction a heart attack.

OPQRRRST memory aid used to help get a good description of pain from the patient; letters stand for onset, provocation, quality, region, radiation, relief, severity, and time.

pacemaker a device that emits electrical discharges to the heart in order to trigger contractions.

palpitations a sensation of throbbing or fluttering of the heart.

pneumonia a term used to describe a group of illnesses characterized by lung infection and fluid- or pus-filled alveoli.

respiratory distress shortness of breath or a feeling of air hunger with labored breathing.

silent myocardial infarction a heart attack without pain.

status asthmaticus a severe, life-threatening, prolonged asthma attack.

tripod position a position in which the patient is sitting upright, leaning forward, fighting to breathe.

Knowledge Check

1. **Which one of the following is NOT a part of First Responder care for a responsive patient in respiratory distress?**
   a. Comfort and reassure the patient.
   b. Place the patient in a prone position.
   c. Assist ventilations if breathing is inadequate.
   d. Administer oxygen by way of a nonrebreather mask.

2. **Which one of the following questions will help you determine if the patient's pain radiates?**
   a. Did anything cause or start the pain?
   b. On a scale of 1–10, how bad is the pain?
   c. What were you doing when the pain started?
   d. Does it begin in one place and travel elsewhere?

3. **Which one of the following statements about cardiac emergencies is TRUE?**
   a. Patients with chest pain rarely experience respiratory distress.
   b. Carry the AED to all potential cardiac events, even if the patient is conscious.
   c. Use the memory aid OPQRRRST to gather a good past medical history of the patient.
   d. Pain caused by a heart attack frequently extends down to the left lower extremity.

4. **First Responder care for a patient who is hyperventilating may include which one of the following?**
   a. Insist on administering nitroglycerin tablets.
   b. Administer oxygen by way of a nonrebreather mask.
   c. Attach the AED and provide three consecutive shocks.
   d. Have him breathe deeply with a paper bag over his mouth.

5. **Respiratory distress may be a symptom of an injury or an illness.**
   a. True
   b. False

6. **First Responder care for either a cardiac or respiratory emergency is to ensure adequate breathing and to help keep the patient as calm and as comfortable as possible until advanced care arrives on scene.**
   a. True
   b. False

7. Do NOT assist an angina patient with nitroglycerin without first getting the approval of medical direction.
   a. True
   b. False

8. List six of the major cardiac risk factors.

   _____   _____

   _____   _____

   _____   _____

9. List the signs of ADEQUATE breathing.

   _____

   _____

   _____

   _____

Scenario

You and your partner have been called to the scene of a 58-year-old man who "doesn't feel well." All this tells you is that you should probably expect a medical rather than a trauma patient, but even that isn't a sure thing. You decide to bring your jump kit and the AED, just in case.

a. What is the first thing you should do when you arrive on scene?

   _____

   _____

b. You and your partner are met at the door of the house by a woman. "I'm Mrs. Kennedy," she tells you. "My husband, Patrick, is in the bedroom." After introducing yourselves and ensuring that it is safe to enter the house, what should you ask her?

   _____

   _____

c. Mrs. Kennedy reports that her husband's chief complaint is nausea and a "heavy weight on his chest." When you get to the patient's side, you observe that the patient is sitting in an easy chair. He looks pale, sweaty, and in some distress. What should you do next?

   _____

   _____

d. You have determined that this is a possible cardiac emergency and have administered oxygen via nonrebreather mask. Before you do anything else, you should:

   _____

   _____

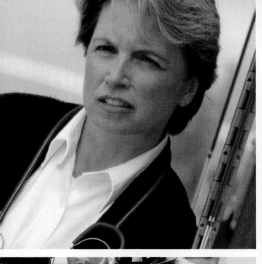
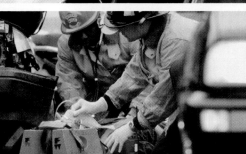
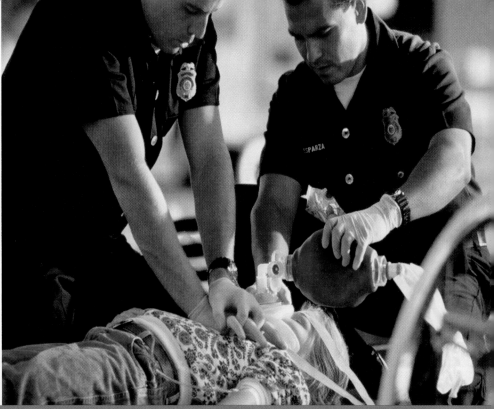

15 | Medical Emergencies

Objectives

From the U.S. Department of Transportation (DOT) 1995 "First Responder: National Standard Curriculum." Material supplemental to the DOT curriculum is listed under "Enrichment."

Cognitive

5-1.1 ▶ Identify the patient who presents with a general medical complaint. (p. 267)

5-1.2 ▶ Explain the steps in providing emergency medical care to a patient with a general medical complaint. (pp. 267–268)

5-1.3 ▶ Identify the patient who presents with a specific medical complaint of altered mental status. (p. 268)

5-1.4 ▶ Explain the steps in providing emergency medical care to a patient with an altered mental status. (pp. 268–269)

5-1.5 ▶ Identify the patient who presents with a specific medical complaint of seizures. (pp. 274, 276)

5-1.6 ▶ Explain the steps in providing emergency medical care to a patient with seizures. (p. 276)

Affective

5-1.15 ▶ Attend to the feelings of the patient and/or family when dealing with the patient with a general medical complaint. (p. 267)

5-1.16 ▶ Attend to the feelings of the patient and/or family when dealing with a specific medical complaint. (pp. 269, 274, 276)

5-1.18 ▶ Demonstrate a caring attitude toward patients with a general medical complaint who request emergency medical services. (p. 267)

5-1.19 ▶ Place the interests of the patient with a general medical complaint as the foremost consideration when making any and all patient care decisions. (pp. 268, 270)

5-1.20 ▶ Communicate with empathy to patients with a general medical complaint, as well as with family members and friends of the patient. (p. 267)

5-1.21 ▶ Demonstrate a caring attitude toward patients with a specific medical complaint who request emergency medical services. (pp. 269, 274, 276)

5-1.22 ▶ Place the interests of the patient with a specific medical complaint as the foremost consideration when making any and all patient care decisions. (pp. 269, 270, 274, 276, 278)

5-1.23 ▶ Communicate with empathy to patients with a specific medical complaint, as well as with family members and friends of the patient. (pp. 269, 274, 276)

Psychomotor

5-1.27 ▶ Demonstrate the steps in providing emergency medical care to a patient with a general medical complaint. (pp. 267-268)

5-1.28 ▶ Demonstrate the steps in providing emergency medical care to a patient with an altered mental status. (pp. 268–269)

5-1.29 ▶ Demonstrate the steps in providing emergency medical care to a patient with seizures. (pp. 274, 276)

Enrichment

▶ Recognize the relationship between airway and breathing care and the patient with altered mental status. (p. 269)

▶ Describe assessment and care of the patient with a diabetic emergency. (pp. 269–272)

▶ Describe assessment and care of the patient with an altered mental status and a loss of speech, sensory, or motor function. (pp. 272–274)

▶ Identify the three components of the Cincinnati Prehospital Stroke Scale. (pp. 273–274, 275)

▶ Describe how to use the Cincinnati Prehospital Stroke Scale on a patient with altered mental status. (pp. 273–274, 275)

▶ Recognize the common signs and symptoms of a generalized seizure. (p. 276)

▶ Explain the assessment and emergency care of a seizing patient. (p. 276)

▶ Identify the signs and symptoms of abdominal pain or distress. (pp. 276–278)

▶ Describe assessment and care of a patient with abdominal pain or distress. (pp. 276–278)

▶ List various ways that poisons enter the body. (p. 278)

▶ List signs and symptoms of poisoning. (pp. 278–281)

▶ Describe the assessment and care of a patient with suspected poisoning. (pp. 278–281)

▶ Recognize the need for medical direction in caring for the patient with poisoning. (pp. 278–281)

Introduction

A medical complaint is any chief complaint that is not caused by trauma. There will be many such calls in your career. They may involve abdominal pain, altered mental status, or even complaints such as "I don't feel well." As with any patient, your responsibility in the emergency care of these patients is to follow your patient assessment plan from scene size-up to patient hand-off.

Section 1 General Medical Complaints

As a First Responder, you will be called to the scenes of patients with specific medical complaints, such as "my chest hurts" or "I can't breathe." Every once in a while, however, your medical patient will have a nonspecific complaint such as "I feel weak" or "I don't feel well."

Note that these patients may be just as frightened and worried as patients with more specific problems. Consider their feelings as you assess and care for them. Be gentle and empathetic. If the family is present, they may be very concerned and ask you to tell them "what's wrong." Be truthful and kind. For example, you might say that though you do not know exactly what the problem is, you are doing all that is possible. Reassure them. Let them

know you have arranged for the patient to be transported to a hospital.

Patient Assessment

First Responder assessment of patients with a general medical complaint is the same as for any other patient. After your scene size-up, complete an initial assessment and treat any life-threatening conditions you observe. Perform a physical exam as needed, and be especially thorough gathering the patient's history. It could provide important clues to the underlying problem. ■

First Responder Care

To provide care to a patient with a general medical complaint for which you are unable to determine a more

THE CALL

Dispatch My partner and I were making rounds on the trails when a group of hikers stopped us. It seems that an older gentleman was suppose to have packed out that day. Several hikers remarked that he had looked sick. They asked us to check on him. We did.

Scene Size-up As we approached the man's lean-to, we saw a supine body. We quickly did a scene size-up. There were no mechanisms of injury or obvious dangers, so we put on our gloves and approached the patient.

Initial Assessment Our general impression was poor. He was responsive to verbal stimuli, but his speech was slurred and he was unable to respond appropriately to our commands. His breathing was adequate, and his radial pulse was slow, strong, and regular. There was no evidence of external bleeding, but he was very pale. We were worried. We radioed our office to request immediate air medical evacuation.

Why did these First Responders believe their patient to be a high priority for transport? (You may want to review the "First on Scene" on page 221.) Consider their decision as you read Chapter 15. What else might be done to assess and care for this patient?

---

specific complaint or to obtain a pertinent history, do the following:

1. *Monitor the patient's ABCs.* Be sure both breathing and circulation are adequate.
2. *Position the patient.* If the patient is conscious and there are no suspected spine injuries, allow the patient to get in a position of comfort.
3. *Perform an ongoing assessment* until the incoming EMTs take over patient care. Be sure to report any changes in the patient's condition. ■

 1. What is First Responder care for a patient whose chief complaint is "I don't feel well"?

Section 2 Altered Mental Status

A change in a patient's normal level of responsiveness or a loss of the ability to understand is called an **altered mental status.** An altered mental status can occur quickly or slowly. It can range from disoriented to com-bative to unresponsive. There are many medical reasons for a change in mental status. A few examples are:

- Hypoxia (decreased levels of oxygen in the blood).
- Diabetic emergencies.
- Stroke (loss of blood flow to part of the brain).
- Seizures.
- Fever, infection.
- Poisoning, including drug and alcohol poisoning.
- Head injury.
- Psychiatric conditions.

As a First Responder, you do not need to figure out why your patient has an altered mental status. Your job is to recognize it as soon as possible and to support the patient appropriately.

Patient Assessment

After ensuring scene safety and taking the appropriate BSI precautions, proceed with patient assessment. Ensure an open airway, adequate breathing, and adequate circulation. Since a patient with altered mental status can deteriorate rapidly, gather an accurate history as soon as possible. If you wait too long, the patient's history—and any clues to the cause of the emergency—could be lost to the EMTs and hospital staff who take over care. ■

First Responder Practice

✓

An altered mental status can range from slightly confused to totally unresponsive. Although this condition has many possible causes, one important fact applies to all: Patients who have an altered mental status may not be able to maintain their own airway and must be monitored carefully.

First Responder Care

To provide care to a patient with altered mental status:

1. *Closely monitor the patient's airway and breathing.* These patients may not be able to protect their own airways. It is up to you to be aware of this danger. If the patient is unresponsive, secure the airway with an adjunct. Suction as needed.

2. *Position the patient.* If there is no reason to suspect head or spine injury, place the patient in the recovery position. Continue to monitor the patient's breathing closely.

3. *Administer high-flow oxygen.* One of the most common causes of altered mental status is hypoxia. If the patient is breathing adequately, apply high-flow oxygen by nonrebreather mask. If the patient is not breathing adequately, assist with a pocket face mask or bag-valve-mask device attached to an oxygen source. ■

Note that a patient with an altered mental status may be aware of his condition. This can be very frightening. If the underlying cause is a seizure, the patient could lose control of his bowels and bladder, which adds to embarrassment and anxiety. A caring attitude on your part, as well as helping the patient maintain some privacy, will help.

The patient's condition may be very upsetting to the family, too. Take time, if possible, to make sure they understand that you are caring for the patient and that an ambulance is on the way.

Specific Related Conditions

As mentioned above, many medical conditions can cause an altered mental status. Some of the most common include diabetic emergencies, stroke, and seizures.

Diabetic Emergencies

Sugar is the body's primary fuel. For the body to metabolize (use) sugar for energy, the pancreas secretes a hormone called **insulin**. People with diabetes either do not make enough insulin or, for some reason, the insulin does not do its job (Figure 15-1). Often they take a medication—also

NORMAL VS. DIABETIC USE OF SUGAR

NORMAL

⬇ Food is eaten.

Digestion begins in the stomach.

Food is broken down into simple sugars in the small intestine.

Sugars enter the bloodstream. Insulin is released by the pancreas.

Sugar enters body cells with aid of insulin.

DIABETIC

⬇ Food is eaten.

Digestion begins in the stomach.

Food is broken down into simple sugars in the small intestine.

Sugars enter the bloodstream. Little or no insulin is released by the pancreas or the body's cells are resistant to the effects of insulin.

Sugar cannot enter the cells, stays in bloodstream, and finally is eliminated with urine.

FIGURE 15-1 Diabetes has long been recognized as a serious disorder.

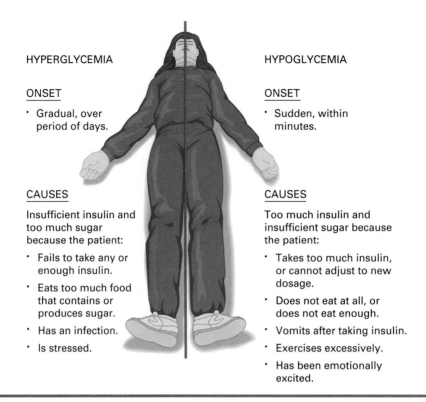

HYPERGLYCEMIA

ONSET

- Gradual, over period of days.

CAUSES

Insufficient insulin and too much sugar because the patient:

- Fails to take any or enough insulin.
- Eats too much food that contains or produces sugar.
- Has an infection.
- Is stressed.

HYPOGLYCEMIA

ONSET

- Sudden, within minutes.

CAUSES

Too much insulin and insufficient sugar because the patient:

- Takes too much insulin, or cannot adjust to new dosage.
- Does not eat at all, or does not eat enough.
- Vomits after taking insulin.
- Exercises excessively.
- Has been emotionally excited.

FIGURE 15-2 Causes of hyperglycemia and hypoglycemia.

called *insulin*—that can help them control blood sugar. However, blood sugar can still get too low or too high. When this happens, the body reacts. The most common reaction is altered mental status.

Two types of related emergencies are associated with diabetes: **hyperglycemia** and **hypoglycemia** (Figure 15-2). To give you greater understanding, the following paragraphs describe each one. However, you will not be required to distinguish one from the other, because emergency care is the same for both conditions.

Hyperglycemia is basically a case of too much blood sugar and too little insulin. Common causes of hyperglycemia include infection, increased or prolonged stress, failure of the patient to take insulin or to take a sufficient amount, and eating too much food that contains or produces sugar. Although a hyperglycemia emergency is sometimes called "diabetic coma," the patient is not usually found in a coma.

Signs and symptoms of hyperglycemia may include (Figure 15-3):

- Sweet, fruity, or acetone-like breath.
- Flushed, warm, dry skin.
- Hunger and thirst.
- Rapid, weak pulse.
- Altered mental status.

- Intoxicated appearance, staggering, slurred speech.
- Frequent urination.
- Reports that the patient has not taken the prescribed diabetes medications.

The onset of severe hyperglycemia is gradual. In most cases it develops over 12 to 48 hours. At first, the patient experiences excessive hunger, thirst, and urination. The patient appears extremely ill and becomes sicker and weaker as the condition progresses. If left untreated, the patient may die. With treatment, improvement is gradual, occurring 6 to 12 hours after insulin and intravenous fluids are administered.

Hypoglycemia, or low blood sugar, is the result of too much insulin or too little sugar. This occurs less frequently than hyperglycemia, but its onset is sudden and

First Responder Practice

Never jump to conclusions. Consider all patients who exhibit an altered mental status or unusual behavior as having a medical problem. Never assume that the patient is drunk, drugged, or mentally ill.

SIGNS AND SYMPTOMS OF A DIABETIC EMERGENCY

Hyperglycemia

Altered mental status.

Sweet, fruuity, or acetone-like breath.

Hunger and thirst.

Intoxicated appearance, staggering, slurred speech.

Rapid, weak pulse.

Frequent urination.

Reports that patient has not been taking prescribed medications.

Hypoglycemia

Headache, hunger.

Rapid onset of altered mental status.

Intoxicated appearance, staggering, slurred speech.

Seizures.

Cool, clammy skin.

Rapid pulse rate.

FIGURE 15-3 Diabetic emergencies may include a wide range of signs and symptoms.

often more dramatic. People with diabetes can suffer from low blood sugar. So can alcoholics, people who have ingested certain poisons, and people who are ill.

Some common causes of low blood sugar are skipped meals, particularly for a patient with diabetes; vomiting, especially with illness; strenuous exercise; physical stress from extreme heat or cold; and emotional stress, such as at weddings or funerals. The most recognized cause of low blood sugar is the accidental overdose of insulin. (After a time, diabetes can inflict a degree of blindness in patients. This can make it very hard for them to give themselves the proper amount of insulin. The result can be an accidental overdose.)

Signs and symptoms of hypoglycemia may include (Figure 15-3):

- Rapid onset of altered mental status.
- Intoxicated appearance, staggering, slurred speech.
- Rapid pulse rate.
- Cool, clammy skin.
- Hunger.
- Headache.
- Seizures.

When you gather the history of a patient with altered mental status, try to find out about the onset of the emergency. Be sure to ask, "Do you have diabetes?" If he or she says yes, ask: "Have you eaten today? Did you take your medication (insulin injections or oral medications)?" Also ask about any current illness, stress, and problems with medications.

Look for a medical identification tag during the physical exam. If the police are present, ask them to check the patient's wallet, too. If the patient is at home, check the refrigerator for diabetes medications such as insulin. Also check around the house for needles and syringes. Special needle containers are often present in the house.

Proceed with emergency care as you would for any patient with altered mental status. However, if you suspect hypoglycemia or hyperglycemia (you don't have to distinguish one from the other, because care is the same), alert the incoming EMS crew immediately. While waiting for them, monitor the airway closely. Note that this patient may suddenly have a seizure. Be prepared. (See "Seizures" later in this chapter.)

Your EMS system may permit you to help a diabetic patient take some sugar. (You will not harm a hyperglycemic patient with sugar, and you could save the life of a patient with hypoglycemia. Follow local protocols.) If the patient is awake and able to control his own airway, he may benefit from one of the following:

- Dissolve some sugar in a glass of water or juice.
- Pour a drink that is naturally rich in sugar, such as orange juice. If using a prepared juice or beverage product,

First Responder Practice

Giving sugar (glucose) to a patient who has low blood sugar can cause a rapid and seemingly miraculous recovery. But remember that giving any medication to a patient is a very serious responsibility. Never give an oral medication to any patient who cannot swallow or who does not have a gag reflex.

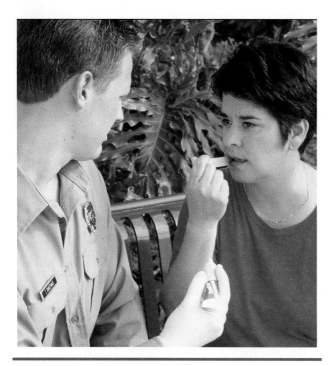

FIGURE 15-4 Your EMS system may allow you to help a patient self-administer oral glucose. Follow local protocols.

be sure it contains sugar. Some contain artificial sweeteners, which will not help the hypoglycemic patient.

■ Squeeze a commercially prepared **glucose** paste onto a tongue depressor (Figure 15-4). Then, assist the patient in placing the tongue depressor between his cheek and gums. The glucose will be quickly absorbed. In the event the patient becomes unresponsive or unable to control his own airway, the tongue depressor can be easily removed. Note that a tube of glucose should be used for a single patient only and then discarded.

Never give a patient who cannot control his own airway anything to eat or drink. He could aspirate the substance into his lungs. This can have grave results, including death. If you are in doubt, call for medical direction. If sugar or glucose is administered, be sure to tell the EMTs who take over care. Report any changes in mental status that occurred while the patient was in your care.

Stroke

A patient may suffer a **cerebrovascular accident (CVA)**, or **stroke,** when an area of the brain is deprived of blood. This can occur when a blood clot (thrombus) blocks an artery, when matter (embolus) lodges in an artery, or when an artery bursts (aneurysm) (Figure 15-5). The National Stroke Association refers to a stroke as a "brain attack."

Strokes are the third leading cause of death in the U.S. and a leading cause of adult disability. They are more common in people over the age of 65 but can affect anyone. Patients at risk for heart attack may also be in danger of having a stroke. They include patients with high blood pressure or diabetes, and patients who smoke tobacco.

The signs and symptoms of stroke are the result of several factors. Among them are the location and amount of brain damage. Signs and symptoms may be mild or life-threatening. Sometimes they are temporary. Temporary ones indicate a "mini-stroke," or **transient ischemic attacks (TIAs)**. These mini-strokes are often warning signs of an impending larger stroke.

Signs and symptoms of stroke include (Figure 15-6):

■ *Altered mental status.* This can range from a change in personality to seizures and unresponsiveness.

■ *Inability to communicate.* The patient may either fail to speak or fail to understand what others say.

■ *Impairment in one part of the body.* For example, loss of muscle control on one side of the face or loss of movement on one entire side of the body. If the patient's limb seems paralyzed, handle it carefully. You could injure it without knowing. The patient also may unintentionally cause it to strike an object.

After your initial assessment, try to gather a history from the patient, family, or bystanders. Be sure to find out if there is a medical history of stroke, high blood pressure, diabetes, or heart disease.

About 50% of stroke patients have an elevated blood pressure during a stroke. However, the combination of an elevated blood pressure, slow pulse, and rapid or irregular breathing is a sign of a major stroke. Be prepared if the patient should convulse suddenly.

Identification of stroke in the prehospital setting has become more reliable by the addition of specific prehospital tests. One of the most common is called the *Cincinnati*

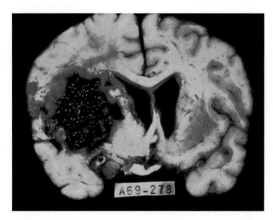

a. *A stroke from cerebral hemorrhage.*

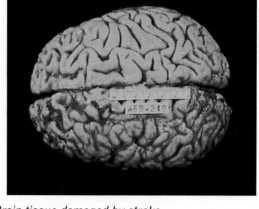

b. *Brain tissue damaged by stroke.*

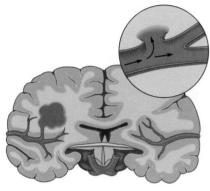

c. *Cause of stroke: a blood vessel in the brain ruptures (cerebral hemorrhage).*

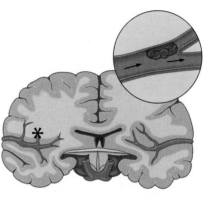

d. *Cause of stroke: a clot or foreign body forms in the body and travels to the brain (cerebral embolism).*

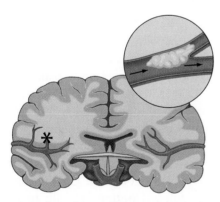

e. *Cause of stroke: a blood clot forms in the brain (cerebral thrombosis).*

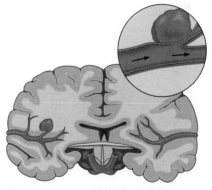

f. *Cause of stroke: a compression injury.*

FIGURE 15-5 Also called a cerebrovascular accident (CVA), a stroke refers to the interruption of blood flow to a portion of the brain.

Prehospital Stroke Scale (Figure 15-7). Through the three components of the exam—facial droop, arm drift, and speech—this scale tests nerves commonly affected by stroke. Report any abnormalities to the EMTs when they arrive.

To perform the Cincinnati Prehospital Stroke Scale exam, look for each of the following in your patient:

■ *Facial droop.* Look at the patient's face. Observe for asymmetry (drooping on one side and not the other). Ask the patient to give you a big smile that shows his teeth. Notice the evenness of the mouth and cheeks while the patient smiles. A normal finding is symmetry (both sides are even, or there is no droop). An abnormal

SIGNS AND SYMPTOMS OF STROKE

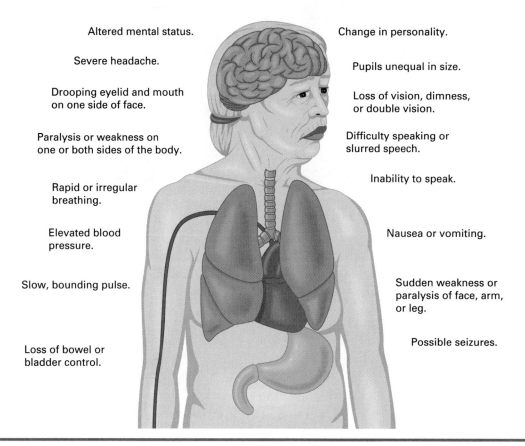

Altered mental status.

Severe headache.

Drooping eyelid and mouth on one side of face.

Paralysis or weakness on one or both sides of the body.

Rapid or irregular breathing.

Elevated blood pressure.

Slow, bounding pulse.

Loss of bowel or bladder control.

Change in personality.

Pupils unequal in size.

Loss of vision, dimness, or double vision.

Difficulty speaking or slurred speech.

Inability to speak.

Nausea or vomiting.

Sudden weakness or paralysis of face, arm, or leg.

Possible seizures.

FIGURE 15-6 **One or more signs or symptoms may indicate a stroke.**

finding is asymmetry, or drooping on one side and not the other.

- *Arm drift*. Have the patient place both arms straight out in front of his body, palms down. Then ask him to close his eyes and hold his arms in position for about 30 seconds. Watch to see if one arm, and not the other, begins to fall or drift. A normal finding is arms remain even and in place or they drift evenly together. An abnormal finding is one arm drops or raises, while the other arm remains in position.

- *Speech*. Listen for slurred speech while the patient talks. You may also ask the patient to say something specific, such as "The quick brown fox jumped over the lazy dog's back." (This will reveal a problem faster than yes or no answers.) A normal finding is clear speech. An abnormal finding is slurred speech or the inability to accurately repeat a phrase.

First Responder care for a suspected stroke patient is the same as for any patient with altered mental status. However, once a stroke is suspected, you should try to determine from the patient or from bystanders the exact time signs or symptoms appeared. This is crucial information on which patient care will depend. Be especially alert to the airway of a patient who has difficulty speaking or slurred speech. Never give a suspected stroke patient anything to eat or drink. Be prepared to assist ventilations.

Note that the loss of a mental or motor function is a frightening reality for stroke patients. Try to remain calm and never express surprise about abnormal physical findings. Instead, maintain a professional attitude. Reassure the patient. Do not make any statements about long-term disability. Continue to talk to the patient even if he or she cannot speak. These patients often can hear very well. Explain to them what you are doing. Do not talk down to them or treat them like children.

Seizures

There are many causes of seizures. Sometimes the cause is unknown. All of the conditions described in this chapter can lead to seizures. Common causes include chronic medical conditions, epilepsy, hypoglycemia, poisoning (including alcohol and drug poisoning), stroke, fever (most common in children), infection, head injury or brain tumors, hypoxia (decreased levels of oxygen in the blood), and complications of pregnancy.

SKILL SUMMARY *Cincinnati Prehospital Stroke Scale*

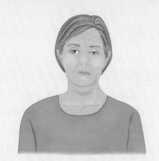

FIGURE 15-7A *Assess for facial droop.*

FACIAL DROOP

Normal   Both sides of the face move equally.

Abnormal   One side of the face does not move equally with the opposite side or it doesn't move at all.

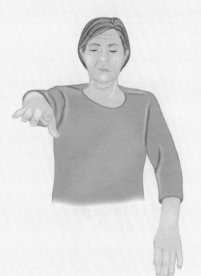

FIGURE 15-7B *Assess for arm drift.*

ARM DRIFT

Normal   Both arms move equally or can be held steady.

Abnormal   One arm drifts compared to the other.

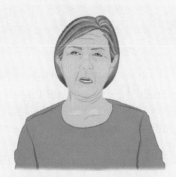

FIGURE 15-7C *Assess for speech difficulties.*

SPEECH

Normal   Patient uses correct words with no slurring.

Abnormal   Words are slurred, inappropriate, or the patient is unable to speak.

A **seizure** is the result of a nervous system malfunction. It may last five minutes or it may be prolonged. Its symptoms can range from a twitch of a limb to whole body muscle contractions. Most patients become unresponsive. Typically, patients are tired and sleep afterwards. Seizures are rarely life-threatening, but they do indicate a very serious condition.

You will probably be called most often to a *grand mal,* or generalized seizure. There are four phases to this type of seizure:

- *Aura phase*—the patient becomes aware that a seizure is coming on. The aura is often described as an unusual smell or a flash of light. It usually lasts a split second.

First Responder Practice

During your scene size-up, ask yourself if the seizure patient might have been injured when he or she fell to the ground. Pay careful attention to the potential for spine or head injury. If you suspect either one, take the appropriate precautions immediately.

■ *Tonic phase*—the patient becomes unresponsive and collapses to the ground. Then, all of the muscles of the body contract. This can force a scream out of the patient. It also can force out sputum, which can look like foam. During this phase, the patient may stop breathing briefly.

■ *Clonic phase*—the patient's muscles alternate between contraction and relaxation. The patient may become **incontinent** of urine (unable to retain it). Because the patient may bite the tongue and cheek, there may be blood in the mouth.

■ *Postictal phase*—the patient gradually regains responsiveness. At first, the patient is confused and even combative. Gradually, the patient becomes aware of his or her surroundings.

If the patient is still seizing when you arrive on scene, just wait. Stay calm. Seizures are usually over in a few minutes. While waiting, prevent any further injury by moving objects away from the patient (Figure 15-8a). If they cannot be moved, put something between them and the patient or drag the patient a few feet away from the danger. If possible, place padding, such as a coat or blanket, under the patient's head. Remove the patient's eyeglasses. Do not force anything into the patient's mouth. Do not try to restrain the patient.

When the seizure has stopped, assess and monitor the patient's airway and breathing closely. If there is no reason to suspect head or spine injury, place him in the recovery position (Figure 15-8b). If you are allowed, administer high-flow oxygen. If you suspect he was injured during a fall, use a jaw-thrust to open the airway. As the patient recovers, offer comfort and reassurance. Remember that he will have muscle soreness as well as fatigue.

While you wait for the EMTs to arrive on scene, consider the patient's feelings. Often, he is embarrassed. Consider asking onlookers to move away to provide the

patient with some privacy. If there was incontinence, place a sheet or towel over the patient's body.

When you give your hand-off report to the EMTs, be sure to include a description of the seizure. It may be important in determining its cause.

Note: A continuous seizure, or two or more seizures without a period of responsiveness, is called *status epilepticus.* This is a true medical emergency, which can be fatal. Complications include aspiration, hypoxia, hyperthermia (fever), and heart problems. If you suspect this type of seizure, advise responding EMS units immediately. Transportation must not be delayed. While waiting, position the patient on his or her side and suction if possible. If breathing is inadequate, assist ventilations with a bag-valve mask attached to 100% oxygen.

Q: 1. What is First Responder care for a patient with a chief complaint of altered mental status?

2. What is First Responder care for a patient with diabetes whose chief complaint is an altered mental status?

3. What specific signs would lead you to suspect stroke in a patient with an altered mental status?

4. How can you help prevent a patient from injuring himself during a seizure?

Section 3 Abdominal Pain and Distress

The abdominal cavity contains many different organs and blood vessels. Therefore, complaints of pain or discomfort could actually be caused by a number of problems or conditions. Do not try to determine the cause of abdominal pain. Instead, follow your patient assessment plan and be sure to gather a thorough patient history.

Abdominal emergencies require aggressive care to prevent shock and to save lives. So all abdominal pain should be taken seriously.

Patient Assessment

Any abdominal pain that is persistent or is significant enough for the patient or family to call for assistance should be considered an emergency. A patient with

SKILL SUMMARY *Caring for a Seizure Patient*

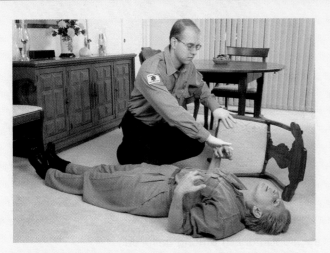

FIGURE 15-8A *Move objects away from the seizure patient to help prevent injury.*

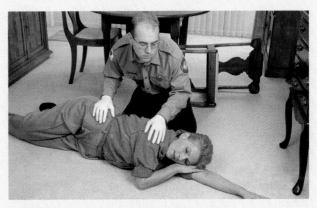

FIGURE 15-8B *When the seizure stops, position the patient to allow drainage of saliva and vomit.*

abdominal distress or pain will appear very ill. Signs and symptoms include:

- Abdominal pain, local or diffuse.
- **Colicky pain** (cramps that occur in waves).
- Abdominal tenderness, local or diffuse.
- Anxiety, reluctance to move.
- Loss of appetite, nausea, vomiting.
- Fever.
- Rigid, tense, or distended abdomen.
- Signs of shock.
- Vomiting blood, bright red or like coffee grounds.
- Blood in the stool, bright red or tarry black. ■

A patient with acute abdominal distress often "guards" his abdomen with knees drawn up (Figure 15-9). This position reduces tension on the muscles of the abdomen, which in turn helps reduce pain. In assessing a patient with acute abdominal distress, the initial assessment is the first priority. Even after ensuring the patient's ABCs, stay alert for signs of shock, which include a rapid and thready pulse, restlessness, cold clammy skin, and falling blood pressure. Shock is common with internal bleeding or with prolonged vomiting and diarrhea.

As with all medical patients, gather a good patient history. It may identify clues to the patient's condition,

such as prior similar problems and factors that may have caused the pain.

During the physical exam, determine whether the patient is restless or quiet. Find out if movement causes pain. Check to see if the abdomen is distended, and ask the patient to confirm your observation. Note if the patient can relax the abdominal wall when asked to do so. Palpate the abdomen gently to determine if it is rigid or soft. If you know one area is causing pain, examine that area last.

Do not spend too much time on assessment before making sure the EMS system has been activated. Too

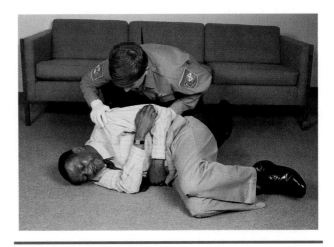

FIGURE 15-9 A patient "guarding" a painful abdomen.

much palpation can worsen the pain. It also can aggravate the medical condition that caused it.

First Responder Care

To provide care to a patient with acute abdominal distress, your goals are to prevent any possible life-threatening complications, to make the patient comfortable, and to arrange transport as quickly as possible.

In addition, maintain an open airway. Be alert for vomiting and possible aspiration. If the patient is nauseated, position the patient on his or her left side if this does not cause too much pain. Administer oxygen by way of a nonrebreather mask at 10 to 15 liters per minute. Be alert for shock.

If vital signs and other observations point to shock, position the patient on his or her back with legs elevated. If there are no signs of shock, allow the patient to get into a position of comfort. Protect the patient from any rough handling. Never give anything by mouth. Do not allow the patient to take any medications. They could mask symptoms and complicate the physician's diagnosis and treatment. ■

1. What does a patient who "guards" his abdomen look like? Describe the position.

2. What is First Responder care for a patient with a chief complaint of abdominal pain and distress?

Section 4 Poisoning

Though poisonings can occur in a variety of settings, many poisoning emergencies occur in the relative safety of the home (Figure 15-10). There are four routes of exposure, or ways that a poison can enter the body. They are **ingestion, inhalation, absorption,** and **injection:**

■ *Ingestion*—a poison can be introduced into the digestive tract by way of the mouth. Every year in the U.S. there are over eight million reported ingested poisons. Drugs such as aspirin and alcohol are among the top offenders.

■ *Inhalation*—a poison in gaseous or aerosol form is breathed into the body. A common source of poisonous gas is fire. The product of incomplete combustion, carbon monoxide is the most common type of poison gas. Poison gases from fire also may contain cyanide, a by-product of burning certain plastics. But fire is not the only source of poison gases. Large amounts of carbon

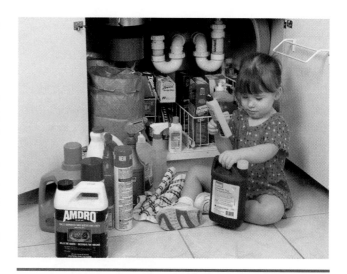

FIGURE 15-10 Poisoning is a leading cause of accidental death among children.

dioxide can come from sewage treatment plants or industrial sites. Even the chlorine gas in swimming pools can be deadly.

■ *Absorption*—a poison enters the body by way of contact with the skin. Examples of natural sources include poison ivy, sumac, and oak (Figure 15-11). Other sources of absorbed poisons are corrosives, insecticides, herbicides, and cleaning products.

■ *Injection*—a poison can enter the body by way of an object that pierces the skin. Hypodermic needles, as well as the bites and stings of insects and other creatures, can inject poisons into the body.

Note that not all poisonings are intentional or involve illegal or dangerous substances. Some of the poisonings you may be called to could involve a senior citizen's accidental overdose of his or her own prescribed medications.

Patient Assessment

The first rule of EMS is safety. Do not enter a scene where you suspect a poisonous gas or any poison to which you could come in contact. As soon as you suspect a poisoning emergency, make sure that EMS has been activated. Keep scene safety your top priority. A poison can affect you, just as easily as it affected your patient.

When it is safe to approach your patient, take special care to protect yourself. Remember that an ingested poison on the lips of your patient or an absorbed poison on your patient's skin could affect you, too. Be sure to put on all appropriate personal protective equipment. Perform a complete patient assessment including vital signs, when it is safe to do so.

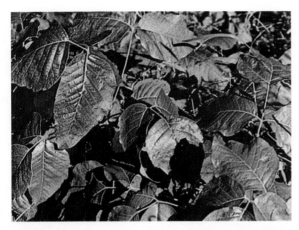

a. *Poison ivy.*

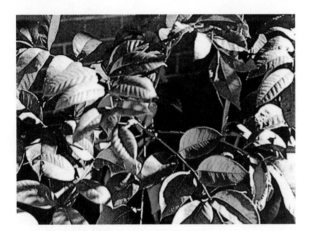

b. *Poison sumac.*

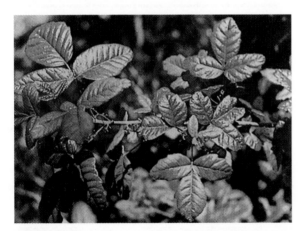

c. *Poison oak.*

FIGURE 15-11 Some natural sources of absorbed poisons.

An altered mental status is one of the most common signs of poisoning. Other signs and symptoms depend on the source of the poison. (See specific signs and symptoms of for each type of poison discussed later in this chapter.)

Whenever you suspect a poisoning, try to answer these questions:

- What substance is involved?
- How much is involved?
- When did the poisoning occur?
- What has the patient or others done to relieve symptoms? ■

First Responder Care

To provide care to a patient with a poisoning emergency, proceed just as you would for any patient with an altered mental status, no matter what the source of a poisoning. Focus your efforts on maintaining the patient's ABCs. Your local protocols may also require you to contact medical direction or your area's poison control center for specific instructions. ■

Specific Types of Poisonings

Ingested Poisons

During scene size-up and after, try to identify the ingested poison. Be alert for clues such as an overturned or empty pill box, scattered pills, chemical containers, household cleaners, empty alcohol bottles, or overturned plants.

As you perform your initial assessment, keep in mind that patients who are poisoned often vomit. So be alert to airway obstruction and breathing difficulty. They can lead to hypoxia and death.

In addition to altered mental status, signs and symptoms of an ingested poisoning may include a history of ingested poisons and:

- Burns around the mouth.
- Odd breath odors.
- Nausea, vomiting.
- Abdominal pain.
- Diarrhea.

The signs and symptoms of an ingested poison follow the path of ingestion. Start at the mouth. Look for chemical burns. Notice any chemical odor on the breath (Figure 15-12). Then, see if there has been any nausea, vomiting, abdominal cramps, or diarrhea.

Often poisons will affect the central nervous system. You may see dilated or constricted pupils, or you may hear the patient complain of double vision. There may be excessive saliva or foaming at the mouth. There may be excessive tearing or sweating. Finally, the patient may become unresponsive or have seizures.

To help limit the damage a poison can cause, make sure the EMS system is activated. Your local protocols

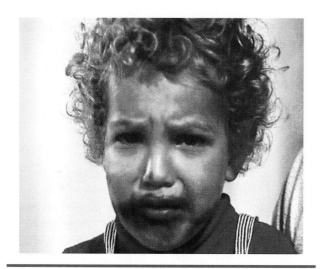

FIGURE 15-12 Burns or stains around the mouth may indicate poisoning.

may also direct you to contact medical direction or a poison control center for instructions. They may include giving the patient either activated charcoal or syrup of ipecac.

Activated charcoal (Figure 15-13) is a finely ground charcoal that is very *adsorbent*. (Activated charcoal binds with the poisons in the stomach and then passes through the body harmlessly.) It may be effective in reducing poisons for up to four hours after ingestion. *Use it only by order of poison control or according to your local protocols.* Most activated charcoal is premixed with water. If it is dry, mix two tablespoons of it in a glass of water to make a slurry. Be careful. It stains most clothing easily.

If the patient swallows an acid, corrosive, or petroleum product, you may have to dilute the poison. You may be instructed to use either several glasses of water or milk. Since emergency care for different poisons varies widely, contact medical direction or poison control before attempting to dilute the poison and before administering any medication. Whatever the situation, always follow local protocols.

Inhaled Poisons

Don't forget that many poison gases are colorless, odorless, and tasteless. You may not know you are in danger until it is too late. Look out for hazardous materials. Pay constant attention to the nature of the incident and the dangers it might contain. Protect yourself and keep others away from the scene.

It is imperative for you to give special attention to this patient's airway. Once in a safe location, open the airway. Then inspect the mouth and nose. Be careful to note the presence of soot, burns, or singed hair. Other signs and symptoms include a history of inhaling poisons and:

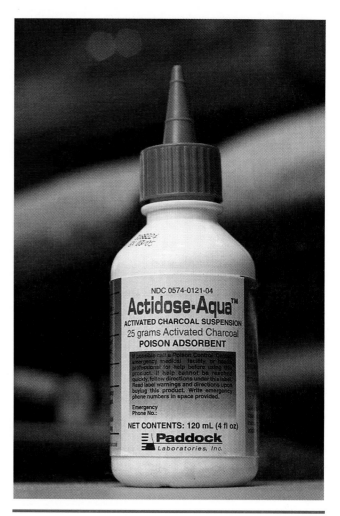

FIGURE 15-13 Activated charcoal.

- Breathing difficulty.
- Chest pain.
- Cough, hoarseness, burning sensation in the throat.
- Cyanosis (bluish discoloration of skin and mucous membranes).
- Dizziness, headache.
- Seizures, unresponsiveness (late findings).

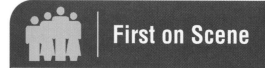

First on Scene

At the scene of an inhalation poisoning, safety should be your foremost concern. If an inhaled substance was able to hurt your patient, it can hurt you, your partner, and other rescue personnel. If necessary, call for the fire department and hazmat teams to make the scene safe. Never enter an unsafe scene.

Carbon monoxide is a poison gas that is especially lethal. Kerosene heaters, hot water heaters, and car exhaust fumes are some of the most common sources. Be particularly alert to carbon monoxide poisoning if several members of a household have the same signs and symptoms. Also suspect it if they say they are only sick when they are in a certain location. Be alert if the family pet seems sick as well. Signs and symptoms of carbon monoxide poisoning include:

- Throbbing headache and agitation.
- Nausea, vomiting.
- Confusion, poor judgment.
- Diminished vision, blindness.
- Breathing difficulty with rapid pulse.
- Dizziness, fainting, unresponsiveness.
- Seizures.
- Paleness.
- Cherry-red color to skin (very late sign).

The first rule of EMS is safety. You must protect yourself. Do not enter a scene where a poisonous gas is suspected. Call dispatch for specialized rescue teams who will have the appropriate safety equipment, including a self-contained breathing apparatus.

When it is safe to do so, quickly remove the patient from the source of the poison. Administer oxygen at 10–15 liters per minute via nonrebreather. Then proceed as you would for any patient with altered mental status. Verify that an ambulance is en route. Consider helicopter evacuation, if it would be quicker.

Note that all patients who are exposed to carbon monoxide need medical care, even those who seem to recover.

Absorbed Poisons

In general, signs and symptoms include a history of exposure and:

- Liquid or powder on the skin.
- Burns.
- Itching, irritation.
- Redness, rash, blisters (Figure 15-14).

Once a poison is identified, advise the incoming EMS units. If hazardous materials are suspected, follow local protocols. Note that an oil-based poison can spread easily from person to person. Protect yourself. Gloves are essential. Also consider wearing a gown, mask, and eye protection.

General guidelines for emergency care of a patient with an absorbed poison are as follows: Remove the clothing

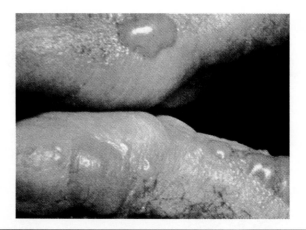

FIGURE 15-14 Blisters from poisonous plant contact.

that came in contact with the poison. Then, with a dry cloth, blot the poison from the skin. If the poison is a dry powder, brush it off. After as much as possible has been removed, flood the area with copious amounts of water. A shower or garden hose are ideal for this purpose. Continue until other EMS units arrive. Follow instructions from poison control and medical direction.

Continually monitor the patient's vital signs. Be alert for sudden changes. Seizures and shock are not uncommon.

The eyes are especially vulnerable to absorbed poisons. If ordered, flood the eyes with copious amounts of water. If only one eye is affected, be sure to avoid running contaminated water into the other eye. Advise incoming EMS units of the patient's condition. Follow local protocol.

Injected Poisons

An injected poison may be an illegal drug that enters the body by way of a hypodermic needle. (For more information on overdose emergencies, please see Chapter 17.) Injected poisons may also be the result of bites and stings from insects, spiders, snakes, and marine animals. The venom of these creatures can cause serious allergic reactions, even death. (For more information on this type of emergency, see Chapters 16 and 18.)

1. What precautions should you take to protect yourself when responding to a suspected poisoning emergency?

2. How is First Responder care for a patient with an ingested poisoning different from care for an inhaled or absorbed poisoning? Explain your answer.

The Call Follow-up

At the beginning of this chapter, you read that First Responders found a hiker lying in a lean-to beside a hiker trail. His level of responsiveness seemed to be verbal only. To see how chapter skills apply, read the following. It describes how the call was completed.

Patient History As near as we could tell from the scene, the patient was probably eating breakfast when this all started. In response to slow and careful questioning, he began to communicate. He indicated that he had no allergies and he was taking medication. We found high blood-pressure meds in his pack. The labels told us the patient's name was William Johnson. He denied any other medical conditions. The patient also tried to describe the event and indicated that his head hurt. Then he passed out. When he woke, he found he could not move the right side of his body.

Physical Examination We quickly performed a head-to-toe exam of the patient and a Cincinnati Stroke Scale exam. He had definite weakness on the right side of his body. He had no deformities, no open injuries, no signs of tenderness or swelling. We found that his pulse was 64 strong and regular and his respirations were 18 and adequate. His pupils reacted equally and his skin was cool and dry. We didn't have a BP cuff in our light packs.

Ongoing Assessment Our impression was that the patient may have had a stroke. Aware that he could get worse, we continued to perform the initial assessment as well as vital signs. Our patient appeared to be somewhat anxious. Who wouldn't be? So we tried to comfort and reassure him. We told him more help was on the way and that he would be in the hospital soon.

Patient Hand-off When the Medflight team arrived, we gave them a hand-off report, including the physical findings and the history we were able to gather (see below). The flight team took it from there. I have to say that this guy was lucky. If he had been left alone much longer, he might have died from exposure.

Hand-off Report

"This is William Johnson. He's 67. Others on the trail saw him and called us. We arrived to find him with difficulty speaking and weakness on his right side. His face is drooping a bit, too. He complained of a headache and reports losing consciousness prior to our arrival. He has high blood pressure meds in his pack. Denies any other history. We don't have a BP cuff, but his pulse is 64, strong, and regular, respirations are 18 and adequate, skin cool and dry, pupils equal and react to light. We'll give you a hand getting him on a stretcher."

The Last Word *Whether or not you know the cause of a medical emergency in your patient, your job is the same. Assess, care for, and monitor the airway until the EMTs arrive to take over.*

Be prepared to provide basic life support if needed. And try to get as complete a patient history as possible from the patient, the family, or bystanders.

Chapter Review

Focus on the EMS Team

This chapter covered a wide range of medical problems—from general complaints to specific types of poisoning. Remember that it is never necessary for you to diagnose a patient's medical problem. It is not practical to do so in the field. Even in the hospital, with all the tests and procedures available to physicians, diagnosis can be difficult.

However, there are many things you can do for your medical patients. You know you must treat any life-threatening problems in the initial assessment. A history is extremely important to a medical patient, too. It will provide the clues to the patient's condition, which will help you, the EMTs, and hospital personnel determine proper care.

Summing Up

- Assessment for a general medical complaint, such as "I don't feel well," is the same as for any other patient. Follow your patient assessment plan and be especially thorough gathering a patient history. First Responder care consists of monitoring the patient's ABCs, allowing the patient to get into a position of comfort, and reporting any changes in the patient's condition when the EMTs take over care.

- Altered mental status may be caused by a number of medical conditions, including diabetes, stroke, and seizure. Whatever the cause, guidelines for First Responder assessment and care generally remain the same: Closely monitor the patient's airway and breathing, keeping the airway open and clear with an adjunct and suctioning as necessary. If there is no reason to suspect head or spine injury, place the patient in the recovery position. Administer oxygen. Do your best to gather a thorough patient history.

- In the case of a patient with a chief complaint of abdominal pain and distress, make the initial assessment your first priority. Arrange transport as quickly as possible. Stay alert for signs of shock, administer oxygen, and gather a good patient history.

- For a patient with a possible poisoning, First Responder care is the same as for any patient with an altered mental status. However, you must pay special attention to personal and scene safety. And you must try to determine what poisonous substance and how much of it was involved, when the poisoning may have occurred, and what anyone has been done to try to relieve symptoms. Note that local protocols may require you to contact medical direction or your area's poison control center for specific instructions.

Key Terms

absorption a route of exposure whereby a poison enters the body upon contact with the skin.

activated charcoal a finely ground charcoal that is very adsorbent (binds with harmful substances) and may be used as an antidote to some ingested poisons.

altered mental status a change in a patient's normal level of responsiveness.

cerebrovascular accident (CVA) See *stroke*.

colicky pain cramps that occur in waves.

glucose a simple sugar.

hyperglycemia increased blood sugar.

hypoglycemia low blood sugar.

incontinent unable to retain; loss of control, especially of urine or feces.

ingestion a route of exposure whereby a poison is introduced into the body by way of the mouth.

inhalation a route of exposure whereby a poison is introduced into the body by way of the respiratory system.

injection a route of exposure whereby a poison enters the body by way of an object that pierces the skin.

insulin a hormone secreted by the pancreas to metabolize sugar; a medication used by people with diabetes to perform the same function as the hormone.

seizure a convulsion caused by a sudden discharge of electrical activity in the brain.

stroke a sudden loss of neurological function caused by an interruption of blood flow to a portion of the brain. *Also called* cerebrovascular accident (CVA) *or* brain attack.

transient ischemic attack (TIA) a kind of stroke that resolves within 24 hours, but may be a warning sign of an impending larger stroke. *Also called* mini-stroke.

Knowledge Check

1. The term "hypoglycemia" refers to:
- a. high blood pressure.
- b. low blood sugar.
- c. seizures.
- d. stroke.

2. Patients with altered mental status who have a history of diabetes should receive oral glucose or sugar solution if they are:
- a. awake and NOT able to control their own airway.
- b. awake and able to control their own airway.
- c. unresponsive and NOT able to swallow.
- d. unresponsive but able to swallow.

3. First Responder care for the seizing patient includes all of the following EXCEPT:
- a. placing padding under the patient's head.
- b. moving dangerous items away from the patient.
- c. monitoring the patient's airway and breathing.
- d. placing something in the mouth to prevent injury.

4. First Responder care for a patient who has absorbed a poisonous chemical powder through his skin includes:
- a. brushing off the poison and flushing the skin with water.
- b. administering activated charcoal to absorb the poison.
- c. leaving the patient's clothes on to absorb the poison.
- d. neutralizing the chemical with an alkaline agent.

5. Which one of the following statements about stroke is FALSE?
- a. Stroke patients may have weakness on one side of the body.
- b. Prompt identification and treatment of stroke is critical.
- c. Patients rarely delay seeking medical care for stroke.
- d. Stroke is sometimes referred to as a "brain attack."

6. Your patient is an 18-year-old who has had a sudden onset of altered mental status. Her airway is patent and her breathing is adequate. She has a rapid pulse; cool, clammy skin; and a headache. There is no reason to suspect a head or spine injury. She has no history of medical problems. You should:
- a. treat her for low blood sugar and administer glucose.
- b. monitor her ABCs closely and administer oxygen.
- c. manually stabilize her head and neck.
- d. administer activated charcoal.

7. All of the following are common causes of seizures EXCEPT:

   a. stroke.
   b. allergic reaction.
   c. alcohol poisoning.
   d. complications of pregnancy.

8. Your patient has been found unconscious, with no suspected trauma. His wife tells you that he has diabetes. What should you do first?

   a. Assist in administering oral glucose.
   b. Ensure an open airway and adequate breathing.
   c. Get permission to administer an antidote.
   d. Question bystanders about a possible overdose.

9. Your adult patient tells you that he has ingested an unknown number of pills he bought illegally. You should ask all of the following questions EXCEPT:

   a. What kind of pills and how many did you take?
   b. Has anyone tried to treat you with anything?
   c. Who sold the pills to you? What is his name?
   d. What time was it when you took the pills?

10. A patient with a diabetic emergency might appear to be intoxicated.

    a. True
    b. False

11. Another term for a minor seizure is status epilepticus.

    a. True
    b. False

12. Insulin is the primary fuel for the body's cells.

    a. True
    b. False

13. Hyperglycemia is the condition in which there is too little insulin and too much blood sugar.

    a. True
    b. False

14. You are caring for a conscious diabetic patient with an altered mental status. She has a gag reflex and is able to swallow. You do not have oral glucose paste but wish to give her sugar. How else could you provide sugar?

    _____

    _____

15. List the three components of the Cincinnati Prehospital Stroke Scale.

    _____

    _____

    _____

16. Your patient's general medical complaint is "I feel so bad!" Outline your plan for First Responder assessment and care of this patient.

    _____

    _____

    _____

    _____

Scenario

You are called to an unconscious patient. When you arrive on scene, you find a male patient, about 45 years old, who is lying on the ground. He does not respond to your voice but moans when you pinch the webbing between his thumb and index finger. His wife says she found him that way a short time ago. She also tells you that he is a diabetic and has been since childhood. He takes insulin but lately has been having trouble keeping his blood sugar at normal levels.

a. What initial assessment steps would you take for this patient?

b. Would you consider giving glucose to the patient? Explain your answer.

c. In your update to the incoming ambulance, would you describe this patient as unstable (in serious condition)? Explain your answer.

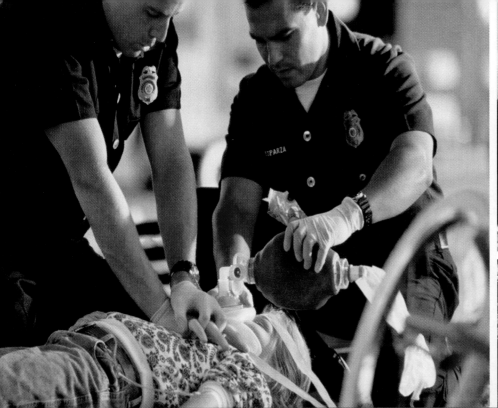
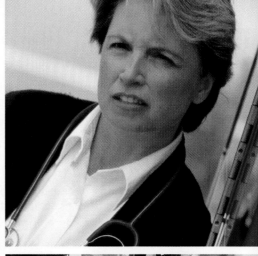
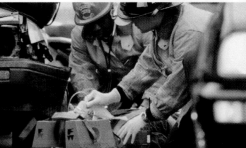

16 | Environmental Emergencies

OBJECTIVES

From the U.S. Department of Transportation (DOT) 1995 "First Responder: National Standard Curriculum." Material that is supplemental to the DOT curriculum is listed under "Enrichment."

Cognitive

5-1.7 ▶ Identify the patient who presents with a specific medical complaint of exposure to cold. (pp. 289–293)

5-1.8 ▶ Explain the steps in providing emergency medical care to a patient with an exposure to cold. (pp. 289–293)

5-1.9 ▶ Identify the patient who presents with a specific medical complaint of exposure to heat. (pp. 294–296)

5-1.10 ▶ Explain the steps in providing emergency medical care to a patient with an exposure to heat. (pp. 294–296)

Affective

5-1.16 ▶ Attend to the feelings of the patient and/or family when dealing with the patient with a specific medical complaint. (pp. 291, 293, 298)

5-1.21 ▶ Demonstrate a caring attitude towards patients with a specific medical complaint who request emergency medical services. (pp. 291, 293, 298)

5-1.22 ▶ Place the interests of the patient with a specific medical compliant as the foremost consideration when making any and all patient care decisions. (pp. 290–291, 293, 296, 298)

5-1.23 ▶ Communicate with empathy to patients with a specific medical complaint, as well as with family members and friends of the patient. (pp. 291, 293, 298)

Psychomotor

5-1.30 ▶ Demonstrate the steps in providing emergency medical care to a patient with an exposure to cold. (pp. 289–293)

5-1.31 ▶ Demonstrate the steps in providing emergency medical care to a patient with an exposure to heat. (pp. 294–296)

Enrichment

▶ Describe the various ways that the body creates and loses heat. (pp. 288–289)

- Describe how to rewarm a patient with hypothermia and a patient with a local cold injury. (p. 293)
- Describe how to cool a patient with hyperthermia. (p. 296)
- Recognize the signs and symptoms of bites or stings, including allergic reactions to them. (pp. 297–306)
- Describe the guidelines for emergency care of patients with bites or stings, including those who have allergic reactions. (pp. 297–306)

- Identify the signs and symptoms of poisonous snakebites. (pp. 298–301)
- Identify the signs and symptoms of poisoning by common marine life. (pp. 303–306)
- Describe the proper method of applying a constricting band to an extremity. (p. 300)
- Describe how to remove a stinger embedded in a patient's skin. (pp. 298, 303, 304)

Introduction

Environmental emergencies can occur in any setting—wilderness, rural, suburban, and urban areas. They include exposure to heat and cold, as well as bites and stings from insects, spiders, snakes, and marine life. Just as important as First Responder care in these emergencies is recognizing that the cause of the emergency may put you at risk. Always be certain to ensure your own safety and the safety of your crew.

Section 1 Cold Emergencies

Body Temperature

Heat and cold can produce a number of emergencies. To respond to them appropriately, you need a basic understanding of how people adjust to heat and cold.

The body produces and conserves heat mainly through the process of **metabolism** (all the physical and chemical changes that occur in the body, including digestion). In cold, the body holds onto its heat by constricting blood vessels near its surface. Hair also erects, thickening the layer of warm air trapped near the skin. The body can produce more heat, if needed,

THE CALL

Dispatch It was 9 a.m. and we were on our way to 153 Western Avenue for a "woman down." Rescue 3 was dispatched to assist with an ETA of 15 minutes.

Scene Size-up The person who called EMS was there to greet us. "Mrs. Downe and I have tea every morning at 7 a.m.," she told us. "She's not answering the door. I just know something is wrong." We approached the neat little cottage. I knocked and then yelled through the door, "EMS. Can we help you?" We heard a faint voice from the back of the house.

We entered through the back door and immediately saw the patient. She appeared to be about 80. She was lying supine on the kitchen floor, calling out weakly. The contents of a garbage bag were spilled on the floor beside her. We could see dried blood in her hair and under her head.

This patient is injured. But might she have problems other than an injured head? What else might the First Responders have to think about as they proceed with her assessment and care? Consider this patient as you read Chapter 16.

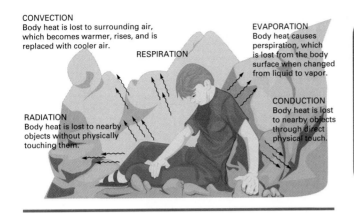

CONVECTION
Body heat is lost to surrounding air, which becomes warmer, rises, and is replaced with cooler air.

RESPIRATION

EVAPORATION
Body heat causes perspiration, which is lost from the body surface when changed from liquid to vapor.

RADIATION
Body heat is lost to nearby objects without physically touching them.

CONDUCTION
Body heat is lost to nearby objects through direct physical touch.

FIGURE 16-1 Mechanisms of heat loss.

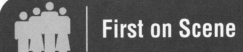

First on Scene

When you perform scene size-up and patient assessment, remember that the very young and old are especially susceptible to hypothermia. These patients may require a higher ambient temperature than you do. So even if the air is comfortable for you, consider the possibility of hypothermia.

by shivering and by producing certain hormones such as epinephrine.

In general, the body loses heat in five ways (Figure 16-1):

- *Convection.* This occurs when moving air passes over the body and carries heat away. (See "wind chill index," Figure 16-2.)

- *Conduction.* This occurs when direct contact with an object carries heat away. For example, a swimmer is in direct contact with water. If it is cooler than the body, the water will take away the swimmer's body heat. It can do so 25 times faster than air.

- *Radiation.* This method involves the transfer of heat to an object without physical contact. Most heat loss is from the head and neck, areas rich in blood and blood vessels.

- *Evaporation.* The process by which sweat changes to vapor has a cooling effect on the body. Note that

evaporation stops when the relative humidity of the air reaches 75%.

- *Respiration.* This occurs when a person breathes in cold air and breathes out air that was warmed inside the body.

Exposure to cold can cause two kinds of emergencies. One is a generalized cold emergency, or generalized **hypothermia.** It involves an overall reduction of body temperature, which can be deadly. The other kind of emergency is called a **local cold injury,** or damage to body tissues in a specific (local) part of the body.

Generalized Hypothermia

Exposure to extreme cold for a short time or moderate cold for a long time can cause hypothermia. There are several risk factors you should know about. The first is the medical condition of the patient. Any underlying problem—such as shock, head or spine injury, burns, infection, diabetes, and hypoglycemia—can weaken the body's responses to heat and cold.

WIND SPEED (MPH)	WHAT THE THERMOMETER READS (degrees °F.)											
	50	40	30	20	10	0	−10	−20	−30	−40	−50	−60
	WHAT IT EQUALS IN ITS EFFECT ON EXPOSED FLESH											
CALM	50	40	30	20	10	0	−10	−20	−30	−40	−50	−60
5	48	37	27	16	6	−5	−15	−26	−36	−47	−57	−68
10	40	28	16	4	−9	−21	−33	−46	−58	−70	−83	−95
15	36	22	9	−5	−18	−36	−45	−58	−72	−85	−99	−112
20	32	18	4	−10	−25	−39	−53	−67	−82	−96	−110	−121
25	30	16	0	−15	−29	−44	−59	−74	−88	−104	−118	−133
30	28	13	−2	−18	−33	−48	−63	−79	−94	−109	−125	−140
35	27	11	−4	−20	−35	−49	−67	−82	−98	−113	−129	−145
40	26	10	−6	−21	−37	−53	−69	−85	−100	−116	−132	−148
	Little danger if properly clothed			Danger of freezing exposed flesh			Great danger of freezing exposed flesh					

Source: U.S. Army

FIGURE 16-2 Wind-chill index.

STAGES OF HYPOTHERMIA

Stage 1: **Shivering** is a response by the body to generate heat. It does not occur below a body temperature of 90°F.

Stage 2: **Apathy and decreased muscle function.** First, fine motor function is affected, then gross motor functions.

Stage 3: **Decreased level of responsiveness** is accompanied by a glassy stare and possible freezing of the extremities.

Stage 4: **Decreased vital signs,** including slow pulse and slow respiration rate.

Stage 5: **Death**.

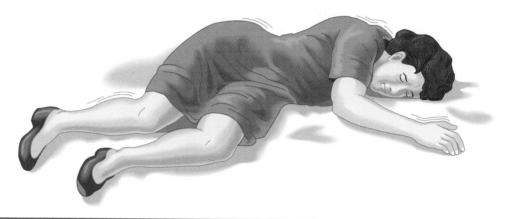

FIGURE 16-3 Hypothermia can be a progressive condition.

The second risk factor is use of drugs or alcohol and exposure to poisons. Any one of these can impede the body's ability to maintain body temperature. Many outdoor clubs and organizations discourage or even ban the use of alcohol. The momentary flush of warmth felt after a drink actually increases heat loss. That along with impaired judgment can quickly turn a walk in the woods into a deadly excursion.

Finally, the third risk factor is the age of the patient. Very young or very old patients are especially at risk. Infants are at risk because of their anatomy. The head is large in proportion to the body. The body surface is large compared to the mass. The result is that infants lose more heat more rapidly than do adults. Infants also have an immature nervous system, which means they cannot shiver well enough to warm themselves when needed.

Elderly people are at risk, too. If they are on a fixed income, for example, they may not be able to afford to heat their homes properly. Sudden illness or injury can limit their ability to escape the cold. Impaired judgment due to a medication or limited mobility due to a medical condition can also contribute to their risk for hypothermia.

Patient Assessment

During scene size-up, notice the location of the patient. Ask yourself these questions: Does the environment suggest the possibility of generalized hypothermia? How long has the patient been exposed to those conditions? If scene size-up suggests the possibility of a cold emergency, put your hand on the patient's abdomen during the physical exam. If the skin is cool or cold, treat for hypothermia. ■

Note that if left unchecked hypothermia is a progressive condition (Figures 16-3 and 16-4). At first the patient will shiver. When shivering stops, he may appear clumsy, confused, and forgetful. He may even appear intoxicated. Often witnesses will say that the patient had mood swings, one moment calm and the next animated or even combative.

Finally, the patient's level of responsiveness decreases. He becomes less communicative and is difficult to rouse. He may display poor judgment and do things like remove his clothing while still in the cold. There may be muscle stiffness, a rigid posture, and loss of sensation. The most ominous sign of a life-threatening condition is unresponsiveness. These patients are unstable and need immediate transport if they are to survive.

First Responder Care

To provide care to a patient with generalized hypothermia (Figure 16-5):

1. *Remove the patient from the cold environment.* Move him to a shelter, away from the cold wind or water. If

SIGNS AND SYMPTOMS OF HYPOTHERMIA

	Below 68°F (20°C)	68°F to 82°F (20°C to 28°C)	82°F to 86°F (28°C to 30°C)	86°F to 90°F (30°C to 32°C)	90°F to 95°F (32°C to 35°C)	95°F to 98°F (35°C to 37°C)

CORE TEMPERATURE

Fixed, dilated pupils.
Coma.
Flaccid muscles.
Slow respiration.
Slow or rapid heart rate.
Possible cardiac arrest.

Cold, pale skin.
Alert and shivering.
Poor muscle coor-
  dination.
Rapid breathing.
Rapid heart rate.

Cyanosis.
Fixed, dilated pupils.
Unresponsiveness.
Barely detectable
  vital signs.
Irregular pulse.
Cardiac arrest.

Dilated pupils.
Diminished reflexes.
Stupor or coma.
Rigid muscles.
Slow breathing rate.
Hypotension.
Slow heart rate.

Cold, waxy skin.
Puffy face, possibly pink.
Confusion.
Muscle rigidity, no shivering.
Slow heart rate.

FIGURE 16-4 **Signs and symptoms of hypothermia vary according to body temperature.**

the patient is on the ground, get him off the ground or put a blanket between him and the ground.

2. *Administer oxygen,* if you are allowed to do so. If possible, it should be warm and humidified.

3. *Remove all wet clothing,* and cover the patient with a blanket. A thin layer of dry clothing or even just a blanket is better than a thick layer of wet clothing.

4. *Handle the patient very gently.* Rough handling can make the patient's condition worse and even cause injuries. Do not massage the extremities. Do not allow the patient to walk or exert himself. Do not allow the patient to eat or drink stimulants.

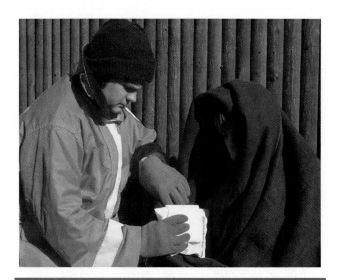

FIGURE 16-5 **A patient with generalized hypothermia needs to be rewarmed.**

5. *Comfort, calm, and reassure the patient.* Tell him that everything that can be done will be done. Communicate with empathy. ∎

Mild Hypothermia

The patient with mild hypothermia will present with cold skin and shivering. He will still be alert and oriented. Signs and symptoms may include:

- Increased breathing rate.
- Increased pulse rate and blood pressure.
- Slow, thick speech.
- Staggering walk.
- Apathy, drowsiness, incoherence.
- Sluggish pupils.
- Uncontrollable shivering.

If the patient is alert and able, allow him to drink warm fluids. A good test of the patient's ability to protect his own airway is to have him hold the cup. If he drops the cup or is unable to get it to his mouth, for example, do not allow him to drink. Never give a confused or lethargic patient anything to drink. The danger of aspiration is too great. Never give coffee, tea, or other caffeine drinks such as cola. Do not allow the patient to smoke. Stimulants promote heat loss.

Cover the patient with a warm blanket. Remember that heat loss is greatest from the head and neck. An old sailor's saying is "When your feet are cold, put on a hat." Cover the patient's head, and wrap a blanket around him.

First Responder Practice

In severe hypothermia there is no shivering, which could cause you to overlook this life-threatening condition. Do not be fooled by the lack of shivering. If you see a patient who has been in the cold and is unresponsive, be sure to suspect hypothermia.

If heat packs are available, consider using them. (Be sure to follow local protocol.) Apply the packs to the patient's neck, armpits, and groin. Remember that the patient may have a decreased sense of touch. So check the skin beneath the heat packs periodically to be sure they are not burning it.

Severe Hypothermia

Patients with severe hypothermia may become unresponsive. This is a true medical emergency that can lead to death. Signs and symptoms may include:

- Extremely slow breathing rate.
- Extremely slow pulse rate.
- Unresponsiveness.
- Fixed and dilated pupils.
- Rigid extremities.
- Absence of shivering.

Consider using a nasopharyngeal airway to secure the airway of an unresponsive patient. Administer high-concentration oxygen. If breathing is adequate, administer oxygen with a nonrebreather mask. If breathing is not adequate, assist ventilations with a BVM and supplemental oxygen.

When assessing circulation, you may find no pulses in the patient's limbs. Remember that the body is a "metabolic icebox" at this stage. It does not need normal circulation to sustain life, because everything is slowed down. A slow pulse is not deadly and may actually be protective.

Assess the carotid pulse for about one minute before starting CPR. If it is cold outside, remember that your sense of touch may be less than it should be. Consider putting your fingers in your armpits or your groin before taking a pulse. Handle the patient gently. Any rough handling can induce ventricular fibrillation or sudden cardiac death.

If the patient is breathless and pulseless, begin CPR. Even if he has all the signs of death—including fixed pupils and stiff extremities—begin CPR. The rule of thumb in EMS is: "You're not dead until you're warm and dead." That means you cannot consider resuscitation a failure until the heart has been given a chance to re-start at a near normal temperature.

Rewarming in the field is not recommended for patients with severe hypothermia. These patients need special attention in a hospital. Arrange for transport to the nearest medical facility as soon as possible. (Follow your local protocols.)

Local Cold Injuries

Cold emergencies also can result from the cooling of parts of the body, most commonly the face, nose, ears, hands, fingers, feet, and toes (Figure 16-6). This type of emergency is called a *local cold injury* or *frostbite*. When a

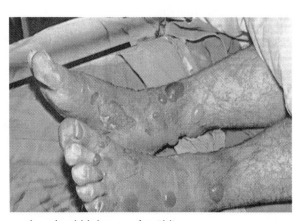

a. *Local cold injury, or frostbite.*

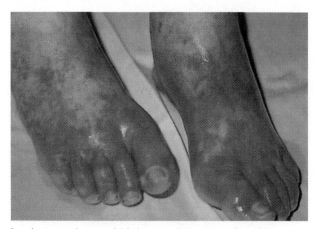

b. *Late or deep cold injury, or late-stage frostbite.*

FIGURE 16-6 The term "local cold injury" refers to the freezing or near freezing of a body part.

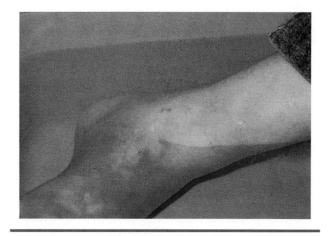

FIGURE 16-7 Active rewarming of a local cold injury.

body part is exposed to intense cold, blood flow to that part is limited by the constriction of blood vessels. When this happens, tissues freeze. Ice crystals can form in the skin, and in the most severe cases, **gangrene** (localized tissue death) can set in and ultimately lead to the loss of the body part.

Patient Assessment

A local cold injury, or frostbite, is usually easy to identify. With early or superficial frostbite, light skin will redden. Dark skin will turn pale. When the skin is depressed gently, it will blanch and then return to its normal color. The patient often will complain of loss of feeling and sensation in the injured area.

In the later stages of frostbite (called "late or deep cold injury"), the skin may appear waxy. It also may be firm to the touch. As freezing continues, it becomes **mottled** or blotchy. Finally, the area becomes swollen, blistered, and white.

When the injured parts begin to thaw, skin color changes. It may appear flushed with areas of purple and blanching, or it may be mottled and cyanotic. ■

First Responder Care

To provide care to a patient with a local cold injury:

1. *Remove the patient from the cold environment.* Do not allow him to walk on a frostbitten limb.

2. *Administer oxygen,* if you are allowed to do so.

3. *Remove all wet clothing.*

4. *Protect the frostbite area from further injury.* If the injury is to an extremity, manually stabilize it. If the injury is superficial, cover it with a blanket. If it is late and deep, cover it with a dry cloth or dressings. Do not rub or massage the area. Ice crystals under the skin could damage the fragile capillaries and tissues, making the injury worse.

5. *Comfort, calm, and reassure the patient.* Tell him everything that can be done will be done.

6. *Monitor the patient* for signs of hypothermia. ■

Rewarming

If transport will be delayed, consider rewarming the affected area. Never rewarm an area with late or deep frostbite. Never rewarm an area if there is a chance that it may refreeze. The injury from the second freezing would be much worse than the original one.

Warm the entire frostbite area in tepid water (about 100°F to 105°F). The water should feel comfortable to the normal hand. Be sure to pick a container that permits the entire area to be immersed (Figure 16-7). Continue to support the injured limb during rewarming. Do not allow the injured area to touch the bottom or side of the container. If the water starts to cool, remove the patient. Then, add more warm water. As the area rewarms, the patient may complain of tingling and shooting pains. In this case, some EMS systems allow First Responders to help an alert patient self-administer an **analgesic** such as Tylenol®. Follow local protocol.

When the injured area is rewarmed, the tissues will be fragile. To protect them, cover the injury with dry sterile gauze. If the injury is to the fingers or toes, place gauze between them, too. Consider padding the entire area with a large bulky dressing.

 :

1. Which will take away a person's body heat faster, air or water? How much faster?

2. How can you minimize the effects of hypothermia in your patient?

3. What is First Responder care for a local cold injury?

Section 2 Heat Emergencies

When a person cannot lose excessive heat, he or she develops **hyperthermia**. Left untreated, hyperthermia can lead to organ damage and death. The major heat-related medical conditions are commonly called **heat cramps**, **heat exhaustion**, and **heat stroke**. Heat stroke, the most serious, is life-threatening.

Heat cramps involve acute spasms of the muscles of the legs, arms, or abdomen (Figure 16-8). This may be the result of losing too much salt during profuse sweating. Heat cramps usually follow hard work in a hot environment. Hard work in a hot, humid environment also can affect blood flow. This can result in a mild state of shock, or heat exhaustion.

If the patient does not stop work, move to a cool environment, and replace lost fluid, his condition will get worse. The result can be heat stroke, which is very serious and life-threatening. It occurs when the body becomes overheated and, in many patients, sweating stops. If left untreated, brain cells begin to die, causing permanent disability or death. (See Figure 16-9.)

Contributing Factors

Several factors contribute to the risk of hyperthermia. One involves heat and humidity. High air temperature

First Responder Practice

With heat emergencies, the temperature of the patient's skin is one indicator of severity. A patient with cool skin and a normal mental status is less severely ill than a patient with hot skin. Be sure to get any patient experiencing a heat emergency out of the sun and to a place with cooler temperatures. Cool the patient, but prevent chilling or very sudden reduction of body temperature.

can reduce the body's ability to lose heat by radiation. High humidity can reduce its ability to lose heat by way of evaporation. (See "Heat and Humidity Risk Scale," Figure 16-10.) Exercise and strenuous activity also play a part. Each can cause a person to lose more than one liter of sweat (fluid and essential salts) per hour.

Other risk factors for a heat emergency include age, medical condition, and certain drugs and medication. That is, very young and very old patients may be unable to respond to overheating effectively. Any number of medical conditions, such as heart or lung disease, diabetes, **dehydration** (fluid loss), obesity, fever, and fatigue

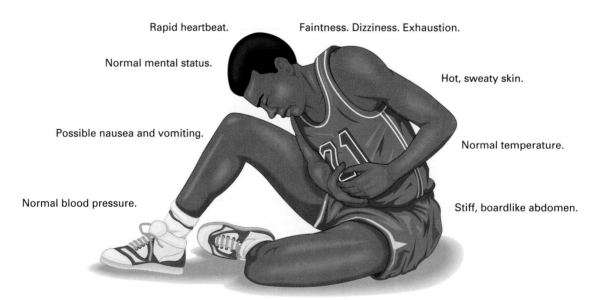

SIGNS AND SYMPTOMS OF HEAT CRAMPS

Rapid heartbeat.

Normal mental status.

Possible nausea and vomiting.

Normal blood pressure.

Faintness. Dizziness. Exhaustion.

Hot, sweaty skin.

Normal temperature.

Stiff, boardlike abdomen.

Severe muscular cramps and pain, especially of the arms, fingers, legs, calves, and abdomen.

FIGURE 16-8 Heat cramps are the most common but least serious heat emergency.

SIGNS AND SYMPTOMS OF HEAT STROKE

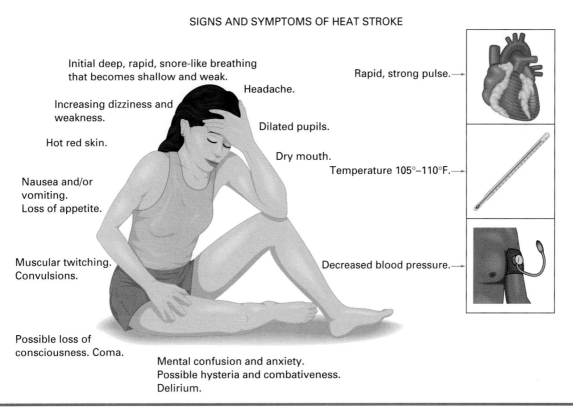

Initial deep, rapid, snore-like breathing that becomes shallow and weak.

Headache.

Increasing dizziness and weakness.

Hot red skin.

Dilated pupils.

Dry mouth.

Rapid, strong pulse. →

Temperature 105°–110°F. →

Nausea and/or vomiting.
Loss of appetite.

Muscular twitching.
Convulsions.

Decreased blood pressure. →

Possible loss of consciousness. Coma.

Mental confusion and anxiety.
Possible hysteria and combativeness.
Delirium.

FIGURE 16-9 Heat stroke is a life-threatening emergency.

can inhibit heat loss. And alcohol, cocaine, barbiturates, hallucinogens, and other drugs can affect heat loss in many ways, including through side effects such as dehydration (fluid loss).

Patient Assessment

When you suspect a heat emergency, feel the patient's abdomen to check the body temperature. Keep in mind that the chief characteristics of heat stroke are hot skin

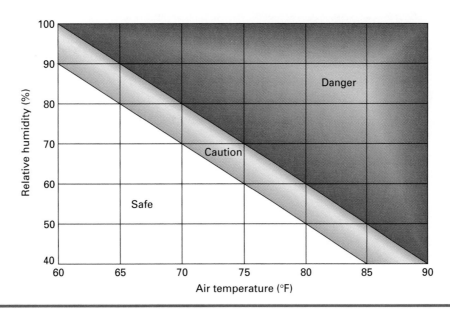

FIGURE 16-10 Heat and Humidity Risk Scale.

and a change in mental status. General signs and symptoms of a heat emergency include the following:

- Muscle cramps.
- Weakness, exhaustion.
- Dizziness, faintness.
- Rapid pulse rate that is strong at first, but becomes weak as damage progresses.
- Headache.
- Seizures.
- Loss of appetite, nausea, vomiting.
- Altered mental status, possibly unresponsiveness.
- Skin may be moist, pale, and normal-to-cool in temperature ("heat cramps" or "heat exhaustion"). Or it may be hot and dry or hot and moist ("heat stroke"). ■

First Responder Care

To provide care to a patient with a heat emergency:

1. *Remove the patient from the hot environment.* Place him in a cool one, if possible. If the source of heat is the sun, place the patient in the shade.

2. *Administer oxygen,* if you are allowed to do so. If breathing is adequate, administer oxygen with a nonrebreather mask. If breathing is not adequate, assist ventilations with a BVM and supplemental oxygen.

3. *Cool the patient* (Figure 16-11). First, loosen or remove his clothing. Then:
   —If the patient has moist, pale, and normal-to-cool skin, fan the surface of his body while applying a light mist of water. Be careful not to cool the patient so fast that he becomes chilled.
   —If the patient has hot and dry or hot and moist skin, apply cold packs to his neck, armpits, and groin. Keep the skin wet by applying water with wet towels or a sponge. Fan the patient aggressively, or direct an electric fan at him.

4. *Position the patient.* Place him in a supine position with legs elevated 8 to 12 inches, if there is no indication of spine or lower extremity trauma.

5. *Monitor the patient.* Take vital signs frequently. Advise the incoming units if the patient develops signs of shock.

If the patient is alert and not nauseated, encourage him to drink about one-half glass of cool water or sport drink every 15 minutes or so. (Follow local protocol or consult with medical direction.) ■

: 1. What are the signs and symptoms of a heat-related emergency?

2. What is First Responder care for a patient with a heat-related emergency?

SKILL SUMMARY   *Caring for a Heat Emergency Patient*

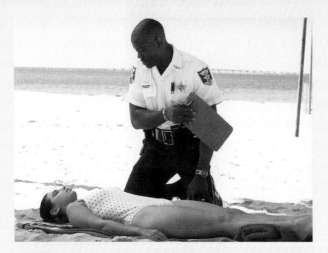

FIGURE 16–11A *For a patient with normal-to-cool skin temperature, cool by fanning.*

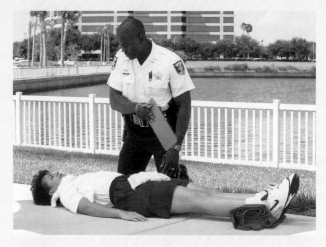

FIGURE 16–11B *For a patient with hot skin, cool by applying cold packs.*

Section 3 Bites and Stings

First Responder assessment and care of a patient with a bite or sting are described in the general guidelines below. NOTE: An allergic reaction to bites and stings can lead to **anaphylactic shock,** an emergency that generally has a rapid life-threatening affect on the airway and breathing. Respiratory distress and shock can develop rapidly. (Read more about shock in Chapter 18.)

You may wish to note that allergic reactions are especially common following the stings of wasps, hornets, yellow jackets, and fire ants. Bites or stings from deer flies, gnats, horse flies, mosquitoes, cockroaches, and miller moths also can cause an allergic reaction. Venom from snakes and spiders can, too.

Patient Assessment

As always, your priority during scene size-up is to protect yourself. If your patient has been bitten or stung, you could be bitten or stung, too. Exercise caution. Do not become a victim. As you size up the scene, ask yourself: Is an insect nest visible in a nearby tree, under the eaves of a house, or in the ground nearby? Are there signs that the patient was engaged in activity such as clearing underbrush or gardening that might have disturbed snakes or insects? Was the patient working in a garage, basement, attic, or shed where spiders and other insects might nest? Are there dead insects on the ground near the patient?

General signs and symptoms of bites and stings include:

- History of bites or stings.
- Bite mark or stinger embedded in the skin.
- Immediate pain that is severe or burning.
- Numbness at the site after a few hours.
- Redness or other discoloration of the skin around the bite or sting.
- Swelling around the site, sometimes spreading gradually.

If the patient has an allergic reaction, any combination of a range of signs and symptoms may develop. They include the following (Figure 16-12):

- Skin:
  —Warm, tingling feeling in the mouth, face, chest, feet, and hands.
  —Itching, **hives,** and flushing.
  —Swelling of the tongue, face, neck, hands, and feet.
- Respiratory system:
  —Tightness in the throat or chest.
  —Cough, **hoarseness** (losing the voice).
  —Rapid or labored breathing.
  —Noisy breathing, stridor, **wheezing.**
- Circulatory system:
  —Increased heart rate.
  —Decreased blood pressure.

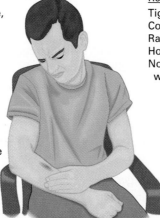

ALLERGIC REACTIONS

<u>Skin</u>
Tingling in the mouth, face,
  chest, feet, and hands
Itching of mouth, ears
Red skin (flushing)
Hives
Swelling to tongue,
  face, neck, hands, feet

<u>Circulatory System</u>
Increased heart rate
Decreased blood pressure

<u>Respiratory System</u>
Tightness in the throat or chest
Cough
Rapid or labored breathing
Hoarseness (losing the voice)
Noisy breathing, stridor,
  wheezing

<u>General Findings</u>
Itching, watery eyes
Headache
Sense of impending doom
Runny nose
Decreasing mental status

NOTE:
Signs and symptoms of shock or
respiratory distress indicate a
life-threatening condition.

FIGURE 16-12 Allergic reactions to bites and stings can cause a variety of signs and symptoms.

- General findings:
  —Itchy, watery eyes.
  —Headache.
  —Runny nose.
  —Sense of impending doom.
  —Decreasing mental status.

If you suspect an allergic reaction, inform EMS dispatch immediately, monitor the patient's airway and breathing continually, and be prepared to assist ventilations.

During your assessment, be alert to the possibility that insects may have become trapped in the patient's clothing. When you gather a patient history, be sure to ask the patient to identify any allergies he may have. Also, if possible and if it is safe to do so, try to identify what bit or stung your patient. During your ongoing assessment, continually monitor the patient's ABCs. Be prepared to deliver basic life support if it is needed. ■

First Responder Care

To provide care to a patient with bites or stings:

1. *Treat all life threats.* If you suspect an allergic reaction, maintain the patient's airway. Insert an airway adjunct if appropriate. Suction as needed.

2. *Administer oxygen,* if you are equipped and allowed to do so. If breathing is adequate, administer oxygen with a nonrebreather mask. If breathing is not adequate, assist ventilations with a BVM and supplemental oxygen.

3. *Position the site of the bite or sting.* It should be slightly below the level of the patient's heart. Manually stabilize a bitten or stung extremity until it can be immobilized.

4. *Remove any constricting objects* such as jewelry as soon as possible. Ideally, this should happen before swelling begins.

5. *Inspect the bite or sting site.* If a stinger is present, remove it by scraping along the surface of the skin with the edge of a credit card or a knife. Make sure you remove the venom sac.

6. *Wash the area around the bite or sting.* Be very gentle. Use soap and water. Then, irrigate with clean water. (Follow local protocol.)

7. *Apply a cold pack* (Figure 16-13). It will help relieve pain, itching, and swelling. Do not apply cold to snakebites or marine animal bites.

8. *Keep the patient calm and warm,* and limit physical activity.

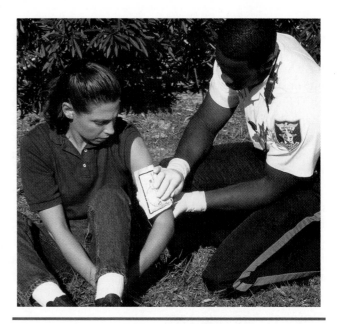

FIGURE 16-13 Apply a cold pack to an insect bite or sting to help relieve pain and swelling.

If at any time during emergency care you suspect an allergic reaction, inform EMS dispatch immediately. (You can read more about First Responder care of a patient in anaphylactic shock in Chapter 18.) Demonstrate a caring attitude towards your patient. Place his or her interests first in any patient-care decision. Remember to communicate with empathy with patients and their family members or friends. ■

Specific Bites and Stings

Snakebite

About 20 of the 120 species of snake in the U.S. are poisonous. They include rattlesnakes, coral snakes, water moccasins or cottonmouths, and copperheads (Figure 16-14). Snake venom contains some of the most complex poisons known. It can affect the central nervous system, heart, kidneys, and blood. Simply stated, a snake's venom is its digestive enzyme. It "digests" any tissue into which it is injected.

Most poisonous snakes have the following distinctive characteristics:

- *Two large, hollow fangs that work like hypodermic needles.* Nonpoisonous snakes (and the poisonous coral snake) have small teeth.

- *Elliptical pupils.* That is, the pupils look like vertical slits, much like those of a cat. Nonpoisonous snakes (and the poisonous coral snake) have round pupils.

- *Presence of a pit.* Certain poisonous snakes have a telltale pit between the eye and the mouth. That is why

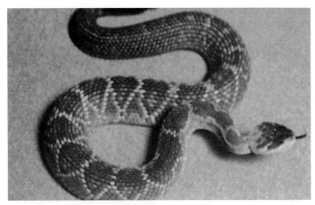

a. *Rattlesnake.*

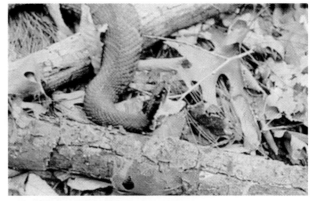

b. *Water moccasin or cottonmouth.*

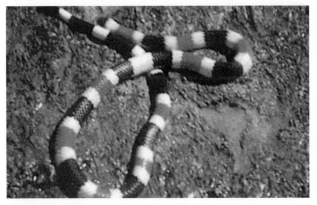

c. *Coral snake.*

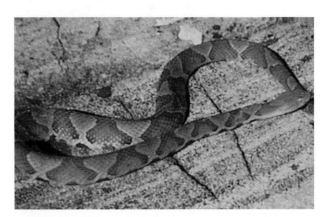

d. *Copperhead.*

FIGURE 16-14 **About 20 of the 120 species of snakes in the U.S. are poisonous. These are some of the most common.**

they are called "pit vipers." The pit is a heat-sensing organ. It allows the snake to strike a warm-blooded animal accurately, even if the snake cannot see it.

- *Special markings.* Poisonous snakes are marked with shapes on a background of pink, yellow, tan, gray, or brown skin. The exception is the small coral snake, which is ringed with red, yellow, and black.

- *Triangular head* larger than the neck.

Poisonous snakebites cause medical emergencies. However, only about one-third of all bites cause symptoms. When symptoms do develop, they usually occur immediately after a person is bitten. Signs and symptoms of a poisonous snakebite include puncture wounds, swelling, discoloration, and severe pain and burning at the bite site. (See Figures 16-15 and 16-16.) In addition, the venom of a coral snake affects the central nervous system. One to eight hours after the bite, the patient will experience symptoms that progressively worsen, including: blurred vision, drooping eyelids, drowsiness, slurred speech, increased

salivation and sweating, nausea, vomiting, weakness, paralysis, seizures, and unresponsiveness.

Always make sure EMS has been activated if you suspect any kind of snakebite. When you gather a patient history, be sure to note how much physical activity the

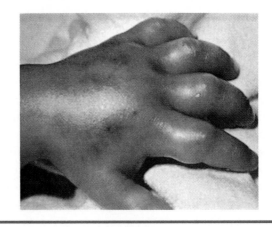

FIGURE 16-15 Snakebite to the hand.

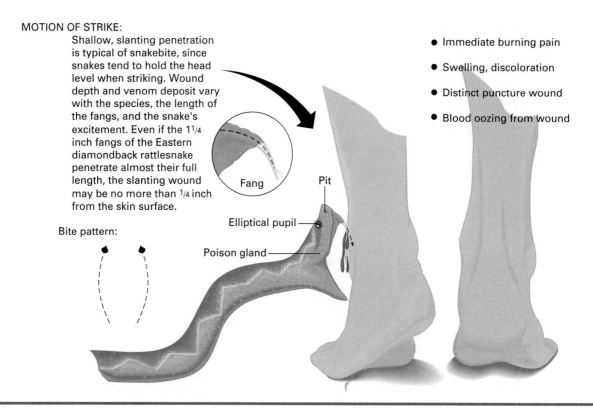

MOTION OF STRIKE:
Shallow, slanting penetration is typical of snakebite, since snakes tend to hold the head level when striking. Wound depth and venom deposit vary with the species, the length of the fangs, and the snake's excitement. Even if the 1¼ inch fangs of the Eastern diamondback rattlesnake penetrate almost their full length, the slanting wound may be no more than ¼ inch from the skin surface.

Bite pattern:

Fang

Pit

Elliptical pupil

Poison gland

- Immediate burning pain
- Swelling, discoloration
- Distinct puncture wound
- Blood oozing from wound

FIGURE 16-16 Poisonous snakebites.

patient engaged in after the bite. (Activity helps to spread the venom.) Also find out when the patient last had a tetanus vaccine.

First Responder care for a patient with a snakebite is the same as for a patient with any bite or sting (described earlier in this chapter). However, if your EMS system allows, you also might want to apply a constricting band and suction the wound.

The use of constricting bands is controversial. Some say they should be used only within 30 minutes of the time of the bite. Others say a constricting band should not be used at all. Constricting bands are used only on extremities. Never place a constricting band around a joint or around the head, neck, or trunk. Follow all local protocols.

To apply a constricting band, first find the fang marks. Then wrap a flat band about two to three inches wide around the extremity (Figure 16-17). Place it two to four inches above (proximal to) the fang marks between the bite and the patient's heart. The band should be snug, but not too tight. You should be able to slip two fingers between it and the patient's skin. You may adjust the constricting band as swelling occurs so that it does not become too tight. But leave it in place until a physician checks the patient.

The use of suction also is controversial. Recent medical research has called the device's effectiveness into question. Follow local protocols. If permitted, apply suction to the wound directly over the fang marks. An extractor from a snakebite kit is ideal. Never use your mouth to provide suction. Suction must be strong and must be applied within the first five minutes to be effective. After 30 minutes, the venom is diffused and

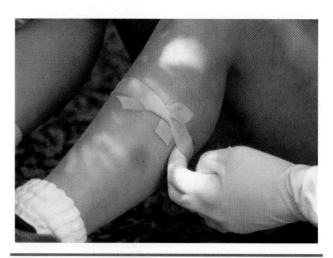

FIGURE 16-17 Follow local protocol regarding the use of a constricting band.

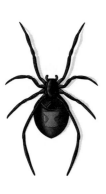 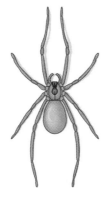 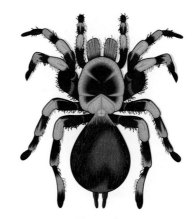

Black Widow   Brown Recluse   Tarantula

FIGURE 16-18 Poisonous spiders.

cannot be removed by suction. Note, never suction a coral snake bite.

Insect Bites and Stings

For assessment and First Responder care of patients with insect bites and stings, follow the general guidelines described earlier in this chapter. The discussion below provides details on specific insects and spiders.

Black Widow Spider. The black widow spider is characterized by a shiny black body, thin legs, and a crimson red mark on its abdomen the shape of an hour glass or two triangles. (See Figure 16-18.) Its bite is a leading cause of death from spiders in the U.S. Fourteen times more toxic than rattlesnake venom, black-widow venom results in pain and muscle spasms within 30 minutes to three hours. Severe bites cause respiratory failure and death. Those at highest risk for developing severe symptoms are children under 16 years old, adults over the age of 60, and anyone with a chronic disease or hypertension (high blood pressure).

The most serious sign of a black-widow bite is high blood pressure. Other signs and symptoms, which last for 24 to 48 hours, include:

- Brief pinprick sensation at the bite site. It becomes a dull ache within 30 to 40 minutes. There is almost never a local reaction, although in some cases there may be some swelling or a **wheal** (a raised, round, red mark).

- Flushing, sweating, and grimacing of the face within 10 minutes to two hours.

- Pain and spasms in the shoulders, back, chest, and abdominal muscles within 30 minutes to three hours. These gradually spread over the entire body within one to six hours.

- Rigid abdomen with cramping.

- Agitation, restlessness, anxiety.

- Lack of coordination.

- Weakness, headache, which may last for months.

- Profuse salivation, tearing, or sweating.

- Fever, rash.

- Nausea, vomiting.

The antivenom for the black-widow spider bite is generally used only for high-risk patients. If you can do so safely, find the spider. The patient's physician will be able to identify it, even if it is crushed, and will not have to guess about treatment.

Brown Recluse Spider. The brown recluse spider can range in color from yellow to dark chocolate brown. The characteristic marking is a brown, violin-shaped mark on the upper back. Its bite is not often serious. However, about 10% of the time, the bite does not heal and the patient needs a skin graft. A small percent of patients develop kidney failure and die.

Brown-recluse bites are rare. They most often occur when spiders are trapped in clothing. Unfortunately, most victims are unaware that they have been bitten, since the bite often is at first painless. There may be a slight stinging sensation and itching. The most severe reactions are among children.

If the patient is going to react, the following signs and symptoms may occur:

- Within a few hours, the bite is surrounded by sunken tissue. There is a bluish area with white edges, gradually becoming surrounded by a red halo (a bulls-eye pattern). Two tiny puncture marks may be apparent.

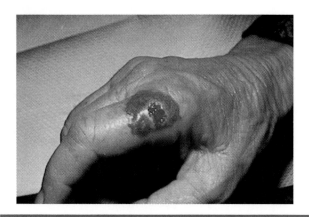

FIGURE 16-19 Soft-tissue injury from a brown recluse spider several days after initial bite.

- Within 72 hours, if there is a severe reaction, the bite becomes a large **ulcer** (Figure 16-19). The following also sometimes occur: a fever of 103°F, joint pain, nausea, vomiting, and chills.

Again, it is important for you to identify the spider so that physicians may begin appropriate treatment as soon as possible.

Tarantula. Although the tarantula looks more menacing than the black widow and the brown recluse, its bite usually causes only moderate pain. Other symptoms from tarantula bites are rare.

Scorpion. In the U.S., three species of scorpion sting and inject venom (Figure 16-20). Only one species—the Bark Scorpion—can deliver a potentially fatal sting. Of all scorpion stings, 90% occur to the hands.

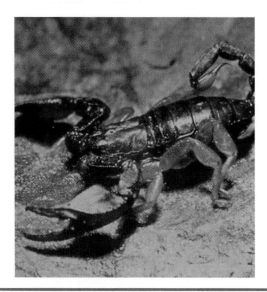

FIGURE 16-20 Scorpion.

In addition to the general signs and symptoms, those for scorpion bites include nausea and vomiting, drooling, poor coordination, incontinence, and seizures.

If you are allowed, apply a flat constricting band to the extremity about two inches above the sting. The band should be snug, but not too tight. You should be able to slip two fingers between it and the patient's skin. Leave it in place until a physician checks the patient. (Follow local protocols.)

Fire Ants. Fire ants are most common in the southeastern U.S. They get their name not from their color (which ranges from red to black) but from the intense, fiery, burning pain their bites cause.

Fire ants bite downward as they pivot. The result is a characteristic circular pattern of bites, which produce extremely painful **vesicles** (small blisters). At first, the fluid in the vesicles is clear. Later, it becomes cloudy. The bitten extremity usually becomes red, swollen, and painful. Within 24 hours, the bites develop **pustules** (raised areas filled with pus) on a red, swollen base (Figure 16-21).

Mites. Mites are most common in the southern part of the U.S. However, since they feed on tall grasses and grains, they are found in rural and agricultural areas throughout the country. Many types of mites bite humans. The most common are the scabies mite and chigger mite.

Mites embed themselves in the skin, generally without the patient realizing it. As soon as they are engorged with blood, the mites drop off or are brushed off. If the patient sees the mite at all, it is in the center of a red lesion. Most bites are on the legs and ankles or under tight-fitting clothing such as waistbands. Bite sites often enlarge into nodes that last for two to three weeks.

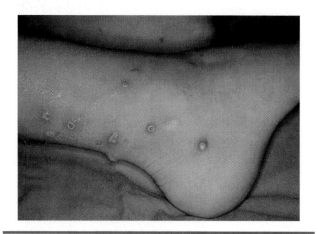

FIGURE 16-21 Fire-ant bites.

Ticks. Ticks can cause a serious problem because they can carry tick fever, Rocky Mountain spotted fever, Lyme disease, and other bacterial diseases. A prolonged attachment of a female tick can cause progressive paralysis.

Tick bites are painless. The patient does not notice the bite until he or she finds an engorged tick, which can be as large as a pea (Figure 16-22). Ticks are visible after they have attached themselves to the skin. They often stay attached for more than 10 days. However, since they often choose warm, moist areas, you should carefully inspect the patient's scalp and other hairy areas such as the armpits, groin, and skin creases. If a tick is brushed off, the mouth parts may stay embedded in the skin, causing infection or an allergic reaction. Never pluck an embedded tick head out of the skin. You may force infected blood into the patient.

If you are providing emergency care in an isolated area, local protocol may permit you to remove a tick. If so, remove it as soon as you discover it. The longer the tick remains attached to the skin, the more likely it is that an infection will result. To remove a tick, follow these guidelines:

1. *Take BSI precautions and use tweezers.* Do not touch the tick; you may contaminate yourself. If you do not have tweezers, do not wait to look for an appropriate implement.

2. *Grasp and pull.* Grasp the tick as closely as possible to the point where it is attached to the skin. Then pull firmly and steadily until the tick is dislodged. Do not twist or jerk the tick, since that may result in incomplete removal. Avoid squashing an engorged tick during removal. Infected blood may spurt into your eyes, mouth, or cut on the surface of your skin.

3. *Clean up.* Once the tick is removed, wash your hands and the bite area thoroughly with soap and water. Apply an antiseptic to the area to prevent a bacterial infection. Carefully note any residual parts of the tick that may be left behind.

Have the patient mark the date of removal on a calendar. This will document the exact time of exposure and will serve as a reminder if he or she needs to seek medical care. If the patient develops fever with chills, headache, or muscle aches after being exposed to a tick, immediate treatment from a physician should be sought.

Bee, Wasp, or Hornet Stings. A patient with an insect sting should see a physician if the bite is on the face or if he receives multiple stings, even if there seems to be no allergic reaction. If the patient has an allergic reaction, ensure an open airway and adequate breathing and arrange for him to be transported to a hospital immediately. (See Figure 16-23.)

First Responder care is the same as described for bites and stings at the beginning of this chapter. However, if you are allowed, proceed with the following:

1. *Position the sting site.* Lower the affected part below the heart.

2. *Apply a constricting band.* Place it above the sting site if it is on an extremity. The band should be snug, but not too tight. You should be able to slip two fingers between it and the patient's skin. Remember that the use of a constricting band is controversial. Follow local protocols.

3. *Remove the stinger.* Gently scrape against it with the edge of a knife or a credit card (Figure 16-24). Be careful not to squeeze the stinger. If you do, you could inject additional venom into the area. Make sure you remove the venom sac. It can continue to secrete venom for up to 20 minutes.

If you know the patient is allergic to stings, do not wait for signs or symptoms to develop. Delay can be fatal. If the patient has a history of severe allergic reactions and has an insect sting kit, assist in the administration of the kit's contents. (See Chapter 18.) *Follow all local protocols.*

Marine-Life Bites and Stings

See Figure 16-25 for common sources of marine animal stings and wounds. In general, First Responder care is as follows (follow all local protocols):

1. *Clean the wound site.* Use forceps to remove any material that sticks to the sting site on the surface of the

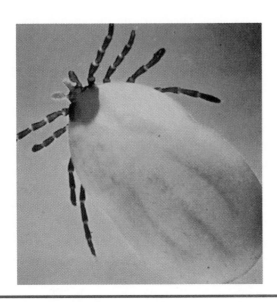

FIGURE 16-22 Engorged tick.

WASPS, BEES, AND FIRE ANTS

The following members of this group commonly attack humans, causing local pain, redness, swelling, and subsequent itching. Always consider the possibility of an allergic reaction.

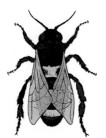

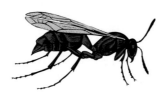

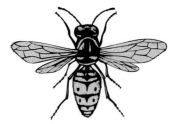

HONEYBEE: Found throughout the United States at any time of year, except in colder temperatures when they remain in their hives. In the Northeast and Midwest, they are major insects causing sting reactions. Hives are usually found in hollowed out areas such as dead tree trunks. Honeybees principally ingest nectar of plants, so they are often seen in the vicinity of flowers. The honeybee with its barbed stinger will self-eviscerate after a sting, leaving the venom sac and stinger in place.

WASPS: The most likely insect to cause sting reactions in the Southeast and Southwest. Wasps tend to nest in small numbers under the eaves of houses and buildings. Carnivores that are found in picnic areas, garbage cans, and food stands, they can deliver multiple stings at one time.

YELLOW JACKET: A principal insect causing sting reactions in the Northeast and Midwest. Yellow jackets tend to dominate in late summer and fall. Nests are located in the ground. Often seen in picnic areas and garbage cans, yellow jackets are ill-tempered and aggressive and can deliver multiple stings at one time. They will often sting without being provoked.

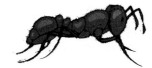

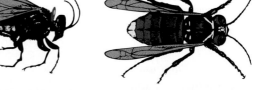

FIRE ANT: Can range from red to black and lives in loose dirt mounds. It is found throughout the southern states as far west as New Mexico. Fire ants may cause serious illness and/or allergic reactions. The ant attaches itself to the skin by its strong jaws and swivels its tail-position stinger about, inflicting repeated stings.

YELLOW HORNET AND WHITE-FACED OR BALD-FACED HORNET: Seen mainly in the spring and early summer. Nests usually found in branches and bushes above ground. Carnivores that are seen in picnic areas, garbage cans, and food stands, they can deliver multiple stings at one time.

Adapted from: John W. Georgitis. "Insect Stings – Responding to the Gamut of Allergic Reactions," *Modern Medicine*

FIGURE 16-23 Always consider a possible allergic reaction to the bites of wasps, bees, and fire ants.

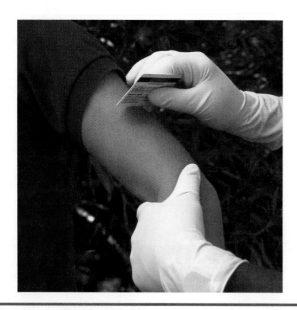

FIGURE 16-24 If the insect stinger is still present, remove it.

patient's skin. Then, irrigate the wound thoroughly with water. If the skin is unbroken, wash the wound with an antibacterial agent. Do not scrub the area. Make sure that washings flow away from the body.

2. *Remove stingers and barbs.* Remove them the same way you would remove a bee stinger. If you are unable to remove one without excessive force, then bandage it in place. Stabilize the area to keep the venom from spreading.

3. *Apply heat.* Maintain the injured area at a temperature of 110°F to 114°F for thirty minutes or until the EMTs take over care. Follow local protocol.

4. *Activate the EMS system,* if that has not already been done. Arrange for immediate transport of the patient.

Tentacle Stings. Tentacle stings can be inflicted by jellyfish, corals, hydras, and anemones (Figure 16-26). To care for such a patient, first remove the patient from the

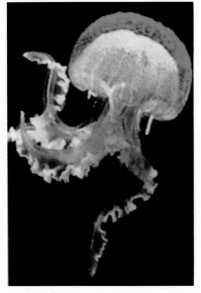

a. *Jellyfish.*

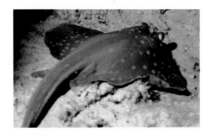

b. *Stingray.*

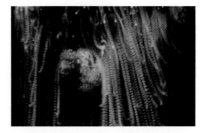

c. *Tentacles of the Portuguese man-of-war.*

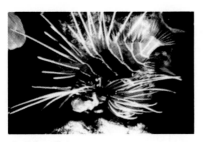

d. *Lion fish.*

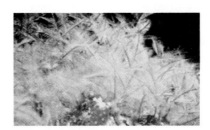

e. *Feather hydroid.*

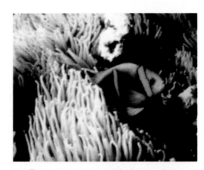

f. *Sea anemone and clown fish.*

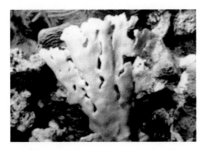

g. *Fire coral.*

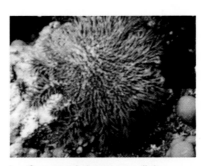

h. *Crown-of-thorns starfish.*

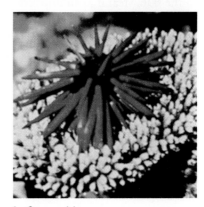

i. *Sea urchin.*

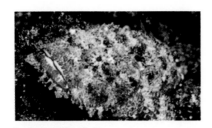

j. *Scorpion fish.*

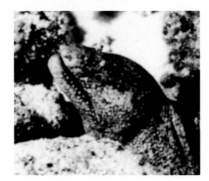

k. *Moray eel.*

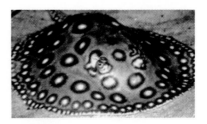

l. *Stingray.*

FIGURE 16-25 Common sources of marine life bites and stings.

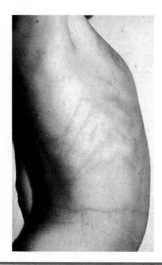

FIGURE 16-26 Jellyfish sting.

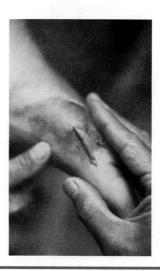

FIGURE 16-27 Stingray sting.

water. With gloved hands, carefully remove dried tentacles if possible. Immediately rinse the wounds with sea water for 30 minutes until pain is relieved. If possible, pour vinegar on the affected area. Arrange for immediate transport of the patient to a hospital.

Puncture Wounds. To treat puncture wounds caused by stingray spines and spiny fish (Figure 16-27), first remove the patient from the water. If a spine is embedded in the skin, treat it as an impaled object and stabilize it in place. Prevent any movement of the injured part. Apply a sterile dressing and bandage the area. Arrange for immediate transport of the patient to a hospital.

Large Bites. Bites from sharks or other marine life should be treated the same way you would treat any major injury. Perform an initial assessment and treat life

threats. Be especially attentive to the control of external bleeding and the treatment of shock. Arrange for immediate transport of the patient to a hospital. If possible, try to identify the animal that caused the injury.

1. What are the general signs and symptoms of bites and stings?

2. What are the signs and symptoms of an allergic reaction in a patient with a bite or sting?

3. What are the general guidelines for First Responder care of a patient with a bite or sting?

The Call Follow-up

At the beginning of this chapter, you read that First Responders were on scene with "a woman down." Their first impression was of an elderly woman who had fallen and has a bleeding head wound. To see how chapter skills apply to this emergency, read the following. It describes how the call was completed.

Initial Assessment My partner got in position and manually stabilized the patient's head. I got down on my knees, introduced myself, and asked her what was wrong. She told us that last night at about 9 p.m. she tripped over her cat and fell. She was sore all over, but her hip hurt most. I was glad to note that she was awake and alert. Her airway was open, breathing was good, and all bleeding appeared to have stopped.

It appeared at first that Mrs. Downe was a trauma patient, the fall being her mechanism of injury. However, we found that her skin was ice cold and she was shivering. We reported our initial findings to dispatch, then continued the assessment.

Physical Examination I performed a complete physical exam on Mrs. Downe. In addition to the open head wound, my findings included a swollen, painful deformity in her right hip, plus bruises to her hips, knees, and ankles. I also noticed she had been incontinent of urine during the night. Her shivering continued.

Mrs. Downe had been lying on a cold, wet floor for nearly 12 hours. I suspected hypothermia. After completing the physical exam, we placed a warm blanket over her. We didn't want to move her because of her injuries and the ambulance was less than five minutes away.

Patient History Mrs. Downe told us she had no allergies and that she took several medications, including aspirin, digitalis, and insulin. She had a long history of circulatory problems. She had not eaten for 12 hours. Unable to get up from the floor, she had called out for help until she lost her voice.

Ongoing Assessment We monitored Mrs. Downe's mental status and vital signs. We kept her head stabilized and tried to keep her as warm as possible.

Patient Hand-off When the Rescue 3 team arrived, we gave them our hand-off report (see below). Later that week, I ran into Rescue 3's crew chief. He said that Mrs. Downe had suffered a broken hip and hypothermia. She was treated successfully at the hospital but would likely go to a nursing home after discharge.

Hand-off Report

"We have an 80-year-old female who fell 12 hours ago and remained down until we arrived. Her chief complaint is pain in her right hip. She also hit her head when she fell. There was minor bleeding, and we manually stabilized her cervical spine. Her pulse is 100, respirations 18. We also felt that she could be hypothermic, so we warmed her with a blanket."

The Last Word *Heat and cold emergencies often occur in isolated areas to such people as campers, hikers, skiers, and mountain climbers. But as you can see, they also can happen in our own neighborhoods. Always consider the environmental conditions as soon as you get your call. Early recognition and the appropriate care can save a life.*

Chapter Review

Focus on the EMS Team

Even though most people—including rescuers—are aware of the effects of environmental hazards, they still fall victim. People in the cold with wet clothes and people in the heat who do not maintain their fluid levels can be overcome quickly. Even those exposed to moderate temperatures for long periods of time can be stricken. Though bites and stings are a mere annoyance for most people, they can be life-threatening.

If you live and work in an area with extreme temperatures or if you have poisonous snakes or other dangerous species in your area, learn about them. Find out what EMS personnel can do to stay safe. First Responders and other EMS providers can make a difference to patients with environmental emergencies, but not if they become victims, too. Never forget scene safety and your own well-being.

Summing Up

- The body produces heat mainly through the process of metabolism. It holds onto heat by constricting blood vessels near its surface and by raising hairs. In a cold environment, it can produce additional heat by shivering and with hormones such as epinephrine. The body loses heat through convection, conduction, radiation, evaporation, and respiration.

- Exposure to cold can cause two kinds of emergencies: generalized hypothermia and local cold injury (frostbite).

- To assess a patient for cold injury, consider the temperature of the environment and how long the patient has been exposed to it. If the environment suggests a possible cold injury, pay special attention to skin color, temperature, and condition. If the patient's abdomen is cold, suspect hypothermia. If a body part appears abnormal (discolored, lack of sensation, swollen or blistered), suspect frostbite.

- First Responder care of a cold injury includes removing the patient from the cold environment, ensuring an open airway and adequate breathing, removing all wet clothing, and covering with a blanket. Also avoid any rough handling. If there is frostbite, the affected body part should be stabilized and covered to protect it from further injury. Follow local protocols for rewarming.

- When a person cannot lose excessive heat, he or she develops hyperthermia. Heat-related emergencies include heat cramps, heat exhaustion, and heat stroke. Heat stroke, the most serious, is life-threatening.

- For a heat emergency, consider contributing and risk factors, including the environmental temperature and humidity, the patient's level of activity, age, medical condition, and the use of

any drugs or medications. If the skin of the abdomen is hot, suspect a severe heat emergency.

- First Responder care of a heat emergency includes removing the patient from the hot environment, ensuring an open airway and adequate breathing, cooling the patient, and placing him in a supine position with legs elevated. If allowed and appropriate (follow local protocol), encourage the alert patient to drink some water or a sport drink.

- In cases of bite or sting emergencies, be especially careful during scene size-up. Be alert for signs that the insects or animals remain on scene and pose a danger to you or others.

- If possible and if it is safe to do so, try to identify what bit or stung your patient. Knowing can help health-care providers determine proper treatment.

- Bites or stings can lead to anaphylactic shock, an emergency that can have a rapid life-threatening affect on the airway and breathing. Respiratory distress and shock may develop rapidly. If you suspect an allergic reaction, inform EMS immediately, monitor the patient's airway and breathing, and be prepared to assist ventilations. If the patient has a history of severe allergic reactions and has an insect sting kit, assist in the administration of the kit's contents *(follow all local protocols).*

- First Responder care of a bite or sting includes maintaining an open airway and adequate breathing. Also, manually stabilize the bite site, position it slightly below the level of the heart, remove any constricting objects before swelling begins, and limit the patient's physical activity. If a stinger is present, remove it and wash the injured area gently with soap and water. If the injury is not a snakebite or marine animal bite, apply a cold pack.

Key Terms

analgesic a medication that relieves pain.

anaphylactic shock an acute allergic reaction with severe bronchospasm and vascular collapse, which can be rapidly fatal. *Also called* anaphylaxis.

dehydration excessive loss of body fluids.

gangrene localized tissue death.

heat cramps muscle cramps in the lower limbs and abdomen, associated with fluid loss and possibly salt loss while active in a hot environment.

heat exhaustion prolonged exposure to heat, which produces moist, pale skin that may feel normal or cool to the touch.

heat stroke prolonged exposure to heat, which produces dry or moist skin that may feel warm or hot to the touch; associated with elevation of core body temperature.

hives slightly elevated red or pale areas of the skin that also may be itchy.

hoarseness losing the voice.

hyperthermia fever or raised body temperature.

hypothermia a overall reduction of body temperature.

local cold injury freezing or near freezing of a specific body part. *Also called* frostbite.

metabolism all the physical and chemical changes that occur in the body, including digestion.

mottled many colors or discolorations.

pustules raised areas on the skin that are filled with pus.

ulcer a patch of skin or mucous membrane marked by redness, possible infection, and loose dead skin.

vesicles small blisters.

wheal a raised, round, red mark.

wheezing whistling breathing sounds.

Knowledge Check

1. **If your patient is found in the cold, not shivering, with a diminished level of responsiveness, you should suspect:**
   a. mild hypothermia.
   b. severe hypothermia.
   c. mild hyperthermia.
   d. severe hyperthermia.

2. **Which one of the following signs is NOT seen in severe hypothermia?**
   a. rigidity or freezing of the extremities
   b. slow or irregular pulse rate
   c. increased respiratory rate
   d. dilated pupils

3. **First Responder care for a late (deep) local cold injury to an extremity includes:**
   a. rubbing and massaging the affected part.
   b. covering the affected area with a dry dressing.
   c. actively rewarming the part to prevent tissue damage.
   d. allowing the patient to walk to maintain circulation.

4. **A responsive patient who is suffering from a heat emergency has cool, moist skin. She is most likely suffering from:**
   a. mild hypothermia.
   b. severe hypothermia.
   c. mild hyperthermia.
   d. severe hyperthermia.

5. **Which one of the following factors does NOT directly contribute to the risk of a heat-related emergency?**
   a. patient's age
   b. strenuous activity
   c. patient's mental status
   d. patient's medication and drug use

6. **All of the following are common names for heat-related emergencies EXCEPT heat:**
   a. cramps.
   b. stroke.
   c. exhaustion.
   d. anaphylaxis.

7. **You suspect that your patient is suffering from severe hypothermia. During assessment, she becomes unresponsive and stops breathing. Before starting CPR, you must palpate the carotid pulse point for:**
   a. 45 seconds.
   b. one full minute.
   c. 30 seconds, and multiply by 2.
   d. 15 seconds and multiply by 4.

8. **Your severely hypothermic patient is showing signs of death. What rule of thumb can guide you in your decision to continue—or stop—performing CPR on this patient?**
   a. You're not dead until you're warm and dead.
   b. Rely on the chain of survival.
   c. Airway! Airway! Airway!
   d. OPQRRRST

9. **Your patient has a particularly painful insect bite on his upper right arm. He also tells you that his face feels tingly and his eyes are getting watery and itchy. Upon hearing this, you determine that you should be prepared for:**
   a. stroke or seizures.
   b. other imaginary symptoms.
   c. respiratory difficulties.
   d. drug or alcohol poisoning.

10. **Applying a cold pack to the site of a bite or sting can help relieve pain, itching, and swelling.**
    a. True
    b. False

11. **Position the site of the bite or sting slightly above the level of the patient's heart.**
    a. True
    b. False

12. **List the stages of hypothermia in order.**

_____

_____

_____

13. **List six risk factors for hyperthermia.**

_____   _____

_____   _____

_____   _____

14. List 10 signs or symptoms of an allergic reaction to a bite or sting.

_____   _____

_____   _____

_____   _____

_____   _____

_____   _____

Scenario

It's your summer vacation and you and your friend Pat are hiking through the state park. You are both in good physical condition. After a while, you notice that she is trailing behind. You backtrack and in just a few minutes spot her stopped and standing just to the side of the path.

a. As you approach, what should you do first?

_____

_____

b. When you are at Pat's side, you ask her: "Are you okay? Why have you stopped?" She looks you straight in the eye, smiles shyly, and says, "I'm fine. I just want to rest for a second. I'm not used to trekking uphill with a full backpack." You notice that she is sweating a little harder than you'd like, but her breathing and color seem to be fine. As you observe your friend, you bring to mind the signs and symptoms of a heat emergency. What are they?

_____

_____

_____

_____

c. When Pat felt she had rested enough, you both went on with your hike without any further incident. But if Pat had been experiencing a heat emergency, what could you have done for her?

_____

_____

_____

_____

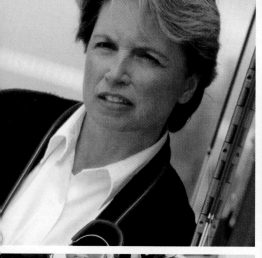
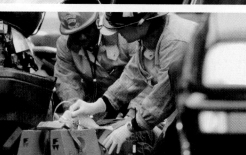
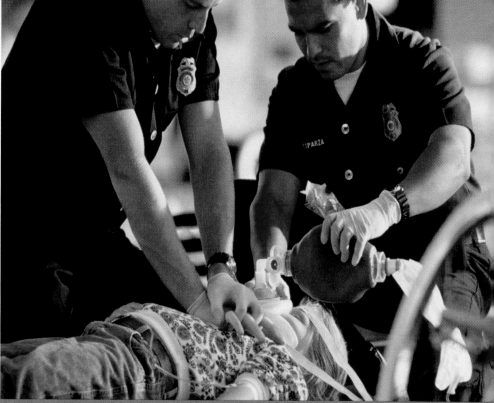

17 | Psychological Emergencies and Crisis Intervention

Objectives

From the U.S. Department of Transportation (DOT) 1995 "First Responder: National Standard Curriculum." Material supplemental to the DOT curriculum is listed under "Enrichment."

Cognitive

5-1.11 ▶ Identify the patient who presents with a specific medical complaint of behavioral change. (pp. 313–315)

5-1.12 ▶ Explain the steps in providing emergency medical care to a patient with a behavioral change. (p. 315)

5-1.13 ▶ Identify the patient who presents with a specific complaint of a psychological crisis. (pp. 313–315)

5-1.14 ▶ Explain the steps in providing emergency medical care to a patient with a psychological crisis. (p. 315)

Affective

5-1.17 ▶ Explain the rationale for modifying your behavior toward the patient with a behavioral emergency. (pp. 313–314)

5-1.24 ▶ Demonstrate a caring attitude toward patients with a behavioral problem who request emergency medical services. (pp. 314, 315–316, 320)

5-1.25 ▶ Place the interests of the patient with a behavioral problem as the foremost consideration when making any and all patient care decisions. (p. 316)

5-1.26 ▶ Communicate with empathy to patients with a behavioral problem, as well as with family members and friends of the patient. (pp. 314, 315–316, 320)

Psychomotor

5-1.32 ▶ Demonstrate the steps in providing emergency medical care to a patient with a behavioral change. (p. 315)

5-1.33 ▶ Demonstrate the steps in providing emergency medical care to a patient with a psychological crisis. (p. 315)

Enrichment

▶ Discuss the guidelines for restraining patients with a behavioral emergency. (pp. 316–317)

▶ List the legal considerations involved in providing emergency care to a patient with a behavioral emergency. (p. 317)

▶ Identify the signs and symptoms of a patient with a drug or alcohol emergency. (p. 319)

▶ Describe management of a patient with a drug or alcohol emergency. (pp. 317–320)

▶ Discuss the four general stages of rape trauma syndrome. (pp. 320–321)

▶ Describe the proper management of a rape scene. (p. 321)

Introduction

In emergency care for physical problems, you can usually see the wounds you care for. You can assess, dress, and bandage them and often get to see the positive results of your efforts. In contrast, you cannot easily see what is causing a behavioral patient's emergency. In addition, you may not see the comfort your words or presence provides to someone who is panicked or depressed. Understand that the care you give to patients in behavioral emergencies can save lives, too.

Section 1 Behavioral Emergencies

Behavior is the manner in which a person acts or performs. A **behavioral emergency** is a situation in which a patient exhibits "abnormal" behavior, or behavior that is unacceptable or intolerable to the patient, family, or community. Such an emergency may be due to extremes of emotion, a psychological condition such as a mental illness, or even a physical condition such as lack of oxygen or low blood sugar.

It is best to consider all patients who exhibit unusual or bizarre behavior as having an altered mental status. This means that they are not acting as they would normally. It also acknowledges the fact that the behavior could be caused by a number of conditions. Consider a classic example:

Because a patient slurred his words and waved his arms wildly, EMS providers and police assumed he was intoxicated and did not transport him to a hospital. After they left the scene, the patient experienced a seizure and fell into a coma. Later, everyone learned that the behavioral emergency had been caused not by alcohol abuse, but by dangerously low blood sugar (hypoglycemia).

Never assume a patient is simply intoxicated until you consider hidden medical conditions or injuries. Keep in mind that there are a number of factors that can cause a change in a patient's behavior. They include situational stresses, which can occur in the aftermath of the death of a loved one, for example. Illness and injury (such as head

trauma, lack of oxygen, inadequate blood flow to the brain, low blood sugar in a person with diabetes, or excessive heat or cold) also are factors. Mind-altering substances—such as alcohol, depressants, stimulants, psychedelics, and narcotics—are common causes of behavioral emergencies. So too are psychiatric problems, such as phobias (irrational fears of specific things), depression, paranoia, and schizophrenia.

Patients with behavioral emergencies may act in unusual and unexpected ways. They can pose a danger to themselves through self-inflicted injuries or suicide. They also can pose a danger to others through violence or actions they are not able to understand.

Keep the following basic principles in mind whenever you are on the scene of a behavioral emergency:

■ Identify yourself. Let the patient know you are there to help.

First on Scene

Your communication and interpersonal skills are your equipment for handling a patient with a behavioral emergency. Splints stabilize injured extremities and dressings control bleeding, but for the patient with a behavioral problem, the way you communicate will help the patient the most.

THE CALL

Dispatch I was driving home from my shift at the fire department when I saw a man running along the road. He was naked. He stopped every few hundred feet or so to throw punches in the air.

Scene Size-up I realized this person might be dangerous. So I called the police on a cell phone from my car. I stayed there, observing the patient, until they arrived.

Initial Assessment After the man was restrained by the police, I offered my help. They were careful not to restrict the man's breathing. They also covered him with an emergency blanket to keep him warm. He was screaming at the police officers, so I knew he had adequate breathing. There were no indications of airway problems or external bleeding. My general impression was that of a patient with an altered mental status, possibly from a psychiatric emergency, alcohol, or drugs. We called for an ambulance.

This First Responder was correct to call for the assistance of the police. (Remember: Safety first!) Consider this patient as you read Chapter 17. Could he consent to care? If so, will he? If not, what may be done to assess and treat his condition?

- Inform the patient of exactly what you are doing. Uncertainty will make the patient more anxious and fearful.

- Ask questions in a calm, reassuring voice. Speak directly to the patient. Stay polite. Use good manners. Show respect. Make no unsupported assumptions.

- Without being judgmental, allow the patient to tell you what happened.

- Show you are listening by rephrasing or repeating part of what is said. Ask questions to show you are paying attention. Also use gestures such as a nod of the head or verbal responses such as "I see" or "Go on."

- Acknowledge the patient's feelings. Use phrases like, "I can see that you are very sad and upset" or "I am not surprised that you feel frightened."

- Assess the patient's mental status by asking specific questions. Try to determine whether or not the patient is oriented to time, person, and place. Watch the patient's appearance, level of activity, and speech patterns.

Patient Assessment

Consider the need for law enforcement during your scene size-up and throughout the call. If you suspect that the patient is a threat to others or to himself, arrange for backup law enforcement at the scene. The following guidelines may help you determine if your patient is likely to become violent:

- During scene size-up, look around. Locate the patient before approaching (Figure 17-1). Look for any

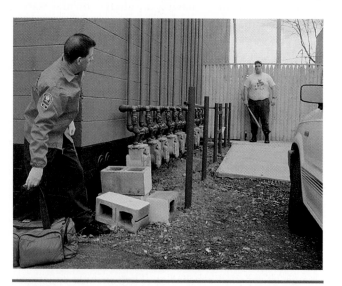

FIGURE 17-1 Locate the patient before approaching and look for any weapons.

weapons or items that could be used as weapons such as a knife or blunt object. If you see any of these, assume that the patient may use them to hurt you or himself. Overturned furniture or other signs of chaos also can indicate violent behavior.

- If the patient's family members, friends, or bystanders are at the scene, ask if the patient has a history of being aggressive or combative. Also find out if the patient has been violent or has threatened violence at the scene.

- Expect violence if the patient is standing or sitting in a way that threatens anyone (including himself). Clenched fists, even when the patient is holding them at his side, may be a sign.

- Listen to the patient. Expect violence if he is yelling, cursing, arguing, or verbally threatening to hurt someone.

- Signs of possible violence in a patient include moving toward you, carrying a heavy or threatening object, making quick or irregular movements, and muscle tension. ■

First Responder Care

While caring for a patient who has a behavioral emergency, be sure to comfort, calm, and reassure the patient as you proceed. Never leave the patient alone. All such patients are escape risks, and violence is a real possibility. Once you have responded to a behavioral emergency, the patient's safety is legally your responsibility until someone with more training arrives on scene. Even if the patient pleads to be alone for just a few minutes, do not do it. Firmly explain that you could get in trouble if you did.

If you suspect the patient may have overdosed, provide emergency medical care as described in Chapter 15 for a poisoning patient. Give any medications or drugs you find on scene to the transporting EMS personnel. ■

Methods to Calm Patients

Situations presented by behaviorally disturbed patients are often difficult. However, the following techniques can help:

- Acknowledge that the patient seems upset and restate that you are there to help.

- Inform the patient of exactly who you are and what you are going to do to help.

- Ask questions in a calm, reassuring voice. Speak directly to the patient.

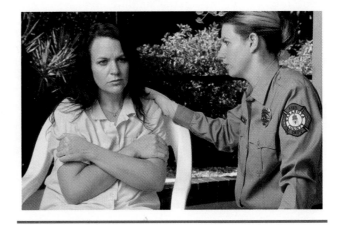

FIGURE 17-2 With the patient's consent, touch may be comforting.

- Maintain a comfortable distance between you and the patient. Many patients are threatened by physical contact. Unwanted touching could set off a violent response. After you have established some rapport with the patient, get his or her permission before moving in any closer (Figure 17-2).

- Encourage the patient to tell you what is troubling him or her. Ask the patient to explain the problem.

- Never assume that you cannot communicate with the patient until you have tried, even if others insist it is impossible.

- Do not make any quick movements. Act quietly and slowly. Let the patient see that you are not going to make any sudden moves.

- Respond honestly to the patient's questions. Instead of saying, for example, "You have nothing to worry about," say something like "Even with all the problems you told me about, you seem to have lots of people around who really care about you."

- Never threaten, challenge, belittle, or argue with disturbed patients. Remember that the patient is ill. His or her comments are not about you personally.

- Always tell the truth. Never lie to a patient.

- Do not "play along" with a patient's visual or auditory disturbances. Instead, reassure the patient that they are temporary and can clear up with treatment.

- Involve the patient's family members or friends when you can. Some patients are calmed and reassured by their presence. However, others may be upset or embarrassed. Let the patient decide.

- Be prepared to stay at the scene for a long time.

- Avoid unnecessary physical contact. Enlist the help of law enforcement if you are unable to maintain control on your own.

First Responder Practice

Monitor a restrained patient constantly. If he becomes quiet after being agitated, you must be sure that his condition has not deteriorated. The sudden change could be due to unconsciousness or respiratory arrest.

■ Maintain good eye contact with the patient. It communicates your control and confidence. Also, the patient's eyes can reflect his emotions. They may tell you if the patient is terrified, confused, struggling, or in pain. The eyes can telegraph intentions, too. If a patient is about to reach for a weapon or make a dash, the eyes may alert you.

Always place the interests of the patient first in all patient-care decisions. Communicate with empathy with the patient and with his or her family and friends.

Restraining Patients

Restraining the patient should be avoided unless he poses a danger to himself or others. Restraining patients may require police authorization in your EMS system. Seek medical direction and follow local protocol. If you are not authorized by state law to use restraints, wait for someone with the authority to do so. If you are authorized to use restraints, work in conjunction with the police and other EMS providers. (See Figure 17-3.)

Be aware that a violent physical struggle usually is brief. However, after a struggle, some apparently calm patients may cause unexpected and sudden injury to themselves and others.

Avoid using unreasonable force. Never inflict pain or use unnecessary force in restraining a patient. Use only as much force as needed for restraint. **Reasonable force** refers to the amount of force needed to keep a patient from injuring himself or someone else. It depends on:

■ *Size and strength of the patient.* What may seem reasonable force for a 275-pound athlete may not be reasonable for a 150-pound homemaker.

■ *Type of abnormal behavior the patient is exhibiting.* You would not expect to use the same kind of force against a frightened patient who is huddling quietly

in a corner as you would against an angry patient who is loudly threatening to kill you.

■ *Mental state of the patient.* It may be reasonable to use more force on a patient who is loud and threatening than on a patient who is quiet and subdued.

■ *Method of restraint you are using.* Soft leather or cloth straps are called "humane restraints." They are generally considered reasonable. Metal cuffs are not.

Asphyxia is a lethal condition caused by an insufficient intake of oxygen. Use extreme caution when restraining patients to prevent **positional asphyxia.** It has been associated with hog-tie or hobble restraints, which are suspected of decreasing respiratory effort. Alcohol and drug use also may play a role. Careful and frequent monitoring of all restrained patients will help prevent this condition from occurring.

A restrained patient should always be placed in a face-up position. While caring for him, monitor his airway and breathing carefully. Note that it is common for a patient to resist being restrained, to struggle against restraints, and then appear to stop struggling and calm down. In some cases, that patient may have actually stopped breathing and died. So, be very alert for any changes in any restrained patient's mental status–especially from agitated to calm. Reassess him frequently.

In any case, a good rule of thumb is to involve the chain of command and seek medical direction before you restrain a patient. This may be the best way to protect yourself legally. Follow local protocols.

Remember that law enforcement personnel also should be involved when you need to restrain a patient, when you need to give care without consent, and when there is any threat of violence. Law enforcement personnel can help protect you from injury, and they can serve as credible witnesses if a legal case arises.

The best way to protect yourself against false accusations by a patient is to carefully and completely document everything that happens during the call. Failure to document the care you provide implies to a judge and jury that it was not done. This can have serious legal consequences.

Another source of protection is witnesses, preferably throughout the entire course of treatment. Emotionally disturbed patients can wrongfully accuse medical personnel of sexual misconduct. To protect yourself against such allegations, involve other EMS providers who can testify that there was no misconduct. Use EMS responders who are the same gender as the patient and involve third-party witnesses whenever possible.

SKILL SUMMARY   *Assisting with the Combative Patient*

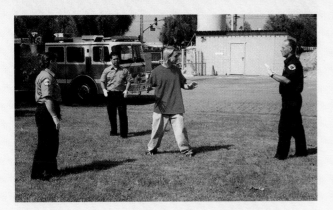

FIGURE 17-3A *If asked to assist other EMS providers, stay beyond the range of the patient's arms and legs.*

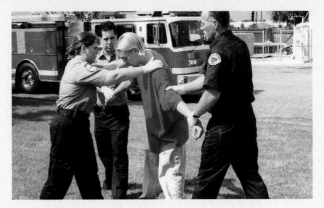

FIGURE 17-3B *If restraining is needed, work in conjunction with an adequate number of other EMS providers.*

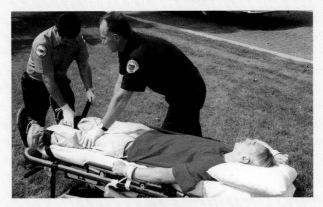

FIGURE 17-3C *You also may be asked to assist the EMTs when they apply ankle and wrist restraints.*

Legal Considerations

Your legal problems are greatly reduced if an emotionally disturbed patient consents to care. However, such patients commonly refuse treatment—especially patients who are intoxicated or who have taken a drug overdose. They may even threaten you or others. Unless the patient is considered mentally incompetent, legally he or she must provide consent before you can treat. Remember, the patient—not concerned family members—must consent to care.

Generally, you may provide care against a patient's will only if the patient threatens to hurt him- or herself or others and only if you can demonstrate reason to believe that the patient's threats are real. A good rule of thumb to follow is to consult with medical direction and involve law enforcement.

Q:

1. What is a behavioral emergency?

2. What are some conditions that can cause a behavioral emergency?

3. How can you ensure your own safety during a call for a behavioral emergency?

4. How can a rescuer prevent positional asphyxia in a restrained patient?

5. May you provide emergency care in a behavioral emergency against the patient's will? Explain your answer.

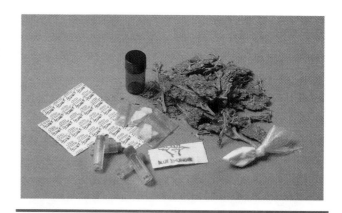

FIGURE 17-4 Examples of illegal drugs.

Section 2 Drug and Alcohol Emergencies

Drug abuse is the self-administration of one or more drugs in a way that differs from approved medical or social practice. An **overdose** is an emergency that involves poisoning by drugs or alcohol. The term **withdrawal** refers to the effects on the body that occur after a period of abstinence from the drugs or alcohol to which the body has become accustomed. Note that withdrawal—especially from alcohol—can be as serious as an overdose emergency.

Many drug overdoses involve drug abuse by long-time drug users. (See Figure 17-4.) However, a drug overdose also can be the result of miscalculation, confusion, use of more than one drug, or a suicide attempt.

Various drugs can cause changes in respiration, heart rate, blood pressure, and central nervous system function. In addition, several major medical problems can result from a drug or alcohol overdose or from sudden withdrawal (Figure 17-5). Among them are respiratory problems, internal injuries, seizures, hypothermia or hyperthermia, and cardiac arrest.

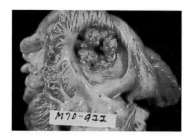

a. *Fungal-damaged heart related to drug injections.*

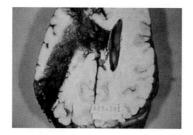

b. *Bullet wound to the brain, from alcohol-related shooting.*

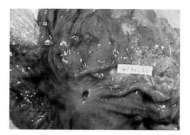

c. *Chronic gastric ulcer from alcohol abuse.*

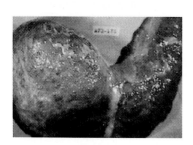

d. *Alcoholic cirrhosis of the liver.*

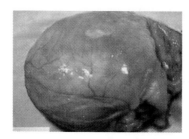

e. *Enlarged weak heart, alcohol-related.*

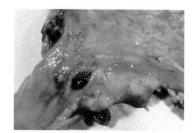

f. *Ruptured vein in esophagus, alcohol-induced.*

FIGURE 17-5 Major problems, even death, can result from overdose or abuse of alcohol and other drugs.

SIGNS OF A DRUG OR ALCOHOL EMERGENCY

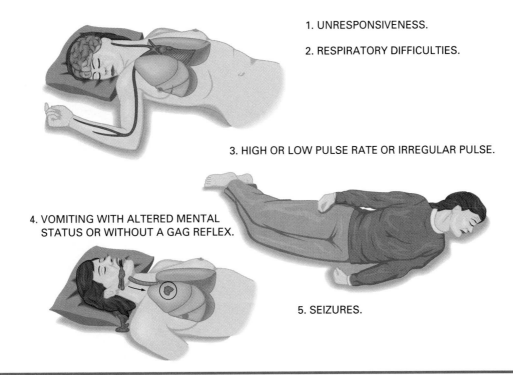

1. UNRESPONSIVENESS.

2. RESPIRATORY DIFFICULTIES.

3. HIGH OR LOW PULSE RATE OR IRREGULAR PULSE.

4. VOMITING WITH ALTERED MENTAL STATUS OR WITHOUT A GAG REFLEX.

5. SEIZURES.

FIGURE 17-6 Drug and alcohol emergencies can present with a variety of signs.

Patient Assessment

Signs and symptoms that indicate a life-threatening emergency include (Figure 17-6):

- Unresponsiveness.
- Breathing difficulties or inability to maintain an open airway.
- Abnormal or irregular pulse.
- Vomiting with an altered mental status (including unresponsiveness).
- Seizures.

If these signs and symptoms are present, your patient is a high priority for transport. Report to dispatch immediately. Additional signs and symptoms will vary widely. They may include:

- Altered mental status.
- Extremely low or high blood pressure.
- Sweating, tremors, and hallucinations (with alcohol withdrawal).
- Digestive problems, including abdominal pain and bleeding.
- Visual disturbances, slurred speech, uncoordinated muscle movement.
- Disinterested behavior, loss of memory.

- Combativeness.
- Paranoia.

If your patient is unresponsive and you suspect a drug or alcohol emergency, after your initial assessment proceed with the following:

- With a gloved hand, check the patient's mouth for partially dissolved pills or tablets. If you find any, remove them so they cannot block the patient's airway.
- Smell the patient's breath for traces of alcohol. Do not confuse the smell of alcohol with a musky, fruity, or acetone odor. Those three can indicate an emergency related to diabetes.
- Ask the patient's friends or family members what they know about the incident.

Because signs and symptoms vary so widely and are so similar to many medical conditions, the most reliable indications of a drug- or alcohol-related emergency are likely to come from the scene and the patient history. ■

First Responder Care

To care for a patient with a drug or alcohol emergency, your immediate goals are to protect your own safety, maintain the patient's airway, and manage life-threatening conditions (Figure 17-7). After taking BSI precautions, if you believe the patient has overdosed, follow the instruction offered below and in Chapter 15 for poisoning.

ALCOHOL EMERGENCIES

CAUTION: Do not immediately decide that a patient with apparent alcohol on the breath is drunk. The signs may indicate an illness or injury such as epilepsy, diabetes, or head injury.

SIGNS OF INTOXICATION
• Odor of alcohol on the breath.
• Swaying and unsteadiness.
• Slurred speech.
• Nausea and vomiting.
• Flushed face.
• Drowsiness.
• Violent, destructive, or erratic behavior.
• Self-injury, usually without realizing it.

EFFECTS
• Alcohol is a depressant. It affects judgment, vision, reaction time, and coordination.
• When taken with other depressants, the result can be greater than the combined effects of the two drugs.
• In very large quantities, alcohol can paralyze the respiratory center of the brain and cause death.

MANAGEMENT
• Give the same attention as you would to any patient with an illness or injury.
• Monitor the patient's vital signs constantly. Provide life support when necessary.
• Position the patient to avoid aspiration of vomit.
• Protect the patient from hurting him- or herself.

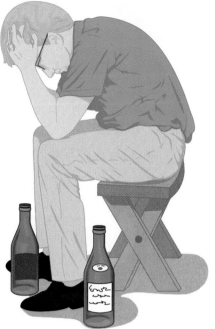

FIGURE 17-7 For an alcohol emergency, your immediate goals are your own safety, patient airway care, and care of life-threats.

1. *Establish and maintain an open airway.* Remove anything from the unresponsive patient's throat or mouth that might obstruct the airway, including loose-fitting false teeth, blood, or mucus. In case of vomiting, turn the patient's head to the side for drainage (unless trauma is suspected).

2. *Administer oxygen* to the patient by nonrebreather mask. If the patient is breathing inadequately, assist ventilations. Overdoses of narcotic medications, such as heroin, oxycontin, other pain medications, cause significantly reduced respiratory effort. Provide artificial ventilation to nonbreathing patients.

3. *Monitor the patient's mental status and vital signs frequently.* Overdose patients can be alert one minute and unresponsive the next. Be prepared to provide basic life support if needed.

4. *Maintain the patient's body temperature.* If the patient is cold, cover him with blankets.

5. *Take measures to prevent shock,* which can result from vomiting, profuse sweating, or inadequate fluid intake. Also be alert for allergic reactions.

6. *Manage the emergency as described earlier in this chapter.*

7. *Support the patient.* Comfort, calm, and reassure him while waiting for additional EMS personnel to arrive.

If the patient is responsive, try to get him to sit or lie down. Do not restrain a patient unless he poses a risk to safety—his, yours, or that of others. If the patient is unresponsive and you suspect trauma, begin emergency care by immediately stabilizing the patient's head and neck. If there is vomiting, carefully roll the patient as a unit to facilitate drainage. ■

Q: 1. Are drug emergencies always caused by drug abuse? Explain your answer.

2. What are the signs and symptoms of a life-threatening emergency in a patient with a drug or alcohol emergency?

3. Briefly, what are your emergency care goals for a patient with a drug or alcohol emergency?

Section 3 Rape and Sexual Assault

Rape is one of the most devastating crises that can occur in a person's life. It involves both emotional and physical trauma. Legally, **rape** is defined as sexual intercourse that is performed without consent and by compulsion through force, threat, or fraud. **Sexual assault** is defined as any touch that the victim did not initiate or agree to and that is imposed by coercion, threat, deception, or threats of physical violence.

Such crimes often are committed by someone the victim knows, such as a relative, friend or classmate, date, neighbor, or a friend of the parents.

Rape Trauma Syndrome

An intensely personal experience under forced or terrifying circumstances can destroy a person's inner defenses. Most rape victims go into acute emotional shock during or shortly after the attack. Common physical reactions to rape include:

- Struggling and screaming to avoid penetration.
- Physical and psychological paralysis.
- Pain and shock from penetration or physical abuse.
- Choking, gagging, nausea, vomiting.
- Urinating.
- Hyperventilating.
- Dazed state, unresponsiveness.

Following rape, most patients experience a great deal of disorganization in their lives. This emotional trauma follows a pattern described as **rape trauma syndrome.** It involves four general stages. The first is acute (impact) reaction, which takes effect immediately after the rape and continues for several days. The second is outward adjustment, which lasts for weeks or months after the rape. Depression is third; it is recurring for days and months after the rape. Finally, there is acceptance and resolution, which takes months or years.

Rape is a difficult and complex problem. It involves physical and emotional trauma, as well as significant legal issues. Supporting the patient is of critical importance, especially during the acute reaction stage. When you care for such a patient, remember that his or her coping system has already been stressed to the limit by the attack.

Note that too often the seriousness of rape is equated with physical damage alone. This is a mistake. Even if there are no external visible injuries, the rape victim will suffer profound emotional trauma.

Managing the Rape Scene

Keep the following considerations in mind:

- Be sure EMS has been activated.
- Your immediate reaction to the patient is important. Do not impose your own feelings. Instead, try to find out the patient's emotional state.

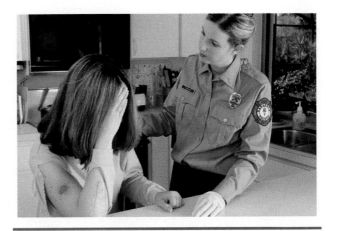

FIGURE 17-8 It may be best for a First Responder of the same gender to assist the rape patient.

- Action can minimize the helplessness the patient may be feeling. Tell the patient what can and should be done immediately.
- The patient might be comforted by a rescuer of his or her own gender (Figure 17-8).
- Perform patient assessment and care as you would for any patient. Also, check for trauma, especially around the thighs, lower abdomen, and buttocks. If vaginal bleeding is significant, give appropriate care.
- Do not clean the patient. Keep him or her from showering or bathing, brushing teeth, gargling, douching, or urinating. Cleaning could destroy important evidence.
- When you have cared for the patient's injuries, check the scene for evidence. If the police are present, they will handle evidence collection. If you must leave the scene with the patient before the police arrive, evidence should be preserved. Isolate and bag items separately to prevent cross contamination. Then, turn the evidence bags over to the police at the hospital. Follow local protocols.

Note that your documentation of the call should include the patient's chief complaint, information about the incident that relates to your care for injuries, and your objective observations and physical findings. Your notes may be used later as evidence in court.

1. What are some of the common physical reactions to rape?

2. What should your documentation of a call involving a suspected rape include?

The Call Follow-up

At the beginning of this chapter, you read that an agitated, naked male patient found wandering along a road has been restrained by the police. To see how chapter skills apply, read the following. It describes how the call was completed.

Physical Examination I spoke to the patient. He was beginning to calm down a little. He consented to care and then denied any injuries. Knowing that some conditions can affect mental status, I did a head-to-toe exam. It had to be quick, since the patient was still quite agitated. Pulse was 88 and bounding. His respirations were 20 and deep.

Patient History When the patient was quieter, I tried to gather a history. He was talking in a very confused manner. One minute he said he was a god. The next he was crying like a baby. He didn't have any medical identification tags on him. Since he had no clothes, he certainly didn't have a wallet I could check.

One of the officers said he thought he knew the patient's name from a prior call. The dispatcher checked the police computer and found that the man had done this several times before. He was a frequent patient at the psychiatric center in the next county.

Ongoing Assessment While the dispatcher's information answered some questions, I still felt that I should monitor the patient in case there was an underlying medical problem. However, the patient soon became agitated again, so I couldn't recheck vitals. There was really no other change that I could see.

Patient Hand-off When the EMTs arrived on scene, I gave them my report (see below). The EMTs asked the police to ride along with them to the hospital. Later, I found out that the hospital transferred the patient back to the psychiatric center. It seemed that whenever he stopped taking his medications, incidents like this would occur.

 Hand-off Report

"This is John Schmidt, a 38-year-old man, whom I found naked and walking along the road about 35 minutes ago. I called the police. When they arrived, they found out that a man by that name is an outpatient of Greystone Psychiatric Center and has had several similar incidents. I was able to do a quick head-to-toe exam and found no injuries. Vital signs: respirations, 20 and deep; and pulse, 88 and bounding. He told me he is God, and I observed some big emotional swings from happiness to crying."

The Last Word *Your patient's well-being is your responsibility. However, your own well-being is important, too. Call for law enforcement and for additional EMS resources whenever they are needed at the scene. Remember, a patient with a behavioral emergency may have a medical problem such as diabetes or overdose. Monitor these patients carefully.*

Chapter Review

Focus on the EMS Team

Keep in mind that many medical causes can lead to unusual behavior. Never assume the emergency is due to alcohol or other drugs. But remember: safety first. Not all patients with behavioral emergencies will want to harm you, but you must be cautious. Even when there is an underlying medical condition, such patients can be dangerous, if only to themselves. Don't hesitate to call for assistance when you need it.

When a behavioral emergency patient needs care, it's time to take out your best communication skills to get consent and to help keep him calm. Empathize, listen, and watch your body language. At the same time, your partner should be continually alert for any signs of danger. If there are signs, both of you should retreat and radio for law enforcement.

If the patient must be restrained, work in conjunction with the police and other EMS providers. And consult with medical direction. Do not attempt to restrain a patient yourself unless you are trained to do so and there are enough trained personnel on scene to help you.

Summing Up

- A behavioral emergency may be due to extremes of emotion, a psychological condition such as a mental illness, a medical condition such as lack of oxygen or low blood sugar, as well as abuse of alcohol or other drugs.

- Patients with behavioral emergencies may act in unusual and unexpected ways. They can pose a danger to themselves through self-inflicted injuries or suicide. They also can pose a danger to others through violence or actions they are not able to understand.

- Consider the need for law enforcement during your scene size-up and throughout the call. If you suspect that the patient is a threat to other or to him- or herself, arrange for backup law enforcement at the scene.

- Assess the patient's mental status by asking specific questions to determine whether or not the patient is oriented to time, person, and place. Watch the patient's appearance, level of activity, and speech patterns. And stay alert to any possible signs of danger. If possible, find out if the patient has been violent or has threatened violence at the scene.

- First Responder care includes calming and reassuring the patient, never leaving the patient alone, and providing the appropriate emergency care for any injuries.

- Restraining a patient should be avoided unless the patient poses a danger to himself or others. If restraint is needed, call for the police. And be sure extreme caution is used to prevent positional asphyxia. Seek medical direction and follow local protocol.

- If a patient refuses care, provide it only if the patient threatens to hurt himself or others and only if you can demonstrate reason to believe that the patient's threats are real. Consult with medical direction and involve law enforcement.

- Document everything that happens during a behavioral emergency call. Involve third-party witnesses whenever possible.

- Because signs and symptoms of drug and alcohol emergencies vary so widely and are so similar to many medical conditions, the most reliable indications are likely to come from the scene and the patient history. However, if there is unresponsiveness, breathing difficulties, abnormal or irregular pulse, vomiting with an altered mental status, and seizures, immediately arrange for rapid transport.

- For a patient with a drug or alcohol emergency, your immediate goals are to protect your own safety, maintain the patient's airway, and manage life-threatening conditions. When you suspect trauma in the unresponsive patient, manually stabilize the head and neck.

- Most rape victims go into acute emotional shock during or shortly after the attack. Supporting them is of critical importance, as is care for any injuries.

- Do your best to preserve evidence at a rape scene. Also document the call objectively and carefully.

Key Terms

behavior the manner in which a person acts or performs.

behavioral emergency a situation in which a patient exhibits abnormal behavior, or behavior that is unacceptable or intolerable to the patient, family, or community.

drug abuse the self-administration of one or more drugs in a way that differs from approved medical or social practice.

overdose an emergency that involves poisoning by alcohol or other drugs.

positional asphyxia suffocation caused by the position a patient is in, usually face-down; associated with hog-tie or hobble restraints.

rape sexual intercourse that is performed without consent and by compulsion through force, threat, or fraud.

rape trauma syndrome a reaction to rape that involves four general stages: acute (impact) reaction, outward adjustment, depression, and acceptance and resolution.

reasonable force refers to the amount of force needed to keep a patient from injuring himself or someone else.

sexual assault any touch that the victim did not initiate or agree to and that is imposed by coercion, threat, deception, or threats of physical violence.

withdrawal refers to the effects on the body that occur after a period of abstinence from the drugs or alcohol to which the body has become accustomed.

Knowledge Check

1. **Which one of the following is a good way to calm a behavioral emergency patient?**
   a. Lie if it seems like the truth will upset him.
   b. Talk about anything except the current problem.
   c. Use a calm, reassuring tone when you speak to him.
   d. Pat him on the back, touch his elbow, and stay close.

2. **Which one of the following statements is FALSE?**
   a. Psychiatric patients are usually restrained.
   b. Use only reasonable force to restrain a patient.
   c. Restrained patients should be constantly monitored.
   d. Patients should be restrained in a face-up position.

3. **Until there is more information available, First Responders should consider a patient who is acting in a bizarre way as having a(n):**
   a. allergy to alcohol.
   b. alcohol abuse problem.
   c. psychiatric condition.
   d. altered mental status.

4. **First Responder care for an intoxicated patient includes:**
   a. placing him in a prone position in case he vomits.
   b. protecting him from hurting himself and others.
   c. exposing him to cold weather so he will sober up.
   d. restraining him in case he decides to get violent.

5. **Signs and symptoms of a life-threatening drug or alcohol emergency include all of the following EXCEPT:**
   a. vomiting with an altered mental status.
   b. inability to maintain an open airway.
   c. unresponsiveness and abnormal pulse.
   d. loss of memory and slurred speech.

6. **Withdrawal—especially from alcohol—can be as serious as an overdose emergency.**
   a. True
   b. False

7. When your patient is having a behavioral emergency, his or her safety is legally the responsibility of law enforcement.

   a. True
   b. False

8. List six signs that can help you determine if your patient is likely to become violent.

   _____   _____

   _____   _____

   _____   _____

9. List three ways to let the behavioral emergency patient know you are listening to what he or she is telling you.

   _____

   _____

   _____

Scenario

You are called to a college dormitory where you are met by several young men. They tell you that one of their friends must have had too much alcohol and is passed out on the floor of their communal bathroom. You and your partner are then led to the scene.

a. On the way, you bring to mind your most immediate goals for this type of emergency. What are they?

   _____

   _____

   _____

b. You determine that the scene is safe to enter. You find the patient lying nearly prone on the tile floor in the open space between the sinks and the urinals. There is a large pool of vomit beside him and more vomit trailing from his mouth. What should you do for the patient first?

   _____

   _____

   _____

c. While you wait for the EMTs to arrive on scene, what else should you do for the patient?

   _____

   _____

   _____

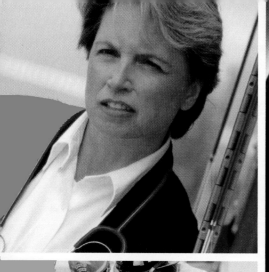
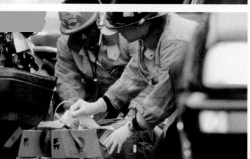
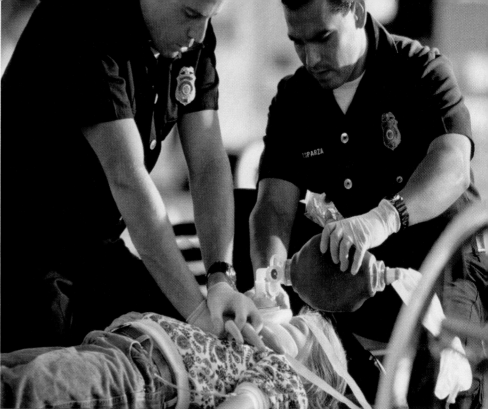

18 | Bleeding and Shock

Objectives

From the U.S. Department of Transportation (DOT) 1995 "First Respon-der: National Standard Curriculum." Material supplemental to the DOT cur-riculum is listed under "Enrichment."

Cognitive

5-2.1 ▸ Differentiate between arterial, venous, and capillary bleeding. (pp. 328–330)

5-2.2 ▸ State the emergency medical care for external bleeding. (pp. 330–334)

5-2.3 ▸ Establish the relationship between body substance isolation and bleeding. (p. 327)

5-2.4 ▸ List the signs of internal bleeding. (p. 334)

5-2.5 ▸ List the steps in the emergency medical care of the patient with signs and symptoms of internal bleeding. (p. 334)

Affective

5-2.15 ▸ Explain the rationale for body substance isolation when dealing with bleeding and soft tissue injuries. (p. 327)

5-2.16 ▸ Attend to the feelings of the patient with a soft tissue injury or bleeding. (pp. 330, 334, 338)

5-2.17 ▸ Demonstrate a caring attitude toward patients with a soft tissue injury or bleeding who request emergency medical services. (pp. 330, 334, 338)

5-2.18 ▸ Place the interests of the patient with a soft tissue injury or bleeding as the foremost consideration when making any and all patient care decisions. (pp. 330, 334, 338)

5-2.19 ▸ Communicate with empathy to patients with a soft tis-sue injury or bleeding, as well as with family members and friends of the patient. (pp. 330, 334, 338)

Psychomotor

5-2.20 ▸ Demonstrate direct pressure as a method of emergency medical care for external bleeding. (pp. 330, 331)

5-2.21 ▸ Demonstrate the use of diffuse pressure as a method of emergency medical care for external bleeding. (pp. 330–334)

5-2.22 ▸ Demonstrate the use of pressure points as a method of emergency medical care for external bleeding. (pp. 330, 331, 332)

Introduction

Bleeding associated with trauma can be a significant, life-threatening emergency. If bleeding is left untreated, your patient could deteriorate rapidly, go into shock, and die. Control of severe external bleeding is performed during the initial assessment. Only airway and breathing have a higher priority. Internal bleeding is more difficult to detect and may be even more deadly than external bleeding. Both internal bleeding and shock are treated immediately following the initial assessment.

Section 1 Bleeding

Protection Against Infection

Always take steps to protect yourself from diseases that can be transmitted by way of blood and body fluids. This is especially urgent when your patient has external bleeding. Body substance isolation (BSI) precautions are your best defense. (This may be a good time to review Chapter 2, "Well-Being of the First Responder.")

Briefly, BSI precautions include keeping a barrier between you and the patient's blood and body fluids. That is, at a minimum, wear a pair of disposable protective gloves. When you provide ventilations, use a face mask with a one-way valve. Wear an approved face shield, or protective eyewear and mask plus gown if there is spurting or splashing of blood or the potential for it. Keep all of the patient's open wounds covered with dressings. Never touch your mouth, nose, or eyes or handle food while you are giving emergency care, and wash your hands properly as soon as you have finished treating the patient. Decontaminate or properly dispose of any item that has been in contact with the patient's blood or body fluids. (Follow all local protocols.)

How the Body Responds to Blood Loss

Blood is part of the body's circulatory system (Figure 18-1). The natural response of the body to bleeding—external or internal—is blood vessel constriction and blood clotting.

When a serious injury prevents that response, uncontrolled bleeding may be the result.

The sudden loss of one liter (1,000 cc) of blood in an adult is serious. About one-half liter (500 cc) of blood loss is serious in a child. In an infant 100 cc to 200 cc blood loss can be serious. (See Figure 18-2.) Just how severe bleeding is depends on other factors, too. They are:

■ Size of the blood vessel and how fast it is bleeding.

■ Whether the blood is flowing from an artery or a vein. (Bleeding from an artery is faster and more profuse.)

■ Whether the bleeding is external or internal.

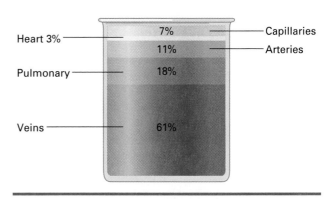

DISTRIBUTION OF BLOOD IN THE BODY

Heart 3% — 7% — Capillaries
11% — Arteries
Pulmonary — 18%
Veins — 61%

FIGURE 18-1 Blood is part of the circulatory system.

THE CALL

Dispatch Our first-response unit was dispatched to a call for a laceration.

Scene Size-up When we arrived on scene, we parked at the curb. A woman opened the door of the house and approached our vehicle. She told us that she had been installing linoleum in her kitchen. She slipped with a knife and was bleeding badly from her arm. There were no dangers or hazards we could see, so we exited our vehicle. We put on our gloves and face shields right away.

Initial Assessment We saw that the woman was holding a blood-soaked towel to her arm. She appeared to be alert and oriented. She had no airway problems and was breathing adequately. Blood was still flowing from beneath the towel.

What steps would you take to control this woman's bleeding? How much blood has she lost? At what point could her bleeding become critical? Consider this patient as you read Chapter 18.

- Whether or not the bleeding is a threat to respiration. (Bleeding in the patient's airway could compromise breathing.)
- Patient's age, weight, and general physical condition.

In general, bleeding is considered severe when the patient's pulse quickens, level of responsiveness falls, breathing rate increases, and skin becomes pale. Eventually, the blood pressure will drop, but this is a late sign of severe blood loss. Uncontrolled bleeding or significant blood loss can lead to shock and, possibly, death. (Read about shock later in this chapter.)

First on Scene

As soon as you learn that your patient is a trauma patient, get out your gloves. They are always required. Wear all appropriate personal protective equipment when you are controlling bleeding. And don't forget to protect your eyes and mouth (mucous membranes of the face) from splashing or spurting blood and other body fluids. On those occasions, wear a face shield, or protective eyewear and a mask, plus gloves and gown.

External Bleeding

There are three types of external bleeding—**arterial, venous,** and **capillary.** Each type can be life-threatening.

Patient Assessment

Each of the three types of bleeding has its own characteristics (Figure 18-3). They are:

- **Arterial bleeding**—Bright red blood spurting from a wound usually indicates a severed or damaged artery. The blood is bright red because it is rich in oxygen. Spurting generally coincides with the patient's pulse or contractions of the heart. Because blood in the arteries is under high pressure, this type of bleeding can be more difficult to control than any other. As the patient's blood pressure drops, the arterial spurting also may decrease (a late sign of shock).

- **Venous bleeding**—Dark red blood that flows steadily from a wound usually indicates a severed or damaged vein. The blood is dark red because it holds little or no oxygen. It flows steadily because it is under less pressure than blood in the arteries. Venous bleeding may be profuse, but it is usually easier to control than arterial bleeding.

- **Capillary bleeding**—Dark red blood that oozes slowly from a wound usually indicates damaged capillaries. In most cases, this type of bleeding clots spontaneously and is controlled easily. However, if the body surface

THE FOUR STAGES OF HEMORRHAGE

CLASS 1	CLASS 2	CLASS 3	CLASS 4
Up to 15% blood loss	Up to 30% blood loss	Up to 40% blood loss	More than 40% blood loss

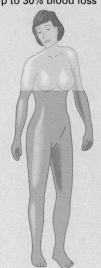
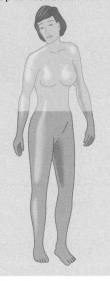
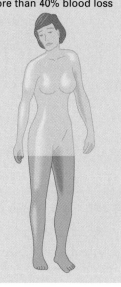

HOW THE BODY RESPONDS

The body compensates for blood loss by constricting blood vessels (vasoconstriction) in an effort to maintain blood pressure and delivery of oxygen to all organs of the body.

EFFECT ON PATIENT

• Patient remains alert.
• Blood pressure stays within normal limits.
• Pulse stays within normal limits or increases slightly; pulse quality remains strong.
• Respiratory rate and depth, skin color, and temperature all remain normal.

*The average adult has 5 liters (1 liter = approximately 1 quart) of circulating blood; 15% is 750 ml (or about 3 cups). With internal bleeding 750 ml will occupy enough space in a limb to cause swelling and pain. With bleeding into the body cavities, however, the blood will spread throughout the cavity, causing little, if any initial discomfort.

• Vasoconstriction continues to maintain adequate blood pressure, but with some difficulty.
• Blood flow is shunted to vital organs, with decreased flow to intestines, kidneys, and skin.

EFFECT ON PATIENT

• Patient may become confused and restless.
• Skin turns pale, cool, and dry because of shunting of blood to vital organs.
• Diastolic pressure may rise or fall. It's more likely to rise (because of vasoconstriction) or stay the same in otherwise healthy patients with no underlying cardio-vascular problems.
• Pulse pressure (difference between systolic and diastolic pressures) narrows.
• Sympathetic responses also cause rapid heart rate (over 100 beats per minute). Pulse quality weakens.
• Respiratory rate increases because of sympathetic stimulation.
• Delayed capillary refill.

• Compensatory mechanisms become overtaxed. Vaso-constriction, for example, can no longer sustain blood pressure, which now begins to fall.
• Cardiac output and tissue perfusion continue to decrease, becoming potentially life threatening. (Even at this stage, however, the patient can still recover with prompt treatment.)

EFFECT ON PATIENT

• Patient becomes more confused, restless, and anxious.
• Classic signs of shock appear—rapid heart rate, decreased blood pressure, rapid respiration and cool, clammy extremities.

• Compensatory vasoconstriction now becomes a complicating factor in itself, further impairing tissue perfusion and cellular oxygenation.

EFFECT ON PATIENT

• Patient becomes lethargic, drowsy, or stuporous.
• Signs of shock become more pronounced. Blood pressure continues to fall.
• Lack of blood flow to the brain and other vital organs ultimately leads to organ failure and death.

FIGURE 18-2 Learn the signs and symptoms of blood loss.

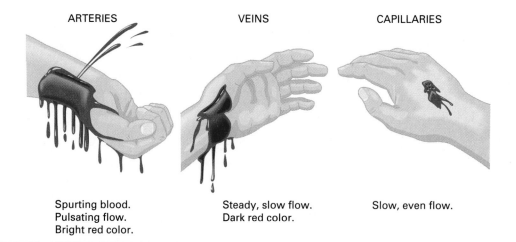

ARTERIES   VEINS   CAPILLARIES

Spurting blood.
Pulsating flow.
Bright red color.

Steady, slow flow.
Dark red color.

Slow, even flow.

FIGURE 18-3 **Types of external bleeding.**

involved is large, bleeding may be profuse and threat of infection may be great.

Note that pulse oximetry has only a limited value when there is blood loss. Instead, you can determine the patient's perfusion status by assessing level of responsiveness, pulse rate, and skin color. ■

First Responder Care

To provide care to a patient with external bleeding, first be sure you have taken BSI precautions. Then, follow these directions (Figure 18-4):

1. *Apply direct pressure to the wound.* If profuse bleeding is discovered during the initial assessment, apply pressure to the bleeding site with your gloved hand until dressings can be applied. As soon as possible, place a sterile gauze pad or dressing over the bleeding wound. If the wound is small, apply pressure directly over the point of bleeding using the flat part of your fingertips. If it is large and gaping, pack the wound with sterile gauze and apply direct hand pressure.

2. *Elevate the bleeding extremity.* As you apply direct pressure, lift the bleeding arm or leg above the level of the heart. This should slow the flow of blood and aid in clotting. NOTE: If you suspect a possible bone or joint injury, do *not* elevate the extremity.

3. *Assess bleeding.* If the wound has bled through the dressing, apply another dressing on top of it. Then, reapply direct pressure.

4. *Use pressure points.* If the bleeding in an extremity persists, apply pressure to the arterial pulse point to help reduce blood flow (Figure 18-5).

   —For bleeding in the arm, find the brachial pulse point. Then, use the flat surfaces of your fingers to compress the artery against the bone.

   —For bleeding in the leg, find the femoral pulse point. Use the heel of one hand to compress it.

   Because a number of arteries supply each extremity, you may need to use a pressure point at the same time you apply direct pressure to the wound. Always reassess bleeding immediately after using a pressure point to make sure that it has been controlled.

5. *Support your patient* while you wait for additional EMS personnel to arrive. Communicate with empathy. Comfort, calm, and reassure him or her. Keep safety and patient care your main priorities. ■

> ✓ | **First Responder Practice**
>
> Management of life-threatening bleeding must occur during the initial assessment. Only a patient's airway and breathing take precedence. In some cases, you may need to care for a patient's airway and breathing at the same time you control bleeding.

Other Methods of Bleeding Control

Two other methods of bleeding control are the use of a **splint** and the use of a **tourniquet.** Be sure to follow local protocols.

Splints.   Bleeding can be life-threatening in an open wound to an extremity that also has a bone or joint injury. If left unsplinted, the bone ends or bone fragments can move, damaging soft tissues and blood vessels and causing more bleeding. Immobilizing the extremity with a splint

SKILL SUMMARY *Controlling Bleeding*

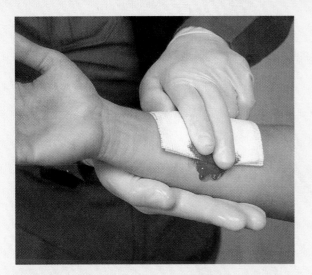

FIGURE 18-4A *Apply direct pressure.*

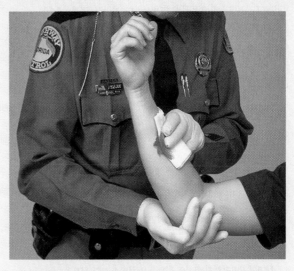

FIGURE 18-4B *Elevate the extremity.*

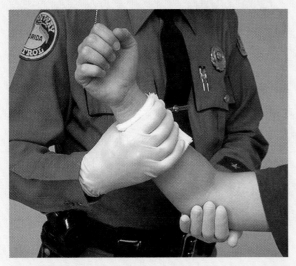

FIGURE 18-4C *Assess bleeding and apply additional pressure if needed.*

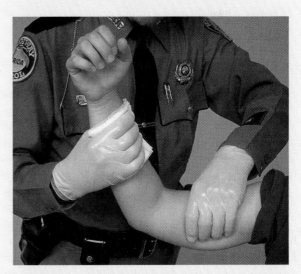

FIGURE 18-4D *If bleeding persists, use a pressure point.*

can help to avoid these problems. (For information on splinting, see Chapter 25.)

A special splint is used in some EMS systems. An *air splint* (also called a "pressure splint") can exert pressure to an extremity to help provide additional bleeding control. It may be effective over a wound larger than your hand, which would be difficult to control with direct pressure. Note that an air splint will not provide enough pressure to control arterial bleeding or other types of severe bleeding.

To apply pressure to a bleeding wound with an air splint, be sure the wound is dressed and bandaged first. (See Chapter 25 for information on how to apply an air splint.)

Tourniquets. A tourniquet should be used only as a last resort to control life-threatening bleeding when all other methods have failed. Because it can stop all blood flow to an extremity, use a tourniquet only as a last resort. A tourniquet can cause permanent damage to nerves, muscles, and blood vessels, and it can result in the loss of the affected extremity. Always seek medical direction before using a tourniquet and follow local protocols.

To apply a tourniquet (Figure 18-6), first select a bandage four inches wide and six to eight layers deep. Wrap it around the extremity twice at a point above but as close to the wound as possible. Tie a knot in the

Arterial pulse points are places where an artery lies close to the skin or passes over a bony prominence. When an artery is so located, it can be palpated, or felt with gentle fingertip pressure. Since most body parts are supplied by more than one artery, the use of arterial pressure points alone rarely controls hemorrhage. However, compression of arterial pulse points *in addition to direct pressure* can sometimes help to control severe bleeding. Major arterial pulse points include:

- **Carotid arteries** are located on each side of the neck next to the larynx. These two arteries supply blood to the head. *Do not exert pressure on the carotid pulse points.*

- **Maxillary arteries** supply much of the blood to the face. One can be palpated on each side of the face on the inner surface of the lower jaw.

- **Temporal arteries** supply part of the blood supply to the scalp. One can be palpated on each side of the face just above the upper portion of the ear.

- **Brachial arteries,** located on the inner arms just above the elbows, supply blood to the arms.

- **Radial** and **ulnar arteries,** located in the wrist, also supply blood to the arms and hands.

- **Femoral arteries,** which pass through the groin, supply blood to the legs.

- **Posterior tibial artery,** which passes through the ankle, and the **dorsalis pedis artery,** on the front surface of the foot, can determine circulation to the feet.

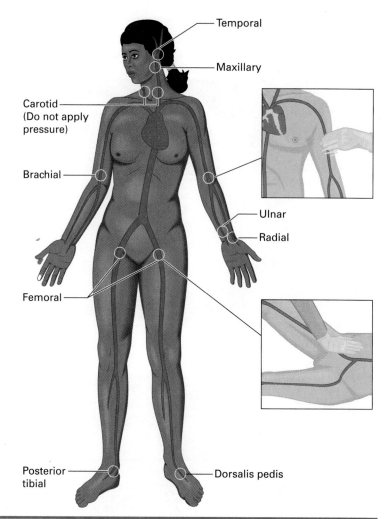

FIGURE 18-5 Arterial pulse points.

bandage material. Then, place a stick or rod on top of the knot. Tie the ends of the bandage again in a square knot over the stick. Twist the stick until the bleeding stops. Secure the stick or rod in position. Note the time. Finally, notify the EMTs who take over patient care that you have applied a tourniquet.

In some cases an inflated blood pressure cuff may be used as a tourniquet until bleeding stops. If you choose to do this, you need to monitor the cuff continuously to make sure pressure is maintained.

When using any type of tourniquet, take the following precautions:

- Always use a wide bandage and secure it tightly. Never use a wire, belt, or any other material that could cut the skin or underlying soft tissues.

- Once applied, never loosen or remove a tourniquet unless you are directed to do so by medical direction.

- Never apply a tourniquet directly over a joint.

- Always make sure the tourniquet is in open view. A tourniquet covered by clothing or bandages may be overlooked, resulting in permanent tissue damage.

Nosebleeds

Nosebleeds are a relatively common source of bleeding. They can result from an injury, disease, activity, the environment, or other causes. Generally, they are more annoying than serious. However, enough blood can be lost to cause shock. In an unresponsive patient, a nosebleed also can be a serious threat to respiration.

In most cases a nosebleed may be treated as follows (Figure 18-7): First, position the patient. Keep him still and calm. Have him sit leaning forward in order to prevent aspiration of blood into the lungs. (Do not let the patient lean so far forward that the head is below the heart.) If sitting is impossible because of other injuries, have the patient lie down with head and shoulders elevated. Then, if you do *not* suspect a nasal fracture, pinch

USING A TOURNIQUET

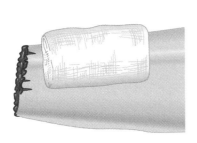

1. Apply pad

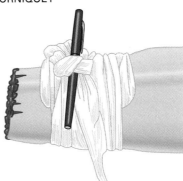

2. Tighten tourniquet

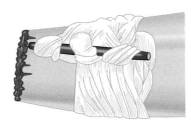

3. Fix in place

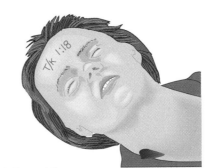

4. Record time

FIGURE 18-6 Apply a tourniquet only as a last resort.

the nostrils together to apply pressure. Finally, apply cold compresses to the nose and face.

When the bleeding has stopped, instruct the patient to avoid blowing his or her nose for several hours. This could dislodge the clot and restart bleeding. If bleeding continues and is severe enough, activate the EMS system if this has not already been done.

Note: If a fractured skull is suspected, do not try to stop a nosebleed. To do so might increase pressure on the brain. Cover the nasal opening loosely instead. Use

SKILL SUMMARY *Controlling a Nosebleed*

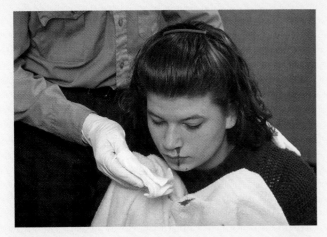

FIGURE 18-7A *Keep the patient quiet and leaning forward in a sitting position.*

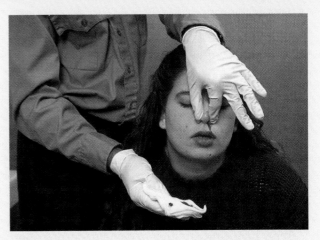

FIGURE 18-7B *Apply pressure by pinching the nostrils. Also apply cold compresses if needed.*

dry, sterile dressings. Do not apply pressure. Treat the patient for skull fracture as outlined in Chapter 23.

Internal Bleeding

When internal organs are injured or damaged, they may bleed. This type of bleeding, which is concealed inside the body, is called **internal bleeding.** It may result from a variety of causes including blunt trauma, abnormal clotting, rupture of a blood vessel, or a fracture (especially a pelvic fracture). Because it is not visible, internal bleeding can result in severe blood loss with rapid progression to shock and death—all in a matter of minutes.

The two most common sources of internal bleeding are injured or damaged internal organs and fractured extremities (especially fractures of the femur and pelvis). The severity of internal bleeding depends on the patient's overall condition, age, and the source of the bleeding.

Patient Assessment

Suspect internal bleeding if the mechanism of injury suggests it and if there is evidence of scrapes and bruises, swelling, deformity, or impact marks. Always suspect it if there are penetrating wounds to the skull, chest, or abdomen. Always suspect it in cases of unexplained shock. The signs and symptoms of internal bleeding are:

- Discolored, tender, swollen, or hard tissue.
- Increased respiratory and pulse rates.
- Pale, cool, clammy skin.
- Nausea and vomiting bright red blood or blood the color of dark coffee grounds.
- Thirst.
- Changes in mental status including anxiety, restlessness, or combativeness.
- Dark, tarry stools or stools that contain bright red blood.
- Tender, rigid, or distended abdomen.
- Weakness, faintness, or dizziness. ■

First Responder Care

If you suspect internal bleeding in your patient, update the incoming EMS personnel. This patient is a priority for immediate transport. Be sure you have taken BSI precautions. Then follow these steps:

1. *Maintain an open airway and adequate breathing.* Apply high-concentration oxygen by way of a nonrebreather mask, if allowed. If breathing is inadequate, assist ventilation by way of a BVM with supplemental oxygen. Provide artificial ventilation if needed.

2. *Control any external bleeding* with direct pressure, elevation, and pressure points when necessary.

3. *Keep the patient warm,* but be careful not to overheat him or her.

4. *Treat for shock* as described in the next section.

5. Always support, comfort, calm, and reassure the patient. Do not provide anything by mouth. ■

Q:

1. What precautions against infection should you take with a patient who is bleeding?

2. What amount of blood loss is considered serious in adult, child, and infant patients?

3. What are five methods of external bleeding control?

4. In addition to obvious blood loss, what are the signs of severe bleeding in a patient?

Section 2 Shock

Perfusion refers to the circulation of blood throughout a body organ or structure. Perfusion delivers oxygen and other nutrients to the body's cells and removes waste products. When the cells of the body do not receive the oxygen and other nutrients they need, they begin to fail and die. **Shock,** or *hypoperfusion,* is a condition that results from the inadequate delivery of oxygenated blood. If the condition persists, cell failure, organ failure, and death will follow. It is therefore imperative to survival for shock to be recognized and treated promptly.

Shock (hypoperfusion) can be caused by failure of the heart, abnormal dilation of blood vessels, or blood volume loss:

- *Failure of the heart.* Conditions that cause the heart to fail to provide oxygenated blood to the body include heart attack, coronary artery disease, heart-valve disease, pulmonary embolism (a blood clot), tension pneumothorax (air leaking from a lung into the chest cavity), and cardiac tamponade (fluid leaking into the sac around the heart).

- *Abnormal dilation of the blood vessels.* This is usually the result of a spine or head injury that causes the nervous system to lose control over the blood vessels. The blood vessels dilate (enlarge), causing blood pressure to drop and blood to pool in the outer areas of the body, away from vital organs.

- *Blood volume loss.* This is caused either by external or internal bleeding. It also may result from a profound

HYPOVOLEMIC SHOCK

Watch for shock in all trauma patients. They can lose fluids not only externally through hemorrhage, vomiting, or burns, but also internally through crush injuries and organ punctures.

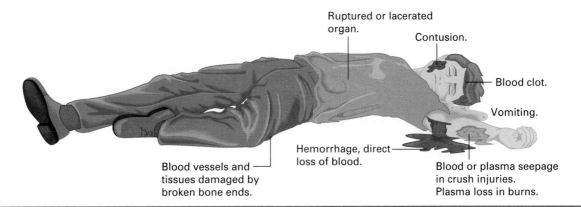

Ruptured or lacerated organ.

Contusion.

Blood clot.

Vomiting.

Hemorrhage, direct loss of blood.

Blood or plasma seepage in crush injuries. Plasma loss in burns.

Blood vessels and tissues damaged by broken bone ends.

FIGURE 18-8 Loss of blood and body fluids can be both external and internal.

fluid loss that occurs during illness or injury (Figure 18-8). One example is **plasma** loss due to burns. Another is **dehydration** due to diarrhea, vomiting, or excessive urination.

Patient Assessment

Shock passes through three stages: compensatory, decompensated, and irreversible (Figure 18-9). As it progresses, the body works hard to make sure oxygen reaches its cells.

First Responder Practice

Capillary refill testing and pulse oximetry are often considered in assessing trauma patients. However, both can lead to false conclusions:

- *Capillary refill*—delayed reaction may indicate shock, but it also may indicate hypothermia or a patient with poor circulation.
- *Pulse oximetry*—in cases of shock, the patient may have 100% oxygen saturation. But if the patient has lost 30%, 20%, or even 10% of his blood volume, the oximetry reading has little value.

Often, better tests are available. The patient's mental status, respirations, pulse, and skin condition are still the best and most reliable indications of shock.

However, if shock is severe or prolonged, it may become irreversible and end in death.

- **Compensatory shock**—In this first stage of shock, the body uses its defenses to try to maintain normal function. If the injury does not get worse, the body could overcome the condition. The signs and symptoms of shock at this stage are subtle. They include pale skin, slightly rapid heart rate, blood pressure in the normal range, restlessness or anxiety, and delayed capillary refill in the infant or child. Even though it is difficult to identify shock at this stage (be sure to consider the patient's mechanism of injury), it is vital that you recognize and treat shock early. You must prevent progression to the next more serious stage.

- **Decompensated shock**—At this stage, the body can no longer make up for reduced perfusion. Without medical intervention, further decline occurs. The body tries to keep vital organs perfused with oxygenated blood. It shunts blood away from arms, legs, and abdomen and directs it to the brain, heart, and lungs. As a result, tissues in the extremities and abdomen produce toxic by-products. Signs and symptoms include major changes in mental status, extreme thirst, rapid heart rate, decreased blood pressure, cool moist skin that is pale, gray, or bluish and mottled. (See Figure 18-10.) Decreased blood pressure is a very late sign of shock. Note that infants and children can maintain their blood pressure until blood volume is cut almost in half. Then, their condition suddenly and rapidly deteriorates. Dropping blood pressure in an infant or child is an ominous sign.

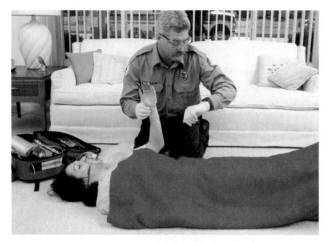

a. *Compensatory shock: slight increase in pulse.*

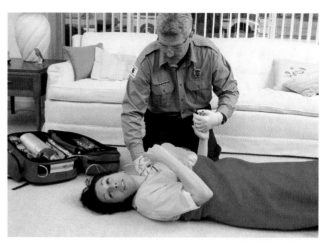

b. *Compensatory shock: restlessness or anxiety.*

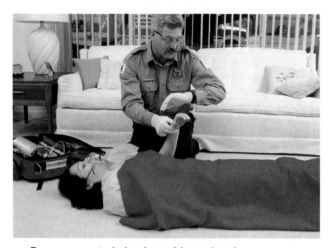

c. *Decompensated shock: rapid, weak pulse.*

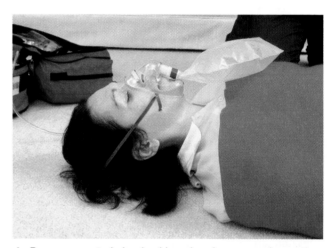

d. *Decompensated shock: skin color changes and sweating.*

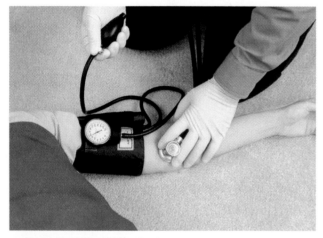

e. *Decompensated shock: decreasing blood pressure.*

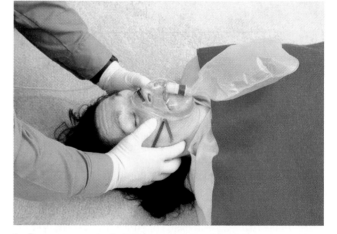

f. *Decompensated shock: unresponsiveness.*

FIGURE 18-9 As shock progresses, signs show that the body is working hard to get oxygen to the cells. If shock is prolonged, it can become irreversible and end in death.

SIGNS OF SHOCK

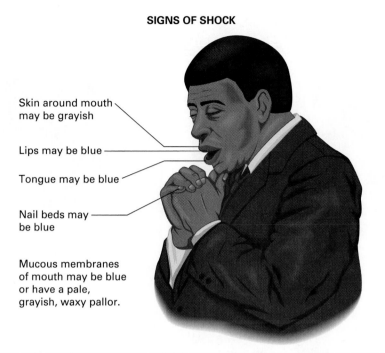

Skin around mouth may be grayish

Lips may be blue

Tongue may be blue

Nail beds may be blue

Mucous membranes of mouth may be blue or have a pale, grayish, waxy pallor.

FIGURE 18-10 Additional signs of shock in a dark-skinned patient.

- **Irreversible shock**—Blood flow is so low that body cells are dying. The main signs are very low blood pressure and extremely rapid pulse. At this stage, blood is shunted away from the liver and kidneys to the heart and brain. The liver and kidneys then die. Blood vessels can no longer sustain pressure, so blood begins to pool away from vital organs. Even with treatment, damage to vital organs is permanent. The inevitable result of irreversible shock is death. ■

Trauma is a major cause of shock in patients. You may recall from Chapter 1 that the **Golden Hour** refers to the urgency with which care must be given. It is based on the belief that seriously injured patients have the highest survival rates when they are on the operating table within 60 minutes of injury.

 First Responder Practice

By the time a patient exhibits signs and symptoms of shock, he is already in serious condition. The body is able to compensate for blood loss for some time, so when you finally see blood pressure drop, it is already very late. Watch for earlier signs of shock (mechanism of injury, altered mental status, elevated pulse, and skin color) and treat for shock immediately.

Your role as a First Responder is vital. The general rule is for an ambulance to remain on scene no longer than 10 minutes. You can help keep time to a minimum by identifying serious trauma patients, performing initial assessments and treatment, and preparing patients for transport. Be sure you have taken BSI precautions.

First Responder Care

To provide care to a patient with signs of shock, follow these steps (Figure 18-11):

1. *Maintain an open airway.* If breathing is adequate, administer oxygen by way of nonrebreather mask at 15 liters per minute. If breathing is inadequate, assist ventilation by way of a BVM with supplemental oxygen. Be prepared to provide artificial ventilation, if needed.

2. *Prevent further blood loss.* Control external bleeding through direct pressure, elevation, and pressure points if necessary.

3. *Elevate the lower extremities* about 8 to 12 inches. If there are serious injuries to the head, neck, spine, chest, abdomen, pelvis, or to the lower extremities, do *not* elevate them.

4. *Keep the patient warm,* but do not overheat him or her. Try to maintain normal body temperature. Use a blanket over and under the patient, if necessary, to help prevent loss of body heat.

5. *Provide care for specific injuries* while waiting for EMS crews to arrive.

SKILL SUMMARY   *Caring for a Patient with Signs of Shock*

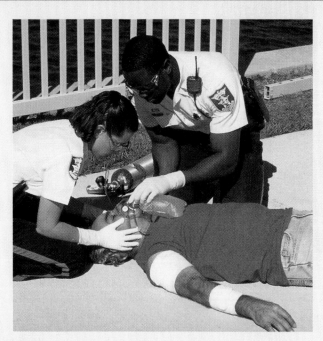

FIGURE 18-11A *After ensuring an open airway, administer oxygen, if you are allowed.*

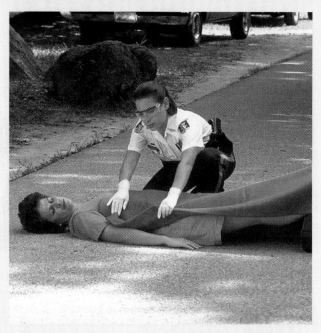

FIGURE 18-11B *Prevent any further blood loss. Then, when appropriate, elevate the shock patient's feet 8 to 12 inches. Also be sure to keep the patient warm.*

Be sure to comfort, calm, and reassure the patient while you wait for the EMTs to arrive on scene. Never give the patient anything to eat or drink. During the ongoing assessment, assess the patient's vital signs every five minutes and monitor for changes in mental status. Report your observations to the EMS crew when they take over patient care. ∎

Anaphylactic Shock

Anaphylactic shock results from a severe allergic reaction to a foreign protein. It can be caused by an insect sting, food, medicine, pollen, or some other inhaled, ingested, or injected substance. The most common causes of anaphylactic shock are drugs, foods such as peanuts, and bee stings (Figure 18-12). At least 1% of the general population is at risk for developing anaphylactic shock from bee stings alone.

Not every allergic reaction is anaphylactic shock. Patients who experience hives, itching, and blotchy skin may not develop more severe signs or symptoms. For an allergic reaction to be considered anaphylactic, there must be respiratory compromise, circulatory compromise (shock), or both.

Anaphylactic shock is a life-threatening medical emergency. A reaction can occur within seconds after a sting or other exposure. Immediate treatment is required to prevent death. Note that the shorter the time between exposure and the appearance of signs and symptoms, the greater the risk of a fatal reaction.

Note that an allergic reaction can occur 30 minutes or more after an exposure. All patients experiencing an allergic reaction of any type should be urged to seek medical care.

Patient Assessment

Anaphylactic shock is a life-threatening emergency involving the respiratory and/or circulatory systems and may involve any combination of the following signs and symptoms:

- Skin:
  —Warm, tingling feeling in the mouth, face, chest, feet, and hands.
  —Itching, hives, and flushing.
  —Swelling of the tongue, face, neck, hands, and feet.
  —Cyanosis.
  —Paleness.

ANAPHYLACTIC SHOCK

A grave medical emergency.
Anaphylactic shock is a severe allergic reaction to an injected, inhaled, or ingested foreign protein. Onset can occur within minutes, even seconds.

Early signs and symptoms.
• Flushing, itching. Skin rash
• Sneezing. Watery eyes and nose.
• Airway swelling.
• Cough. "Tickle" or "lump" in the throat that cannot be cleared.
• Gastrointestinal complaints.

The signs and symptoms of anaphylactic shock may swiftly lead to:

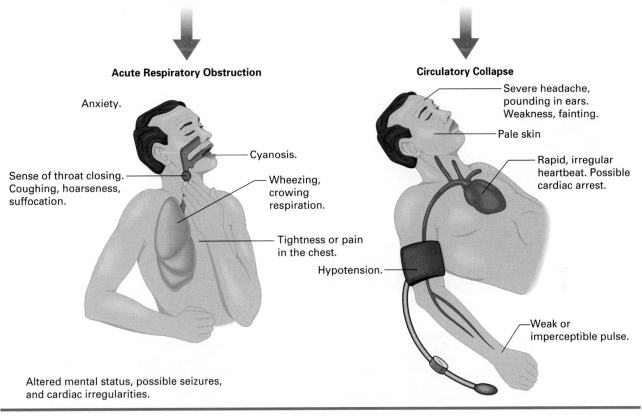

Acute Respiratory Obstruction

Anxiety.

Cyanosis.

Sense of throat closing. Coughing, hoarseness, suffocation.

Wheezing, crowing respiration.

Tightness or pain in the chest.

Altered mental status, possible seizures, and cardiac irregularities.

Circulatory Collapse

Severe headache, pounding in ears. Weakness, fainting.

Pale skin

Rapid, irregular heartbeat. Possible cardiac arrest.

Hypotension.

Weak or imperceptible pulse.

FIGURE 18-12 The most common causes of anaphylactic shock are drugs and bee stings.

■ Respiratory system:
— Swelling of the mouth, tongue, or throat leading to airway obstruction.
— Painful, squeezing sensation in the chest.
— Cough, hoarseness (losing the voice).
— Rapid or labored breathing.
— Noisy breathing, stridor, wheezing.
■ Circulatory system:
— Increased heart rate.

— Decreased blood pressure.
— Dizziness.
— Restlessness.
■ General findings:
— Itchy, watery eyes.
— Headache.
— Runny nose.
— Sense of impending doom.
— Decreasing mental status. ■

SKILL SUMMARY *Managing an Anaphylactic Reaction*

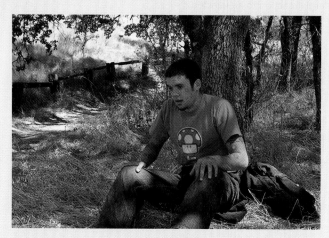

FIGURE 18-13A *Recognize the anaphylactic shock patient and perform an initial assessment.*

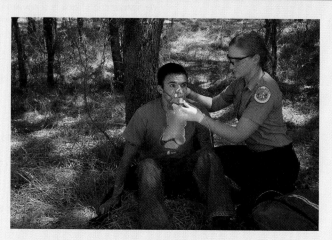

FIGURE 18-13B *Provide high-concentration oxygen by nonrebreather mask. If breathing is inadequate, assist ventilations by way of a BVM with supplemental oxygen.*

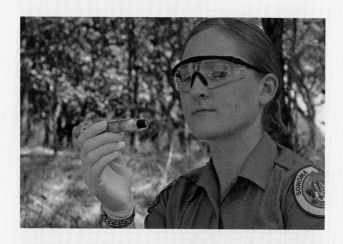

FIGURE 18-13C *If the patient has his own pre-scribed epinephrine auto-injector, check the expiration date and for cloudiness or discoloration. If allowed by medical direction, assist the patient in administration of the epinephrine.*

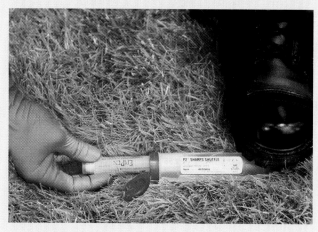

FIGURE 18-13D *Dispose of the used injector in a portable biohazard container.*

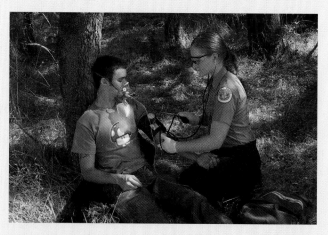

FIGURE 18-13E *Monitor the patient closely until the EMTs arrive on scene.*

First Responder Care

To provide care to a patient in anaphylactic shock, be sure EMS has been activated. The patient needs to be transported rapidly for further life-saving treatment. Arrange for advanced life support (ALS) care, if it is available. Then follow these steps (Figure 18-13):

1. *Perform an initial assessment.* Treat all life-threats. Be prepared to provide basic life support if it is needed.

2. *Administer 100% high-flow oxygen,* if you are equipped and allowed to do so. If breathing is adequate, deliver it by way of a nonrebreather mask. If breathing is inadequate, deliver it by way of BVM with supplemental oxygen. If the patient needs artificial ventilation, use supplemental oxygen.

3. *Assist the patient with his or her medications,* but only if local protocol allows you to do so. Medications may include an epinephrine auto-injector.

Note: Epinephrine is a medication that causes dilation (opening) of lung passages and constriction (narrowing) of blood vessels. That makes it the ideal drug to administer for anaphylaxis. The auto-injector dose is predetermined at 0.3 ml for adults and 0.15 ml for pediatric patients. It is administered in the lateral thigh and easily injects through clothes. Be sure to dispose of the auto-injector properly. Remember that epinephrine auto-injectors are used for anaphylaxis, not for simple, non-life-threatening allergic reactions. *Follow all local protocols.*

First Responder Practice

Assisting in the administration of any medication of any kind is an extreme responsibility. Always follow all local protocols.

If the patient's reaction is due to an insect sting or injection, local protocol may direct you to place a constricting band between the injection site and the heart. (See Chapter 16 for more specific directions.) During your ongoing assessment of the patient, monitor the patient's ABCs continually. Be prepared to deliver basic life support if it is needed. ■

1. What are the three stages of shock?

2. What is the "Golden Hour"? How does it affect First Responder care of an injured patient?

3. What is First Responder care for a patient with signs of shock?

▶▶ The Call Follow-up

At the beginning of this chapter, you read that First Responders were on scene with a woman who had what appeared to be serious bleeding from an arm. To see how chapter skills apply to this emergency, read the following. It describes how the call was completed.

Initial Assessment *(continued)* I saw blood flowing steadily from beneath the towel. This—combined with the amount of blood at the scene—indicated severe bleeding. I removed the towel, applied a sterile dressing and direct pressure to the wound. The bleeding stopped in two or three minutes. I kept up the pressure for a bit longer to make sure the bleeding stayed under control. Lian, my partner, updated the EMTs by radio.

Physical Examination The patient claimed to have slipped with her knife still in her hand. She denied injuring any other part of her body. My partner scanned the patient's body and saw that this appeared to be true. The patient did not fall to the ground or lose consciousness. There was no need to do a more detailed assessment. My partner took vitals. Pulse was 92, strong, and regular. Respirations were 16 and adequate. Blood pressure was 118/84. The patient's skin was cool and dry.

Patient History The patient claimed to be in good health. She took no medications, had no medical problems she knew of, and had a physical examination last year. She denied any allergies. She had lunch about two hours before the incident.

Ongoing Assessment We took another set of vitals. Pulse was 88, strong, and regular. Respirations were 16 and adequate. Blood pressure was 120/78. Her skin was cool and dry. We rechecked the status of her wound, which was stable (there was no more bleeding). We applied a pressure bandage to be sure it did not start again. We were careful not to cut off the patient's circulation. The EMTs arrived shortly after.

Patient Hand-off We advised the EMTs that the bleeding was under control in our hand-off report (see below). The EMTs took over care and applied oxygen to the patient. They transported her to the hospital. It was one of the worst cases of bleeding I had seen. I was glad we were able to get it under control. We saw the EMTs later. They told us that the patient's wound took a lot of stitches. She was considering another hobby.

Hand-off Report

"This is Jill Romano, 27 years old. She slipped with her knife while installing linoleum. The knife caused about a four-inch laceration to her left arm. The bleeding was steadily flowing on our arrival but was quickly brought under control by direct pressure. She did not lose consciousness or suffer any further injuries. Jill has no past medical history, no meds, no allergies. Her most recent vitals are pulse 88 strong and regular, respirations 16, blood pressure 120/78, skin cool and dry. Jill had lunch about two hours ago. We applied a pressure bandage. The bleeding is controlled and there is good circulation distal to the bandage."

The Last Word *A patient's blood can be an unnerving sight, especially if bleeding is profuse. One way to stay clear-headed is to stick to your patient assessment plan. Always start with scene size-up.*

Move to initial assessment and treatment. And continue, if you can, with a physical exam, a patient history, and ongoing assessment. Remember, your patient's well-being depends on it.

Chapter Review

Focus on the EMS Team

Severe bleeding is controlled during initial assessment and treatment. The only other problems that take priority concern the airway and breathing. Be assured, however, that even severe bleeding can be controlled by the simple methods described in this chapter—direct pressure, elevation, and pressure points. Experienced First Responders and EMTs will tell you that these methods work. Use them appropriately and confidently.

Keep in mind that whenever you suspect serious injury, it is critical to get the patient to the hospital as quickly as possible. This is because in many cases only surgery will correct internal bleeding and other life threats. As a First Responder, you can help save time on scene by quickly notifying incoming EMS units, by maintaining the patient's ABCs, and by assisting the EMTs in the backboarding process and in any other way required.

Summing Up

- Take BSI precautions with every patient to prevent exposure to blood and body fluids. Wash your hands after every call (it's one of the best ways to protect yourself against infection). Finally, decontaminate or properly dispose of any item that has been in contact with the patient's blood or body fluids.

- Sudden loss of one liter or 1,000 cc of blood is serious in an adult, half of that is serious in a child, and 100 cc to 200 cc is serious in an infant. In general, bleeding is considered severe when the patient's pulse quickens, level of responsiveness falls, breathing rate increases, and blood pressure drops.

- There are three types of external bleeding—arterial, venous, and capillary. Arterial bleeding is bright red, spurting, and pulsating. Venous bleeding is steady, slow, and dark red. Capillary bleeding is a slow, even ooze.

- To control external bleeding, apply direct pressure to the wound, elevate the bleeding extremity (unless there is a possible bone or joint injury), and use pressure points if necessary. Two other methods of bleeding control are splints and tourniquets. (Use a tourniquet only as a last resort.)

- To control a nosebleed, have the patient sit and lean forward. Then pinch the nostrils together and apply cold compresses. Note that a nosebleed in an unresponsive patient can threaten the airway.

- Suspect internal bleeding if the mechanism of injury suggests it and if there is evidence of scrapes and bruises, swelling, deformity, or impact marks. Always suspect it if there are penetrating wounds to the skull, chest, or abdomen and in cases of unexplained shock.

- First Responder care of a patient with internal bleeding includes maintaining an open airway and adequate breathing, controlling any external bleeding, and treating for shock.

- Shock (hypoperfusion) is a condition that results from the inadequate delivery of oxygenated blood. If the condition persists, cell failure, organ failure, and death will follow. It is therefore imperative to survival for shock to be recognized and treated promptly.

- To provide care to the patient with signs of shock, maintain an open airway and adequate breathing, prevent further blood loss, elevate the lower extremities if appropriate, and keep the patient warm. Comfort, calm, and reassure the patient. Never give anything to him to eat or drink. During the ongoing assessment, assess vital signs every five minutes and monitor for changes in mental status.

- Anaphylactic shock is a life-threatening medical emergency. Immediate treatment is required to prevent death. First Responder care includes treating all life-threats, administering oxygen, and being prepared to provide basic life support with supplemental oxygen if needed. The First Responder may also be allowed to assist the patient who carries his own medication (epinephrine auto-injector).

Key Terms

anaphylactic shock an acute allergic reaction with severe bronchospasm and vascular collapse, which can be rapidly fatal. *Also called* anaphylaxis.

arterial bleeding recognized by bright red blood that spurts and pulsates from a wound.

capillary bleeding recognized by dark red blood that slowly and evenly oozes from a wound.

cc cubic centimeters.

compensatory shock the first stage of shock, during which the patient's body is still able to maintain perfusion.

decompensated shock the second stage of shock, during which the patient's body can no longer maintain perfusion. Without medical intervention, further decline occurs.

dehydration excessive loss of body fluids.

external bleeding bleeding that occurs on the outside of the body.

Golden Hour a term trauma experts use to refer to the belief that severely injured patients have the highest survival rates when they are on the operating table within 60 minutes of injury.

internal bleeding bleeding that occurs inside the body.

irreversible shock the last stage of shock, during which the body's cells are dying. Even with treatment, damage to vital organs is permanent.

perfusion refers to the circulation of blood and delivery of oxygen throughout the body's organs and other structures.

plasma the fluid that surrounds the blood cells.

shock a life-threatening progressive condition that results from the inadequate delivery of oxygenated blood throughout the body. *Also referred to as* hypoperfusion.

splint any rigid device used to immobilize a body part.

tourniquet a constricting band used as a last resort on an extremity to apply pressure over an artery in order to control bleeding.

venous bleeding recognized by dark red blood that flows steadily and slowly from a wound.

Knowledge Check

1. **Which one of the following shows the steps for bleeding control in the correct order?**
   a. direct pressure, elevation, pressure point, tourniquet
   b. pressure point, elevation, tourniquet, direct pressure
   c. direct pressure, tourniquet, elevation, pressure point
   d. elevation, pressure point, direct pressure, tourniquet

2. **What BSI precautions, if any, are needed for a patient who is spitting blood from a wound on his face?**
   a. gloves
   b. gloves and eye protection
   c. gloves plus eye and face protection
   d. No BSI precautions are required.

3. **Signs of shock in a patient include all of those listed below EXCEPT:**
   a. decreasing pulse rate.
   b. increasing respiration rate.
   c. altered mental status.
   d. low blood pressure.

4. **Dark red blood that flows steadily from a wound usually indicates ___ bleeding.**
   a. compensated
   b. capillary
   c. arterial
   d. venous

5. Which one of the following pulse points is NOT used for bleeding control?
   a. brachial
   b. carotid
   c. radial
   d. femoral

6. Which one of the statements below BEST describes why prompt transport of seriously injured patients is necessary?
   a. They cannot be helped by First Responders.
   b. Injured limbs may have to be amputated.
   c. External bleeding is a life-threat.
   d. They have higher survival rates.

7. In general, a sudden blood loss of ___ liter in an adult and ___ liter in a child is considered serious.
   a. one, one-half
   b. one-half, one-third
   c. one-third, one-fourth
   d. one-fourth, one-eighth

8. When should you NOT use elevation as a method of bleeding control for an injured limb?
   a. if an artery lies close to the injury
   b. if you suspect a possible bone or joint injury
   c. when you use both direct pressure and a pressure point
   d. when you have to remove a dressing to reassess bleeding

9. First Responders should be especially careful when assessing infant and child patients for shock because these patients:
   a. have a capillary refill time twice that of an adult.
   b. compensate for blood loss longer than adults can.
   c. deteriorate slowly with plenty of warning time.
   d. do not respond well to artificial ventilation.

10. What takes precedence over management of life-threatening bleeding?
    a. gathering a pertinent past medical history
    b. performing a head-to-toe physical examination
    c. ensuring an open airway and adequate breathing
    d. dressing and bandaging both major and minor wounds

11. Management of life-threatening bleeding must occur during the initial assessment of your patient.
    a. True
    b. False

12. List four ways other than using barrier devices that can help protect you against infection.

_____

_____

_____

_____

13. List at least 10 signs or symptoms of internal bleeding.

_____   _____

_____   _____

_____   _____

_____   _____

_____   _____

Scenario

You are called to respond to an emergency at a butcher shop where one of the butcher's assistants dropped a large knife onto his foot and sustained a deep cut. You are told that bleeding is profuse.

a. Before you arrive on scene, you review in your mind what you will do. Briefly describe the patient assessment plan for this patient.

_____

_____

_____

_____

b. After you determine that the scene is safe, you enter to find the patient sitting in the owner's office. His foot is wrapped in a large towel. You can see no bleeding, but his hands and his pant legs are covered with blood. Your general impression of the patient is that he looks "sick" (skin looks grayish and moist and he seems tense). How should you proceed?

_____

_____

_____

_____

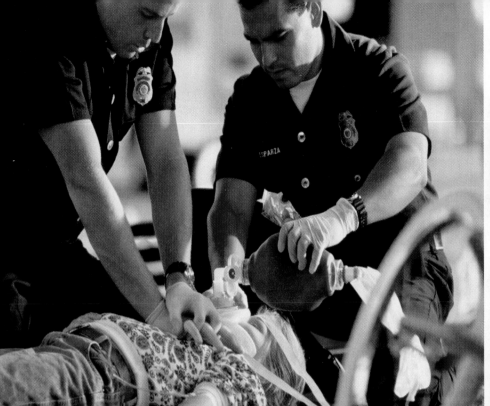
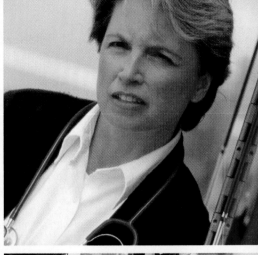
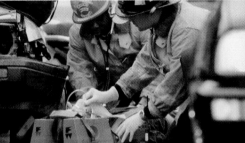

19 | Soft-Tissue Injuries

Objectives

From the U.S. Department of Transportation (DOT) 1995 "First Responder: National Standard Curriculum." Material supplemental to the DOT curriculum is listed under "Enrichment."

Cognitive

5-2.6 ▶ Establish the relationship between body substance isolation (BSI) and soft tissue injuries. (p. 349)

5-2.7 ▶ State the types of open soft tissue injuries. (pp. 350–353)

5-2.8 ▶ Describe the emergency medical care of the patient with a soft tissue injury. (p. 353)

5-2.9 ▶ Discuss the emergency medical care considerations for a patient with a penetrating chest injury. (p. 353)

5-2.10 ▶ State the emergency medical care considerations for a patient with an open wound to the abdomen. (p. 355)

5-2.11 ▶ Describe the emergency medical care for an impaled object. (pp. 353–355)

5-2.12 ▶ State the emergency medical care for an amputation. (pp. 355, 357)

5-2.14 ▶ List the functions of dressing and bandaging. (pp. 358–360)

Affective

5-2.15 ▶ Explain the rationale for body substance isolation when dealing with bleeding and soft tissue injuries. (p. 349)

5-2.16 ▶ Attend to the feelings of the patient with a soft tissue injury or bleeding. (p. 353)

5-2.17 ▶ Demonstrate a caring attitude towards patients with a soft tissue injury or bleeding who request emergency medical services. (p. 353)

5-2.18 ▶ Place the interests of the patient with a soft tissue injury or bleeding as the foremost consideration when making any and all patient care decisions. (pp. 349, 355)

5-2.19 ▶ Communicate with empathy to patients with a soft tissue injury or bleeding, as well as with family members and friends of the patient. (p. 353)

Psychomotor

5-2.24 ▶ Demonstrate the steps in the emergency medical care of open soft tissue injuries. (p. 353)

5-2.25 ▶ Demonstrate the steps in the emergency medical care of a patient with an open chest wound. (p. 353)

5-2.26 ▶ Demonstrate the steps in the emergency medical care of a patient with open abdominal wounds. (p. 355)

5-2.27 ▶ Demonstrate the steps in the emergency medical care of a patient with an impaled object. (pp. 353–355)

5-2.28 ▶ Demonstrate the steps in the emergency medical care of a patient with an amputation. (pp. 355, 357)

5-2.29 ▶ Demonstrate the steps in the emergency medical care of an amputated part. (pp. 355, 357)

Enrichment

▶ Describe the emergency medical care for a patient with a large open neck wound. (p. 355)

▶ State the general principles of dressing and bandaging soft-tissue injuries. (pp. 358–360)

Introduction

Injuries to a patient's skin, muscles, nerves, and blood vessels are among the most common you will care for. Some will be minor cuts, scrapes, and bruises. Others may be life-threatening. Whatever your patient's soft-tissue injuries may be, your priorities will include controlling bleeding, preventing further injury, and reducing the risk of infection.

Section 1 Soft-Tissue Injuries

Soft-tissue injuries are injuries to the skin, muscles, nerves, and blood vessels. They are often dramatic, but they are rarely life-threatening. They can be serious, however, if they lead to airway or breathing problems, uncontrolled bleeding, or shock.

A soft-tissue injury is commonly referred to as a **wound.** Wounds may be classified as open or closed, single or multiple. They also are classified by location (head wounds or chest wounds, for example).

In general, First Responder care for soft-tissue injuries focuses on controlling bleeding, preventing further injury, and reducing the risk of infection. Unless a life-threat, a soft-tissue injury is usually cared for after the initial assessment.

Closed Wounds

In a **closed wound,** soft tissues beneath the skin are damaged (Figure 19-1). The skin itself is not broken. Generally, a closed wound is caused by **blunt trauma.** It

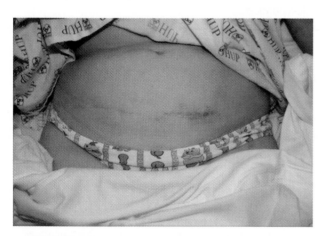

a. *Contusions.*

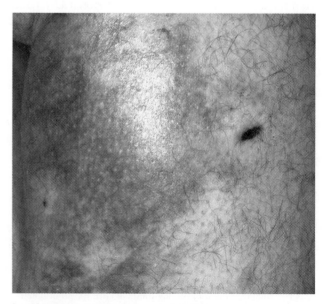

b. *Hematoma. (Charles Stewart M.D. & Associates)*

FIGURE 19-1 In a closed wound, soft tissues beneath the skin are damaged. Blunt trauma is usually the cause.

THE CALL

Dispatch I work as a lathe operator at the mill. I'm also a First Responder. One day, the emergency signal broke into the noise of the machines. I called in and was told to report to Building B.

Scene Size-up My partner and I arrived at the main entrance, where a guard directed us to the injury site. He advised us that there were no dangers. A worker had a piece of wood impaled in one hand. We put on protective gloves and glasses and approached the scene.

Initial Assessment The patient was standing near a workbench. We saw that mental status, airway, and breathing were okay because she was swearing quite loudly about her injury. We approached and identified ourselves. There was surprisingly little bleeding coming from the wound. We calmed the woman down and asked her to sit while we assessed the injury. We reported the patient's status and the nature of the injury to the incoming EMTs. Their ETA was 10 minutes.

What kind of assessment and care should these First Responders provide to their patient? Should they remove the piece of wood from the patient's hand? What could happen if they did? Consider this patient as you read Chapter 19.

---

may be due to anything from being struck by a car to dropping a block on the foot. Either way, blunt trauma can cause serious internal injuries, including organ rupture, with few external signs. A patient may look fine at first and then very quickly slip into shock. The result can be decompensated shock and death. For this reason, always suspect internal injuries with blunt trauma.

Closed wounds include contusions, ecchymosis, and hematomas. A **contusion**, or bruise, is a closed wound characterized by swelling and pain at the injury site. If small blood vessels have been broken, the patient will have **ecchymosis** (black-and-blue discoloration). If there is a larger collection of blood under the skin, a **hematoma** is evident as a lump with bluish discoloration.

First on Scene

Treat life-threats first! Even when wounds are big and gross, exercise self-control. A compromised airway, inadequate breathing, and severe uncontrolled bleeding must be your first priorities. Your patient's life may depend on it.

Patient Assessment

Closed wounds may be minor, severe, or somewhere in between. Just because they are not bleeding externally, do not be fooled into thinking they are not serious. Use the DOTS memory aid to observe for signs of closed injury. Also be sure to consider the mechanism of injury and check vitals for any signs of shock. ■

First Responder Care

To provide care to a patient with closed wounds, first take BSI precautions and then consider the following:

- Small contusions generally do not need treatment. Use cold compresses help to relieve pain and reduce swelling in moderately sized contusions.

- Large contusions or large areas of discoloration of the skin can indicate serious internal bleeding. A bruise the size of a fist, for example, could mean a 10% blood loss. If the patient has a large contusion, or if the mechanism of injury suggests blunt trauma, treat the patient for internal bleeding. Be sure to assess carefully for broken bones, especially when swelling or deformity is present.

- If you are ever in doubt about the seriousness of a closed wound, treat the patient for internal bleeding, including administering oxygen. ■

OPEN WOUNDS

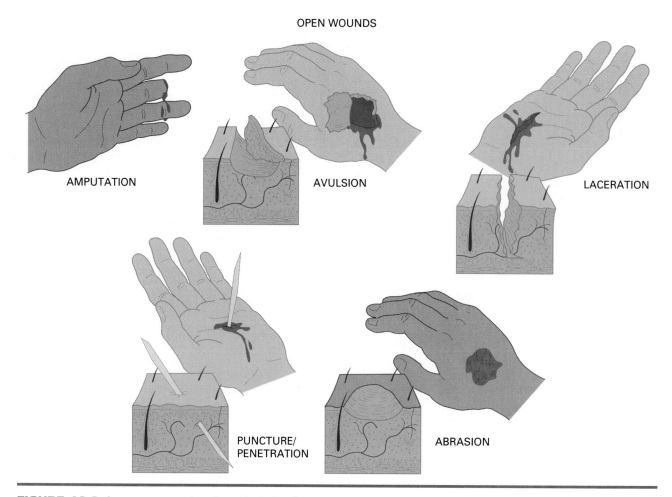

AMPUTATION   AVULSION   LACERATION

PUNCTURE/
PENETRATION   ABRASION

FIGURE 19-2 In open wounds, the skin is broken.

Open Wounds

When injured skin breaks, the break is referred to as an **open wound** or open injury. (See Figure 19-2.) Open wounds place the patient at risk for contamination, which can lead to infection. Open wounds also may be the first indicators of a deeper, more serious injury such as a fracture. They include abrasions, lacerations, and penetration/puncture wounds.

First Responder Practice

Take appropriate BSI precautions when you care for a patient with open wounds. Wear protective gloves. Protect your face and eyes, and wear a disposable gown, as necessary. After patient assessment and care, wash your hands—even if you wore gloves. Handwashing is the most important thing to do to prevent the spread of infection.

Abrasions

An **abrasion** is an open wound caused by scraping, rubbing, or shearing away of the epidermis (outermost layer of skin). Even though an abrasion is considered a superficial injury, it is often very painful because of exposed nerve ends. Though there may be no bleeding at all from an abrasion, in most cases there is capillary bleeding.

Small abrasions usually are not life-threatening. Large ones, however, may be cause for concern. For example, a motorcycle rider who is thrown and slides across the pavement will sustain head-to-toe abrasions ("road rash"). Bleeding in such a case may not be serious, but contamination, infection, and the potential for underlying injuries may be.

Lacerations

A **laceration** is a break of varying depth in the skin. It may occur in isolation. It also may occur with other types of soft-tissue injuries (Figure 19-3). Lacerations are caused by forceful impact with a sharp object. Bleeding may be severe, especially if an artery is involved.

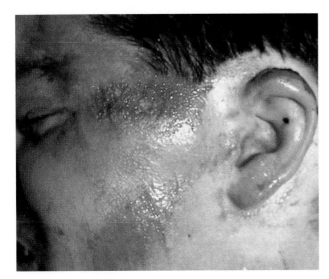

a. *Facial abrasions.*

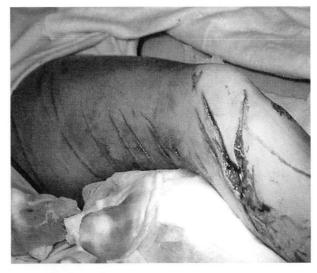

b. *Lacerations to the leg.*

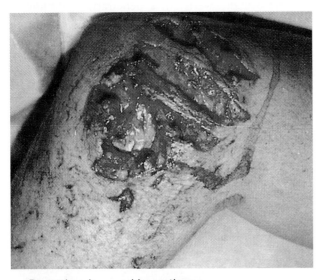

c. *Deep abrasions and lacerations.*

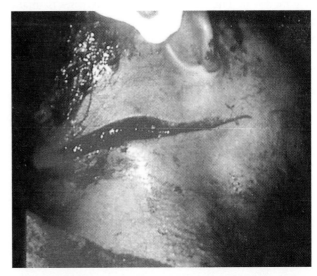

d. *Laceration to the neck.*

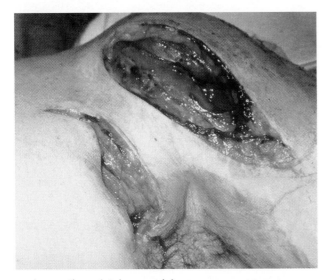

e. *Lacerations (stab wounds).* (Shout Picture Library)

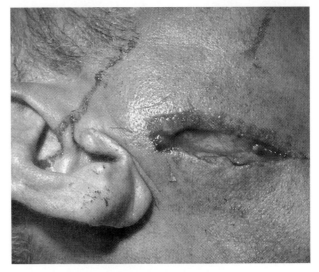

f. *Laceration to the face.* (Shout Picture Library)

FIGURE 19-3 Two types of open wounds are abrasions and lacerations.

The edges of a laceration may be regular or irregular. Regular lacerations are usually caused by a knife or razor. They may heal better because their edges are smoother. Irregular lacerations are commonly caused by a blunt object, serrated knife, or broken bottle. The edges of the wound are jagged, and healing is usually prolonged.

Penetration/Puncture Wounds

A **penetration/puncture wound** is usually the result of a sharp, pointed object being pushed or driven into soft tissues. This type of injury may have both an entry wound and an exit wound. The entry wound may be small, and there may be little or no external bleeding (Figure 19-4). However, such injuries may be deep damaging and cause severe internal bleeding. A gunshot injury is an example (Figure 19-5). The entry wound in many cases is smaller than the exit wound. If the patient was shot at close range, the entry wound may be surrounded by powder burns. The larger exit wound generally bleeds more profusely.

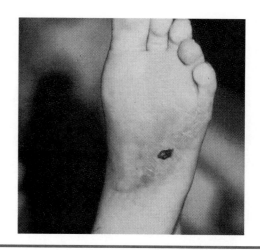

FIGURE 19-4 Puncture wound to the foot.

The overall severity of a penetration or puncture wound depends on the following factors: location, size of the penetrating object, and the forces involved in creating the injury. It can be difficult to determine the

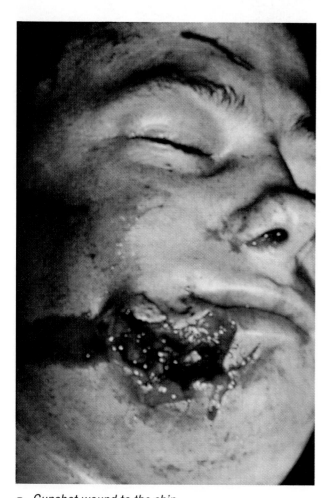

a. *Gunshot wound to the chin.*

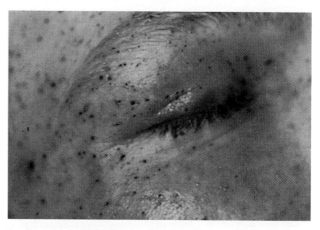

b. *Powder burns from a gunshot.*

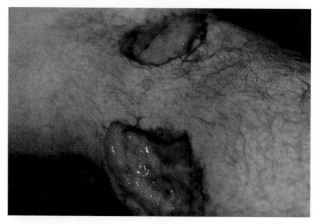

c. *Entrance and exit gunshot wounds.*

FIGURE 19-5 Gunshot injuries can involve a variety of wounds, including entry and exit wounds.

extent of these injuries based only on external signs. So treat penetration and puncture wounds with great caution.

Patient Assessment

Examine the mechanism of injury and take BSI precautions as you size up the scene. As you begin to assess your patient, remember that open wounds that can cause bleeding into the mouth, nose, or pharynx require your immediate attention. Be alert for signs of shock (altered mental status, increased breathing and pulse rate, and poor skin color). Keep in mind that the patient may have injuries below the surface, such as fractures or damage to internal organs.

Complete a head-to-toe exam to identify any additional wounds or injuries, especially in the case of a gunshot wound. (Often multiple gunshot wounds are involved.) ■

First Responder Care

To care for a patient with an open soft-tissue injury:

1. *Assess and treat all life-threats.* Maintain a patent airway and adequate breathing. If breathing is adequate, administer oxygen by way of a nonrebreather mask. If breathing is inadequate, assist ventilation by way of a BVM with supplemental oxygen. Provide artificial ventilation if needed.

2. *Expose the entire injury site.* Cut away clothing, if needed. Then, clear the area of blood and debris with sterile gauze or the cleanest material available.

3. *Control bleeding.* Begin with direct pressure and elevation. If bleeding still is not controlled, use a pressure point.

4. *Prevent further contamination.* Keep the wound as clean as possible. If there are loose particles of foreign matter around the wound, wipe them away from the wound, never toward it. Never try to pick embedded particles or debris out of the wound.

5. *Dress and bandage the wound.* Apply a dry sterile dressing. Then, secure it with a bandage. Check distal pulses both before and after applying the bandage to make sure it is not cutting off circulation.

As you care for a patient's soft-tissue injuries—especially open bleeding ones—be careful what you say and do. Do not alarm the patient by your reaction to the wounds. In fact, you will help the patient significantly if you do your best to be comforting, calming, and reassuring. If possible, also keep the patient's family informed and reassured. ■

Special Considerations

Some open wounds need special consideration. First Responder care is the same as for all other open wounds, but there are certain exceptions, which are described below. In all of these cases, administer oxygen by way of a nonrebreather mask. If breathing is inadequate, assist ventilation by way of a BVM with supplemental oxygen. Provide artificial ventilation if needed.

Chest Injuries

A penetrating chest wound can prevent a patient from breathing adequately. Such a wound is sometimes called a *sucking chest wound,* because it can bubble and make a sucking noise when the patient breathes. In this case, apply an **occlusive dressing.** (This is a special type of dressing used to make an airtight seal. It may be commercially prepared or it can be created from a strong plastic bag or other similar material.) Secure the dressing with tape on three sides (Figure 19-6). Leave one side untaped to allow air to escape as the patient exhales. This will help to prevent a condition called **tension pneumothorax,** a severe build-up of air that compresses the lungs and heart toward the uninjured side of the chest.

Let the patient assume a position of comfort, if you do not suspect spine injury. Generally, the patient will favor the position that allows for the greatest chest expansion. Assume spine injury if there is any significant mechanism of injury to the chest, including a gunshot wound.

Impaled Objects

An **impaled object** is an object embedded in an open wound. It should never be removed in the field unless it is through the patient's cheek or it interferes with airway management or CPR.

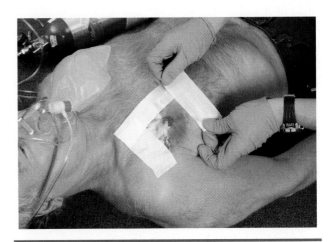

FIGURE 19-6 Seal three sides of an occlusive dressing for an open chest wound.

SKILL SUMMARY *Stabilizing an Impaled Object*

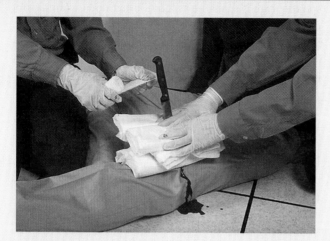

FIGURE 19-7A *Bulky dressings can help stabilize an impaled object.*

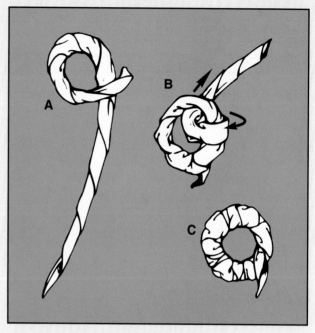

FIGURE 19-7B *An alternative is to use a doughnut-type ring pad to stabilize an impaled object.*

To provide emergency care to a patient with an impaled object, you must first prevent the object from moving. Manually secure it, keeping in mind that any movement could cause further damage and bleeding. Then expose the wound area by removing clothing from around it. Remember to take care not to move the object at all. Finally, control the bleeding. Apply direct pressure to the edges of the wound only. Avoid putting pressure directly on the impaled object. Once bleeding has stopped, stabilize the object. Surround it entirely with a bulky dressing. Pack more dressings around the object, and tape them all securely in place. A ring or doughnut pad may be used (Figure 19-7).

When an object is impaled in a patient's cheek, bleeding can interfere with breathing. If this should occur, you must remove the object (Figure 19-8). First, while maintaining an open airway, feel inside the patient's mouth with gloved fingers to find out if the object has penetrated completely. Then, remove the object in the direction in which it entered. Control bleeding from the outside of the cheek and dress the wound. If the object penetrated the cheek completely, pack sterile gauze between the cheek wall and the teeth. Continue to monitor the airway, suctioning when necessary.

You may encounter resistance when you try to remove an impaled object from the cheek. If so, maintain an open airway and suction as needed. Stabilize the object

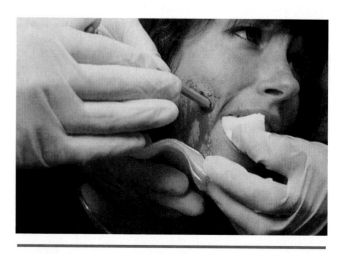

FIGURE 19-8 An impaled object in the cheek.

while you wait for the EMTs to arrive on scene. Position the patient on his or her side for drainage.

Large Open Neck Wounds

Severe bleeding from a wound involving a major blood vessel of the neck is a serious emergency. In addition to the possible loss of a great deal of blood, there is danger of air being sucked into a neck vein and carried to the heart. This can be lethal. Also suspect spine injury with any significant injury to the neck.

In this case, control of bleeding and prevention of an **air embolism** (air bubble) are your major goals. As soon as you recognize the wound, place a gloved hand over it to control the bleeding. Apply an occlusive dressing, making sure it extends beyond the wound on all sides. (This will prevent it from being sucked in.) After taping the occlusive dressing on all four sides, cover it with a regular one. Apply only enough pressure to control the bleeding.

Once bleeding is under control, apply a pressure dressing. Do not restrict air flow or compress major blood vessels. Do not apply a dressing that circles the neck.

Eviscerations

An **evisceration** occurs when internal organs protrude from an open wound. This most commonly occurs with abdominal wounds. When you care for a patient with an

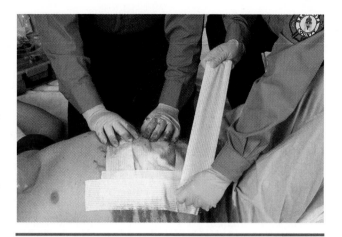

FIGURE 19-9 Cover an abdominal evisceration with a thick, moist, sterile dressing and an occlusive covering.

evisceration, never try to replace protruding organs and never touch them. You could cause further damage and contaminate both the organs and the cavity from which they protrude.

Cover the exposed organs with a thick, moist, sterile dressing. You can moisten the dressing with sterile water or saline. The dressing should be large enough to cover all protruding organs. Sterile gauze is preferred. Never use absorbent materials such as toilet tissue or paper towels, which can shred and cling to the organs. Loosely cover the moistened dressing with an occlusive (airtight) dressing. (See Figure 19-9.)

Maintain the temperature of the wound area by covering the dressing with layers of a more bulky dressing such as a particle-free bath blanket or towel. The dressings may be held loosely in place with a bandage or clean sheet.

Amputations

In an **amputation,** a body part has been completely severed from the body (Figure 19-10). This is the result of ripping or tearing forces, often from an industrial accident or motor-vehicle crash. Massive bleeding usually is present. In some cases, however, the elasticity of the blood vessels helps them to contract and bleeding is minimal. Care for an amputation in the same way you care for all open injuries.

First provide emergency care to the patient. Do not spend time looking for the amputated body part. If possible, have other First Responders or support personnel search for it. Once the body part is found, care for it (Figure 19-11). That is, wrap the amputated part in sterile gauze moistened with sterile saline. Place it in a plastic bag and label the bag with the patient's name, date,

First Responder Practice

Amputations are gruesome injuries that can intimidate any EMS provider. Remember these few basic concepts to make sure you give the best care to your patient:

- Always treat the patient before the amputated part. Recovering the part is very important, but it is not as important as assessing and treating life-threatening conditions.

- Control bleeding, although many limbs with an amputated part do not bleed as freely as you might expect.

- When preparing the amputated part, do not allow the part to come in direct contact with ice, to freeze, or to become immersed in water.

- Notify the incoming units and the dispatcher if an amputation is present, since it may affect transport decisions. The hospital also may wish to be notified early.

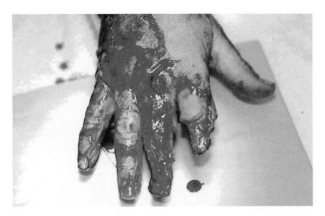

a. *Finger amputation.*

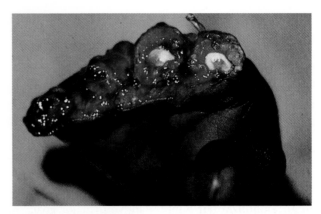

b. *Finger amputation.*

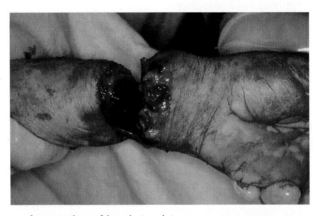

c. *Amputation of hand at wrist.* (Charles Stewart M.D. & Associates)

FIGURE 19-10 In an amputation, a body part has been completely severed from the body.

SKILL SUMMARY   *Caring for an Amputated Part*

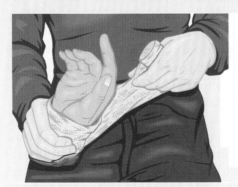

FIGURE 19-11A *Wrap completely in saline-moistened sterile dressings.*

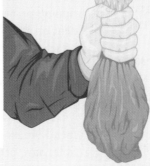

FIGURE 19-11B *Place in plastic bag and seal shut.*

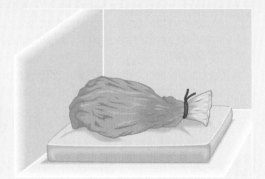

FIGURE 19-11C *Place sealed container on top of a cold pack or another sealed bag of ice. Do not allow the tissue to freeze.*

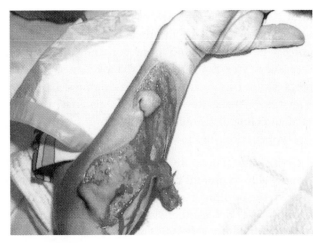

a. *Avulsion to the forearm.*

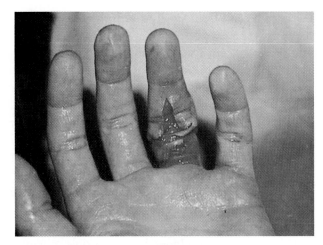

b. *Ring avulsion.*

FIGURE 19-12 An avulsion is a flap of skin or soft tissue that has been torn loose or pulled off completely.

and time the part was bagged. Never immerse the part in water. Keep the bagged part cool by putting it in a larger bag or container of ice and water. Do not use ice alone. Never use dry ice. Never place the part directly on ice. Mark the container with the patient's name, date, and body part. Give the packed part to arriving EMS personnel, so they can transport it with the patient to the hospital.

Note that if the amputation is partial, never complete it. Care for the injury as you would any other soft-tissue injury. Make sure that the partially amputated part is not twisted or constricted.

Avulsions

An **avulsion** is a torn flap of skin or soft tissue that has been torn loose or pulled off completely. (See Figure

19-12.) Healing generally is prolonged and scarring may be extensive.

Avulsions are most commonly the result of accidents with industrial or home machinery and motor vehicles. They commonly involve the fingers, toes, hands, feet, forearms, legs, ears, and nose. The seriousness of the injury depends on how well blood can circulate to the avulsed skin. If it is still attached and the flap is folded back, circulation may be compromised severely. If this is the case, emergency care includes making sure the flap is lying flat and aligned in its normal position.

Bites

Bite wounds can be quite serious (Figure 19-13). Even when they look minor, soft tissues may be badly lacerated

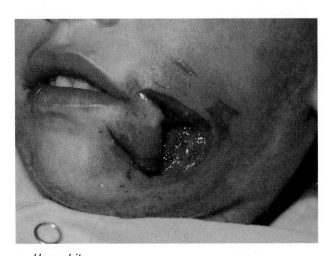

a. *Horse bite.*

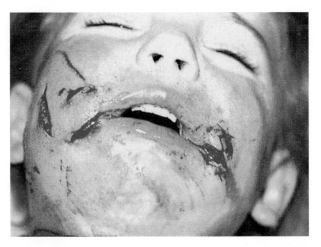

b. *Dog bite.*

FIGURE 19-13 Bite wounds can be serious, even when they seem minor.

and the threat of infection is usually high. During emergency care, if possible, wash a bite wound with plenty of warm, soapy water. Check it for any teeth fragments, too.

Note that you should not kill the animal who bit your patient unless absolutely necessary to stop an attack. If you do kill the animal, call an animal control officer and request that the corpse be examined for *rabies,* a viral infection that affects the nervous system. If you do not kill the animal, try to trap it in some kind of enclosure so that it can be examined for rabies. Take care not to injure the animal's head. Remember to protect yourself.

If the animal is not present, find out where it can be located. If getting an address is not possible, obtain a description of the animal, where it was encountered, and whether or not the attack might have been provoked. Follow local protocols on reporting requirements.

1. What is a closed wound? What is it usually caused by?

2. What BSI precautions, if any, should you take before caring for a patient with closed wounds?

3. Is an abrasion ever considered a serious injury? Explain your answer.

4. How should you care for a patient with a minor laceration?

5. Briefly, what special care should you give to a patient with an open chest injury? An impaled object? An abdominal evisceration? An amputation?

Section 2 Dressing and Bandaging Wounds

The basic purposes of dressing and bandaging are to control bleeding, prevent further contamination and damage to the wound, keep the wound dry, and stabilize the wound site. Proper wound care also enhances healing. It adds to the comfort of the patient, and it promotes more rapid recovery. Improper wound care can cause infection, severe discomfort, and, in rare cases, result in the loss of a limb.

Dressings

A **dressing** is a covering for a wound (Figure 19-14). It should be **sterile** (free of all microorganisms and spores).

Ideally, a dressing is layered and consists of coarse mesh gauze. It also should be absorbent and large enough to protect the entire wound from contamination. In an emergency, you can use clean handkerchiefs, towels, sheets, cloth, or sanitary napkins as dressings. Never use toilet tissues, paper towels, or other materials that can shred and cling to a wound.

Types of dressings include:

■ *Gauze pads.* These are usually individually wrapped and sealed to prevent contamination. Take care not to touch the portion of gauze that will make contact with the wound. Unless otherwise specified, all gauze dressings should be covered with open triangular, cravat, or roller bandages.

■ *Trauma dressing.* Large and absorbent, this type of dressing is used on larger injuries and when maximum absorbency is needed.

■ *Bandage compress.* This is a gauze pad that is attached to the middle of a strip of bandaging material. The pad can be applied directly to an open wound with virtually no exposure to the air or your fingers. The strips of bandage can be folded back and used to tie it in place. When necessary, the sterile pad may be extended to twice its normal size by continued unfolding.

■ *Occlusive dressing.* Made of plastic wrap, petroleum gauze, or other material, this dressing is used to form an airtight, moisture-proof seal over a wound.

■ *Petroleum gauze.* This is sterile gauze saturated with petroleum jelly to prevent it from sticking to a wound.

Large, thick, layered, bulky pads (some with waterproof surfaces) are also available. They come in several sizes for quick application to an extremity or to a large area of the trunk. They are used to help control bleeding and to stabilize impaled objects. These pads are also referred to as bulky dressings, multi-trauma dressings, trauma packs, general purpose dressings, burn pads, or ABD dressings.

If a commercial bulky dressing is not available, you can improvise one with a sanitary napkin. If purchased in individual wrappers, sanitary napkins have the added advantage of cleanliness.

Bandages

A **bandage** does not make contact with a wound. It is used to hold a dressing in place, create pressure to help control bleeding, or provide support for an injured body part. Properly applied, a bandage promotes healing. It

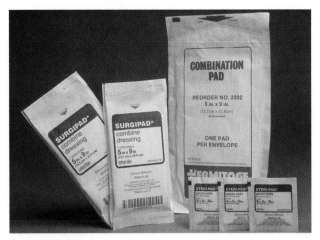

a. *Sterile gauze pads.*

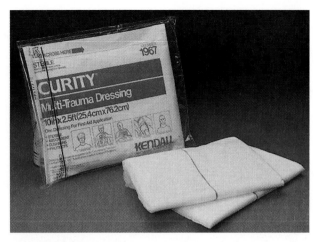

b. *Multi-trauma dressing.*

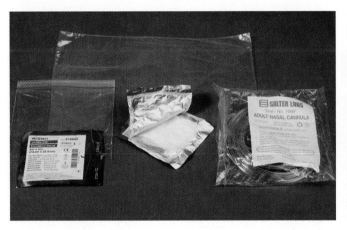

c. *Occlusive dressings.*

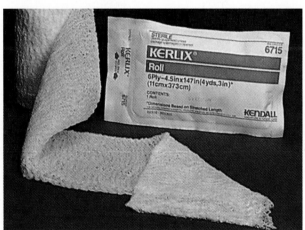

d. *Nonelastic, self-adhering dressing and roller bandage.*

FIGURE 19-14 A dressing is a sterile covering for a wound.

also helps the patient to remain comfortable during transport.

Bandages should be applied firmly and fastened securely. They should not be so tight as to stop circulation. They should not be so loose as to let dressings slip. If a bandage becomes unfastened, the wound could bleed or become infected.

Before bandaging, remove the patient's jewelry and other potentially restricting materials such as tape. Where swelling occurs, these items can restrict circulation. Loosen bandages if the skin around them becomes pale or cyanotic, if pain develops, or if the skin distally is cold, tingly, or numb.

If the pain or discomfort caused by a bandage disappears after several hours, severe damage may have already occurred. Permanent muscle paralysis may result. Please note that improper bandaging can be defined in a court of law as negligence.

Types of bandages include:

- *Triangular bandage.* This is used to support injured limbs, to secure splints, to form slings, and to make improvised tourniquets. It also can be used to bandage the forehead or scalp (Figure 19-15). The standard triangular bandage is made from a piece of unbleached cotton about 40 inches square, which is folded diagonally and cut along the fold. It can be handled and applied easily. If applied correctly, it usually remains secure. In an emergency, one can be improvised from a clean handkerchief or clean piece of shirt.

- *Cravat.* This is a triangular bandage that has been folded (Figure 19-16). For a wide cravat, make a one-inch fold along the base of the triangle. Bring the point to the center of folded base, placing the point under the fold. For a medium cravat, fold lengthwise

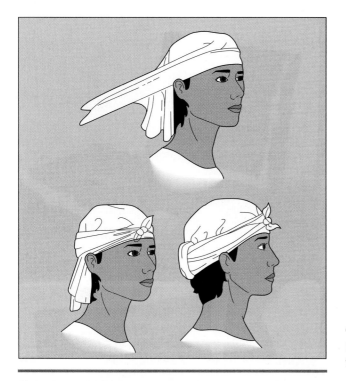

FIGURE 19-15 Triangular bandage for the forehead or scalp.

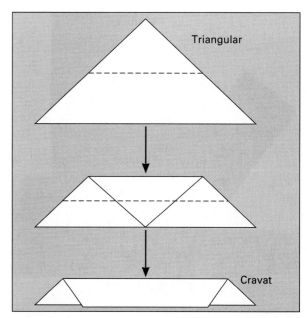

FIGURE 19-16 Creating a cravat by folding a triangular bandage.

along a line midway between the base and the new top of the bandage. For a narrow cravat, repeat folding. To complete the procedure, tie the ends of the bandage securely.

■ *Roller bandage.* The self-adhering, form-fitting, nonelastic roller bandage is the most popular and easy to use. Overlapping wraps cling together and can be cut and tied or taped in place. (See Figure 19-17 for how to apply a roller bandage.) Elastic roller bandages should not be used because a tourniquet effect may result.

To apply a *pressure dressing* to a bleeding wound, first cover the wound with a sterile bulky dressing. Then apply hand pressure over the wound until bleeding stops. Finally, apply a roller bandage, preferably the self-adhering type. It should not be so tight as to restrict circulation. The pressure dressing may be used to hold some manual pressure while you use a pressure point to stop bleeding.

Principles of Application

There are no hard-and-fast rules for dressing and bandaging wounds. Often, adaptability and creativity are far more important. In dressing and bandaging, use materials you have on hand and meet the general conditions listed below (Figure 19-18):

■ Material used for dressings should be sterile. If sterile items are not available, use a cloth that is as clean as possible.

■ Make sure that the dressing is opened carefully. Avoid contaminating it before it reaches the wound surface.

■ The dressing should adequately cover the entire wound.

■ Do not bandage a dressing in place until bleeding has stopped. The exception is a pressure dressing, which is meant to stop bleeding.

■ All edges of a dressing should be covered by the bandage. There also should be no loose ends of cloth or tape.

■ Do not bandage a wound too loosely. Bandages should not slip or shift or allow the dressings beneath to slip or shift.

■ Bandage wounds snugly, but not too tightly. Be sure to ask the patient how the bandage feels. Be careful not to interfere with circulation.

■ If you are bandaging a small wound on an extremity, cover a larger area with the bandage. This will help avoid creating a pressure point, and it will distribute pressure more evenly.

SKILL SUMMARY   *Applying a Roller Bandage*

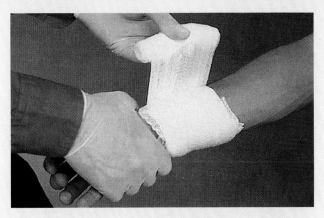

FIGURE 19-17A *Secure a self-adhering roller bandage with several snug, overlapping wraps.*

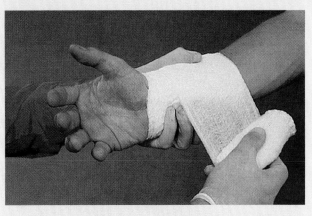

FIGURE 19-17B *Cover an area larger than the wound.*

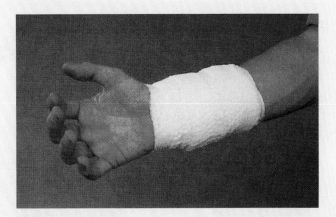

FIGURE 19-17C *Cut and tape or tie the bandage in place.*

SKILL SUMMARY *Bandaging*

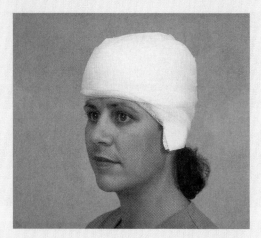

FIGURE 19-18A *Head or ear bandage.*

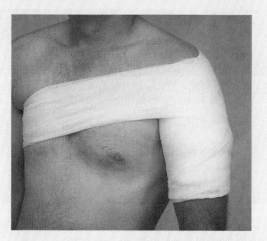

FIGURE 19-18B *Shoulder bandage.*

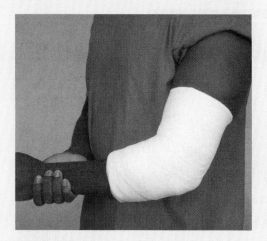

FIGURE 19-18C *Elbow bandage.*

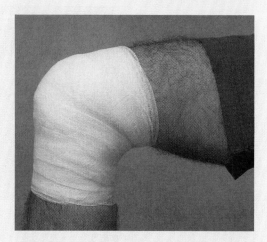

FIGURE 19-18D *Knee bandage.*

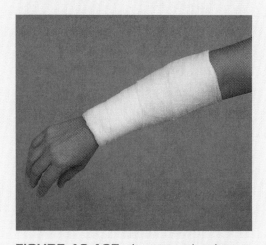

FIGURE 19-18E *Lower arm bandage.*

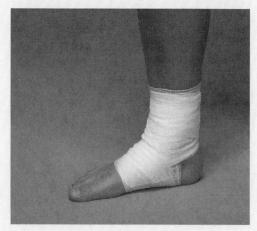

FIGURE 19-18F *Foot or ankle bandage.*

- Always place the body part to be bandaged in the position in which it is to remain. You can bandage across a joint, but do not try bending a joint after the bandage has been applied to it.
- Tape bandages in place or tie them by using a square knot (Figure 19-19).
- Leave fingers and toes exposed when arms and legs are bandaged, so that you can check for problems with circulation.
- Keep the bandage neat in appearance. You will be perceived as more professional, which can result in easier patient management.

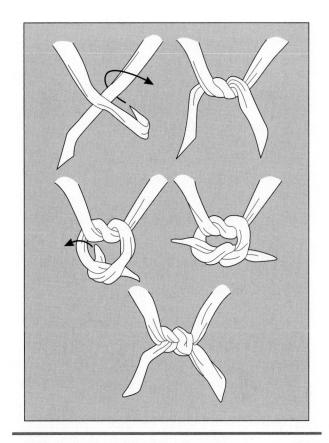

FIGURE 19-19 Tying a square knot.

 Q:

1. What characteristics should a dressing have?

2. What are three types of dressings?

3. Why should a bandage be applied over a dressing?

4. What can happen if a bandage is applied improperly?

▶▶ The Call Follow-up

At the beginning of this chapter, you read that First Responders were on scene with a female patient who had an impaled object in one hand. To see how chapter skills apply to this emergency, read the following. It describes how the call was completed.

Physical Examination A sliver of wood about five inches long had penetrated the palm of the patient's hand. About two inches of it protruded from each side. The patient's name was Victoria Mashot. Vicky hadn't passed out or fallen after the injury. She had sensation in her fingers distal to the injury and felt no numbness or tingling. I didn't ask her to move her fingers, because I didn't want to take the chance of causing further problems. Vicky's pulse was 88, strong, and regular. Her respirations were 18 and adequate. Her skin was cool and dry.

My partner stabilized the impaled object while I obtained a patient history.

Patient History Vicky was still upset that she had been so careless as to let this happen. We were able to find out that she had no allergies to medications or the environment. She was in good health and took no medications. Vicky told us she never missed a day of work. She had a doughnut and coffee from the "roach coach" that came onto the mill grounds about an hour before the injury. She confirmed that she had placed her hand where she wasn't supposed to. She denied any loss of consciousness before or after the object entered her hand.

My partner had done a good job of securing the piece of wood with gauze pads. I continued to stabilize the patient's arm and hand while my partner secured the object in place.

Ongoing Assessment We kept Vicky calm and performed our reassessments. She was still alert. Her airway and breathing were adequate. There was no bleeding from her wound through the bandage. We made sure the bandage wasn't too tight and the object was held securely. Her pulse and respirations were unchanged.

Patient Hand-off When the EMTs arrived, we told them what we had (see hand-off report below). The EMTs took Vicky to the hospital. A plastic surgeon removed the wood from her hand. Fortunately, there was no permanent damage. I heard that Vicky now keeps that sliver of wood over her workbench as a reminder to be more careful.

Hand-off Report

"This is Victoria Mashot. She is 34 years old and has a five-inch sliver of wood impaled in her left hand. She never lost consciousness and hasn't fallen or suffered any other injury. We applied some bulky dressings and bandaged around the object so it wouldn't move. Bleeding was minimal. Vicky has no allergies or medications. She tells us that she has no medical problems. She ate a doughnut and coffee an hour ago. Her pulse is 88, strong, and regular. Her respirations are 18 and adequate."

The Last Word *Whatever your patient's soft-tissue injuries may be, remember your priorities for patient care will always be control of bleeding,* *preventing further injury, and reducing the risk of infection.*

Chapter Review

Focus on the EMS Team

In your experience as a First Responder, you will come across many patients with soft-tissue injuries. Some injuries will be serious. Others won't. As the first medically trained provider on scene, your accurate assessment of the patient's wounds is critical.

Open wounds can be startling and upsetting, even to a trained First Responder. But don't let them distract you. Keep your evaluation of wounds in perspective with the patient's overall condition. If there are serious wounds with profuse bleeding, these are a priority. Only the airway and breathing should take precedence. But if the patient's wound is not a life-threat, it is not a priority. Do not neglect life-saving care for an obvious, even gaping, but nonlethal injury.

In fact, performing life-saving care may be all you can do during a call. When the EMTs arrive, they will be grateful that you knew enough to do so—and so will your patient, who will be alive and able to benefit from more advanced medical care in transit and at the hospital.

Summing Up

- Soft-tissue injuries are often dramatic but rarely life-threatening. They can be serious, however, if they lead to airway or breathing problems, uncontrolled bleeding, or shock.

- Generally, closed wounds are caused by blunt trauma. They include contusions, ecchymosis, and hematomas. First Responder care for closed wounds includes using cold compresses over moderately sized contusions. However, if a contusion is large or you have any doubt about the seriousness of the closed wound, treat for internal bleeding.

- Open wounds include abrasions, lacerations, and penetration/puncture wounds. After ensuring an open airway and adequate breathing, First Responder care includes exposing the injury site, controlling bleeding, preventing further contamination, and dressing and bandaging the wound.

- Treat all soft-tissue injuries as described above, with the following exceptions:

  — *Chest injury.* Apply an occlusive dressing to a penetrating chest wound, taping it on three sides only. This will allow the fourth side of the dressing to act as a pressure relief valve. Assume spine injury with any significant mechanism of injury to the chest.

  — *Impaled object.* Generally, you should stabilize an object manually and then with bulky dressings. If the object is in the cheek, remove it and control bleeding from the outside of the cheek. If the object penetrated the cheek completely, pack sterile gauze between the cheek wall and the teeth. If the object cannot be removed, stabilize it and ensure an open airway by suctioning as needed.

  — *Large open neck wound.* Prevent an air embolism by immediately using your gloved hand to control bleeding. Then apply an occlusive dressing. Cover that with a regular dressing, applying only enough pressure to control bleeding. Once bleeding is under control, apply a pressure dressing. Suspect spine injury with any significant injury to the neck.

  — *Evisceration.* Never try to replace protruding organs and never touch them. Cover the exposed organs with a thick, moist, sterile dressing. Loosely cover them with an occlusive dressing. Maintain the temperature of the wound area with a particle-free bath blanket or towel. Hold all loosely in place with a bandage or clean sheet.

  — *Amputated body part.* Wrap the amputated part in sterile gauze moistened with sterile saline and place it in a plastic bag. Label the bag with the patient's name, date, and time. Place the bag in a container of ice and water marked with the patient's name, date, and body part. Give it to the EMTs to transport with the patient to the hospital.

  — *Avulsion.* Make sure the flap is lying flat and aligned in its normal position.

  — *Bite.* Wash a bite wound with plenty of warm, soapy water. Check it for any teeth fragments, too. If possible, the animal should be checked for rabies.

- Dressing and bandaging control bleeding, prevent further contamination and damage to the wound, keep the wound dry, and stabilize the wound site. Proper wound care also enhances healing and adds to the comfort of the patient. Improper wound care can cause infection, severe discomfort, and in rare cases, result in the loss of a limb.

- For dressing and bandaging, follow the basic principles of application. They include: Dressings should be sterile and cover the wound completely. Bandages should be clean, applied only after bleeding has stopped, and never should interfere with circulation. Before bandaging, place the body part in the position in which it is to remain. Leave fingers and toes exposed when arms and legs are bandaged.

Key Terms

abrasion an injury caused by scraping, rubbing, or shearing away of the outermost layer of skin; a type of open wound.

air embolism gas bubbles in the bloodstream.

amputation an injury that occurs when a body part is severed from the body; a type of open wound.

avulsion an injury characterized by a torn flap of skin or soft tissue that is either still attached to the body or pulled off completely; a type of open wound.

bandage any clean material used to hold a dressing in place.

blunt trauma an injury caused by an object that is not sharp or forceful enough to penetrate the skin.

closed wound an injury to the soft tissues beneath unbroken skin.

contusion a bruise; a type of closed wound.

dressing a sterile covering for a wound.

ecchymosis black-and-blue discoloration of the skin; a type of closed wound.

evisceration the protrusion of internal organs from an open wound; a type of open wound.

hematoma a lump with bluish discoloration caused by a large collection of blood under the skin; a type of closed wound.

impaled object an object embedded in an open injury.

laceration a break of varying depth in the skin; a type of open wound.

occlusive dressing a dressing that can form an airtight and sometimes watertight seal.

open wound an injury that has broken the skin. *Also called* open injury.

penetration/puncture wound the result of a sharp, pointed object being pushed or driven into soft tissues; a type of open wound.

soft-tissue injury an injury to the skin, muscles, nerves, and/or blood vessels.

sterile free of all microorganisms and spores.

tension pneumothorax a severe build-up of air that compresses the lungs and heart toward the uninjured side of the chest.

wound a soft-tissue injury.

Knowledge Check

1. **All of the following are open injuries EXCEPT:**
   a. abrasion.
   b. avulsion.
   c. contusion.
   d. laceration.

2. **An avulsion is best described as a:**
   a. closed wound or lump with bluish discoloration.
   b. sharp object being pushed into the soft tissues.
   c. break of varying depth in the skin and soft tissues.
   d. flap of soft tissue that has been torn from the body.

3. **Which one of the following statements BEST describes the relationship between dressings and bandages?**
   a. Dressings hold bandages in place.
   b. Bandages hold dressings in place.
   c. Bandages are sterile and dressings are not.
   d. Dressings and bandages have the same function.

4. First Responder care for an impaled object in the leg includes:
   a. stabilizing the object in place.
   b. covering it with an occlusive dressing.
   c. pressing on the object to control bleeding.
   d. removing the object if there is external bleeding.

5. After scene safety, your priority for treating a patient with soft-tissue injuries is to:
   a. preserve amputated parts and avulsed tissues.
   b. avoid further damage to underlying tissues.
   c. prevent contamination of the wounds.
   d. assess and treat all life-threats.

6. For an open chest wound, an occlusive dressing should be sealed on ___ side(s).
   a. one   b. two   c. three   d. four

7. For a large open neck wound, an occlusive dressing should be sealed on ___ side(s).
   a. one   b. two   c. three   d. four

8. A large open neck wound is considered a serious emergency for all of the reasons listed below EXCEPT:
   a. it can allow the loss of a great deal of blood.
   b. air may be sucked in and carried to the heart.
   c. a pulse cannot be felt at the carotid artery.
   d. it is a sign of a possible spine injury.

9. You decide to remove an impaled object from your patient's cheek because it is interfering with his breathing. As you proceed, you find you are encountering resistance. You should do all of the following EXCEPT:
   a. continue to try to remove the object.
   b. position the patient for drainage.
   c. stabilize the object in place.
   d. suction the airway as needed.

10. Blunt trauma that has few external signs is NOT likely to be the cause of decompensated shock and death.
    a. True   b. False

11. A contusion can be a sign of serious internal bleeding.
    a. True   b. False

12. List five of the basic purposes for proper wound care.

_____

_____

_____

_____

_____

13. List three consequences of IMPROPER wound care.

_____

_____

_____

Matching

Beside each injury description, write the letter of its proper name.

_____ Knife sticking out of a thigh   **A.** Contusion

_____ Flap of tissue torn away from the body   **B.** Avulsion

_____ Knife-cut with jagged edges down the cheek   **C.** Hematoma

_____ Lump with bluish discoloration on the forehead   **D.** Abrasion

_____ Razor slash with smooth edges across the wrist   **E.** Laceration

_____ Head-to-toe "road rash"   **F.** Impaled object

_____ Exposed abdominal organs   **G.** Evisceration

Scenario

You and your partner are called to the scene of a "bear attack." As you approach the scene, you see several police cars, other emergency vehicles, and a cordoned-off area. An officer motions you toward a spot to park your vehicle.

a. What questions should you ask the officer?

_____

_____

b. Once the scene is safe to enter, you find that your patient is a 14-year-old boy who was bitten by a young, frightened brown bear. (The bear has been caught and is on the way to an observation facility.) Both the boy and his mother are pale and very quiet. The boy is holding a folded towel to his right shoulder. You introduce yourself, get consent, and prepare to perform an initial assessment. How should you proceed?

_____

_____

_____

c. After you administer oxygen by way of a nonrebreather, you begin emergency care for the bite wound. It has bled very little and the puncture wounds are barely visible. There are some claw wounds on the boy's arms as well. Describe your treatment plan.

_____

_____

_____

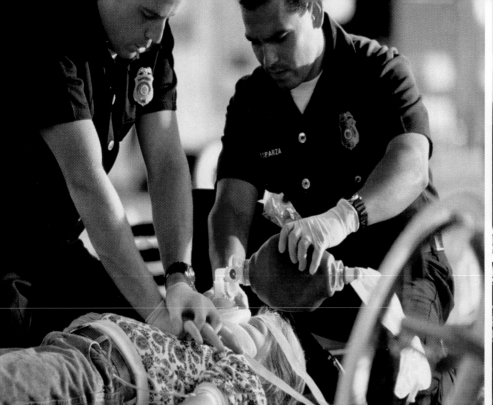
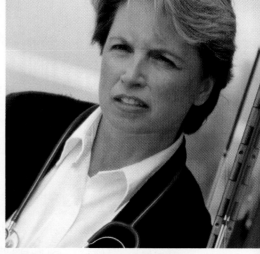
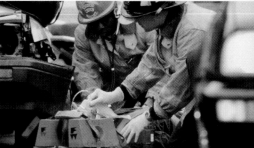

20 | Injuries to the Chest, Abdomen, and Genitalia

Objectives

From the U.S. Department of Transportation (DOT) 1995 "First Responder: National Standard Curriculum." Material supplemental to the DOT curriculum is listed under "Enrichment."

Cognitive

5-2.9 ▶ Discuss the emergency medical care considerations for a patient with a penetrating chest injury. (pp. 374–375)

5-2.10 ▶ State the emergency medical care considerations for a patient with an open wound to the abdomen. (pp. 377–378)

Affective

5-2.16 ▶ Attend to the feelings of the patient with a soft tissue injury or bleeding. (pp. 371–372, 377, 379)

5-2.17 ▶ Demonstrate a caring attitude towards patients with a soft tissue injury or bleeding who request emergency medical services. (pp. 371–372, 377, 379)

5-2.18 ▶ Place the interests of the patient with a soft tissue injury or bleeding as the foremost consideration when making any and all patient care decisions. (pp. 372, 373, 375)

5-2.19 ▶ Communicate with empathy to patients with a soft tissue injury or bleeding, as well as with family members and friends of the patient. (pp. 371–372, 377, 379)

Psychomotor

5-2.25 ▶ Demonstrate the steps in the emergency medical care of a patient with an open chest wound. (pp. 374–375)

5-2.26 ▶ Demonstrate the steps in the emergency medical care of a patient with open abdominal wounds. (pp. 377–378)

Enrichment

▶ Recognize the signs and symptoms of an injured chest. (pp. 370–372)

▶ Discuss common chest injuries, such as flail chest, blunt injuries, compression injuries, and broken ribs. (pp. 373–376)

▶ Describe some complications of chest injuries, such as pneumothorax, hemothorax, and tension pneumothorax. (pp. 373–376)

▸ Recognize the signs and symptoms of an injured abdomen. (p. 377)

▸ Describe emergency care of a male patient with injuries to the genitalia, including blunt trauma, avulsion, and amputation. (p. 379)

▸ Describe emergency care of a female patient with injuries to the genitalia, including special considerations involving sexual assault and the preservation of evidence. (p. 379)

Introduction

Because the chest and abdomen contain organs vital to life, all injuries to these areas should be considered life-threatening until proven otherwise. Injuries to the external genitalia are rarely life-threatening, but they can cause patients considerable pain and embarrassment.

Section 1 Injuries to the Chest

There are two categories of chest injuries—open and closed. As you would expect, an open chest injury occurs when an object passes through the chest wall. A closed chest injury is one in which the skin of the chest is not broken. The main types of chest injury include **blunt trauma** and **penetrating injury.**

Now is a good time for a quick review of the anatomy of the chest (Figure 20-1). A review of the respiratory and circulatory systems as described in Chapter 4 may also be helpful.

Note: Always take BSI precautions when there is any possibility that you will come in contact with a patient's blood or other body fluids. Wear protective gloves at a minimum.

Patient Assessment

Two of the most important signs of chest injury are the patient's respiratory rate and a change in normal breathing pattern. In general, a normal breathing rate is from 12 to 20 breaths per minute. Normal breathing also is done without strain, pain, or difficulty. If a patient breathes more than 20 times per minute and experiences pain with breathing or finds it difficult to take a deep breath, the patient probably has a chest injury.

Whether the injury is open or closed, certain signs and symptoms will occur with chest injury. Many of them may occur simultaneously. The major signs and symptoms include (Figure 20-2):

■ Shortness of breath or difficulty breathing.

■ Pain during breathing.

■ Failure of the chest to expand normally during inhalation.

■ **Sucking chest wound** (an open wound to the chest that bubbles or makes a sucking noise).

■ Reduced or absent breath sounds on one side of chest (when listening with a stethoscope).

■ Cyanosis.

■ Coughing up blood.

■ Distended neck veins.

■ Rapid, weak pulse.

■ Decreasing blood pressure.

■ Bruising to the chest.

■ Chest wall deformity.

■ Pain at injury site.

■ Shock.

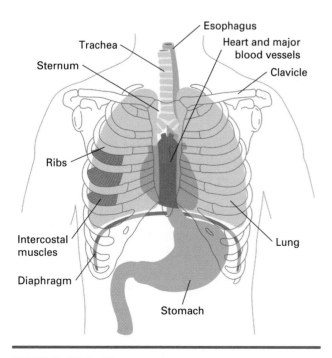

FIGURE 20-1 Chest cavity.

THE CALL

Dispatch My first response unit was called to a "woman down" at the corner of Hamilton and Lake Shore Drive.

Scene Size-up We turned off the lights and sirens before we approached in order to prevent a crowd from being drawn to the scene. The police on scene waved us in. We still were cautious as we pulled up and put on our gloves and eye wear. A woman was lying on the ground. An officer was leaning over her. He reported that the woman had been stabbed, probably during a robbery. As we got nearer to the patient, I saw a hole in her shirt just below the nipple level on the right side of her chest. The woman was moaning and moving around.

What are the immediate priorities for First Responder care of this patient? Is her most obvious injury the one they should be most concerned about? Consider this patient as you read Chapter 20. What should be done to assess and treat her condition?

When you assess the chest, keep in mind that the chest cavity has a front, side, and back. Injuries to the side and back also can penetrate the chest cavity. If the chest is injured, suspect serious underlying damage, even if the skin is not broken. Always assume cardiac damage until it is ruled out. Assume spine injury if there is any significant mechanism of injury to the chest, including a gunshot wound.

Remember that nothing is quite so frightening to a patient as a breathing problem. Be sure to stay calm. Your

SIGNS AND SYMPTOMS OF CHEST INJURY

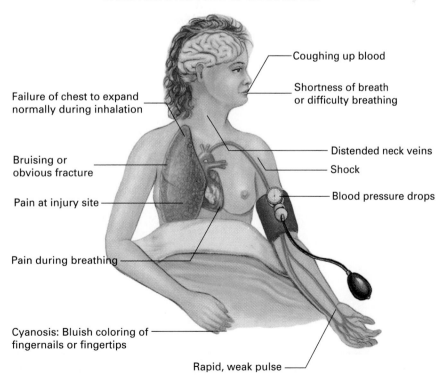

Coughing up blood

Shortness of breath or difficulty breathing

Failure of chest to expand normally during inhalation

Distended neck veins

Shock

Bruising or obvious fracture

Blood pressure drops

Pain at injury site

Pain during breathing

Cyanosis: Bluish coloring of fingernails or fingertips

Rapid, weak pulse

FIGURE 20-2 Chest injuries present with a variety of signs and symptoms.

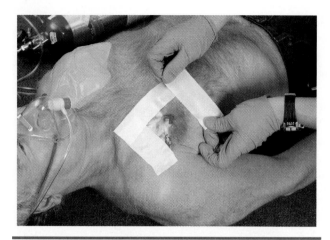

FIGURE 20-3 With any open chest wound (especially a sucking chest wound), suspect penetration into the chest cavity and apply an occlusive dressing.

demeanor will encourage the patient to stay calm, too. Demonstrate a caring, professional attitude to both the patient and the patient's family. ■

First Responder Care

To provide care to a patient with any chest injury, update or activate EMS immediately. The patient must be stabilized and transported as quickly as possible to a medical facility.

1. *Maintain an open airway.* Watch for airway obstruction from foreign objects, blood, mucus, and swelling. Suction when needed.

2. *Monitor breathing constantly.* If it is adequate, administer oxygen via nonrebreather. If it is inadequate, assist ventilations with BVM and supplemental oxygen. Be prepared to provide basic life support, if needed.

3. *Control any external bleeding.* A patient who has a chest injury is likely to have multiple injuries. Be sure you have identified all wounds (e.g., entry and exit wounds). Treat for shock, if appropriate.

4. *Apply an occlusive dressing* to a sucking chest wound or any injury to the chest that could have penetrated the chest cavity. The dressing should be two inches larger than the wound on all sides (large enough *not* to be sucked into the wound). Seal the dressing on three sides only to create a one-way relief valve (Figure 20-3 and 20-4). If the patient develops increased respiratory distress after application of an occlusive dressing, release the seal immediately. Blood may have built up under the dressing, clogging the one-way relief valve and allowing pressure to build up within the chest cavity.

   If you must improvise an occlusive dressing, do not use household plastic wrap. It is not strong enough. If necessary, use material such as a plastic bag. If you have no other choice, use Vaseline® gauze held in place with a pressure dressing.

5. *Allow the patient to get in a position of comfort,* if there is no suspected spine injury. Generally, the patient will favor the position that allows for the greatest chest expansion.

6. *Monitor vital signs.* Since patients with chest injuries are often unstable, monitor them every five minutes.

a. On inspiration, dressing seals wound, preventing air entry.

b. Expiration allows any trapped air to escape through the untaped section of the dressing.

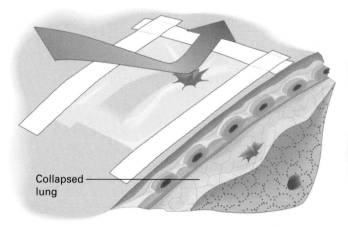

Collapsed lung

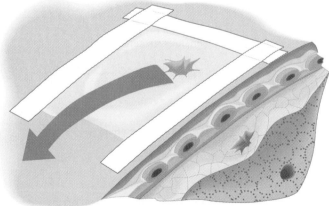

FIGURE 20-4 Sealing an occlusive dressing on three sides creates a one-way relief valve, which allows air to escape but prevents it from entering the chest cavity.

All chest injuries are serious. However, open chest injuries pose an additional problem because they upset the delicate balance of pressure between the inside and outside of the chest. It is vital for you to identify and treat open chest injuries promptly. ■

Specific Conditions

Blunt trauma and penetrating injuries to the chest can result in a number of problems for the patient. For example, blunt trauma can result in traumatic asphyxia, broken ribs, and **flail chest.** Penetrating injuries, such as those caused by stabbing or gunshot, can result in laceration of the great vessels in the chest, massive bleeding, sucking chest wounds, and laceration of the heart and lungs. Either type of injury—blunt trauma or penetrating—can cause a **pneumothorax** or **hemothorax.**

To help improve your understanding of chest injuries, those conditions are described below.

Blunt Trauma and Traumatic Asphyxia

Severe blunt injuries to the chest are life-threatening emergencies. Sudden compression of the chest, such as when a driver is thrown against a steering wheel in a car crash, is an example. Such trauma causes an increase in pressure inside the chest, which can result in internal bruising to the heart and lungs. Signs and symptoms include severe shortness of breath, generalized chest pain, and rapid, sometimes irregular, pulse.

Traumatic asphyxia may occur as a result of blunt trauma to the chest. When it does, blood is forced the wrong way out of the heart—from the right side instead of the left. It is then forced back into the veins, particularly the veins of the head and shoulders. Signs and symptoms include shock, distended neck veins, bloodshot protruding eyes, cyanotic tongue and lips, coughing up or

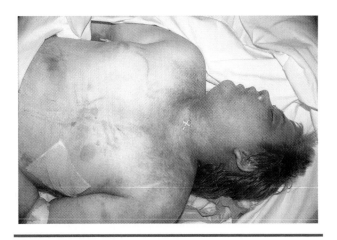

FIGURE 20-5 A patient with traumatic asphyxia.
(Charles Stewart, M.D. & Associates)

vomiting blood, and swollen, cyanotic appearance of the head, neck, and shoulders (Figure 20-5).

Guidelines for First Responder care are the same as described earlier in the chapter. Note that these conditions are dire emergencies. Time is critical. Be sure EMS has been notified and updated.

Broken Ribs

In adults (broken ribs are not common in children), direct blows or blunt trauma to the chest often result in broken ribs. The ribs most often broken are those in the middle of the rib cage. Upper ribs are difficult to break because they are protected by the bony shoulder girdle. When they are broken, suspect severe internal injuries. The lower ribs are "floating." They are not attached to the sternum. So they have more ability to move and a greater ability to withstand impact.

The most common symptom of a broken rib is pain at the fracture site. It usually hurts the patient to move, cough, or breathe deeply. The patient will likely want to hold a hand over the area, since stabilization often offers some pain relief. Other signs and symptoms may include **crepitus** (a grating sound upon palpation), chest deformity, shallow and irregular breathing, a crackling sensation near the suspected fracture site, bruising or lacerations at the suspected fracture site, and frothy blood at the nose or mouth, indicating that a rib may have punctured a lung (Figure 20-6).

Your priority is to make sure the patient can breathe adequately. Upon inspiration, the pain from rib fractures can cause decreased tidal volume. Give the patient a pillow or blanket to hold against the broken ribs for support. Apply a sling and swathe to hold the patient's arm against the injured side of the chest. And monitor breathing carefully.

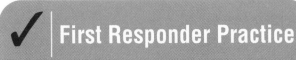

✓ | First Responder Practice

Closed chest wounds can cause significant injury, while leaving little indication on the surface. The chest cavity contains vital organs including the heart, lungs, and large blood vessels. Use the mechanism of injury to help you determine if serious injuries could exist. If you suspect they do, notify incoming units, administer oxygen, and treat for shock.

SIGNS AND SYMPTOMS OF BROKEN RIBS

Pain at fracture site.
Pain on moving, coughing, or breathing deeply.
Shallow, uncoordinated breathing.
Chest deformity.
Bruising or lacerations.
Grating sound upon palpation.
Crackling sensation near site.
Frothy blood at nose or mouth (lung puncture).

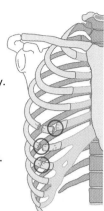

FIGURE 20-6 **Of the signs and symptoms of broken ribs, you may be aware of only the most common symptom—pain.**

If the patient is alert, allow him or her to assume a position of comfort. Some EMS systems recommend placing the patient on the injured side. Do not bind, tape, or use other methods that encircle the chest, as they may impair breathing.

Common complications of rib fracture include:

- *Pneumothorax*—an accumulation of air in the **pleural space.** (The pleural space is the area between the visceral pleura, a membrane that covers the outer surface of the lungs, and the parietal pleura, a membrane that covers the internal chest wall.)

- *Hemothorax*—an accumulation of blood in the pleural space.

- *Subcutaneous emphysema*—a condition in which air escapes into body tissues, especially in the chest wall, neck, and face.

- *Lacerated intercostal vessels*—blood vessels that surround the ribs are torn and cut.

- *Lung contusions.*

- *Injuries to the liver or spleen.*

Flail Chest

A closed chest injury, **flail chest** results when the chest wall becomes unstable due to multiple fractured ribs, fractures of the sternum, or fractures of the cartilage connecting the ribs to the sternum. Flail chest can affect the front, back, or sides of the rib cage. It most often occurs when two or more adjacent ribs are broken, each in two or more places.

In flail chest, an area of chest wall between the broken ribs becomes free-floating. This area is referred to as the *flail segment.* Its motion is opposite the motion of the rest of the chest (Figure 20-7). When the patient inhales, the flail segment collapses or does not expand. When the patient exhales, the flail segment protrudes while the rest of the chest wall contracts. This condition is called **paradoxical breathing.** (You may not notice paradoxical breathing, since the chest muscles may spasm and "splint" the chest.)

Flail chest can be a life-threatening injury. It usually involves bruising of the lung tissues beneath the flail segment. It can lead to inadequate oxygenation of the heart. Fractured ribs also can puncture a lung. Flail chest may involve serious bleeding within the thorax from the arteries and veins between the ribs. This can lead to shock.

Signs and symptoms of flail chest include the following:

- Shortness of breath.

- Paradoxical breathing, which is almost always accompanied by severe pain.

- Swelling over the injured area.

- Signs of shock.

- Increasing airway resistance.

- Patient's attempt to splint the chest wall with hands and arms.

- Possible grating sounds from bone ends rubbing together.

To check for flail chest, have the patient lie on his or her back. Bare the chest. Watch for a seesaw motion of the chest while the patient breathes. Gently place your hands on the patient's chest. Check for symmetry of the sides as

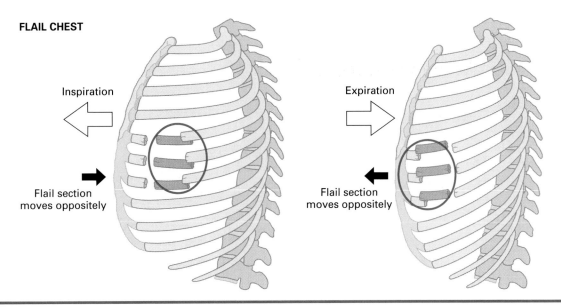

FLAIL CHEST

Inspiration

Flail section
moves oppositely

Expiration

Flail section
moves oppositely

FIGURE 20-7 In flail chest, a free-floating segment of chest wall moves in the opposite direction.

the patient breathes. Note that it can be very difficult to detect flail chest in an obese or muscular patient. Muscles of the chest wall can "splint" the flail segment, restricting movement and making it difficult to observe. Because flail chest can be so painful, the patient may not want to relinquish "guarding" the chest.

In addition to the general guidelines for chest injuries described above, you must also try to splint the chest. It will help to improve respirations. To do so, remove clothing from the chest area. Then tape a small pillow or thick, heavy dressing over the injury site. The dressing should weigh less than five pounds. (See Figure 20-8)

If you suspect internal bleeding or if there is increased pain and discomfort, have the patient lie on the

injured side. However, do so only if there is no possibility of spine injury.

Pneumothorax

Pneumothorax occurs when air from a wound site enters the chest cavity but not the lungs. The pressure of the air in the chest presses against a lung, separating it from the chest wall and causing it to collapse. The volume of the lung is reduced, resulting in respiratory distress.

Air can enter the chest cavity in one of two ways. Air can enter either from the outside, through a sucking chest wound, or air can leak out of a lung laceration. Once the lung is ruptured, it does not expand properly.

In some cases, called *spontaneous pneumothorax,* the lung does not collapse because of injury. It collapses because the patient has a weak area on the surface of the lung that ruptures. The weakened lung loses its ability to expand. The patient then experiences sharp chest

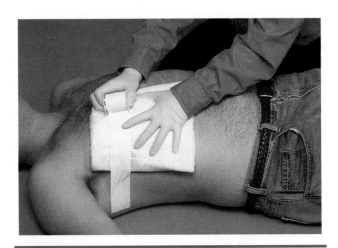

FIGURE 20-8 Stabilize flail chest by applying a pillow or bulky dressing.

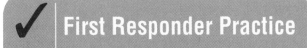

✔ **First Responder Practice**

Open chest injuries are very serious. When they affect the delicate balance in pressures between the inside and outside of the chest, the patient can rapidly deteriorate. The application of an occlusive dressing during the initial assessment will help keep this dangerous situation under control until the patient reaches the hospital.

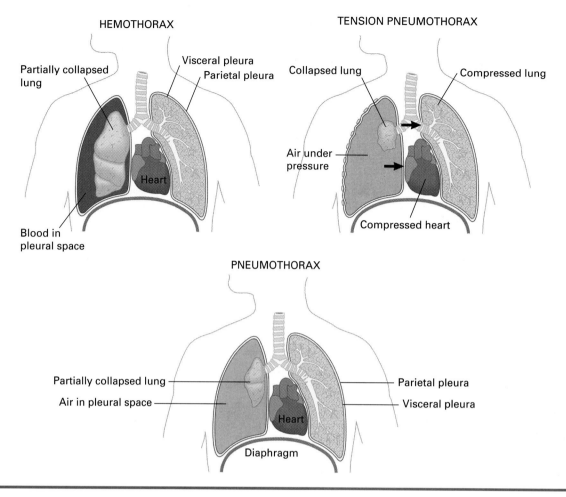

FIGURE 20-9 Complications of chest injuries.

pain and mild to severe respiratory distress. Spontaneous pneumothorax is common among smokers or emphysema patients.

Hemothorax

Hemothorax occurs when the pleural space fills with blood, creating pressure on the heart and lungs (Figure 20-9). The lungs cannot expand, and the same process then occurs as with pneumothorax. In addition, severe bleeding can cause shock.

Hemothorax is the result of blunt or penetrating trauma to the chest. It often accompanies pneumothorax. The blood usually originates from lacerated blood vessels in the chest wall or cavity. In rare cases, it results from a lacerated lung. The severity of the hemothorax depends on the amount of blood lost into the pleural space.

Tension Pneumothorax

Tension pneumothorax is one of the most life-threatening chest injuries. Air continuously leaks out of a lung and becomes trapped in the pleural space. A process of compression starts and worsens with each breath until the lung on the affected side is reduced to the size of a small ball, sometimes only a few inches in diameter.

Even after the lung is as compressed as it can be, air continues to leak into the pleural space. Pressure continues to rise and may then compress major blood vessels, the heart, or the opposite lung. The extreme pressure in the chest cavity prevents blood from returning to the heart through the veins, and the blood is no longer pumped out. Death can occur rapidly.

1. What are the two most important signs of chest trauma in a patient?

2. For First Responders, what are the general guidelines for emergency care of a patient with a chest injury?

3. What is a "sucking chest wound"? What special care does a patient with this type of wound require?

Section 2 Injuries to the Abdomen

A wound that penetrates the skin and abdominal cavity is a dangerous one. Internal bleeding may occur. Bacteria may be introduced into the abdomen from the outside as well as from a penetrated intestine (Figure 20-10). In the presence of open wounds of the abdomen, assume that internal organs have been damaged. Closed abdominal injuries, such as a severe blow or crushing injury, can be extremely dangerous and lead to internal bleeding and shock.

(Now may be a good time to review the four quadrants of the abdomen as described in Chapter 4.)

Patient Assessment

To assess for a closed abdominal injury, have the patient lie down on his or her back. The knees should be flexed and supported. Remove or loosen clothing over the abdomen to expose it. Then look and feel for signs of injury. Look for bruising, lacerations and other open wounds, impaled objects, and protruding organs. Watch how the abdomen moves as the patient breathes. Gently feel all four quadrants. Note rigidity, pain, and tenderness. Also note any guarding, a common reaction to a painful abdomen. If the patient complains of pain in a particular area, palpate that area last. If the area is palpated first, it may prevent accurate palpation of the remaining quadrants.

Suspect abdominal injuries in patients involved in fights, falls, and car crashes. The most common symptom is pain. In addition to open wounds such as an evisceration, general signs and symptoms of an injured abdomen include:

- Distended or irregularly shaped abdomen.
- Bruising of the abdomen, back, or flanks.
- Rigid and tender abdomen.

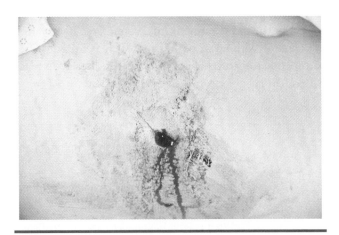

FIGURE 20-10 A patient with an open wound to the abdomen. *(Charles Stewart, M.D. & Associates)*

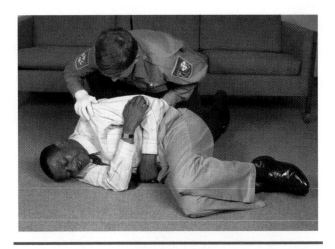

FIGURE 20-11 Patient guarding a painful abdomen.

- Mild discomfort progressing to intolerable pain.
- Pain radiating to a shoulder, both shoulders, or the back.
- Abdominal cramping.
- Lying still with legs drawn up (Figure 20-11).
- Rapid, shallow breathing.
- Rapid pulse, low blood pressure.
- Nausea, vomiting.
- Blood in the urine, vomiting of blood.
- Shock.
- Weakness.
- Thirst.

Remember to communicate with empathy. Your attitude toward the patient will have an impact, so put his or her needs first. Stay calm, cool, and sympathetic. ■

First Responder Care

To provide care to a patient with abdominal injuries, make your top priorities airway, breathing, and circulation. Once the ABCs are assessed and life-threats treated, update or activate EMS immediately to arrange for transport.

1. *Maintain an open airway.* Be alert for vomiting. Position the patient for adequate drainage. Be prepared to suction. Do not give the patient anything to eat or drink.

2. *If breathing is adequate, administer oxygen via nonrebreather.* If it is inadequate, assist ventilations with BVM and supplemental oxygen. Be prepared to provide basic life support, if needed.

3. *Suspect and treat for shock.* Work diligently to prevent it. Keep the patient warm, but do not overheat. Administer high-concentration oxygen, if you are allowed.

4. *Control external bleeding.* Dress open wounds with dry, sterile dressings or follow local protocol.

SKILL SUMMARY *Caring for an Abdominal Evisceration*

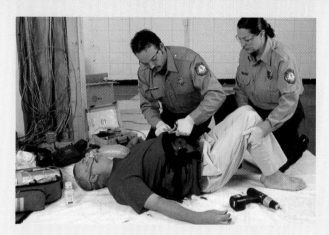

FIGURE 20-12A *Cut away clothing.*

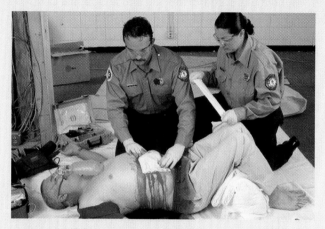

FIGURE 20-12B *Cover the exposed organs with a moist bulky dressing.*

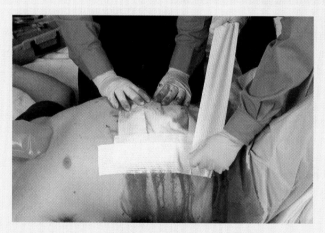

FIGURE 20-12C *Secure an occlusive dressing over the bulky one.*

5. *Position the patient.* The patient usually is most comfortable lying on his or her back with knees flexed. If you suspect a pelvic fracture, prevent movement. Immobilize the patient on a long backboard if possible.

If there is an abdominal evisceration, you must cover the exposed organs (Figure 20-12). Never touch exposed organs. Never try to replace them. Instead, use a thick, moist, sterile dressing to cover them completely. You should moisten the dressing with sterile saline. Never use absorbent materials as dressings, such as toilet tissue or paper towels, which can shred and cling to the organs. Gently and loosely tape the moist dressing in place. Then, loosely cover it with an occlusive dressing. Tape down the edges to help keep the first dressing moist and warm.

Maintain the temperature of the wound area by covering the dressing with layers of dressings such as a particle-free bath blanket or towel. They may be held loosely in place with a bandage or clean sheet. ■

1. What is the most common symptom of abdominal injury?

2. What are three other signs and symptoms associated with abdominal injury?

3. What is First Responder care for a patient with abdominal injuries?

Section 3 Injuries to the Genitalia

While assessing injuries to the male or female genitalia, act in a calm professional way. Protect the patient from onlookers. Be sensitive to the patient's embarrassment as well as his or her pain. Use sheets, towels, or other material as a drape over the area. Provide the same emergency care you would provide for any soft-tissue injury, with the following exceptions.

(Now may be a good time to review the reproductive systems as described in Chapter 4.)

Male Genitalia

Injuries to the external genitalia of a male can cause severe pain, though they are not usually life-threatening.

Penis

The skin of the penis can be torn or avulsed. Such injuries occur most commonly in accidents and assaults. To provide First Responder care, wrap the injured penis in a soft, sterile dressing that is moistened with sterile saline solution. Apply a cold pack to relieve pain and reduce swelling. Never remove impaled objects. Instead, stabilize them and bandage them in place. If you can find avulsed skin, wrap it in sterile gauze that has been moistened with sterile saline and send it with the patient to the hospital.

In some cases, the penis may be partially or completely amputated. Blood loss may be significant. If so, apply a sterile pressure dressing to the remaining stump to control bleeding. Aggressive direct pressure may be needed also. If you can find the amputated penis, follow the usual procedure for preserving and transporting parts with the patient.

Scrotum and Testicles

A direct blow to the scrotum can cause the testes to rupture. It also can result in a pooling of blood, causing tremendous pain and a feeling of pressure. A testicle that ruptures requires surgery. To care for this patient, apply an ice pack to the entire area to reduce swelling and pain. If the scrotal skin becomes avulsed, try to find it. Then, wrap it in moist, sterile gauze. Send it with the patient to the hospital. Dress the scrotum itself in a sterile dressing moistened with sterile saline. Control bleeding with pressure.

Female Genitalia

Injuries to the internal female organs are rare. That is because they are small and well protected, except during pregnancy when the uterus is enlarged. Such an injury can result in serious blood loss and shock.

Injuries to the external female genitalia can follow straddle injuries or sexual assault. Because the area is richly supplied with blood vessels and nerves, injuries can cause severe pain and bleeding. However, they are not usually life-threatening. To provide First Responder care, control bleeding with local pressure, using compresses moistened with sterile saline. Dress wounds and bandage them in place with a diaper-like bandage. Stabilize any impaled objects. Use cold packs over the dressing to relieve pain and reduce swelling. Never place anything inside the vagina. Treat the patient for shock.

If you suspect a sexual assault, protect the patient's privacy. Clear the area of bystanders and provide cover, such as a blanket or sheet. Discretely question the patient about other potential injuries, such as head trauma. Do not touch or examine the genitals unless there is life-threatening bleeding.

To help preserve evidence in case of sexual assault, do not allow the patient to bathe or douche. Discourage the patient from washing her hair or cleaning under her fingernails. If possible, do not clean any wounds. Handle the patient's clothing as little as possible. Bag all items of clothing and other items separately. If there is blood on any item, do not use plastic bags. Follow local protocol.

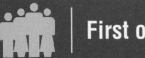

First on Scene

In addition to the physical trauma, the emotional impact of the injuries to the genital region is greater than most. Patients will be hesitant to have this region exposed and examined. Some will be worried about function and disfigurement of the genitalia. Victims of sexual assault will have significant emotional trauma. In all of these cases, your emotional support, understanding, and compassion will be critical.

1. What are the general guidelines for First Responder care of a patient with an injury to the genitalia?

2. What kind of emotional support can you give to the patient with injuries to the genitalia?

The Call Follow-up

At the beginning of this chapter, you read that First Responders were on scene for a female patient with an open chest wound. To see how chapter skills apply to this emergency, read the following. It describes how the call was completed.

Initial Assessment Our immediate priorities were to evaluate the patient's ABCs and seal the chest wound. Fortunately, there were two of us. My partner, Meg, talked to the patient, explaining who we were and what we were doing. The patient was alert but in a lot of pain. Meg applied oxygen by nonrebreather mask. I applied an occlusive dressing.

Our general impression was that of a responsive female patient who was in a potentially serious condition. We updated the EMTs from our portable radio.

Physical Examination The patient reported that she had been struck over the head, stabbed,

and kicked by a gang of teens. We realized that the mechanisms of injury were quite serious, so Meg stabilized the patient's head while I began a head-to-toe exam. I got as far as the abdomen when the EMTs arrived.

Patient History We didn't have time to get much of a history.

Ongoing Assessment The EMTs arrived before we could reassess the patient.

Patient Hand-off We gave the EMTs our hand-off report (see below). The EMTs understood why we couldn't get to the patient's history or vital signs. There were important things to do. They, too, realized the urgency and quickly immobilized the patient and prepared for transport. Meg and I later found out that the woman's wounds were mostly superficial and that she recovered well.

 ## Hand-off Report

"This is Andrea Purne. She is 34 years old and was assaulted during a robbery. Multiple teens struck, kicked, and stabbed her. She is alert with a strong pulse and adequate respirations. She has a good bump on the left side of her skull. She has a stab wound to the chest to which we have applied an occlusive dressing. We just got to her abdomen and found it reddened. It looks like she took some punches or kicks there, too. We applied oxygen. We didn't get to the history or vitals."

The Last Word *Always rely on the mechanism of injury, a high index of suspicion, and a carefully performed patient assessment for any trauma patient. Early recognition and prompt emergency treatment of injuries, especially to the chest and abdomen, can save a life.*

Chapter Review

Focus on the EMS Team

Injuries to the chest and abdomen are potentially very serious. The emergency care you give—such as applying an occlusive dressing—is vital. Quality care also includes immediate transport to a hospital, preferably to a trauma center if one is available. It is your responsibility to recognize the patient's problem quickly and update the incoming EMS unit. The responding crew will begin to get ready even before they reach the scene, so your call will help expedite preparation. You also may be asked to assist with patient immobilization. Do so. The patient must get en route to the hospital as fast as possible.

Remember that the care given on scene is important, but prolonged scene times will hurt rather than help. The care that will ultimately save the patient will occur in the hospital.

Summing Up

- Injuries to the chest include blunt trauma and penetrating injury. Always assume spine injury if there is any significant mechanism of injury to the chest. Two of the most important signs of chest injury are the patient's respiratory rate and a change in normal breathing pattern.

- First Responder care of a chest injury includes getting the patient stabilized and transported as quickly as possible to a medical facility. While on scene, the patient's airway should be maintained and adequate breathing ensured. Bleeding should also be controlled. Treat for shock, if appropriate. If a sucking chest wound or any injury to the chest potentially penetrates the chest cavity, an occlusive dressing should be applied.

- Abdominal injuries can involve internal bleeding, injury to internal organs, bacterial infection, and shock. The most common symptom of an abdominal injury is pain, but suspect it in all patients involved in fights, falls, and car crashes.

- Just as for any patient, First Responder care of a patient with an abdominal injury includes ensuring an open airway, adequate breathing, and bleeding control. Special care for an evisceration involves the application of dressings: first, a thick moist sterile dressing to cover the exposed organs; then, an occlusive dressing; and, finally, a covering such as a particle-free blanket that will help maintain the patient's body temperature.

- In addition to the care provided for any soft-tissue injury, care of injuries to the genitalia includes protecting the patient's privacy and, in the case of sexual assault, helping to preserve any evidence.

Key Terms

blunt trauma an injury caused by an object that is not sharp or forceful enough to penetrate the skin.

crepitus a sound or feeling of broken bones grinding against each other.

flail chest a closed chest injury resulting in the chest wall becoming unstable.

hemothorax the accumulation of blood in the pleural space.

paradoxical breathing a condition in which a segment of the chest moves in the opposite direction to the rest of the chest during breathing; typically seen with a flail segment.

penetrating injury to the chest an injury that occurs when an object passes through the chest wall and into the chest cavity.

pleural space the area between the lungs and the walls of the chest cavity.

pneumothorax an accumulation of air in the pleural space.

sucking chest wound an open wound to the chest that bubbles or makes a sucking noise.

Knowledge Check

1. First Responder care for an open chest injury includes application of a(n) ___ dressing.
   a. moist
   b. trauma
   c. occlusive
   d. encircling

2. The chest cavity is separated from the abdominal cavity by the:
   a. intestines.
   b. diaphragm.
   c. lungs.
   d. liver.

3. A flail chest is best described as:
   a. an open wound.
   b. two rib fractures.
   c. one rib fracture with an underlying lung injury.
   d. two or more ribs, each fractured in two different places.

4. For a sucking chest wound, an occlusive dressing should extend ___ inch(es) beyond the wound edges and be sealed on ___ side(s).
   a. one, four
   b. one, two
   c. two, three
   d. two, two

5. Signs and symptoms of an abdominal injury include all of the following EXCEPT:
   a. hemothorax.
   b. guarding.
   c. cramping.
   d. thirst.

6. First Responder care of an evisceration should NEVER include:
   a. applying a thick, saline-moistened, sterile dressing.
   b. using plastic as an occlusive dressing.
   c. cutting away the clothing from the injured area.
   d. replacing or touching the exposed organs.

7. Your patient had been in a fist fight and took a direct blow to the scrotum. To help reduce the pain and swelling, you should do all of the following EXCEPT:
   a. apply heat to the entire area.
   b. control any bleeding with pressure.
   c. allow him to lie in a position of comfort.
   d. find any avulsed skin and wrap it in moist gauze.

8. Two of the most important signs of chest injury are the patient's respiratory rate and a change in normal breathing pattern.
   a. True
   b. False

9. In the presence of a significant mechanism of injury to the chest, assume cardiac damage and spine injury.
   a. True
   b. False

Scenario

A bicycle and its rider crashed into your patient, hitting her hard in the abdomen before she fell to the ground. There is no bleeding, so you suspect a closed abdominal injury.

a. To assess the injured area, you should:

_____

_____

_____

_____

b. To provide emergency care to this patient, you should:

_____

_____

_____

_____

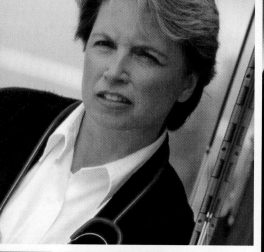
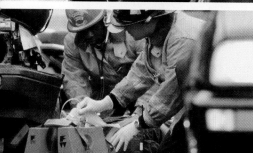
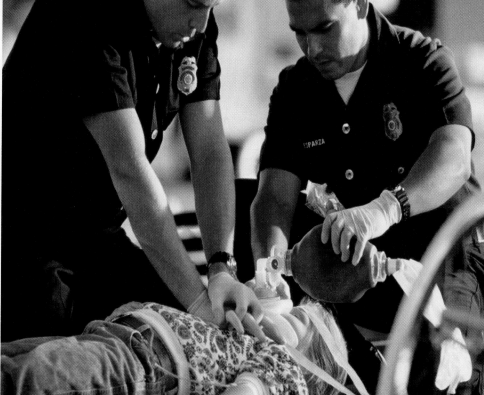

21 | Burn Emergencies

Objectives

From the U.S. Department of Transportation (DOT) 1995 "First Responder: National Standard Curriculum." Material supplemental to the DOT curriculum is listed under "Enrichment."

Cognitive

5-2.6 ▶ Establish the relationship between body substance isolation (BSI) and soft tissue injuries. (p. 389)

5-2.13 ▶ Describe the emergency medical care for burns. (pp. 389–392)

Affective

5-2.17 ▶ Demonstrate a caring attitude towards patients with a soft tissue injury or bleeding who request emergency medical services. (pp. 391–392)

5-2.19 ▶ Communicate with empathy to patients with a soft tissue injury or bleeding, as well as with family members and friends of the patient. (pp. 391–392)

Psychomotor

No objectives are identified by the DOT.

Enrichment

▶ List the classifications of burns. (pp. 385, 386–387)

▶ Define the characteristics of superficial burns, partial thickness burns, and full thickness burns. (pp. 386–387)

▶ Establish the relationship between airway management and patients with burns. (pp. 385, 390, 391, 392–393)

▶ Describe the emergency medical care for a patient with inhalation injuries. (pp. 392–393)

▶ Describe the emergency medical care for a patient with chemical burns. (p. 393)

▶ Describe the emergency medical care for a patient with electrical burns. (pp. 393–395)

Introduction

More than two million burn accidents occur in the U.S. each year. Of those people who are burned, some will die, many more need long-term rehabilitation, and all experience significant pain. In this chapter, you will learn how to assess burns and provide First Responder care. You also will learn about common causes of burns.

Section 1 General Burn Management

The skin is the largest organ of the body. Its outermost layer is the **epidermis,** which contains cells that give the skin its color. The **dermis,** or second layer, contains a vast network of blood vessels. The deepest layers of the skin contain hair follicles, sweat and oil glands, and sensory nerves. Just below the skin is a layer of fat called **subcutaneous tissue.** (See page 66 for an illustration.)

The function of the skin includes protecting the deep tissues from injury, drying out, and invasion by bacteria and other foreign bodies. Skin helps to regulate body temperature and aids in getting rid of water and various salts. It also acts as the receptor organ for touch, pain, heat, and cold. When the skin is damaged by burns, some or all of its functions may be compromised or destroyed.

Patient Assessment

Always make sure the scene of a burn incident is safe before entering. If the emergency involves noxious fumes, chemical spills, or electricity, call for specialized personnel to secure the scene before entering. Never try to rescue people trapped by fire unless you are equipped and trained to do so.

Many burn patients who die in the prehospital setting die from a blocked airway, inhaled smoke and toxins, or other trauma, and not from the burn itself. As with all patients, perform an initial assessment and treat any life-threats you find.

Determine the severity of the patient's burns during the physical exam—after life-threats have been treated. Take into account the depth of burns, extent of **body surface area (BSA)** involved, location of burns, and any complicating factors (Table 21-1). Don't forget to look for other possible injuries as well.

Gather a history of the event if you can. One reason why burns are often critically damaging or even fatal is that some individuals are poorly informed about methods of care. Someone may have tried to treat the patient's burns before you arrived on scene. Find out what they did. Include this information in your patient hand-off report. ■

TABLE 21-1 **Determining Severity of Burns**		
	Adults	**Infants and Children**
Critical Burns	Full-thickness burns involving the hands, feet, face, or genitalia. Burns associated with respiratory injury. Full-thickness burns covering more than 10% body surface area. Partial-thickness burns covering more than 30% body surface area. Burns complicated by painful, swollen, deformed extremity. Burns encompassing any body part, e.g., arm, leg, or chest.	Any full-thickness burns. Any partial-thickness burn greater than 20%, or burns involving hands, feet, face, airway, or genitalia.
Moderate Burns	Full-thickness burns of 2% to 10% body surface area excluding hands, feet, face, genitalia, and upper airway. Partial-thickness burns of 10% to 20% body surface area. Superficial burns of greater than 50% body surface area.	Partial-thickness burns of 15% to 30% body surface area.
Minor Burns	Full-thickness burns of less than 2% body surface area. Partial-thickness burns less than 15% body surface area.	Partial-thickness burns less than 10% body surface area.

THE CALL

 Dispatch It was going to rain hard that day. All the weather reports included storm warnings. As soon as we got back to the station house from our first run, my partner and I checked in and readied our truck for the next call. Before long we were dispatched to a "man hit by lightning."

Scene Size-up Upon arrival at Costanza's farm, we were met by a woman who told us the patient had been moved into the barn. We drove up to the building, located the patient, and took BSI precautions.

✓ **Initial Assessment** My partner immediately stabilized the patient's head

and neck. I found the patient responsive to painful stimuli only. The initial assessment revealed a patent airway, respirations that were adequate and of good quality, and no visible bleeding. We elected to place the patient on oxygen at 15 liters per minute by way of a nonrebreather mask. We also noted a feathery pattern of markings scattered over the patient's left arm.

What injuries might you expect a lightning strike to cause? Are they all as obvious as the burn marks on the patient's arm? Consider this patient as you read Chapter 21. What else should be done to assess and treat him?

Severity of Burns

Severity of a burn depends on many factors, including the depth of the burn, the extent of body surface burned, which part of the body was burned, and other complicating factors.

Depth of Burns

Burns typically are classified by depth (Figure 21-1). A **superficial burn** involves only the first layer of skin. A **partial-thickness burn** involves the epidermis and the dermis. In a **full-thickness burn,** the burn extends through all layers of skin and may involve subcutaneous tissue, muscles, organs, and bone. Note that burns are seldom only one depth. They usually involve a combination of depths.

You can recognize superficial, partial-thickness, and full-thickness burns as follows:

- *Superficial burns* (Figure 21-2). A superficial burn is caused by flash, flame, scald, or the sun. It is the most common of all burns and is considered minor. The patient's skin surface will be dry, and there may be some swelling. Though the skin is red and painful, the burn involves only the epidermis. A superficial burn heals in 2 to 5 days with no scarring. Peeling of the burned skin may occur. Some temporary discoloration may result.

- *Partial-thickness burns* (Figure 21-3). This type of burn usually results from contact with hot liquids or solids,

flash or flame contact with clothing, direct flame from fire, contact with chemicals, or the sun. The skin appears moist and mottled, ranging in color from white to red. The burn area is blistered and intensely painful. It usually requires 5 to 21 days to heal. If infection occurs, healing time can take longer.

- *Full-thickness burns* (Figure 21-4). A full-thickness burn results from contact with hot liquids or solids, flame, chemicals, or electricity. The skin is dry and leathery and may be a mix of colors from white to dark brown to charcoal. Often charred blood vessels are visible. While it can be very painful, the patient may feel little if nerve endings have been destroyed. Small full-thickness burns require

 First Responder Practice

The amount of body surface area burned is significant in evaluating a patient. Even superficial burns when they occur over a large body surface area may require medical attention to reduce pain and to prevent dehydration and infection.

SUPERFICIAL   PARTIAL-THICKNESS   FULL-THICKNESS

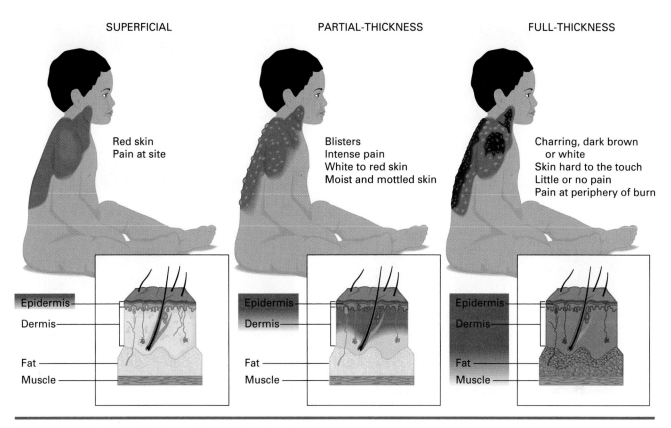

Red skin
Pain at site

Blisters
Intense pain
White to red skin
Moist and mottled skin

Charring, dark brown
or white
Skin hard to the touch
Little or no pain
Pain at periphery of burn

Epidermis
Dermis
Fat
Muscle

Epidermis
Dermis
Fat
Muscle

Epidermis
Dermis
Fat
Muscle

FIGURE 21-1 Classification of burns by depth.

weeks to heal. Large ones, which may need skin grafting and other specialized burn care, can take months or years to heal. These burns often result in scarring.

Extent of Body Surface Burned

The **rule of nines** is a standardized way to estimate the amount of body surface area (BSA) burned. The head and neck region is considered to be 9% of the total body surface area. The posterior trunk is 18%. The anterior trunk is 18%. Each upper extremity is 9%, and each lower extremity is 18%. In an infant, the head is considered to be 18% of BSA and each lower extremity is 14% BSA.

External genitalia are estimated as 1% BSA in all patients. (See Figure 21-5.)

An alternative method is called the **palmar surface method,** or the rule of palms. With this method, use the palm of the patient's hand—approximately 1% of the BSA—to estimate the size of a burn. For example, if a burn area is equal to "7 palms," the burn would be estimated as 7% BSA.

You will find it useful to use the rule of nines to estimate the BSA of larger burn injuries and the palmar surface method for smaller burns. Follow local protocols. However, do not spend time trying to determine a burn's

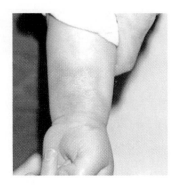

a.

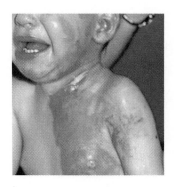

b.

FIGURE 21-2 Superficial burns. This type of burn is usually caused by a flash, flame, scald, or the sun.

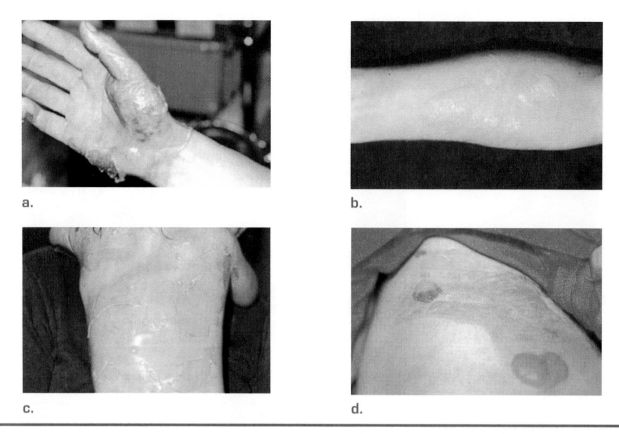

FIGURE 21-3 Partial-thickness burns, which are usually caused by hot liquids or solids, flash or flame contact, chemicals, or the sun.

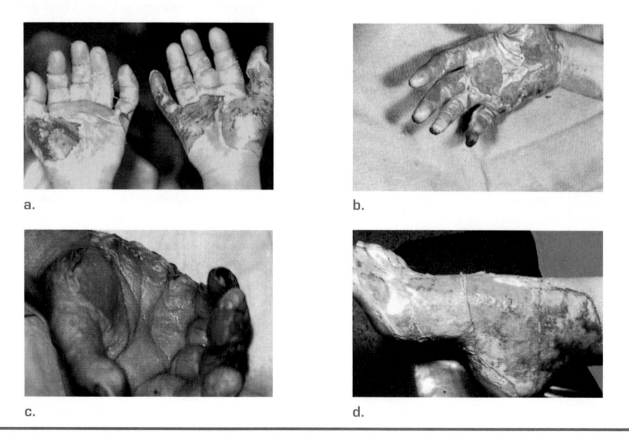

FIGURE 21-4 Full-thickness burns are usually caused by hot liquids or solids, flame, chemicals, or electricity.

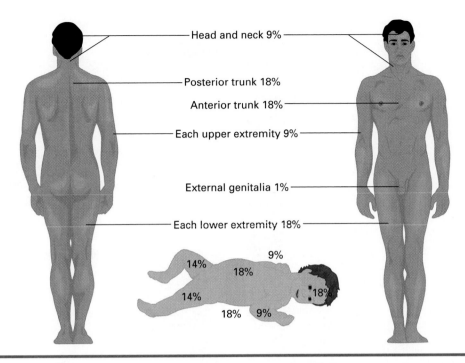

FIGURE 21-5 Rule of nines. This is one method used to estimate the extent of a patient's burns.

exact percent of BSA. Slight differences in percentages will not affect proper First Responder care.

Location of Burns

Burns to certain areas of the body are more critical than others. For example, burns to the face can compromise breathing or cause injury to the eyes (Figure 21-6). Loss of function may be the result of burns to the hands or feet. Burns to the genital area may result in loss or impairment of genitourinary function. Burns that encircle a body part—such as a joint, arm, or leg—are considered critical because of the possibility of blood-vessel and nerve damage. Burns that encircle the chest can limit its ability to expand, which can result in inadequate breathing.

Arrange for patients with burns to any of these areas to be transported to a hospital or burn center immediately.

Complicating Factors

Patients who have other injuries or chronic diseases such as heart disease or diabetes will always react more severely to burns, even minor ones. So try to determine the patient's medical history early in the course of care.

The age of a patient also may be a complicating factor. Children under the age of 5 and adults over the age of 55 tolerate burns poorly. In an elderly patient, a burn covering only 20% of body surface can be fatal. Because the elderly and very young generally have thin skin, they can sustain much deeper burns. Fluid loss from a burn also can affect them more critically. Even a small fluid

loss can result in serious problems. An additional problem concerns the immune system, which is immature in children and usually compromised in the elderly patient.

Please note that burns may be the result of abuse. Look for burn patterns that indicate a patient might have been dipped in scalding water. Cigarettes also are used to burn skin as a form of abuse. Follow local protocols for reporting your observations.

First Responder Care

To provide emergency care to a patient with burns, first the patient must be removed from the source of the burn. Take BSI precautions and then (Figure 21-7):

1. *Stop the burning process.* Run cold water over scald burns. Flush away chemicals with water for 20 minutes or more. Remove any smoldering clothing and jewelry. If you meet resistance, or if you see bits melted into the

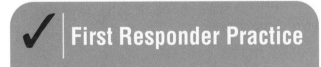

First Responder Practice

The first thing you must do to care for your patient is stop the burning process. Keep in mind that partial- and full-thickness burns can actually continue burning skin and underlying tissues for several minutes after the source of burning has been removed.

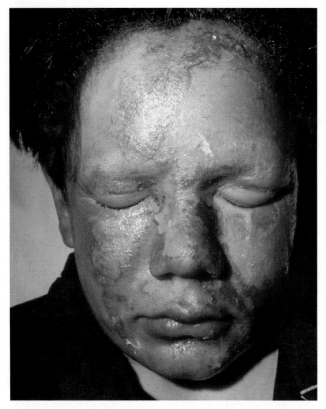

a. *Burns to the face from an exploded gas cylinder.* (Shout Picture Library)

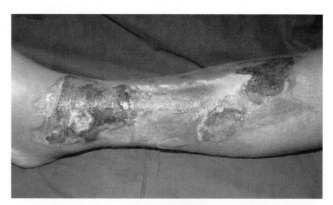

b. *Petroleum burns to the foot and leg.* (Shout Picture Library)

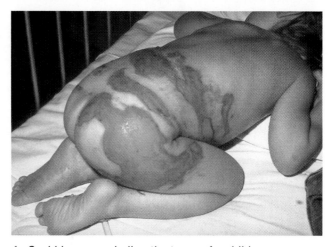

d. *Scald burns encircling the torso of a child.* (Shout Picture Library)

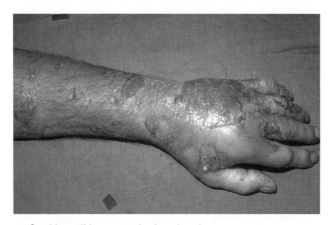

c. *Cooking oil burns to the hand and arm.* (Shout Picture Library)

FIGURE 21-6 Burns to the face, hands or feet, or genitalia, and burns that encircle the body are considered critical.

skin, cut around the area to expose what you can and to prevent additional contamination.

2. *After you have identified and treated all life-threats, administer oxygen.* If breathing is adequate, administer oxygen by nonrebreather. If it is not adequate, provide BVM ventilation with supplemental oxygen. Be prepared to provide basic life support, if needed.

3. *Cover the burns.* Use dry sterile dressings or a disposable sterile burn sheet. Do not use grease or fat, ointment, lotion, antiseptic, or ice on the burns. Do not break any blisters. If a burn involves an eye, be sure to apply dressings to both eyes (Figure 21-8).

4. *Keep the patient warm* and treat other injuries as needed.

SKILL SUMMARY *Caring for a Patient with Burn Injuries*

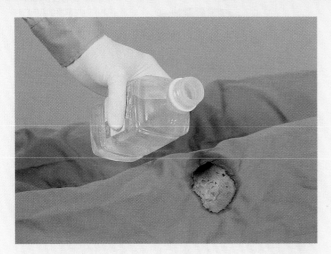

FIGURE 21-7A *Stop the burning process with water . . .*

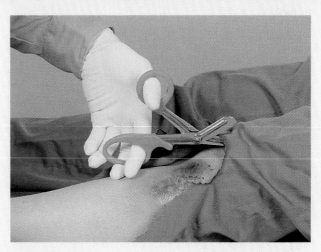

FIGURE 21-7B *. . . and by removing all smoldering clothing.*

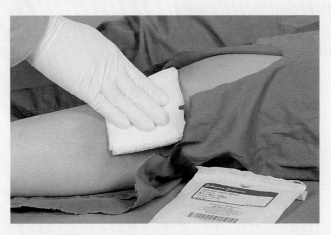

FIGURE 21-7C *After life-threats have been treated and a physical exam completed, cover burns with dry sterile dressings.*

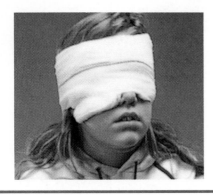

FIGURE 21-8 Apply dressings to both eyes, even if only one is burned.

Proper care of burns must start as soon as possible after the injury. Loss of body fluids, pain contributing to shock, swelling, and infection may quickly follow a burn injury. Be especially alert to any sign of breathing difficulty. If burns were caused by an electrical source, monitor the patient closely for cardiac arrest. Be prepared to administer CPR and, if you are trained and equipped, to apply an automated external defibrillator (AED). Remember that the patient's status can change suddenly, so monitor vital signs continually.

As always, do your best to calm and reassure the patient. He or she may be in a great deal of pain. The patient and family members also may be afraid of permanent scarring and disfigurement. Tell them that you are doing what is necessary to prevent further injury and contamination. Let them know that additional EMS personnel are on the way. ■

Q: 1. Which layers of skin are involved in a superficial burn? Partial-thickness burn? Full-thickness burn?

2. What are the percentages given to each area of an adult's body according to the rule of nines?

3. Using the rule of palms, what is equal to approximately 1% of the patient's body surface area?

4. Briefly, what is First Responder care for a patient who has a burn emergency?

Section 2 Special Types of Burn Injuries

Inhalation Injuries

Greater than half of all fire-related deaths are caused by smoke inhalation. About 80% of those who die in residential fires do so only because they have inhaled heated air or smoke and other toxic gases. Suspect inhalation injury in any patient who was burned in a fire, especially if the patient was confined in an enclosed space.

The severity of an inhalation injury is determined by the following factors: product of combustion (what was burned), degree of combustion (how completely it was burned), duration of exposure (how long the patient was exposed to the smoke or gas), and whether or not the patient was in a confined space.

Most upper airway damage from heat inhalation consists of scorched mucous membranes and swelling, which can block the airway. Specific signs and symptoms include (Figure 21-9):

■ Singed nasal hairs.

■ Burns to the face (Figure 21-10).

■ Burned specks of carbon in the sputum.

■ Sooty or smoky smell on the breath.

■ Respiratory distress.

■ Noisy breathing.

■ Hoarseness, cough, difficulty speaking.

■ Restricted chest movement.

■ Cyanosis.

SIGNS AND SYMPTOMS OF INHALATION BURNS

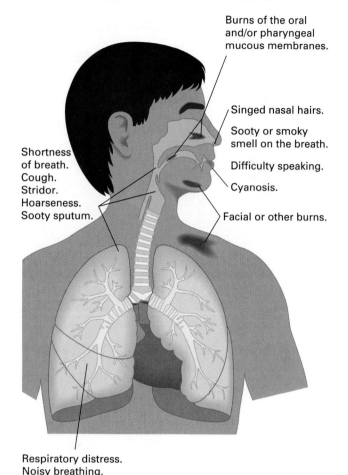

Burns of the oral and/or pharyngeal mucous membranes.

Singed nasal hairs.

Sooty or smoky smell on the breath.

Difficulty speaking.

Cyanosis.

Facial or other burns.

Shortness of breath. Cough. Stridor. Hoarseness. Sooty sputum.

Respiratory distress. Noisy breathing. Restricted chest movement.

FIGURE 21-9 Suspect an inhalation injury in any patient burned in a fire.

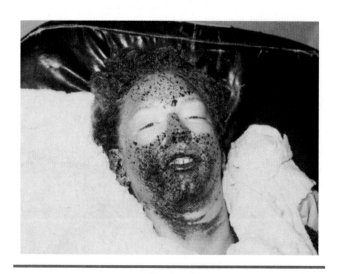

FIGURE 21-10 Burns to the face.

If any of these signs and symptoms are present, administer humidified oxygen if available. Note that this type of injury may appear mild at first and then become more severe. Monitor the patient's airway and breathing closely. Be prepared to assist breathing with artificial ventilation if necessary.

Chemical Burns

It is very difficult to assess the severity of chemical burns in the field. The general guideline is to treat all chemical burns as critical. Speed is essential. The faster you stop the burning process and initiate care, the less severe the burn will be. However, remember scene safety. Make sure that it is safe to approach the patient. If not, wait for trained rescue personnel to arrive. When you can approach your patient, wear protective gear to avoid contamination.

Immediately flush the patient's burns vigorously with water. Do not waste time trying to find an antidote. If the patient is at home, use the shower or a garden hose. Irrigate the area continuously under a steady stream for at least 20 minutes.

If chemical burns affect the eyes, flush them with water (Figure 21-11). Use a faucet or a hose running at low pressure. If necessary, use a pan, bucket, cup, or bottle. Have the patient remove any contact lenses. Minimize further contamination by making sure the water runs away from the injury but not toward any uninjured areas.

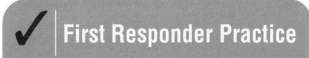

✔ **First Responder Practice**

Recall that carbon monoxide can cause falsely high oxygen saturation readings. All patients with inhalation injuries should receive oxygen regardless of pulse oximeter readings.

Note that you should brush off dry chemicals, such as lime powder, before flushing with water (Figure 21-12). Also wash off phenol or carbolic acid with alcohol first, and then flush the burn with water.

Electrical Burns

In any incident involving a car crash into a power pole, look for downed power lines. Sometimes they are hidden from sight by grass or a bush. Look at the next undamaged pole down the line. Count the number of power lines at the top crossarm. There should be the same number of lines at the top of the damaged pole. If the number is not the same, then proceed as follows:

- If you suspect that lines are down or the power pole has been weakened, notify all rescue personnel of the

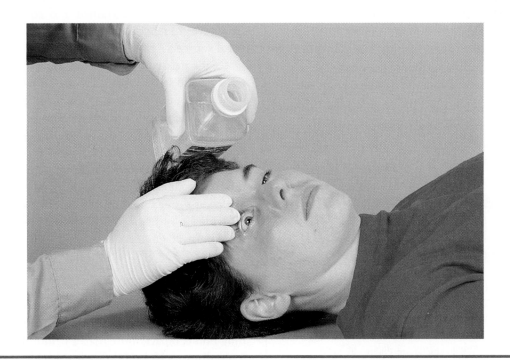

FIGURE 21-11 Flushing chemical burns to the eye.

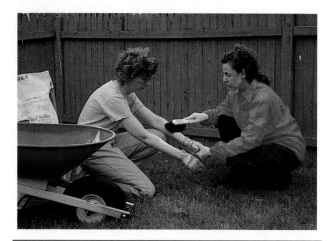

FIGURE 21-12 Lime powder should be brushed off the skin before flushing.

possible danger. Then notify the power company and request an emergency crew.

■ If the soles of your feet tingle when you enter the area, you are already too close. Go no farther. You are entering an energized zone.

■ Assume that a downed power line is live until the power company crew tells you otherwise. Remember that vehicles, guard rails, and metal fences conduct electricity.

■ If the patient's vehicle is in contact with a downed power line, tell the patient to stay inside the car. Maintain a safe distance. Never have a patient try to jump clear unless there is immediate danger of fire or explosion. Do not touch the vehicle and the ground at the same time. If you do, the current can kill you.

■ Never try to remove a power line. Personnel from the electrical company must do it. They have the training and the proper equipment to handle the line safely.

If you approach an emergency scene involving other electrical hazards, make a visual sweep for power cords. Pull the plug before you approach or touch the patient. Remember that a power tool does not have to

First on Scene

At the scene of a car crash, if you suspect that power pole lines are down or a power pole has been weakened, notify all rescue personnel of the possible danger. Then request an emergency crew from the power company. Do not attempt to enter the scene before it is made safe enough to do so.

ELECTRICAL
BURNS

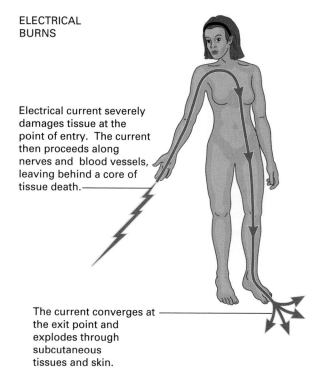

Electrical current severely damages tissue at the point of entry. The current then proceeds along nerves and blood vessels, leaving behind a core of tissue death.

The current converges at the exit point and explodes through subcutaneous tissues and skin.

FIGURE 21-13 For all electrical burns, look for both an entry burn and an exit burn.

be "on" to present a shock hazard. In general, you should never try to remove a patient from an electrical source unless you are trained and equipped to do so. And never touch a patient still in contact with an electrical source.

Signs and symptoms of electric shock may include altered mental status; obvious severe burns; weak, irregular, or absent pulse; shallow, irregular, or absent breathing; multiple fractures due to intense muscle contractions.

Care for a patient with electrical burns the same way you would care for any other patient with burns. However, note that an electric shock can throw a patient a significant distance. So, stabilize the patient's head and neck during assessment and treatment. Also look for both entry and exit burns (Figure 21-13). (See examples of electrical burns, Figure 21-14.)

Lightning Injuries

Thousands of electrical injuries occur each year in the U.S. About 25% of them are lightning injuries. A lightning bolt can pack more than a trillion watts of electricity and up to 100 million volts. Much of the electrical energy from lightning flows around, not through, a

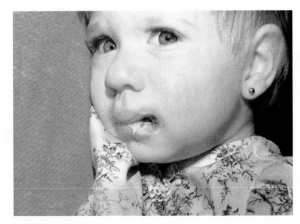

a. *Electrical burn caused by chewing on an electrical cord.*

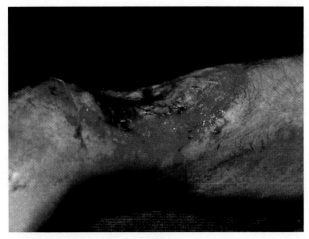

b. *Full-thickness electrical burn.*

FIGURE 21-14 Electrical burns.

strike victim. A patient who has been struck by lightning does not hold a charge. It is safe to approach him or her.

People are struck by lightning most often in open fields, under trees, on or near water, near tractors and heavy equipment, on golf courses, and at telephones. A person may be struck directly by lightning or lightning may "splash" off a nearby object. Whole groups of people can be affected by a ground strike in which lightning hits the ground and electricity ripples outward.

Most victims of lightning are knocked down or thrown. Assume possible spine injury. Also assume that a victim of lightning has sustained multiple injuries. Patients generally sustain the following types of injury:

- *Nervous system.* In many instances of lightning strike, the patient becomes unresponsive. Few actually remember being struck. Some patients suffer partial paralysis. Occasionally, paralysis of the respiratory system causes death.

- *Senses.* Some patients experience a loss of sight, hearing, and ability to speak. Rupture of one or both eardrums (tympanic membranes) occurs in 50% of patients who have been struck by lightning.

- *Skin.* In a lightning burn the skin may appear to be feathery, patchy, or in a scattered pattern resembling flowers. This is called "ferning." The burn may be red, mottled, blue, white, swollen, or blistered. The ferning fades and disappears within days.

- *Heart.* The lightning strike itself can disrupt the heart's rhythm, but the complications that follow are what generally lead to full cardiac arrest.

- *Vascular system.* Within seconds following the lightning strike, the patient may become unresponsive, appear pale and mottled, have cool arms and legs, and lose pulses. If the injury is moderate, the conditions may correct themselves quickly. In case of severe injury, blood may coagulate and tissues in the arms and legs may die, leading to amputation. Kidney failure may result.

Care for lightning burns as you would any other type of burn. In addition, provide manual stabilization of the patient's head and neck. As always, be prepared to provide basic life support. Such measures should continue even if the patient appears lifeless. Victims of lightning have been resuscitated as long as 30 minutes after a strike without lasting damage.

1. What should you always suspect if your patient was burned in a fire?

2. What is First Responder care for a patient with chemical burns?

3. What is First Responder care for a patient with electrical burns?

The Call Follow-up

At the beginning of this chapter, you read that First Responders were on scene with a male patient who had been hit by lightning. To see how chapter skills apply to this emergency, read the following. It describes how the call was completed.

Physical Examination While my partner took spinal precautions and monitored breathing, I conducted a head-to-toe exam. I found an entrance burn on the patient's left arm and a larger exit burn on his left foot. There appeared to be no other injuries. After I took a set of vital signs, which were within normal ranges, the patient moaned and tried to sit up. We encouraged him to lie still and then explained what had happened. I covered the burns with sterile gauze.

Patient History The patient was still somewhat confused, so we interviewed witnesses to the incident. They related that the man had been walking to his barn when he was struck by a lightning bolt. They knew of no medical problems or allergies. We found no medical identification tags or cards.

Ongoing Assessment We took the patient's vital signs every 5 minutes or so until the EMTs arrived. There were no changes noted. His oxygen was continued without resistance. When the patient became more alert, he told us his name was Sam Costanza and gave us a brief medical history.

Patient Hand-off After I gave my hand-off report to the EMTs (see below), they took over patient care. We returned to our duty station and prepared our truck for the next call.

Hand-off Report

"This is Sam Costanza. He is 42. He was struck by lightning as he approached his barn some 20 minutes ago. Initially, he responded only to painful stimuli. He presented with good respirations and strong regular heart rate. During the physical exam, he slowly became responsive. He remembered nothing about what happened to him. The physical exam revealed full-thickness burns on the left arm and left foot. We covered them with dry sterile dressings. He says he has no significant medical history. His respirations are 20 and of good quality, pulse 90 and strong, BP 140/82. His pupils are equal and reactive. His skin is warm and dry."

The Last Word *Treat all burn injuries in basically the same way. Stop the burning process, remove smoldering clothing, and dress the wounds. However, your job may not be finished there. Be sure to perform a thorough physical exam to find and treat other injuries the patient may have. Gather a good patient history. And continue with an ongoing assessment until the EMTs arrive to take over patient care.*

Chapter Review

Focus on the EMS Team

Safety first! The source of the burn (such as flames or chemicals) and a smoke- or vapor-filled environment can be a danger to all rescue personnel—especially to those who enter the emergency scene first. As soon as you suspect or recognize a hazard, make certain that rescuers who are specially trained and equipped have been called. Do not try to enter a hazardous scene yourself unless you are trained and equipped to do so.

When the patient has been removed, the care you provide as a First Responder will be vital for his or her survival. Remember that the most critical complication of burns is the most difficult to observe—burns to the airway. These can cause swelling and obstruction, which lead to inadequate breathing or respiratory arrest. Monitor the patient very carefully for these conditions. If all you can do until more advanced medical personnel arrive is maintain an open airway and adequate breathing in your patient, you have done your job.

Summing Up

- Always make sure the scene of a burn incident is safe before entering. Never try to rescue people trapped by fire unless you are equipped and trained to do so.

- Assessment of a patient with burns is the same as for anyone with soft-tissue injuries, except that you must determine the severity of the burns. Severity depends on the following:
  - *Depth of the burn,* which may be superficial, partial-thickness, full-thickness burns, or some combination of all three.
  - *Extent of body surface burned.* Use the rule of nines to estimate the BSA of larger burn injuries and the palmar surface method for smaller burns.
  - *Which part of the body was burned.* Burns to the face and eyes, hands, feet, or genital area are considered critical. So are burns that encircle a body part.
  - *Other complicating factors,* including other injuries, chronic diseases, and age.

- While gathering a history of the burn incident, find out if and how someone tried to treat the patient's burns before you arrived on scene. Include this information in your patient hand-off report.

- In general, First Responder care of patients with burns includes stopping the burning process, administering oxygen, dressing the burns, and keeping the patient warm. Other injuries should be treated as well.

- Special types of burn injuries include inhalation injuries, chemical burns, electrical burns, and lightning injuries. Though First Responder care for all burns is basically the same, these types of burns require some special attention:
  - *Inhalation injuries.* Suspect inhalation injury in any patient who was burned in a fire. Severity of such an injury is determined by the product of combustion, degree of combustion, duration of exposure, and whether or not the patient was in a confined space. Constant monitoring of this patient's airway is essential.
  - *Chemical burns.* Treat all chemical burns as critical. Immediately flush the patient's burns vigorously with water and continue for at least 20 minutes. Brush off dry chemicals before flushing with water.
  - *Electrical burns.* Assume spine injuries and take the appropriate precautions. Also look for both entry and exit burns.
  - *Lightning injuries.* Assume spine injuries and take the appropriate precautions. Also assume that a victim of lightning has sustained multiple injuries to multiple body systems. Look for both entry and exit burns.

Key Terms

BSA body surface area.

dermis the second layer of skin.

epidermis the outermost layer of skin.

full-thickness burn a burn that extends through all layers of skin and may involve subcutaneous tissue, muscles, organs, and bone.

palmar surface method a way of estimating the amount of body surface area involved in a burn by considering the palm of the patient's hand as 1% of total body surface area. *Also called* rule of palms.

partial-thickness burn a burn that involves both the epidermis and dermis.

rule of nines a way of estimating the amount of body surface area involved in a burn that considers each of 11 regions of the body equal to 9%.

subcutaneous tissue the layer of fat beneath the skin.

superficial burn a burn that involves only the epidermis.

Knowledge Check

1. Using the rule of nines, what is a good estimate of the body surface area of a burn that covers one arm and the front of the torso?
   a. 18%
   b. 22.5%
   c. 27%
   d. 36%

2. Using the rule of nines, what is a good estimate of the body surface area of a burn that covers the front of both legs and the front of the abdomen?
   a. 18%
   b. 22.5%
   c. 27%
   d. 36%

3. Severity of a burn depends on all of the following EXCEPT:
   a. body surface area burned.
   b. level of responsiveness.
   c. part of the body burned.
   d. depth of the burn.

4. Which one of the following characteristics BEST describes a partial-thickness burn?
   a. charred
   b. reddened
   c. charred and painful
   d. reddened with blisters

5. A partial-thickness burn that covers 20% of body surface area may be classified as a ____ burn.
   a. minor
   b. medium
   c. moderate
   d. critical

6. A full-thickness burn involving the hands, feet, face, or genitalia is considered a critical burn.
   a. True
   b. False

7. A superficial burn that covers 63% of body surface area is considered a minor burn.
   a. True
   b. False

8. Use the rule of nines to estimate the body surface area of each region of an ADULT's body.
   a. posterior trunk _____
   b. anterior trunk _____
   c. external genitalia _____
   d. head and neck _____
   e. one upper extremity _____
   f. one lower extremity _____

9. Use the rule of nines to estimate the body surface area of each region of an INFANT's body.
   a. posterior trunk _____
   b. anterior trunk _____
   c. external genitalia _____
   d. head _____
   e. one upper extremity _____
   f. one lower extremity _____

Scenario

You were called to the scene of a "car vs. power pole" at about noon. As you approached the crash site, you noticed that drivers were rubbernecking and slowing down traffic to a crawl. When you finally arrived on scene, you saw about half a dozen cars parked up and down the road and a small crowd of people elbowing each other, pointing, and taking cell cam pictures of the wreck. One or two of them were attempting to move the others away from the scene. Another was pulling at the driver of the wrecked car. That's when you spotted the smoke billowing out from under the badly dented hood of the crashed vehicle.

a. What are the priorities for this emergency scene?

_____
_____
_____
_____

b. The car engine was in flames in a few seconds. By the time the fire service extricated the driver and brought him to you for care, the patient seemed to have been burned on every exposed part of his body. What are the priorities for assessment of this patient?

_____
_____
_____
_____

c. You found the patient was burned on his head, face, both lower arms, and anterior chest. What is the total BSA burned?

_____
_____

d. You then brought to mind the general guidelines for emergency medical care of a burn patient. Briefly, what are they?

_____

_____

_____

_____

e. How would you stop the burning process in this patient?

_____

_____

_____

_____

f. Would you use wet or dry dressings to cover this patient's burns?

_____

_____

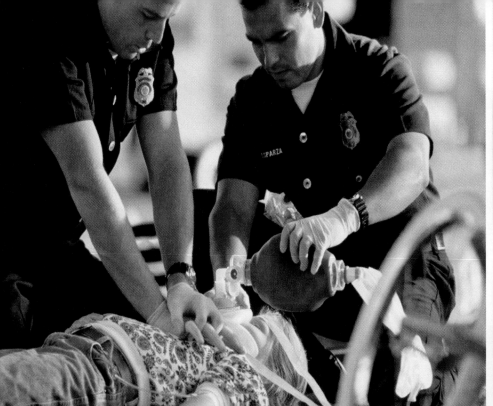
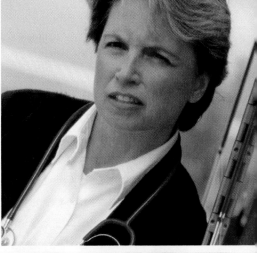
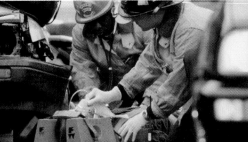

22 | Agricultural and Industrial Emergencies

Objectives

From the U.S. Department of Transportation (DOT) 1995 "First Responder: National Standard Curriculum." Material supplemental to the DOT curriculum is listed under "Enrichment."

Cognitive

No objectives are identified by the DOT.

Affective

No objectives are identified by the DOT.

Psychomotor

No objectives are identified by the DOT.

Enrichment

▸ Discuss the role of First Responders in agricultural and industrial emergencies. (pp. 402–403, 406)

▸ Identify factors involved in the high rate of injury and fatality among farmers. (p. 402)

▸ Discuss common mechanisms of injury among agricultural workers. (p. 403)

▸ Identify common operational controls used on farm machinery. (pp. 403, 406)

▸ Discuss the principles of disentanglement from farm equipment. (pp. 407–408)

▸ Describe how to safely approach an industrial emergency. (pp. 411–413)

Introduction

According to the National Safety Council, farming is considered the nation's most hazardous occupation. The number of accidents per work hour is higher in agriculture than the national average for major industry. You may be interested to learn that farm-type injuries also occur in urban areas. The pizza dough roller works on the same principles as the printing press or the agricultural combine, for example. Workers who do snow removal, construction work, and factory work use similar machinery—and are prone to similar accidents as well.

Section 1 Agricultural Emergencies

Farmers are under a great deal of stress. In fact, farming is rated among the top 10% of the most stressful occupations. They work long hours, often seven days a week. They rarely take breaks or vacations. They are exposed to heat, cold, and excessive noise and vibration. They also must bear the psychological stress of unstable weather conditions and financial difficulties including unfavorable prices at harvest time.

Farming is also a dangerous occupation. In recent years, 44 of every 100,000 farm workers died in work-related accidents. This is more than workers who die in the mining industry, construction trades, or transportation and public utilities. Why are farm accidents so serious? Consider the following:

- Most farm equipment is very complicated. As machinery becomes more sophisticated, the chances of injury increase.

- Some farmers do not use personal protective equipment.

- Farmers often use old, unsafe equipment because of the tremendous cost of replacement.

- Lengthy extrication is often needed when farmers become entangled in equipment. This can increase the severity of injuries.

- Since many farmers work alone in remote areas, they may not be missed for hours. Many farmers die from injuries that would not have been fatal if they had been discovered in time.

- There often is no phone at the scene. Many rural areas have no enhanced 9-1-1 service and no central dispatch.

- Long transport times contribute to the severity of injuries. Farms in rural areas can be long distances from hospitals.

Patient Assessment

There are a wide variety of emergencies possible on a farm—from tractor rollovers and equipment entanglement to exposure to gases that can accumulate in farm storage devices. Whatever the emergency, your approach should always be the same: scene size-up, initial assessment, physical examination, patient history, and patient hand-off. As always, scene safety is your first priority.

In any farm emergency, do not attempt a rescue of a patient unless you are specially trained and equipped to do so. Rescue of the patient should begin only when all of the following have been accomplished:

- Environment is no longer hazardous or toxic.

- Engines have been shut down.

- Farm equipment has been stabilized.

- Other hazards, such as leaking fuel, have been controlled.

When you are certain the scene is safe, begin your assessment of the patient. Special considerations for the assessment and emergency care of specific types of farm emergencies are offered on the pages that follow. ■

First Responder Care

To provide care to a patient with a farm injury, treat him the same way you would treat any injured patient. In the special case of a patient entangled in equipment and in need of rescue:

- Remember the priorities of airway, breathing, and circulation. Disentanglement can take up to an hour. Do not neglect the airway while the patient is being freed. If you are allowed, administer high-flow oxygen throughout the rescue.

- If you cannot apply direct pressure to a bleeding wound, use the nearest pressure point. Sometimes the

THE CALL

Dispatch When the Klaxon alarm goes off, it means that an employee is caught in a baling machine. As soon as I heard it, I made sure that someone called 9-1-1. Then I went to the scene of the accident. I knew that a coworker, Ellen, would meet me with our first-aid kit as we had practiced many times before.

Scene Size-up It was quiet when I got to the scene. All equipment around the patient was shut down. Several employees were working to set the man free. They were experts. They told me it would be a few minutes more. When I got a look at the patient, I saw he was an apprentice. He had been pulled by his sleeve into a baler. The workers who were disentangling him said it looked as if he had one or two amputated fingers.

What can the First Responders do to help the rescuers and their patient—both during and after disentanglement? What are their priorities and responsibilities? Consider this call as you read Chapter 22.

farm equipment itself helps to control bleeding by the pressure it exerts on an injury. In these cases, the patient should be transported while he or she is still entangled in the equipment. Most equipment can be cut to a manageable size.

■ Monitor vital signs constantly, so that you will not lose the patient to an undetected injury.

■ Preserve amputated parts, despite their appearance. If fingers have been injured, stabilize the wrist joint. It probably is injured, too.

As in any emergency, attend to the feelings of the patient as best you can. Explain who you are, what you are doing, and what you plan to do. Keep the patient informed—as well as his or her family, if they are on scene—as you proceed with emergency care. Be the patient's liaison during extrication, too. In addition, be sure to take all safety precautions continuously. Do not let down your guard. ■

Common Equipment Controls and Shutdown

Tractors and other farm equipment have in common a number of mechanisms that can cause injury. (See Figures 22-1 and 22-2.) They include:

■ **Pinch points**—two objects meet to cause a pinching or pulling action.

■ **Wrap points**—an aggressive component moves in a circular motion.

■ **Shear points**—two objects move close enough together to cause a cutting action.

■ **Crush points**—two large objects come together to cause a crushing action.

■ **Stored energy**—the potential for movement even after machinery has been shut down.

Become familiar with those mechanisms and their operational controls. This knowledge can save you time and frustration during rescue. Some manufacturers use different symbols or colors to help an operator quickly identify controls. Color codes include *red,* which indicates combine movement controls (throttle, gearshift, ground speed control). The color *yellow* indicates auxiliary power controls (separator control, cylinder speed control, header drive control). *Black* indicates miscellaneous function controls.

The first step in shutting down farm machinery is to stabilize it. You can use one of several methods: block or chock the wheels, set the parking or operational brakes, or tie the machine to another vehicle. Once the machine is stabilized, your objective is to shut it down. However, if you have any doubt about how to identify and operate the controls, do not touch them. *Wait for help!*

To shut down a machine, first locate the controls. Enter the cab, if possible, and find the ignition switch-on

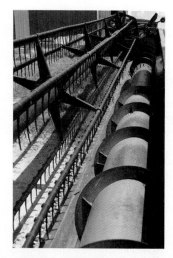

a. *Combine harvester.* (© Ken Kerr)

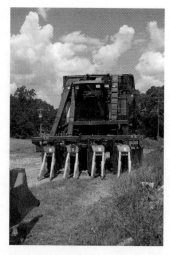

b. *Cotton picker.* (© Ken Kerr)

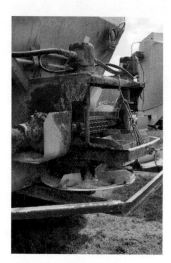

c. *Spreader feed truck.* (© Ken Kerr)

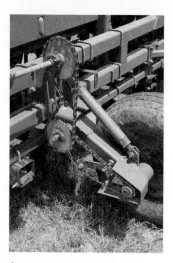

d. *Seed spreader.* (© Ken Kerr)

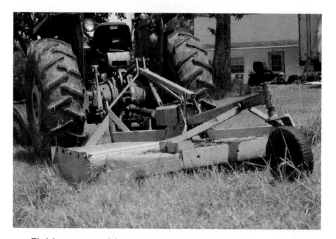

e. *Field mower with power take-off.* (© Ken Kerr)

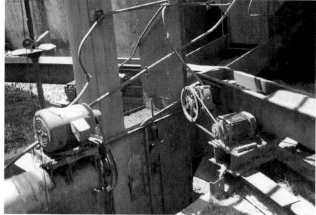

f. *Augers, grain elevator.* (© Ken Kerr)

FIGURE 22-1 Common agricultural equipment.

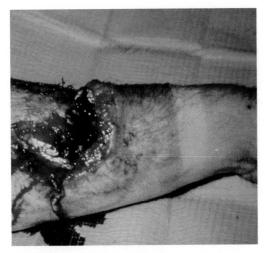

a. *Arm injured in a PTO shaft.*

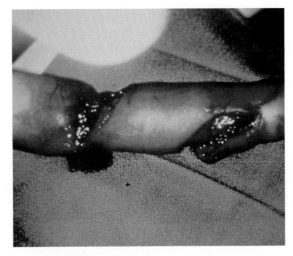

b. *Arm injured in an auger.*

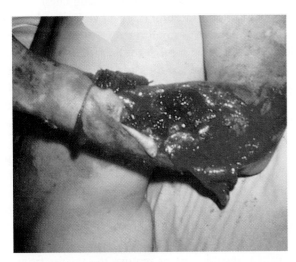

c. *Arm injured in an auger.*

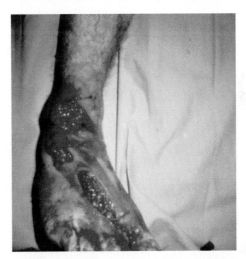

d. *Foot injured in an auger.*

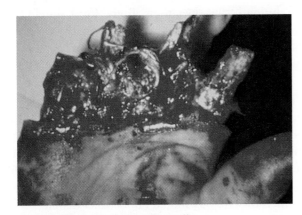

e. *Hand injured in snapping rolls.*

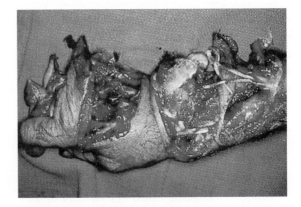

f. *Hand and arm injured in hay baler.*

FIGURE 22-2 First Responder care of patients with farm injuries is the same as for any other trauma patient.

key and throttle lever. Then slow the engine down with the throttle. Switch off the key. If the machine is fueled with diesel, the key may not shut off the engine. If that is the case, locate a fuel or air shutoff lever and pull the knob or lever to shut down the engine. (Again, if you are in doubt, do not touch the lever.)

If you cannot shut down the engine in the cab, try the fuel tank area. As a last resort, locate the fuel line or filters ahead of the fuel pump or injector pump. Interrupt the flow of fuel. Use extreme caution when cutting a fuel line. Large farm machinery can carry up to 300 gallons of fuel.

If the engine is a diesel, loosen the fuel filter. The engine will stall.

If all other attempts at shutting down the machine fail, locate the air intake. Discharge a 20-pound CO_2 fire extinguisher into it. Make sure that you hold the trigger of the extinguisher until the engine comes to a complete stop. *WARNING: This technique can cause extensive damage to the engine.*

Tractors

Tractors are the most common cause of farm-related fatalities. Most involve a tractor turning over backwards or rolling to the side. Of all tractor fatalities, 83% are the result of crushing injuries. The tractors used today fall into two categories: two-wheel drive and four-wheel drive. Engines may be fueled by gasoline, diesel, or liquid propane. Fuel leaks, fires, and explosions can result from tractor accidents. Fire protection is critical during rescue.

Tractor Rollovers and Overturns

Before rescue, a tractor engine must be shut down, the fuel controlled, and the tractor stabilized. If you are unfamiliar with the equipment, call for assistance. Local repair shops and area agriculture workers can be good resources. Rescue teams should be capable of handling fire, since

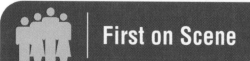

First on Scene

Do not attempt to rescue any patient who is pinned, entangled, or otherwise in need of extrication unless you are specially trained and equipped to do so. Due to the complexity of farm machinery, you must leave that job to trained technicians. Safety first! If you are not properly trained and equipped, attempting the disentanglement yourself will result in personal injury as well as further injury to the patient.

there will almost certainly be spilled fuel and hot hydraulic fluid.

To stabilize a tractor, lock up the rear wheels with two one- or two-ton cable hoists and three chains, even if the tractor is upright. Then wrap one chain around the rear tire and through the high slot in the rim. Wrap the second chain around the same wheel and through the low slot in the rim. Attach a third chain to the front of the tractor and stretch it to a hoist. Attach the other hoist to the two rear chains.

If the tractor does not have slots in the rims, stretch the hoist and chains across the rear tire to a strong point on the rear of the tractor. Make sure you do not lift the secure tire off the ground during hoisting.

For a patient involved in a tractor rollover, suspect possible chest injuries, including sucking chest wounds and pneumothorax (accumulation of air in the chest cavity). Since about 85% of all tractor overturns are to the side, expect crushing injuries to the patient's head, chest, and abdomen, as well as multiple lacerations. Common tractor rollover injuries include burns from spilled engine coolants, transmission fluid, hydraulic fluid, and battery acid. Pay special attention to the eyes and assess for chemical burns.

When it is safe to provide emergency care to the patient, aggressively manage airway, breathing, and circulation. Treat for shock. Then stabilize all injuries. When there are open extremity wounds with possible broken bones, immobilize them in splints if you are trained to do so.

When possible, lift or remove the tractor from the patient once he or she is stabilized. Do not stop patient care during lifting operations. Both efforts should continue at the same time. Be sure to call fire crews, extrication crews, and advance care providers as soon as possible.

Lifting Operations

During any lifting operation, a cross-crib capable of supporting the tractor must be built. This is to protect the patient and other rescuers in case lifting devices fail or the tractor has to be let down and repositioned for another lift.

The crib should be as wide as possible. A safe rule of thumb is the crib box should not be taller than it is wide. Also, the cribbing and lifting devices need a solid surface from which to work and function properly. This is sometimes difficult in a soft field or ditch. The rescue squad should carry several quarter-inch tread plates about 24″ × 24″ each. The plates will serve as a firm lifting surface on soft ground or on blacktop.

High-pressure airbags (approximately 90 to 120 psi) are the best tools available to lift a heavy, irregularly shaped machine. The bags must be placed carefully. Keep in mind the tractor's center of gravity. It is 10″ above and 24″ ahead of the rear axle at the platform area where the operator places his or her feet. About 30% of the tractor's weight is in front of this point and 70% behind.

Even though airbags appear to be indestructible, they are not. Airbags are most efficient during the first three to five inches of lift. They may be stacked (usually limited to two) to get a higher lift, but they become increasingly unstable as they are inflated. Whenever possible, a cross-crib should be built to get the bag within one to two inches of the object. A steel plate should be placed between the bag and the crib to keep the crib from being knocked apart during inflation.

Power spreaders or hydraulic rams also do a good job of lifting. With power hydraulic tools, the steel plate is a must for a good lifting platform. Hydraulic tools move very fast. The operator may have to wait for the crew that is building the cross-crib. The tool operator must continuously take note of the center of gravity. He or she also must watch for unstable conditions, such as changes of angle between the lifting surface of the tool and the tractor, sinking of the tractor on the opposite side of the lift, and so on.

Hand-power hydraulic jacks or manual jacks also can be used to lift a tractor. Use extreme caution if more than one jack has to be used. The cross-crib must be kept as close to the lifting device as possible. If one device becomes overloaded and fails, the other will almost certainly do the same. Cranes, wreckers, and boom trucks also can be used, if readily available, especially if you are dealing with a very large tractor. Regardless, cribs should still be built to protect the patient and rescuers from equipment failure or operator error. A safety officer should be assigned to monitor rescue operations whenever possible.

When lifting or removing the overturned tractor from a patient, follow these basic rules:

- All rescuers should know exactly what their roles will be. They should also know who is responsible for hoisting commands before lifting is done. During any extrication, only one rescuer should give lifting instructions. Instructions from more than one will result in injury to rescuers and patients.

- Always try to determine the tractor's center of gravity. Always build a crib to guard against equipment failures or operator error.

- Watch the patient during the lift to ensure that the part to be lifted is moving properly and that another part is not putting more pressure on the patient. If

conditions change, the rescuer leading the lifting operation should be advised.

- Any time more than one lifting device has to be used, use extra care in coordinating the lift to keep loads from shifting.

Lifting a tractor is not like lifting an automobile. A tractor usually is heavier. (A tractor can weigh up to 15 tons.) It also is difficult to stabilize because of its irregular shape and because many accidents occur on soft ground. To be sure, a tractor rollover presents a difficult challenge. However, if safety precautions are taken and if patient care and extrication are provided at the same time, this complex situation can be handled with confidence.

Power Takeoff Shafts

The power takeoff (PTO) shaft is a high-speed drive shaft that connects a tractor to farm implements such as balers, mowers, corn pickers, forage harvesters, and so on. It is the second most common cause of agricultural fatalities.

PTO-related accidents most often occur in fall or winter when the farmer's heavy clothing gets caught in the shaft and pulls the farmer in. Most of these accidents involve the arms, which are usually amputated. The farmer also can get wrapped around the shaft. PTO shaft injuries are not common. They make up only 8% of farm injuries. However, they usually are fatal.

To shut down a PTO shaft, turn off the source of power—the tractor. Some PTO shafts will free-wheel in either direction when the power is shut off. Some lock up immediately. Take care, because energy can be stored in the shaft.

To disentangle the patient, do the following:

- Always assume that the patient has sustained neck and back injuries. Stabilize the patient's spine as soon as possible. Immobilize him or her before transport.

- If the patient is wrapped on the shaft, determine if clothing could be cut to free the patient. The PTO shaft will wrap the patient's clothing into multiple layers, making cutting difficult and time-consuming. Look for the end of the wrap where clothing is only one layer thick. Cut at this point with rescue knives.

- If you must remove the PTO shaft with the patient, place a fire pry bar (42″ or longer) into the implement side of the PTO shaft to hold the stored energy. If pressure is on the coupling, the shaft will not slide apart. By reversing the shaft one-sixteenth of an inch, the coupling will move. Uncouple the shaft. Slide it apart. Have the patient sent to the hospital with the section.

- If you cannot uncouple the shaft, cut it with a power saw, gasoline-powered circular saw, or hack saw. Cutting should be done if nothing else will extricate the patient. This procedure will release the stored energy in the shaft very quickly. So, when cutting the shaft, take extreme care to prevent it from spinning. Lock the PTO shaft in place with a fire pry bar through the universal joint on both ends.

■ As you remove the patient, make sure that all rescuers and bystanders stand clear to avoid further injury.

■ Locate amputated parts if possible, but do not delay transport. Send parts with the patient.

Because of the energy involved, injuries to the patient can be quite severe. The patient would need rapid treatment and transport. Aggressively control bleeding with trauma dressings at the site of an avulsion or amputation. If advanced care is available (air transport, ground paramedics), call for it as soon as possible.

Other Equipment

Other types of agricultural equipment include the combine, augers and elevators, corn picker, husking beds, and hay baler.

Combines, Snapping Rolls, and Gathering Chains

The combine is a machine used to harvest and thresh all kinds of grain. It is assembled with multiple augers, shafts, belt and pulleys, roller chains, and sprockets. Many times a farmer is injured while doing routine maintenance on the combine, such as greasing bearings or tightening belts. Combines commonly cause partial and complete amputations.

The snapping rolls and gathering chains on an older model combine (two- to four-row units) require power rescue tools and airbags along with wooden wedges to spread the rolls. The rolls on the new models cannot be spread with conventional rescue tools. (See "Corn Pickers, Snapping Rolls, and Gathering Chains" later in this chapter.)

Just behind the combine header, and just ahead of the wheels, is a coupling device that attaches the head to the driving mechanism. This device could be a shaft with a pin in it. It could also be a set of flat gears sitting side by side with a common roller chain wrapped around them. Since it has to be released any time the head is changed, the device will be easy to get to and remove.

If you release the coupling device, you will be able to turn the header backward slowly and keep it under control. However, because of stored energy, you may need to use a pipe wrench or a large channel-lock pliers to move the shaft a sixteenth of an inch forward to

remove the coupling. Once the coupling has been disconnected, manual pressure on the wrench should be released with care.

Never use the self-reversing features on modern combines to remove a trapped person. The reversing feature moves too fast and for too long for you to remove a patient without causing further injury. By turning the shaft backward, you will only reverse the head.

If the patient has been pulled into the feeder-conveyor, where the head attaches to the combine, you will have to disassemble a portion of the head and the shroud that surrounds the conveyor. This should be done by using an air chisel to cut away the sheet metal in the area.

If a torch is used, consider the fire hazards first. One spark could start a fire quickly. A charged fire line should be available after the surrounding area of the field and the combine itself is washed down with water. Any dust standing around the work area should be removed with water. Flush down the inside of the combine header, feeder house, and up into the main combine.

Augers and Elevators

Combines and corn pickers are equipped with augers and elevators that move the grain through the machine. Many augers and elevators have clean-out doors and inspection covers that, if opened while the machine is in operation, become traps to the unwary operator.

Augers are used to move the threshed, separated, and cleaned grain from the cleaning shoe to the wagon or truck for transport. An auger is generally 4 to 12 inches in diameter with flights 3 to 11 inches apart. The elevator has a series of rubber or steel paddles attached to a drive chain that moves at about 350 feet per minute.

The power for the majority of these devices comes from the belt and pulley system on the combine. If a patient becomes trapped in the auger, the drive should be disconnected. Before cutting the belt or chain, place a large pipe wrench on the shaft that drives the auger. This will hold the stored energy and prevent further injuries. After the belt or chain is cut, slowly release the pressure on the shaft. Monitor the patient to be sure no further injury is being done.

Augers can pull in victims with extreme force. They often cause complete amputation, usually of the hands and arms and sometimes of the feet and legs. Auger accidents often involve children who are not experienced enough to avoid an accident. Entanglement in augers is so severe that it often cannot be handled in the field. You may need to cut the auger free and have it transported with the patient.

If amputation is complete, you may be able to slowly rotate the auger in its natural direction until the amputated part emerges at the end. (Never reverse an auger. It can cause increased tissue damage.) If that is not possible, you may have to disassemble the auger.

If the auger tube is held by bolts, remove them first. If not, the tube will have to be split or cut with an air chisel or a reciprocating saw. Do not use a torch. The danger of heat transfer to the patient and the threat of fire is too great. Cut a few feet from the patient. Look for spot welds on the flighting. Cut so the end of the flighting nearest the patient will not spring back to cause further injury. Take care to avoid excessive vibration or movement.

Corn Pickers, Snapping Rolls, and Gathering Chains

Corn pickers can be mounted on a tractor or pulled by a tractor, or they may be self-propelled. Each uses a system of rollers, chains, belts, and blades to remove corn from the stalk and then shear the corn away from the cob. Power for corn pickers is usually taken from the tractor PTO and hydraulic systems.

Corn picker accidents usually involve a hand that is crushed when a farmer tries to free trapped material in the picker. Amputation is rare, but the hand is often lost as a result of damage or infection. Extrication is extremely difficult, since the machinery is in heavy metal housings and cannot be reversed.

Snapping rolls move at a normal speed of 12 feet per second. Generally, they can cause severe crushing injuries to the hand. Often a weed or stalk catches between the rolls and stops them. A farmer who tries to remove the trapped material can cause the snapping rolls to start up with the slightest movement—and the rolls move more quickly than the farmer can pull back.

The majority of snapping rolls on corn pickers can be spread with the use of two wooden wedges plus a small hydraulic wedge. Use the wooden wedges for cribbing the rolls as they are separated by the hydraulic wedge. Insert one wooden wedge from the top of the rolls, while the other wooden wedge is pushed in from below. Equip the bottom wedge with a rope that allows the operator to pull it through from above.

The two wedges are a must. If only one is used and the hydraulic wedge slips or is released, the one wooden wedge will be shot from the machine. If this is allowed to happen, your patient may be further injured and rescuers jeopardized.

Snapping rolls also may be spread with the use of high-pressure airbags and two wooden wedges. The majority of power hydraulic tools may be used with the two wooden wedges. Whatever tool you use, remember these basic rules: Always use the wooden wedges for cribbing. Only open the roll as wide as necessary to remove your patient. Make sure that rescue efforts are coordinated with medical personnel.

Husking Beds

After the ears of corn pass through the snapping rollers, they enter the husking beds, one on each side of a mounted picker. The husking beds pull the leaves from the ear, exposing the kernels of corn still attached to the cob. The ear is then moved to the elevator and dropped in a wagon.

Husking beds present the greatest challenge. They are mounted to the picker with heavy duty bearing housings (normally cast iron) and are held together with strong springs. They are also enclosed by sheet metal, which can be removed by cutting off the bolt heads with an air chisel or just by taking the machine apart with wrenches.

Once the rolls have been reached, take care to avoid uncontrolled release of the springs that hold them together. At this point, you should release the tension-adjusting nuts or bolts. Then remove the bolts that fasten the bearing housings to the husking bed housing, again avoiding explosive release of stored energy in the springs. If you can reach the bearing housings with a power rescue tool, try to break them. However, removing the bolts by hand is the recommended and more controlled method.

Hay Baler

The hay baler compacts straw and hay into bundles. Some are small rectangular bundles. Others are massive rounded ones. The hay baler exerts force of up to 1,300 pounds between spring-loaded rollers. Amputations are often the result. Hay balers also commonly cause compression, avulsion, and wringer injuries. Because the springs can be released and the bolts cut, it is not as difficult to free a patient from a hay baler as it is from other farm equipment.

Agricultural Storage Devices

Grain Tank

Farmers who fall into the grain tanks risk death from suffocation. Always assume that a patient in a grain tank is alive, even if he or she has been trapped there for hours. Turn off electric power to the structure as soon as possible. Call the fire department and extrication teams to the scene. If advanced care providers are available, have them dispatched to the scene as soon as possible. Do not enter the structure without other rescuers to help. Any rescuer entering should be tied to a safety life-line and wearing a disposable mechanical filter respirator rated for dust particles.

Do not use the gravity gate or auger to release the grain. The grain flows from top to bottom, and the patient can be pulled further into the tank. Instead, cut uniform 18″ triangular holes as high as possible but still below the level of the grain. Cut in the middle of the bin sheets, avoiding bolts, seams, and stiffeners. Open the holes simultaneously so that the grain flows out evenly. This will prevent the walls of the tank from collapsing. Once the tank begins to empty, rescuers with shovels, tractors and loads, or skid loaders may be needed to remove grain.

Once the patient is exposed, secure him or her with a lifeline. Then aggressively clear the patient's airway of grain by suctioning. After the airway has been assured, assess for other injuries. Then a trained rescuer must fully immobilize the patient. Move the patient onto a long backboard and position a basket stretcher for extrication. A 24″ × 24″ hole can be cut at the surface of the grain to allow the stretcher to be lowered to the ground. If the grain feels cool or cold, treat the patient for hypothermia.

If the patient is only partially submerged, lower a rescuer on a harness secured with lifelines. Clear the area around the patient's head to make breathing possible and to establish an airway. Use plywood, sheets of metal, or a 55-gallon drum with both ends removed to keep grain away from the patient's face during extrication.

Silo

When crops are stored in silos, gas is formed by natural chemical fermentation. Fermenting crops can release high levels of carbon monoxide, methane, and nitrogen dioxide. These gases can cause serious injury or death. The presence of silo gas may be recognized by any of the following signs:

- Bleach-like odor.
- Yellowish or reddish vapor hovering over the product.
- Stains of red, yellow, or brown on the product or other surfaces touched by the gas.
- Dead birds or insects near the silo.
- Nearby livestock with signs of illness.

The greatest danger of silo gas is just after harvest. However, fumes can persist and occur when a silo is opened months later. Most silo injuries occur when a victim falls into the silo and either becomes trapped in the unloading device or is overcome by gas. Some suffer cardiac arrest in the silo.

Unfortunately, silo gas causes little immediate pain. A victim may not be aware of an injury and die hours later because the injured lungs fill with fluid during sleep. Common reactions to silo gas include:

- Eye irritation.
- Cough, possibly with labored breathing.
- Fatigue.
- Nausea, vomiting.
- Cyanosis.
- Dizziness or sleepiness.

Two teams are usually needed to rescue a patient from a silo. Rescuers should be lowered in, and the patient lifted out through the top on a litter. Always use a self-contained breathing apparatus (SCBA) when doing rescue work at a silo. Place a SCBA with supplementary oxygen on the patient as soon as possible. If the extrication team is delayed or if no SCBA is available, the silo blower may be turned on to purge the air.

Be sure all patients exposed to silo gas are transported to a hospital for monitoring. Complications can develop up to 12 hours after exposure.

Manure Storage Areas

Large livestock facilities handle manure by flushing down the confinement buildings with water. The liquid is then sent to an open pond for storage. In some cases, liquid manure is stored in a structure similar to a silo.

There are two potential injuries from liquid manure: drowning and inhaling toxic fumes. (The liquid manure releases ammonia, carbon monoxide, carbon dioxide, methane, and hydrogen sulfide.) Agitation of a manure pit can cause the sudden release of hydrogen sulfide. Signs and symptoms of hydrogen sulfide poisoning may include:

- Cough.
- Irritation of mucous membranes.
- Nausea.
- Sudden collapse and respiratory paralysis (with high concentrations).

The primary goal of rescue is to provide ventilation to the patient. Always use at least two back-up rescuers. Always wear a self-contained breathing apparatus (SCBA) and lifelines. Provide aggressive airway management to the patient and, if needed, basic life support. Monitor the patient's vital signs. Treat for shock. Place the patient on high-flow oxygen. If advanced care is available (air transport, ground paramedics), call as soon as possible.

After the patient has been pulled from the storage area, remove all clothing from the patient and rescuers. Flush thoroughly with water and wash with green soap. All contaminated clothing must be removed before transport. If not, the clothing will give off fumes that can overcome the ambulance crew.

Q:

1. What are the general guidelines for First Responder care of a patient with a farm-related injury?

2. If a patient is caught in machinery, what four steps must be accomplished before disentanglement begins?

3. Why should medical personnel monitor lifting during rescue of a patient who has debris or machinery on top of him?

Section 2 Industrial Emergencies

As a First Responder, you may be employed at an industrial complex or you may be called to respond to one. The industrial setting is a potentially dangerous one when crisis strikes. This is due to the potential for hazardous materials, toxic environments, explosion, fire, heavy and dangerous machinery, and confined spaces.

When you think of an industrial emergency, you may picture a large petrochemical plant or a factory that spans several acres. It may be easy to overlook some of the most common industrial settings: small locations such as landfills with compactors and improperly disposed of hazardous materials, newspaper publishers with large rolls of paper and high-speed presses, diesel shops and garages with large engines and hoists, and quarries that have conveyors and crushing devices.

Your first priority in responding to the scene of an industrial accident is to protect your own safety. Perform a thorough scene size-up including:

- Determine if there are hazardous materials at the scene before you enter. If you are not familiar with industry operations, check with the staff to determine potential hazards.

- Determine if there are multiple patients and, if so, how many.

- Determine the type of environment the patient or patients are in. For example, is it a confined space, on the machine-room floor, in an elevated location such as a catwalk or tower?

Based on your scene size-up, you should:

- Speak to the industrial safety or management personnel before entering the scene.

- Call for specialized teams that may be needed.

- Determine if the industrial site has an emergency plan and find out if that plan has been activated.

- Initiate the incident command system.

Never enter an industrial area unless you have completed a thorough scene size-up and you are sure that the scene and the areas surrounding it are safe.

Specific Emergencies

Specific emergencies you may find at industrial scenes include:

- *Hazardous materials.* Perhaps one of the most common emergencies at the industrial site involves hazardous materials. These emergencies can cause toxic inhalations, burns, unconsciousness, and death. They are especially hazardous to EMS providers who get caught in the hot zone without appropriate protection or EMS providers who treat contaminated patients.

- *Machinery accidents.* Modern machinery can do amazing things (Figure 22-3). It can also cause horrific injury if proper safety precautions are not taken. Injuries caused by a person being pulled into machinery include soft-tissue and crushing musculoskeletal injuries. If a person is pulled completely into a machine, the injuries may be fatal. Never go into or around machinery until it has been shut down and secured. Trained maintenance workers may be required to disentangle the patient.

First on Scene

Questions to ask when sizing up an industrial emergency include: What is the nature of the incident? Is it a chemical spill, fire, explosion, or entrapment? What is the type and quantity of chemicals involved? Am I safe where I stand now? If I proceed farther, will I be safe? Will the wind or weather affect the situation? Are there injuries or deaths involved? If so, how many? Who do I need to notify?

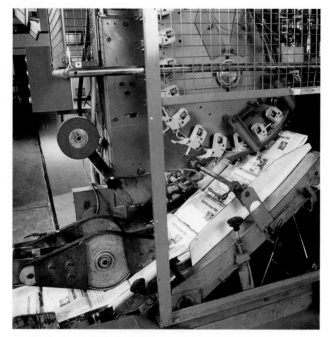

a. *Conveyor belt at a printing plant.* (Maria A. H. Lyle)

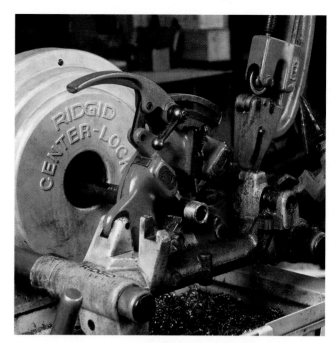

b. *Rigid electrical pipe threader.* (Maria A. H. Lyle)

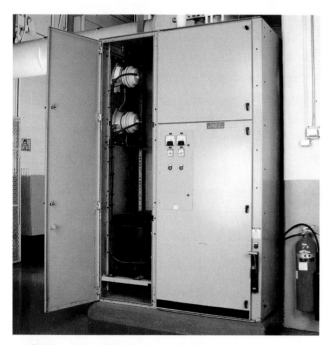

c. *Chiller water system.* (Maria A. H. Lyle)

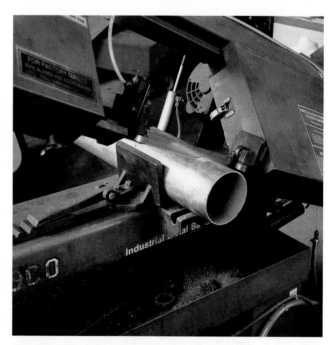

d. *Industrial metal band saw.* (Maria A. H. Lyle)

FIGURE 22-3 Industrial machinery.

- *Confined space and trench emergencies.* Industrial locations and some construction sites may cause emergencies in confined spaces or in cave-ins of excavation sites (Figure 22-4). These types of emergencies are quite dangerous because rescuers may not realize that the confined space is a hazard. While it may appear to be a simple small space, it could easily contain hazardous materials, an oxygen-deprived environment, or an unstable area that could collapse or constrict.

- *Aerial or high-angle rescues.* Facilities with multiple stories, lofts, cranes, and elevated conveyors can cause significant logistical problems. Access to these areas is usually by ladder or very narrow stairs, which make extrication difficult. Patients who are injured or who suffer medical emergencies will require special high-angle rescue teams. Patients who are not seriously injured may be lowered with a harness, while more severely injured patients must be lowered in a basket (Stokes) stretcher.

Industrial emergencies pose great risks for responders—and may cause a significantly greater number of patients at a single emergency scene—due to the materials and locations involved. Be sure to protect yourself at all times. Know what specialized teams are available, and be sure you or your dispatcher knows how to contact them.

Additional information on hazardous materials may be found in Chapter 30. Information on multiple-casualty incidents may be found in Chapter 31. For more detailed information on special rescue situations, see Chapter 34.

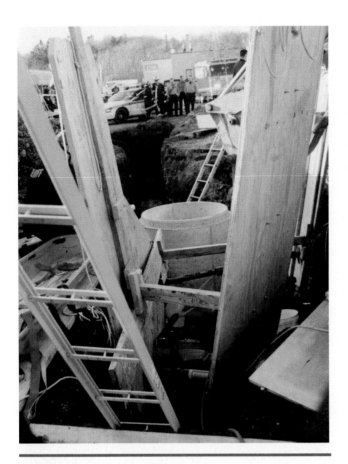

FIGURE 22-4 Industrial trench site. *(Raymond Hughes III)*

Q:

1. What three determinations should you make during your scene size-up of any industrial accident?

2. What are some specific types of hazards involved in an industrial emergency?

▶▶ The Call Follow-up

At the beginning of this chapter, you read that First Responders were on scene with a male patient who was pulled into a baler and as a result may have lost one or two fingers to amputation. To see how chapter skills apply to this emergency, read the following. It describes how the call was completed.

Initial Assessment Ellen and I quickly sorted out our priorities, remembering that the ABCs are always first. When the patient was free and a safe distance away from the machine, we saw that the others had been correct. There were two fingers missing, the hand was badly mangled, and the patient was going into shock. Ellen had him lie down and then positioned him. I assessed his airway and breathing. Ellen applied oxygen as I worked on controlling the bleeding.

Because the plant was so large, I knew that the ambulance crew would need help to find us. Another employee volunteered to go to the main gate to meet them when they arrived.

Physical Examination After bleeding was under control, I performed a quick head-to-toe. I bandaged and splinted the patient's injured hand and wrist. A worker yelled out that he found one of the patient's amputated fingers. I wrapped it in sterile gauze, and instructed him to go to the cafeteria to get some cold packs, a container with a tightly fitting lid, and at least two plastic bags. I wanted to make sure it was stored safely in case it could be reattached.

Patient History The patient reported that he was allergic to penicillin but had no other problems. He answered the rest of our questions, but he was in a lot of pain.

Ongoing Assessment Each time I took vital signs, I wrote them down. I did that a few times. We monitored the patient closely, kept him warm, and kept checking the oxygen until the ambulance crew arrived.

Patient Hand-off When the EMTs arrived, I gave them the hand-off report (see below). We found out later that the doctors were able to reattach the one finger. When we saw him, the apprentice thanked us for saving his life. I don't think we did. He wouldn't have died from his injuries, but I'm real glad we had the training to help him.

Patient Hand-off

"This is Tom Robinson. He is 22. About 15 minutes ago his right arm got pulled into the baler, which amputated two fingers. Tom is responsive. We had him lie down, and applied oxygen. The physical exam did not turn up anything except the injured hand, so we bandaged and splinted it. We wrapped and bagged one of the amputated fingers. The patient had some coffee about two hours ago, nothing else today. He is allergic to penicillin. His vitals are pulse 110, respirations 18. Skin is cool and moist."

The Last Word *No matter where or how your patient is found, follow the First Responder's patient assessment plan—scene size-up through patient hand-off. If special rescue teams are needed to extricate the patient, ensure continued emergency medical care throughout the procedure.*

Chapter Review

Focus on the EMS Team

Like many other emergencies, agricultural and industrial emergencies usually require a team approach. A family member or coworker often finds the injured patient and calls for help. A specially trained team responds to stabilize the scene and disentangle the patient, so that EMS personnel can treat and transport appropriately and safely. All members of the team must be in place to make the system work for your patient.

Summing Up

- Because farm equipment is complicated and often old and unsafe, injuries can be very serious. Lengthy extrications and response times to remote areas often result in increased severity of injuries.

- General guidelines for the assessment and care of these patients are the same as for any other emergency.

- Do not attempt the rescue of a patient who is pinned, entangled, or otherwise in need of extrication unless you are specially trained and equipped to do so. And then only if the equipment has been stabilized, engines have been shut down and all energy expended, other hazards (such as leaking fuel) have been controlled, and the patient has been stabilized.

- Common mechanisms of agricultural injury include:
  — *Tractors,* which are the most common cause of farm-related fatalities. Suspect crushing injuries, multiple lacerations, thermal and chemical burns.
  — *Power takeoff (PTO) shafts* make up only 8% of farm injuries. However, they are the second most common cause of agricultural fatalities. Entanglement injuries, including neck and back injuries, avulsions, and amputations are common.
  — *Combines* commonly cause partial and complete amputations.
  — *Augers* can pull in victims with extreme force, often causing complete amputation of hands, arms, and sometimes feet and legs.
  — *Corn pickers and snapping rolls* can crush a hand. Amputation is rare, but the hand is often lost as a result of damage or infection.
  — *Hay balers* cause amputations, compression injuries, avulsions, and wringer injuries.
  — *Storage devices,* such as grain tanks and silos can cause death from suffocation and poisonous gases. Manure storage areas can cause death by drowning or from toxic fumes.

- The industrial emergency may require you to speak to the industrial safety or management personnel before entering the scene, to call for specialized rescue teams, to determine if the industrial site has an emergency plan and to find out if that plan has been activated, or to initiate the incident command system, as appropriate.

- Specific emergencies at industrial sites include:
  — *Hazardous materials,* which can cause toxic inhalations, burns, unconsciousness, and death.
  — *Machinery accidents,* which are similar to those described for agricultural emergencies, since many of the machines perform similar tasks.
  — *Confined space and trench emergencies,* which can contain hazardous materials, an oxygen-deprived environment, or an unstable area that collapses or constricts.
  — *Aerial or high-angle rescues* from facilities with multiple stories, lofts, cranes, and elevated conveyors.

Key Terms

pinch points two objects meet to cause a pinching or pulling action.

wrap points an aggressive component moves in a circular motion.

shear points two objects move close enough together to cause a cutting action.

crush points two large objects come together to cause a crushing action.

stored energy the potential for movement even after machinery has been shut down.

Knowledge Check

1. What factor does NOT contribute to the severity of injuries to farmers?
   a. long transport times
   b. lengthy extrication times
   c. simplicity of farm equipment
   d. working alone in remote areas

2. First Responder care of a patient with farm injuries:
   a. depends on what the farmer is growing.
   b. is possible only with specialized equipment.
   c. focuses on how to shut down various machinery.
   d. is basically the same as for any other patient.

3. Your patient's arm is entangled in farm equipment. Bleeding is profuse, but you cannot reach it to apply direct pressure. What should you try next?
   a. Elevate the equipment and thereby the arm.
   b. Apply pressure to the nearest pressure point.
   c. Apply tourniquets above the nearest joint.
   d. Apply ice to the areas you can reach.

4. After equipment has been shut down and stabilized, you assess the entangled patient and find possible neck and back injuries. You should immediately:
   a. leave the scene until disentanglement is complete.
   b. be responsible for lifting and moving the patient.
   c. manually stabilize the patient's head and neck.
   d. disentangle and then immobilize the patient.

5. Your patient is pinned in a tractor rollover. If possible, you should stabilize the patient:
   a. before the tractor is lifted and removed.
   b. after patient extrication is complete.
   c. during lifting operations.
   d. before transport.

6. When crops are stored in silos, the fermentation of the grains can release gases that cause serious injury or death.
   a. True
   b. False

7. Industrial areas are regulated by the government as well as worker unions, so you can be sure that the scene of an emergency and the areas surrounding it are safe.
   a. True
   b. False

8. List three types of emergencies you might find at an industrial site.

   _____

   _____

   _____

9. List three types of machinery commonly involved in agricultural emergencies.

   _____

   _____

Scenario

As a community First Responder, you are notified of a "tractor rollover with injuries" just down the way from your farm. The dispatcher tells you that a heavy rescue team and an ALS ambulance have been dispatched from an adjoining town. When you arrive on scene, you find your neighbor has been pinned from the hips down by an overturned tractor. He is responsive and in severe pain.

a. Should you approach and treat this patient? Why or why not?

_____

_____

b. The rescue team has stabilized the tractor and they are working on lifting it off the patient. What can you do for the patient now?

_____

_____

c. Based on the information provided here, do you expect his injuries to be serious? What injuries should you expect?

_____

_____

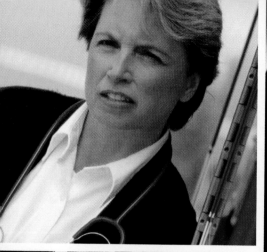
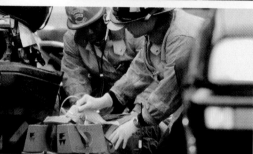
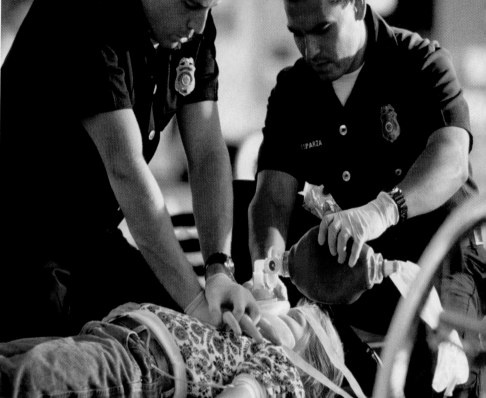

23 | Injuries to the Head, Face, and Neck

Objectives

From the U.S. Department of Transportation (DOT) 1995 "First Responder: National Standard Curriculum." Material supplemental to the DOT curriculum is listed under "Enrichment."

Cognitive

5-3.7 ▶ List the signs and symptoms of injury to the head. (pp. 419–421)

5-3.8 ▶ Describe the emergency medical care for injuries to the head. (pp. 421, 422–423)

Affective

No objectives are identified by the DOT.

Psychomotor

No objectives are identified by the DOT.

Enrichment

▶ Describe the emergency care of injuries to the face, including injuries to the jaw, cheek, nose, and ear. (pp. 423–425)

▶ Establish the relationship between airway management and injuries to the face. (pp. 423, 425)

▶ Describe the emergency care of injuries to the neck. (pp. 426–427)

▶ Describe the emergency care of injuries to the eyes. (pp. 427–433)

Introduction

The head, face, and neck hold very important organs and structures. The head contains the brain, where injuries can cause severe damage to the patient. The head and neck contain many blood vessels, which if injured, can hinder the supply of oxygen to the brain. If the face and neck are injured, the airway also may be compromised. Finally, a mechanism of injury that harms the head, face, or neck also can damage the spine. All these injuries run a high risk of causing life-long complications and even death.

Section 1 Injuries to the Head

A head injury may be open or closed. An *open head injury* is accompanied by a break in the skull, such as that caused by a laceration or an impaled object. It involves direct local damage to tissue. It also can result in brain damage. A *closed head injury* does not involve a break in the skull. Even so, the brain can be seriously injured. The skull holds brain tissue, blood, and **cerebrospinal fluid**. The volume of each can vary, but the total volume cannot. Because the skull is rigid, its capacity is limited. If brain tissue swells or if bleeding occurs, pressure can build up inside the skull causing damage to the brain.

Patient Assessment

The general signs and symptoms of a head injury include the following:

- Altered mental status, from confusion to unresponsiveness.
- Irregular breathing.
- Open wounds to the scalp.
- Penetrating wounds to the head.
- Softness or depression of the skull.
- Blood or cerebrospinal fluid leaking from the ears or nose (Figure 23-1).

✓ First Responder Practice

One of the most significant indications of head injury is the patient's mental status. In head injury, an altered mental status—ranging from agitation and confusion to unresponsiveness—is an early and serious indication of a dangerous underlying problem.

- Facial bruises.
- Bruising around the eyes ("raccoon eyes"), a late sign.
- Bruising behind the ears ("Battle's sign"), a late sign.
- Abnormal findings in an assessment of pulses, movement, and sensation.
- Headache, sudden or severe enough to be disabling.
- Nausea, vomiting.
- Unequal pupil size with altered mental status.
- Seizure activity.

Suspect spine injury in any patient with a head injury (Figure 23-2). If there is an obvious head injury, if the mechanism of injury suggests a head or spine injury, or if a trauma patient is unresponsive, immediately stabilize the patient's head and neck. Maintain manual stabilization until the patient is completely immobilized (Figure 23-3). If you are alone with an injured patient, you may be allowed to place a rigid item on each side of the patient's head to prevent movement. Follow local protocols.

During your initial assessment, use a jaw-thrust maneuver to open, assess, and maintain the airway. Also note

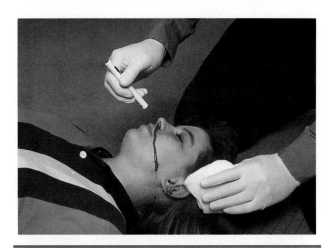

FIGURE 23-1 Blood or cerebrospinal fluid may come from the ears and nose of a patient with head injury.

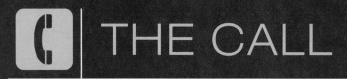

THE CALL

Dispatch Dispatch reported that a man in his 30s had fallen from the second-story roof of a factory supply building and workers "couldn't wake him up."

Scene Size-up Although dispatch did not give us reason to anticipate an unsafe scene, we approached with caution as we were trained to do. The foreman met us at the gate and immediately directed us to the patient's location. The crowd was being controlled by the company security guards. We identified ourselves and approached the patient. He was lying on the grass where he had fallen.

Initial Assessment My partner held the patient's head and neck, while I began the assessment. The patient was not responsive to my voice or painful stimuli. When I assessed his airway, I heard gurgling sounds from his throat. Without delay, I suctioned the mouth, and the gurgling sounds ceased. The patient's respirations appeared to be adequate. We elected to place him on oxygen at 15 liters per minute with a nonrebreather mask. There was no visible bleeding present.

Do you think these First Responders had the correct priorities? What would the mechanism of injury—falling from a two-story building—lead you to suspect? How would you proceed with assessment and care? Consider this patient as you read Chapter 23.

that bleeding from the scalp may be profuse because of the large number of blood vessels there.

During your physical exam of the patient, look for open injuries to the head. Closed injuries may present with swelling or depression of the bones of the skull. Check for cerebrospinal fluid, which appears as a clear liquid, possibly tinged pink with blood. It may be leaking from an open head wound or from the ears or nose.

For the head-injured patient, it is especially important for you to assess pulses, movement, and sensation in the extremities. Note any differences between extremities.

When you take the patient's history, be sure to find out when the injury occurred, if the patient lost consciousness, and if the patient was moved after the injury

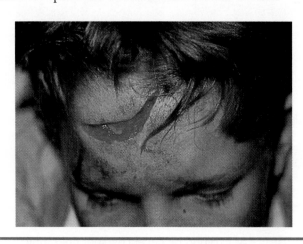

FIGURE 23-2 Always suspect spine injury in a patient with a head injury.

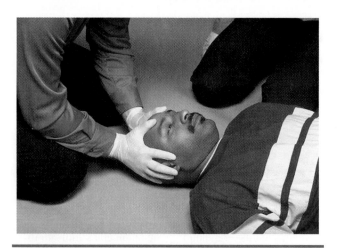

FIGURE 23-3 Maintain manual stabilization until the patient is completely immobilized on a long spine board.

occurred. Details about what happened are crucial to his or her medical care.

During your ongoing assessment, monitor the patient for any change in level of responsiveness. Keep in mind that change in a patient—not the patient's status at any one time—may be the most important sign of how a patient is doing. ■

First Responder Care

To provide care to a patient who has injuries to the head, be sure to update or activate EMS. After taking BSI precautions and establishing manual stabilization of the patient's head and neck, proceed as follows:

1. *Make the airway a top priority.* Note that oxygen deficiency in the brain is the most frequent cause of death following a head injury. So, monitor the airway and breathing closely, and suction as needed. Administer oxygen in high concentrations. If the patient's breathing is adequate, administer oxygen via nonrebreather. If breathing is not adequate, assist with BVM ventilation and supplemental oxygen. Be prepared to provide basic life support.

2. *Control bleeding and dress open wounds.* Scalp wounds may bleed profusely, but they usually are easy to control with direct pressure. NOTE: Never apply direct pressure to a head wound that is accompanied by an obvious or depressed skull fracture. It could drive fragments of bone into brain tissue and cause further injury.

   Do not try to stop a flow of cerebrospinal fluid. If the fluid is leaking from the ears or a head wound, cover the opening loosely with sterile gauze dressings.

   If there is a penetrating object, do not try to remove it. Instead, stabilize it with bulky dressings.

3. *Apply a rigid cervical immobilization device,* if you are trained and allowed to do so. (See Chapter 24 for instructions.) Maintain manual stabilization of the head and neck before, during, and after application and until the patient is completely immobilized on a long backboard.

4. *Monitor vital signs closely.* Watch for any sign of deterioration or change in the patient's status. If the patient has convulsions, protect him from injury.

5. *Calm and reassure the patient.* Continue to talk with him. If you can stimulate the patient, you may be able to prevent loss of consciousness. ■

Specific Head Injuries

Injuries to the head include skull fracture, injuries to the brain, concussion, and penetrating wounds.

First on Scene

Injuries to the central nervous system—the brain and spine—can affect any or all body systems, causing permanent disability or even death. Whenever there is reason to suspect such an injury (obvious head injury, a significant MOI, or unresponsiveness), take all appropriate spinal precautions as soon as you are at the patient's side.

Skull Fracture

The primary function of the skull is to protect the brain from injury. Because of its shape and thickness, the skull usually is broken only by extreme trauma (Figure 23-4). Suspect skull fracture with any significant trauma to the head, even if the injury is a closed one.

A skull fracture accompanied by brain injury is a serious condition that needs immediate management. Signs and symptoms include (Figure 23-5):

■ Damage to the skull, visible through lacerations in the scalp.

■ Deformity of the skull or face.

■ Pain or swelling at the injury site.

■ Clear or pinkish fluid dripping from nose, ears, mouth, or head wound.

■ Unusual size of pupils, or one eye sunken.

■ Purplish bruising under or around the eyes ("raccoon eyes").

■ Purplish bruising behind the ear ("Battle's sign").

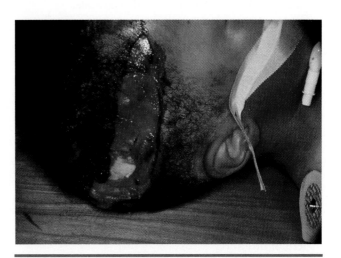

FIGURE 23-4 Lethal open skull fracture. *[Charles Stewart M.D. & Associates]*

SIGNS AND SYMPTOMS OF SKULL FRACTURE

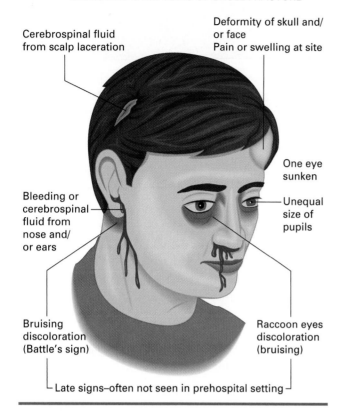

Cerebrospinal fluid from scalp laceration

Deformity of skull and/or face
Pain or swelling at site

One eye sunken

Unequal size of pupils

Bleeding or cerebrospinal fluid from nose and/or ears

Bruising discoloration (Battle's sign)

Raccoon eyes discoloration (bruising)

Late signs–often not seen in prehospital setting

FIGURE 23-5 A patient with a skull fracture may have a variety of signs and symptoms.

Injuries to the Brain

Whether a head wound is open or closed, brain damage can be extensive. In fact, it is often more severe in closed injuries than in open ones. Signs and symptoms include:

- Changes in mental status, ranging from confusion to unresponsiveness. Seizures are also possible.
- Paralysis or flaccidity, usually only on one side of the body.
- Unequal facial movements, squinting, drooping, unequal or unresponsive pupils.
- Disturbances of vision in one or both eyes.
- Rigidity of all limbs (present with severe injury).
- Loss of balance, staggering or stumbling gait.
- Slow, strong heartbeat that gradually becomes rapid and weak (late sign).
- High blood pressure with a slow pulse.
- Rapid, labored breathing or disturbances in the pattern of breathing.
- Vomiting after head injury.
- Incontinence.

Recall that the brain lies within the skull. A brain injury that causes bleeding or swelling within this space is a life-threatening condition. As blood or swelling continues, brain tissue is compressed. If pressure continues to build, the brain can actually be pushed downward and eventually into the *foramen magnum,* the opening at the base of the skull. This is called **herniation**. Signs include:

- Decreasing mental status.
- Decreasing pulse.
- Increasing blood pressure.
- Abnormal or irregular respiratory patterns.
- **Posturing** (a condition in which a patient's limbs exhibit an abnormal flexion or extension either spontaneously or in response to a painful stimulus).
- Sluggish, unequal, or fixed pupils.

Herniation is an ongoing process. Not all signs will appear at first, or appear at all. A classic sign of brainstem injury or brainstem pressure is *Cushing's triad,* which consists of increasing blood pressure, slowing pulse, and erratic respirations. However, in all cases of herniation, a decreasing mental status in combination with several of the signs listed above will be present.

Concussion

A **concussion** is a temporary loss of the brain's ability to function. There is no detectable damage to the brain. A concussion is classified as mild, moderate, or severe, based on the time interval before return to responsiveness. The key distinguishing factor of concussion is that its effects appear immediately or soon after impact. Then, they disappear, usually within 48 hours. If symptoms develop several minutes after impact or do not subside over time, the injury is probably more serious than a concussion. Signs and symptoms of a concussion include:

- Momentary confusion, or confusion that lasts several minutes.
- Inability to recall the period just before and after being injured.
- Repeatedly asking what happened.
- Mild to moderate irritability, uncooperativeness, combativeness, verbally abusive.
- Inability to answer questions or obey commands appropriately.
- Persistent vomiting.
- Incontinence.
- Restlessness.
- Seizures.
- Brief loss of consciousness.

Penetrating Wounds

A penetrating wound occurs when an object passes through the skull and lodges in the brain. It often involves bullets, knives, or ice picks. An extreme emergency, a penetrating wound almost always results in long-term damage.

If an object is impaled in the skull, do not try to remove it. Stabilize it with soft bulky dressings instead. Then, dress the area around it with sterile gauze. If an object has penetrated the skull but you cannot see it, cover the wound lightly with sterile dressings. In both cases, permit blood to drain. Never apply firm pressure to a head injury that might involve a skull fracture.

Q:

1. Can the brain be affected by a closed head injury? Explain.

2. When a patient has a head injury, what are the indications for manual stabilization of the head and neck?

3. In your initial assessment, how should you open the airway of a patient with a head injury?

4. After scene safety and spinal precautions are taken, what is your top priority for care of a patient with a head injury?

Section 2 Injuries to the Face and Neck

Although some injuries to the face and neck are minor, many can be life-threatening (Figures 23-6 and 23-7). They can result from impacts strong enough to cause hidden facial fractures, cervical-spine damage, and skull fractures.

Patient Assessment

For injuries of the face and neck, follow the patient assessment guidelines for injuries to the head described at the beginning of this chapter. Note that the initial assessment is vital to this patient, as injuries to the face and neck can cause bleeding into the airway. ■

First Responder Care

To provide care to a patient with injuries to the face and neck, follow the First Responder care guidelines for injuries to the head described at the beginning of this chapter. Take spinal precautions as appropriate, and remember to keep the airway a priority. Be sure the airway stays clear of fragments of teeth, broken dentures, bits of bone, pieces of flesh, and other possible obstructions. If bleeding into the mouth or throat threatens the airway, roll the patient as a unit onto one side to allow for drainage. Be prepared to monitor the airway and breathing constantly and to suction

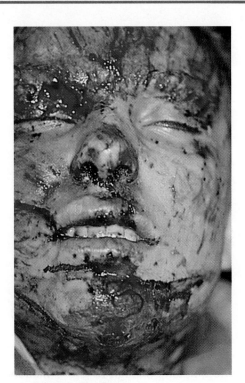

a. *Injury to the face.*

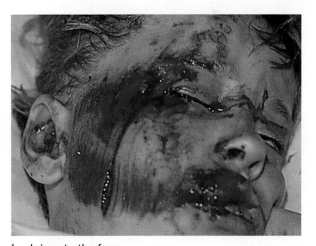

b. *Injury to the face.*

FIGURE 23-6 For all patients with injuries to the face, remember to keep the airway a priority.

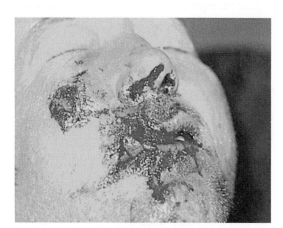

a. *Injury to the cheek, mouth, and jaw.*

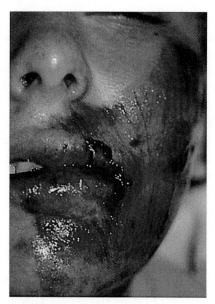

b. *Injury to the cheek, mouth, and jaw.*

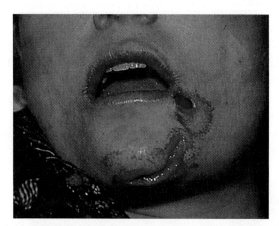

c. *Injury to the mouth and jaw.*

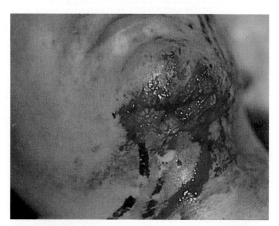

d. *Injury to the jaw.*

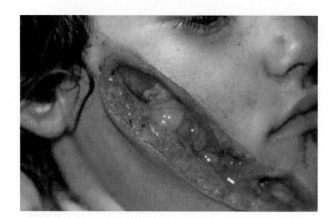

e. *Injury to the cheek and jaw.*

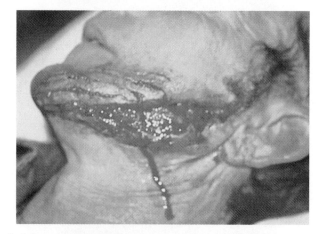

f. *Injury to the jaw.*

FIGURE 23-7 Injuries to the face and neck can result from impacts strong enough to cause hidden face and skull fractures as well as cervical-spine damage.

often. Keep in mind that the patient may be very anxious about possible disfigurement. Reassure him and do your best to help him stay calm. ∎

Specific Facial Injuries

Face

Whenever there are significant soft-tissue injuries to the face, there also may be underlying fractures. Signs and symptoms of facial fractures include:

- Distortion of facial features.
- Numbness or pain.
- Bruising and swelling.
- Bleeding from the nose or mouth.
- Limited jaw motion.
- Teeth that do not meet normally, teeth that are missing.
- Double vision (with fracture of bones around the eyes).
- Asymmetry of bones in face (before swelling).

Jaw

Patients with injuries to the face also may have a broken jaw. Such an injury can cause problems with the airway and breathing. Monitor both closely. Signs and symptoms of injuries to the jaw include:

- Mouth will not open or close.
- Drooling of saliva mixed with blood.
- Difficulty swallowing.
- Pain with talking, or difficulty talking.
- Missing, loosened, or uneven teeth.
- Teeth that do not meet normally.
- Pain in areas around the ears.

If a tooth has been lost, try to find it. Control bleeding from the socket with a gauze pad. If you find the missing tooth, be sure to handle it by the crown, not by the roots. Then, rinse it with tap water and be careful to protect any remaining tissue. Gently pick off debris, and put the tooth in a glass of milk. If milk is not available, wrap the tooth in moistened gauze. Do not allow the tooth to dry. Send it with the patient to the hospital. (These steps will help to maximize the chances for a successful reimplantation.)

If dentures are in place and unbroken, let them stay in place. They can help support the structures of the mouth. If dentures are broken, remove them. Send them with the patient to the hospital so that the surgeon can use them to establish proper alignment.

Cheek

If there is an impaled object in the cheek, stabilize it with bulky dressings. However, if it has penetrated all the way through, it may cause enough bleeding to block the airway. Remove it carefully. Be prepared to suction the airway.

Nose

First Responder care for soft-tissue injuries to the nose (Figure 23-8) is the same as care for other such injuries, with one exception: Take special care to maintain an open airway. Position the patient to prevent blood from draining into the throat.

The nose is the most commonly broken bone in the face. When it is broken, it will swell and appear to be deformed. To treat, apply cold packs to reduce swelling. Arrange for patient transport.

Foreign objects in the nose usually are a problem among small children. Reassure the child and parent, and arrange for transport to a hospital. Do not probe or try to remove the object, because special lighting and instruments are required.

Ear

Soft-tissue injuries to the ear, including avulsions, are common (Figure 23-9). Treat them as you would treat any such injury. Keep in mind that when dressing an injured ear, place part of the dressing between it and the side of the head.

First Responder Practice

One of the most serious complications of a face injury is blood flowing into the airway. Monitor the patient for this life-threatening problem. Make suction as much a part of face injury care as a dressing.

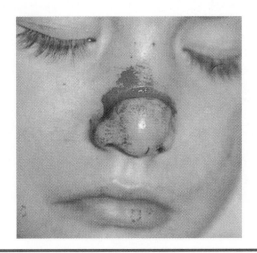

FIGURE 23-8 Injury to the nose.

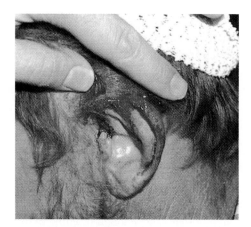
a. *Injury to the ear.*

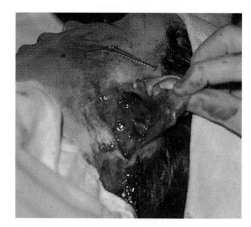
b. *Injury to the ear.*

FIGURE 23-9 Injuries to the ear, including avulsions, are common.

Never probe the ear. Never pack it to stop bleeding from the ear canal. Blood, clear fluid, or blood-tinged fluid draining from the ear may indicate skull fracture. Place a loose, clean dressing across the opening to absorb the fluids. Do not apply pressure.

Foreign objects in the ear, such as beans or peanuts, are common among children. The patient should be transported to the hospital where good lighting and appropriate equipment are available.

Specific Neck Injuries

Common causes of injury to the soft tissues of the neck include hanging (attempted suicide), impact with a steering wheel, or running into a stretched wire or clothesline. (See Figure 23-10.) Large wounds may involve injuries to the major vessels in the neck, which can produce massive,

even fatal bleeding. If a wound to the neck is left uncovered, air may be sucked into the vessels causing an obstruction (air embolism). (For injuries to the neck that affect the cervical spine, see Chapter 24.)

Signs and symptoms of neck injury include:

- Obvious lacerations or other wounds.
- Deformities or depressions.
- Obvious swelling, which sometimes occurs in the face and chest.
- Difficulty speaking, loss of the voice.
- Airway obstruction.
- Crackling sensations under the skin due to air leaking into the soft tissues (subcutaneous emphysema).

If there is bleeding from a neck wound, apply slight to moderate pressure with an occlusive dressing. Tape

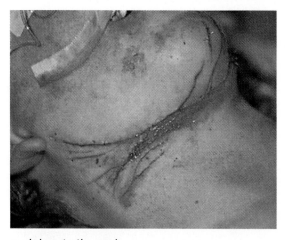
a. *Injury to the neck.*

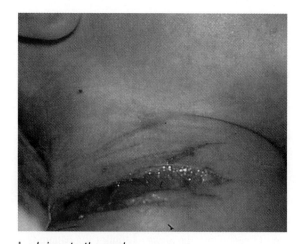
b. *Injury to the neck.*

FIGURE 23-10 Common neck injuries include hanging, impact with a steering wheel, and running into a stretched wire or clothesline.

First Responder Practice

Open injuries to the neck require immediate action to prevent air from being sucked into the wound and into the blood vessels. Air in the circulatory system (called an *air embolism*) can cause serious complications or death. Immediately control bleeding and apply an occlusive dressing over the wound. Seal occlusive dressings to the neck on all four sides to prevent any air from entering.

down the edges of the dressing to form an airtight seal. Add a bulky dressing over the occlusive one (Figure 23-11). Never apply pressure to both sides of the neck at the same time. Never apply a pressure dressing around the neck.

If there is an impaled object in the neck, stabilize it in place with bulky dressings. Do not remove it.

Specific Eye Injuries

When you assess a patient with eye injuries, find out when the injury occurred, whether or not both eyes were affected, and what symptoms the patient first noticed.

SKILL SUMMARY *Caring for Severed Neck Veins*

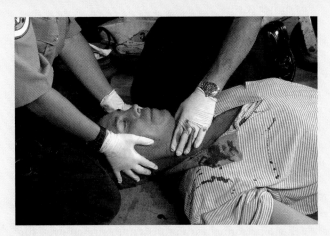

FIGURE 23-11A *Do not delay! Place your gloved palm over the wound.*

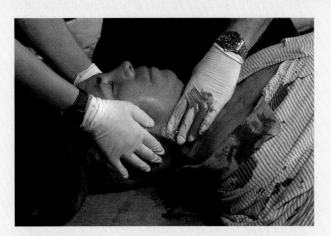

FIGURE 23-11B *Place an occlusive dressing over the wound. It must be two inches larger than the wound on all sides.*

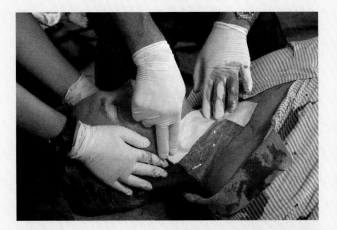

FIGURE 23-11C *Seal the dressing with tape on all four sides.*

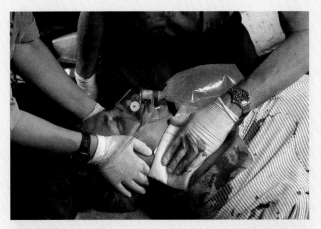

FIGURE 23-11D *Cover the occlusive dressing with a large gauze dressing. Continue to apply pressure to the wound. CAUTION: Do not compress blood vessels on both sides of the neck at the same time.*

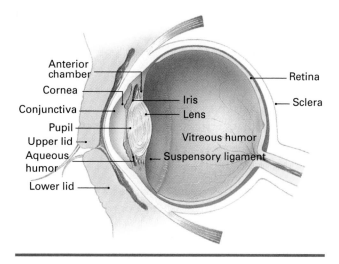

FIGURE 23-12 Anatomy of the eye.

Then, carefully examine the eyes separately and together with a small penlight. (For the anatomy of the eye, see Figure 23-12.) Check the *orbits* (the eye sockets, or bones in the skull that hold the eyeballs) for bruising, swelling, lacerations, tenderness, depression, and deformity. Check the eyelids for bruising, swelling, and lacerations. Mucous membranes should not be red or have pus or any foreign objects. Check the *globes* (eyeballs) for abnormal coloring, laceration, and foreign objects. Check the pupils for size, shape, reactivity, and quality (Figure 23-13). Also check to see that the eyes can move in all directions. There should not be an abnormal gaze or pain upon movement.

Basic rules for First Responder care of an injured eye include the following:

- An eye injury should always be examined by a physician.

- Patch both eyes, even if only one is injured. Eyes move together. Patching both eyes will help keep the injured eye from moving excessively.

- Many EMS systems do not allow flushing of an injured eye unless it has a chemical injury. If the eye has been perforated, damage done during flushing will be irreversible. Follow local protocol.

- Do not put salves or medications in the injured eye.

- Do not remove blood or blood clots from the eye. But you can sponge blood from the face to help keep the patient comfortable.

- Do not try to force the eyelid open unless you have to flush out chemicals.

- Do not let a patient with an eye injury walk without help, especially up or down stairs.

- Do not allow the patient with an eye injury to eat or drink.

- Never panic. It will upset the patient, and you may lose his or her trust.

Foreign Objects

Foreign objects frequently are blown or driven into the eye (Figure 23-14). They include particles of dirt, sand, cinders, coal dust, or fine pieces of metal. If not removed, they can cause inflammation, scarring, or infection. They also may scratch the cornea. Signs and symptoms of foreign objects in the eye include pain, excessive tearing, and abnormal sensitivity to light.

Do not allow the patient to rub his eyes. Rubbing can force a particle with sharp edges into the tissues, making removal difficult. It is always safer for a First Responder to allow EMS personnel with more training to remove a foreign object. However, if removal is necessary and local protocols allow it, there are several ways in which you might proceed. They are as follows:

- Hold the lids apart, and flush the eye with clean water (Figure 23-15). Note that some EMS systems do not

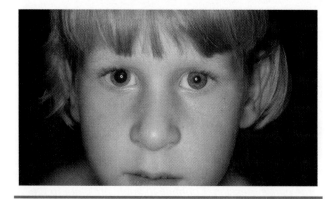

FIGURE 23-13 Unequal pupils. *[Charles Stewart M.D. & Associates]*

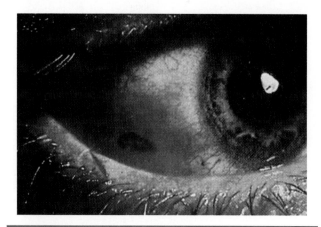

FIGURE 23-14 Foreign object lodged in the eye.

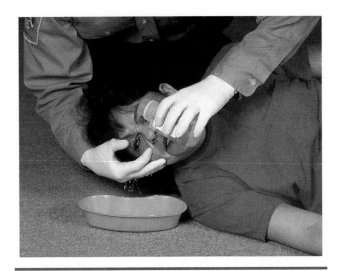

FIGURE 23-15 **Flushing a foreign object from the eye.**

allow flushing except for chemical burns. Follow local protocol.

- If the object is under the lower eyelid, pull down the lower lid to expose the inner surface (Figure 23-16). Then, use the corner of a piece of sterile gauze to remove the object.

- If the object is under the upper lid, grasp the eyelashes of the upper lid. Turn up the lid over a cotton swab. The foreign object then may be carefully removed with the corner of a piece of sterile gauze.

Another method is to draw the upper lid down over the lower lid. When you let it return to its normal position, its undersurface will be drawn over the lashes of the lower lid. The lashes may "sweep" away the foreign object.

Should a foreign object become lodged in the globe, do not try to remove it. If you do, it could be forced deeper into the eye, causing further damage. In this case, place a rigid eye shield over the injured eye. Cover the opposite eye with gauze. Arrange for immediate transport to a hospital. (See Figure 23-17.)

Impaled Objects

Objects impaled in the eye should be removed only by a physician. Your job is to protect the patient from further injury until he can reach a doctor. Begin by having a helper stabilize the patient's head. If no help is available, use your knees or objects such as sandbags to stabilize the head. Keep the patient supine. Then, encircle the eye with a gauze dressing or soft sterile cloth. Do not apply

SKILL SUMMARY *Removing Particles from the Eye*

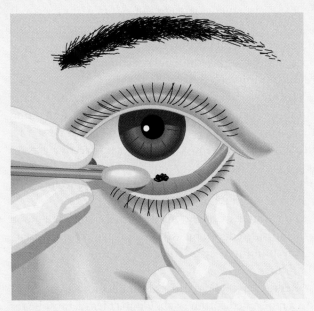

FIGURE 23-16A *For a particle behind the lower lid, pull down the lid while the patient looks up.*

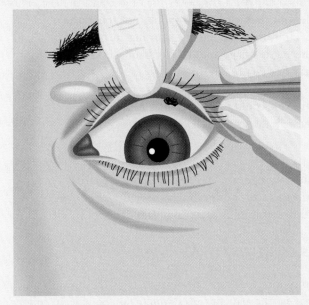

FIGURE 23-16B *For a particle behind the upper lid, pull up the lid while the patient looks down.*

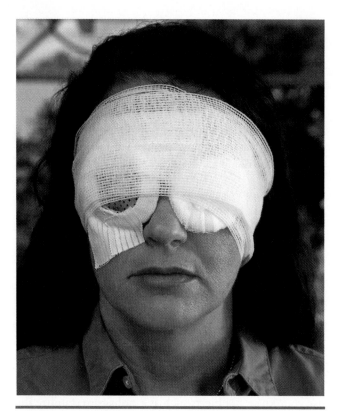

FIGURE 23-17 Place a rigid shield over the eye with the imbedded foreign object. Cover the opposite eye with gauze.

pressure. Cut a hole in a single bulky dressing and slip it over the impaled object. Then, place a metal shield, a crushed cup, or a cone over the object and the eye. The sides of the shield or cup should not touch the object at all. Hold the cup and the dressing in place with a self-adhering bandage and a roller bandage that covers both eyes. (See Figure 23-18.)

After covering the patient's eyes, do not leave him alone. He could panic. Keep him within hand contact so that he knows someone is there.

Orbits

Trauma to the face may result in fracture of the bones that form the orbits, or eye sockets (Figure 23-19). A patient with an orbit injury may complain of double or decreased vision, numbness above the eyebrow or over the cheek, or massive discharge from the nose.

Fractures of the lower part of the orbit are the most common. They can cause paralysis of the upward gaze. That is, the patient's eyes would not be able to follow your finger upward. Patients with an orbit fracture need hospitalization and surgery.

If there is no injury to the globe, place cold packs over the injured orbit to help reduce swelling. However, if the eyeball is injured or if you are in doubt, do not apply cold packs.

Eyelids

Lid injuries include discoloration, burns, swelling or drooping, and laceration (Figure 23-20). Anything that damages the lid also may damage the globe. In general, little can be done for these injuries in the field beyond gentle patching.

To control bleeding from the eyelid, apply light pressure. No pressure should be used if the globe itself is injured.

Never attempt to remove embedded material, such as gravel. Use sterile gauze soaked in saline to keep the wound from drying. If the lid is avulsed, preserve and send it with the patient for later grafting.

Globes

Injuries to the globe (eyeball) include bruises, lacerations, foreign objects, and abrasions. These generally are best treated in the hospital where specialized equipment is available. In the field, keep the patient supine. Lightly apply patches to both eyes since eyes move together. Keep in mind that patients who have both eyes covered need a bit more patience and understanding. This is a very frightening experience for them.

Chemical Burns to the Eye

Chemical burns to the eye are quite common (Figure 23-21). They are the most urgent emergency related to the eyes. Permanent damage can occur within seconds of the injury. The first 10 minutes are crucial to the final outcome. Remember, burning and tissue damage will continue as long as the chemical remains in the eye, even if it is diluted.

To provide First Responder care, begin immediate, continuous irrigation with water. Do not use anything other than water. The water does not need to be sterile, but it must be clean. Be sure to wear protective glasses. Gently hold the patient's eyelid open so that all of the chemical can be flushed away. You may have to force the eyelid open because of the patient's pain.

Pour water from the inside corner across the globe to the outside edge. This will help to avoid contaminating the uninjured eye. Irrigate continuously for 30 to 60 minutes.

Remove any solid particles from the surface of the eye with a moistened cotton swab. Contact lenses must be removed or flushed out. If not, they can trap chemicals between the lens and the cornea. Follow local protocol.

Following irrigation, wash your hands thoroughly. Avoid contaminating your own eyes.

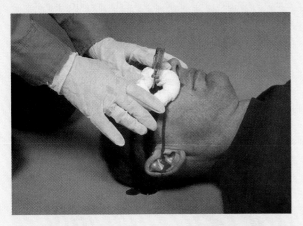

FIGURE 23-18A   *Place padding around the object.*

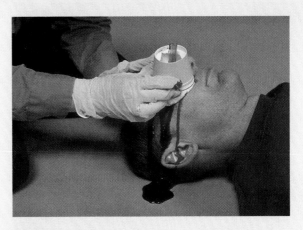

FIGURE 23-18B   *Stabilize the object with a cup.*

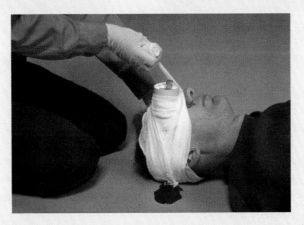

FIGURE 23-18C   *Secure the cup in place.*

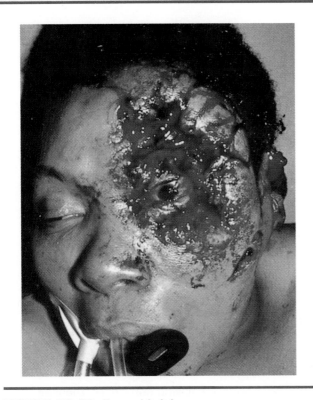

FIGURE 23-19 Eye orbit injury.

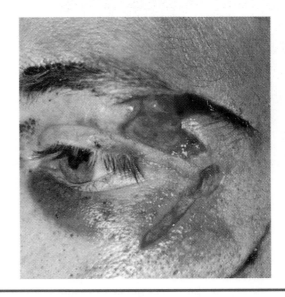

FIGURE 23-20 Eyelid injury.

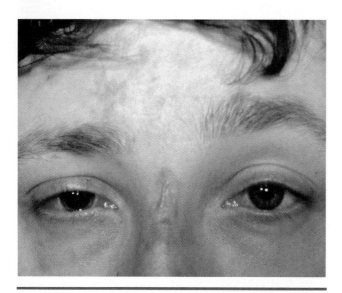

FIGURE 23-21 Chemical burn of the eye. *(Western Ophthalmic Hospital, SPL, Photo Researchers, Inc.)*

Extruded Eyeball

During a serious injury, the eyeball may be knocked out of the socket (orbit), or *extruded* (Figure 23-22). Do not try to replace it. Instead, cover it with a moist dressing and protective cup. Do not apply any pressure. Then, apply a bandage that covers both eyes.

Other Eye Injuries

In all other emergencies involving the eye, patch both eyes and arrange for transport. Such emergencies include eye infections, "black eye," cornea abrasions, light burns, and heat burns. Follow local protocols.

Removing Contact Lenses

Millions of people in the U.S. wear contact lenses. Some may wear a lens in only one eye, so be sure to examine

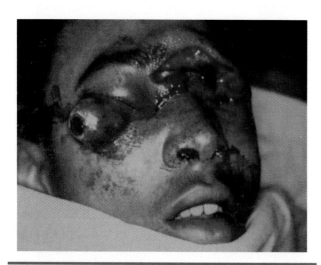

FIGURE 23-22 Extruded globe (eyeball).

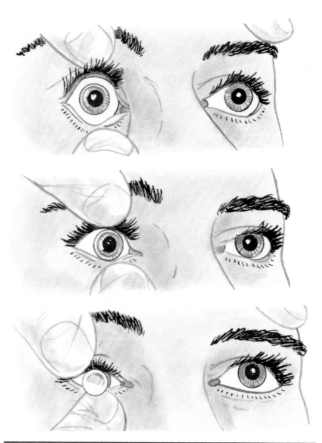

FIGURE 23-23 Removing hard contact lenses.

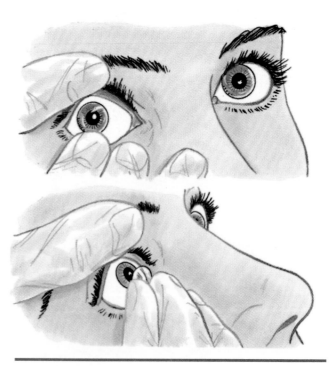

FIGURE 23-24 Removing soft contact lenses.

both eyes carefully. Other patients, especially the elderly, wear both contact lenses and eyeglasses. To detect lenses, shine a penlight into each eye. A soft lens will show up as a shadow on the outer portion of the eye. A hard lens will show up as a shadow over the iris. In general, remove contacts only when there has been a chemical burn to the eye or when it is medically necessary. Always follow local protocols.

To remove hard contact lenses, first separate the eyelids (Figure 23-23). Position the lens over the cornea by manipulating the eyelids. Place your thumbs gently on the top and bottom eyelids, and open the lids wide. Gently press them down and forward to the edges of the lens. Press the lower lid slightly harder, and move it under the bottom edge of the lens. Move the eyelids toward each other, allowing the lens to slide out between them. Finally, remove the lens and put it in a safe place.

To remove soft contact lenses, place several drops of saline onto the lens. Then, gently lift it off by pinching it between your thumb and index finger (Figure 23-24).

Q:

1. What should you do with a tooth that has been knocked out of its socket?

2. If your patient's nose has been injured, is swelling, and appears deformed, what should you do?

3. What bleeding control method may you use for a patient's neck wound? Describe it.

4. How should you assess your patient's injured eyes?

5. What is First Responder care for a patient with a chemical burn to the eye?

▶▶ The Call Follow-up

At the beginning of this chapter, you read that First Responders were on scene with an unresponsive male patient who had fallen more than 15 feet from the roof of a building onto a grassy lawn. To see how the skills in this chapter apply to this emergency, read the following. It describes how the call was completed.

Physical Examination My partner continued to monitor the airway and breathing, while I conducted a head-to-toe exam. I found only a large bruise on the left side of the patient's head. His vital signs were within normal ranges.

During the exam, the patient opened his eyes and responded to my voice. I cautioned him to be very still, told why my partner was holding his head, and explained what I knew of what happened. Although he was somewhat drowsy, he indicated he understood by whispering, "Okay."

Patient History A company personnel officer provided the medical history kept on record. The patient was also able to answer some of our questions. His chief complaint was that he "hurt all over." He had no known allergies and took no medications recently. He had eaten breakfast at 0500. The patient did not remember what happened, but coworkers said he was performing his job when he tripped and flipped over the roof ledge.

Ongoing Assessment The patient required careful monitoring due to changes in his level of responsiveness. We continued oxygen administration. The patient was able to wiggle his toes and fingers, and he continued to respond to questions appropriately.

Patient Hand-off When the EMTs arrived, I gave them the hand-off report (see below). The EMTs then took over care of the patient and told us that we had done a good job. We learned when we started our next shift that Mr. Gonzalez was diagnosed with a concussion and would be released from the hospital the next day.

Hand-off Report

"This is Ray Gonzalez. He is 38 years old. About 15 minutes ago he fell 15–20 feet from the roof of this building onto the grass. No one moved him before or after we arrived on scene. Initially he did not respond to voice or painful stimuli. He presented with adequate respirations but needed suctioning of the airway early in the initial assessment. During the physical exam, he began to respond to our voices. The exam revealed a large bruise to the left side of his head. There was no bleeding at the wound site. There is no record of previous medical problems. His vital signs are pulse 88, respirations 18, blood pressure 130/82, skin warm and dry, and pupils equal and reactive."

The Last Word *By being the first medically trained rescuer on scene, you have the opportunity to really make a difference in the head-injured patient's life. Proper assessment and treatment could save him or her from further injury, permanent disfigurement, and even death.*

Chapter Review

Focus on the EMS Team

Serious head injuries have a real potential for death or life-long disability. Your patient's survival depends on a team effort. Your role is scene safety, to provide for the patient's initial assessment and care, and to activate or update EMS on the severity of the patient's injuries. The EMTs who take over care of your patient will then transport him to the most appropriate health-care facility.

When available, a trauma center or hospital with the ability to perform trauma surgery and care will provide life-saving interventions. When a specialty hospital is not close, an air medical helicopter may be available to transport the patient there promptly.

As a First Responder, your initial care and early recognition of the patient's condition is critical.

Summing Up

- If the patient has an obvious head injury, if the mechanism of injury suggests a head or spine injury, or if a trauma patient is unresponsive, immediately take spinal precautions. That is, manually hold the patient's head and neck in a neutral position. Apply a cervical collar, if you are trained to do so. Maintain manual stabilization until the patient is completely immobilized.

- Assessment of a patient with a possible head, face, or neck injury is the same as assessment for any other patient. However, consider all suspected head injuries to be serious. Also, be sure to use a jaw-thrust maneuver to open the airway; assess pulses, movement, and sensation in the extremities; and find out when the injury occurred, if the patient lost consciousness, and if the patient was moved after being injured.

- First Responder care of a patient with a head, face, or neck injury is the same as for any patient, with the following exceptions:
  - *Head wounds.* Never apply direct pressure to a head wound that is accompanied by an obvious or depressed skull fracture. If cerebrospinal fluid appears to be leaking from the ears or a head wound, do not try to stop the flow. Instead, cover the opening loosely with sterile gauze dressings.
  - *Facial wounds.* Carefully maintain an open airway while providing emergency care. Lost teeth should be found, handled by the crown, rinsed with water, put it in a glass of milk or wrapped in moistened gauze. Broken dentures should be removed. Impaled objects should be stabilized, with one exception: if there is one in the cheek, it may be removed to protect the patient's airway. When dressing an injured ear, place part of a dressing between it and the side of the head.
  - *Neck wounds.* For an open wound to the neck, apply only slight to moderate pressure with an occlusive dressing to control bleeding. Tape down all four edges of the dressing to form an airtight seal. Add a bulky dressing over the occlusive one. Never apply pressure to both sides of the neck at the same time. Never apply a pressure dressing around the neck.
  - *Eye injuries.* Even if only one eye is injured, patch both eyes. Do not put salves or medications in an injured eye. Do not try to force the eyelid open unless you have to flush out chemicals (follow all local protocols for flushing eyes). Do not remove blood or blood clots from the eye. Never attempt to remove embedded material. Remove contacts only when there has been a chemical burn to the eye or when it is medically necessary. Do not let a patient with an eye injury walk without help, especially up or down stairs. Do not allow the patient with an eye injury to eat or drink. Every eye injury should be examined by a physician.

Key Terms

cerebrospinal fluid (CSF) a cushion of fluid that helps to protect the brain and spinal cord from injury.

concussion a temporary loss of the brain's ability to function as a result of a blow or fall.

herniation the displacement of body tissue through an opening.

posturing a condition in which a patient's limbs exhibit an abnormal flexion or extension either spontaneously or in response to a painful stimulus.

Knowledge Check

1. An important indicator of head injury is:
   a. altered mental status.
   b. prior head injuries.
   c. nature of illness.
   d. abdominal pain.

2. You are treating a patient with a closed head injury and observe a clear fluid draining from the left ear. You should:
   a. do nothing.
   b. pack the ear with gauze.
   c. elevate the patient's head.
   d. place a gauze pad outside the ear.

3. Injuries to the neck require an occlusive dressing because:
   a. neck injuries bleed profusely.
   b. it helps to maintain body temperature.
   c. a possible complication is brain injury.
   d. it prevents air from entering the bloodstream.

4. Which one of the following statements about injuries to the face is TRUE?
   a. They have few complications.
   b. They are usually superficial.
   c. They can cause airway problems.
   d. They tend to have only minor bleeding.

5. Closed head injuries are considered serious because bleeding inside the skull can cause:
   a. dilation of the pupils.
   b. softness or deformity.
   c. build-up of pressure.
   d. concussion and death.

6. A closed head injury does NOT involve a break in the skull and therefore cannot cause injury to the brain.
   a. True
   b. False

7. One sign of a possible head injury is irregular breathing.
   a. True
   b. False

8. As part of a First Responder crew, you arrive at the side of a patient with a head injury. You are assigned to the patient's head. What are the responsibilities you would have?

_____

_____

_____

_____

9. List five of the basic rules for First Responder care of an injured eye.

_____

_____

_____

_____

_____

Scenario

You and your partner have been called to the scene of an accident at a lumber yard. When you arrive at the site, you are met by a security guard who tells you that you have only one patient and that he was hit in the head by lumber being lifted by a crane. He also says that the man was unconscious when 9-1-1 was called.

a. Before you approach your patient, what should you find out?

_____

_____

b. When you arrive at your patient's side, your general impression is of a man in his 30s, conscious and looking a little embarrassed, rubbing the back of his head and neck. What is the first thing that you should do? Explain your reasoning.

_____

_____

_____

_____

c. You call dispatch to request an ambulance for this patient. When the patient hears you, he says, "Hey! Don't do that. I'm not even bleeding. Look at me. I'm fine now." Is he correct in judging his condition to be minor? Explain your answer.

_____

_____

_____

_____

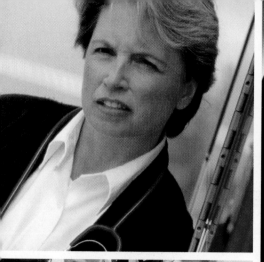
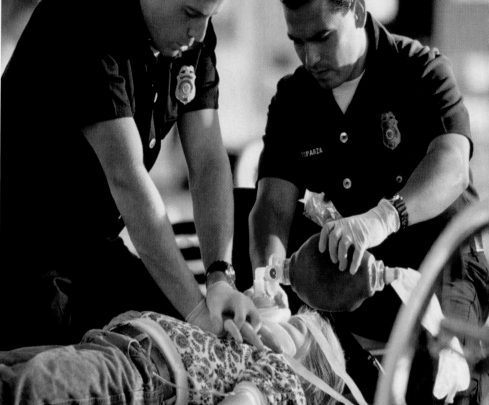
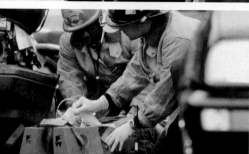

24 | Injuries to the Spine

Objectives

From the U.S. Department of Transportation (DOT) 1995 "First Responder: National Standard Curriculum." Material supplemental to the DOT curriculum is listed under "Enrichment."

Cognitive

5-3.4 ▶ Relate mechanism of injury to potential injuries of the head and spine. (pp. 439, 440, 441)

5-3.5 ▶ State the signs and symptoms of a potential spine injury. (pp. 440, 442)

5-3.6 ▶ Describe the method of determining if a responsive patient may have a spine injury. (pp. 440, 442, 443)

Affective

5-3.10 ▶ Demonstrate a caring attitude towards patients with a musculoskeletal injury who request emergency medical services. (p. 442)

5-3.11 ▶ Place the interests of the patient with a musculoskeletal injury as the foremost consideration when making any and all patient care decisions. (pp. 440, 442, 447)

5-3.12 ▶ Communicate with empathy to patients with a musculoskeletal injury, as well as with family members and friends of the patient. (p. 442)

Psychomotor

5-3.14 ▶ Demonstrate opening the airway in a patient with suspected spinal cord injury. (pp. 440, 442)

5-3.15 ▶ Demonstrate evaluating a responsive patient with a suspected spinal cord injury. (pp. 440, 442)

5-3.16 ▶ Demonstrate stabilizing the cervical spine. (pp. 440, 444)

Enrichment

▶ Describe the implications of not properly caring for potential spine injuries. (pp. 439, 440)

▶ Relate emergency airway techniques to the patient with a suspected spine injury. (pp. 440, 442)

▶ Discuss using a cervical spine immobilization device. (pp. 442, 444)

▶ Describe how to log roll a patient with a suspected spine injury. (pp. 444, 447)

▸ Describe how to secure a patient to a long backboard. (pp. 444–445)

▸ Describe when and how to perform a rapid extrication. (pp. 447–448, 450)

▸ Discuss the circumstances in which a helmet should remain on a patient and when it should be removed. (p. 449)

▸ Explain the preferred methods of removing a helmet. (pp. 449, 451–452)

Introduction

A major goal of EMS has always been the prevention of the problems related to spine injury. So, from the moment you arrive on scene, consider the possibility of spine injury and act accordingly. To appreciate the importance of this task, remember that failing to accomplish it can condemn a patient to a life in a wheelchair or even to death.

Section 1 Anatomy of the Spine

Within the bony spinal column lies the spinal cord. It is responsible for sending signals from the brain to the body and receiving signals from the body and relaying them to the brain. If these signals are interrupted by injury or illness, a person could lose the ability to move, feel, or even breathe. (Now may be a good time to review the musculoskeletal and nervous systems in Chapter 4.)

The spinal column is made up of 33 bones, one stacked on top of another. The vertebrae *articulate,* or fit and move together, so it can bend, turn, and flex.

The spine is divided into five regions—cervical, thoracic, lumbar, sacral, and coccygeal (Figure 24-1).

The **cervical spine** starts at the base of the skull where the spinal cord begins. These seven vertebrae not only house delicate nerve tissue, they also support the substantial weight of the head. This makes them especially vulnerable to injury.

The **thoracic spine** is supported by the rib cage. There are 12 thoracic vertebrae, one for each rib. Because this part of the spine is protected by the ribs, it is less frequently injured.

The next five vertebrae make up the **lumbar spine**. They carry the weight of most of the body. For this reason they are heavier and larger. The discs between the lumbar vertebrae are thicker than in other parts of the spine. Sometimes, a disc can shift, slip, or rupture,

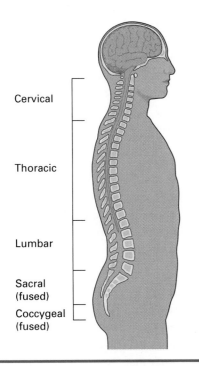

Cervical

Thoracic

Lumbar

Sacral (fused)

Coccygeal (fused)

FIGURE 24-1 Regions of the spine.

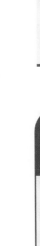

Q:

1. How many vertebrae make up the spinal column?

2. What are the five regions of the spinal column?

3. What is the function of the spinal cord?

First on Scene

If the MOI suggests spine injury, complaints of only minor pain or even no pain at all are not enough to suggest otherwise. Always assume a patient's spine is injured if the MOI suggests it is. The consequences of not doing so are extremely serious.

THE CALL

Dispatch We were on foot patrol at the college football game. Just as the home team receiver looked as if he would score, his lone pursuer dove and hit the post headfirst with full force.

Scene Size-up The coach and team trainer ran out onto the field. Almost immediately the trainer indicated he wanted us there, too. We donned our gloves on the way. When we got to the patient, we saw that the trainer was already stabilizing his head and neck. He quickly told us that the player appeared to be unresponsive. We noticed the helmet was cracked along the top. We called for EMS support immediately.

What are First Responder priorities for this patient? What injuries might you expect to see? Will the patient's football gear prevent the First Responders from providing care? Consider these questions as you read Chapter 24.

resulting in severe lower back pain. Injuries to the lumbar spine cost millions of dollars in medical expenses and lost wages every year. This is also a common area of disabling injury for EMS personnel who do not practice proper lifting and moving techniques.

The last two regions of vertebrae are the **sacral spine** and the **coccygeal spine**. The sacrum has five fused vertebrae. The coccyx has four. Together they form the posterior portion of the pelvis. Because they are fused, these parts of the spine do not bend easily.

Section 2 Spine Injuries

During scene size-up, the First Responder must identify the mechanism that injured the patient. Consider what occurred and what injuries may have resulted. Your index of suspicion for a spine injury should be very high in any of these emergencies: any unresponsive trauma patient; motor-vehicle crashes; pedestrian car crashes; falls; diving accidents; hangings; blunt trauma or penetrating trauma to the head, neck, or torso; any gunshot wounds; any speed sporting accident, such as Rollerblading, bicycling, skiing, surfing, or sledding. (See also Figure 24-2.)

Note that if the mechanism of injury suggests it, proceed as if the patient has a spine injury—even if he says he is not injured at all. The lack of back pain or the ability to walk, move arms and legs, or feel sensation does not rule out spine injury.

Spinal Precautions

Whenever you suspect spine injury in your patient, you must protect the spine from any further injury. Immediately upon completing your scene size-up, stabilize the patient's head and neck. To do so, first place your gloved hands just behind the patient's ears and spread your fingers apart. Then, hold the patient's head firmly and steadily in a neutral, in-line position. *Neutral* means the head is not flexed forward or extended back. *In-line* means the patient's nose is in line with the navel.

If you find the patient's head is not in-line, you must gently put it there. If the responsive patient complains of pain or if you feel resistance in the unresponsive patient, stop at once and stabilize the head in the position in which it was found. Manual stabilization may be released only when the patient is immobilized from head to toe on a long backboard. Have one rescuer maintain manual stabilization, while another provides care.

Spinal precautions also include using a jaw-thrust maneuver to open the patient's airway when necessary (see Chapter 6), as well as the immobilization techniques described in this chapter.

Patient Assessment

To assess a patient with possible spine injuries, manually stabilize his head and neck and assess his ABCs. Be sure to use the jaw-thrust maneuver to open and maintain the airway. Remember that a cervical-spine injury can result in severe breathing problems, even respiratory arrest. So

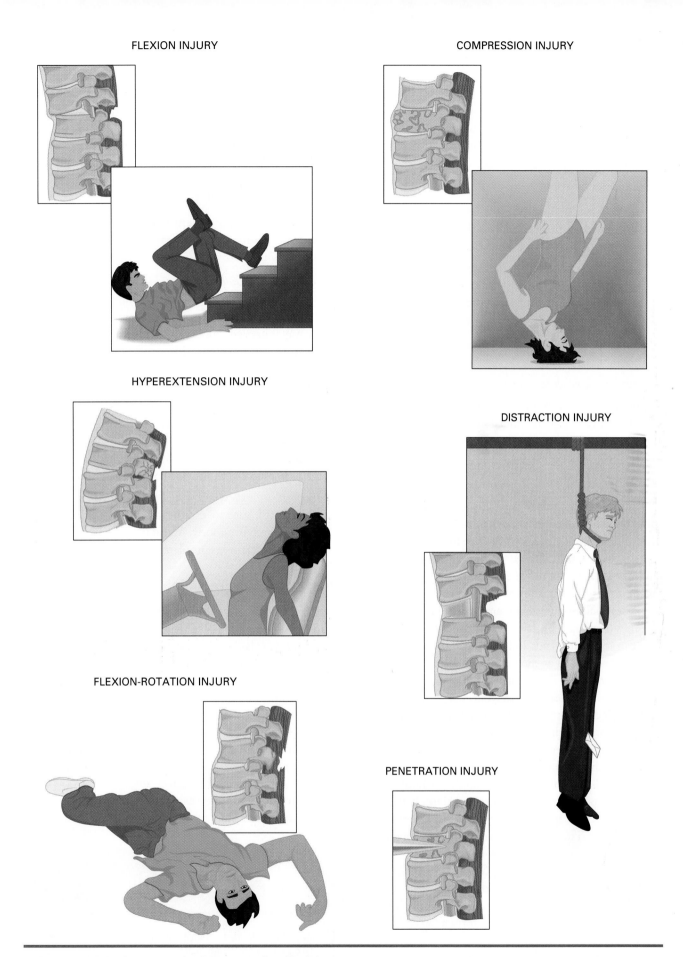

FIGURE 24-2 Common mechanisms of spine injury.

be sure to monitor the patient's airway and breathing continuously.

There may be no signs at all of spine injury. However, when they do appear, they typically include one or more of the following:

- Respiratory distress.
- Tenderness at the site of injury on the spinal column.
- Pain along the spinal column with movement. (Do not move the patient or ask the patient to move to test for this pain.)
- Constant or intermittent pain without movement along the spinal column or in the lower legs.
- Obvious deformity of the spine. (This is rare.)
- Soft-tissue injuries to the head, neck, shoulders, back, abdomen, or legs.
- Numbness, weakness, or tingling in the arms or legs.
- Loss of sensation or paralysis in the upper or lower extremities or below the injury site.
- Incontinence, or loss of bowel or bladder control.
- Priapism, or a constant erection of the penis (a classic sign of cervical-spine injury).

During the physical exam, do not risk moving the spine by taking off the patient's shirt or coat. Cut off the patient's clothes if necessary. Be sure to ask the patient if and where the spine hurts. If the patient complains of pain upon palpation of the spine, stop. Continue the assessment in other areas of the body.

Assess pulses, movement, and sensation in all four extremities (Figure 24-3). To assess movement, ask the patient if he can move his hands and feet. Then, have him squeeze both of your hands at the same time. Gauge the patient's strength and decide if it is equal on both sides. Also have the patient push his feet against your hands. Again, gauge strength and equality. To assess sensation, gently squeeze one extremity and then the other. As you do, ask questions such as: Can you feel me touching your fingers? Can you feel me touching your toes? If the patient is unresponsive or unable to follow your instructions, apply a painful stimulus to check response. Either pinch the webbing between the toes and fingers or apply pressure with a pen across the back of a fingernail. The patient should withdraw from the pain. Note the response to pain in all four extremities.

After the assessment of the front of the patient, perform a log roll so you can assess the back. However, do so only if you are trained in its use and have enough help to do so safely. Details on how to perform a log roll are provided later in this chapter.

Remember that a patient may be uncomfortable, confused, and possibly afraid of paralysis or death. It is important for you to show a caring attitude. As you proceed with the physical exam, for example, be careful how you communicate your findings to your partner. An off-hand remark could terrify the patient. When you speak to his or her family, be honest but do not alarm them unnecessarily. ■

First Responder Care

To provide care to a patient with a suspected spine injury, maintain manual stabilization of the patient's head and neck while you:

1. *Perform an initial assessment and treat all life threats.* Be sure to open and maintain the airway with a jaw-thrust maneuver. Insert an oropharyngeal or nasopharyngeal airway if needed. Suction without turning the patient's head (roll him to the side while maintaining in-line stabilization).

2. *Provide high-concentration oxygen* while maintaining neutral, in-line manual stabilization of the patient's head and neck. If breathing is adequate, administer oxygen with a nonrebreather mask. If breathing is not adequate, assist ventilations with a BVM and supplemental oxygen. Be prepared to provide basic life support.

3. *Perform a physical exam and provide treatment for any injuries.* Be sure to monitor the patient's airway and breathing continuously. Maintain manual stabilization until the patient is completely immobilized. ■

Immobilization Techniques

Many EMS systems allow First Responders to immobilize a suspected spine-injured patient. Even if your system does not, you may be called to assist EMTs. Become familiar with the techniques. They include cervical immobilization, long backboard immobilization, rapid extrication, and helmet removal.

Cervical Immobilization

After an initial assessment, a **rigid cervical immobilization device,** or extrication collar, should be applied to the patient (Figure 24-4). Never use "soft" collars in the field. They are nothing more than cotton-covered foam rings, which do not prevent movement of the head and neck.

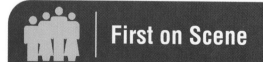

First on Scene

Never attempt to treat or move a spine-injured patient unless you have the proper equipment, training, and personnel.

SKILL SUMMARY   *Assessing Pulses, Movement, and Sensation*

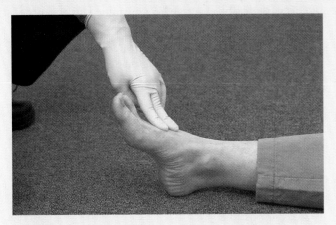

FIGURE 24-3A *Pulses—feel for a pulse in all extremities.*

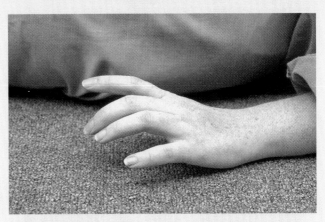

FIGURE 24-3B *Movement—ask the patient if her hands can move.*

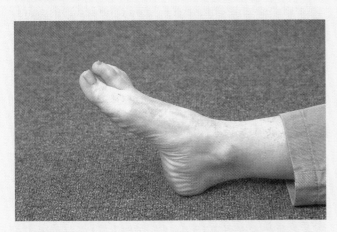

FIGURE 24-3C *Movement—ask the patient if her feet can move.*

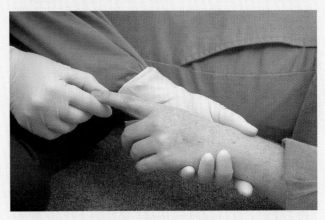

FIGURE 24-3D *Sensation—ask the patient if she can feel you touch her fingers.*

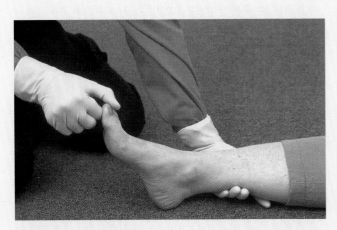

FIGURE 24-3E *Sensation—ask the patient if she can feel you touch her toes.*

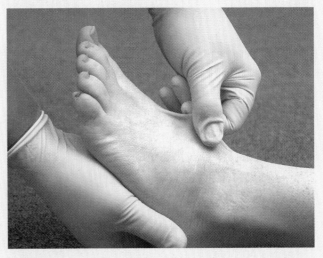

FIGURE 24-3F *In an unresponsive patient, apply painful stimuli to assess response.*

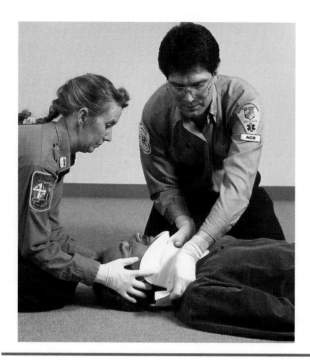

FIGURE 24-4 If allowed, apply a rigid cervical immobilization device to the patient.

Use rigid or hard collars in the field. Various kinds are available (Figure 24-5). They are designed to prevent the patient from turning, flexing, and extending the head. They can restrict movement by up to 70%. The remaining 30% must be accomplished by manual stabilization.

Follow manufacturer's instructions for applying a collar. Though instructions will vary, all collars are supported at the same points: the *maxilla* (jaw), shoulders, and clavicles. Note that failure to fit a patient properly can aggravate the injury.

Before application, be sure that jewelry and long hair have been moved away from the area. Also, examine and palpate the patient's neck before the collar is applied.

In general, to apply a rigid cervical collar to a supine patient (Figure 24-6), first slide the posterior portion of the collar in the gap under the patient's neck. Then, flip the anterior portion over the chin. Finally, secure the collar with the Velcro strap. Be careful not to pull too hard on one end. It can twist the patient's head.

If your patient is sitting, bring the collar up the chest until the chin is trapped. Then slide the posterior portion around the back of the neck and fasten it.

Whatever position your patient is in, you must maintain manual stabilization of the head and neck. Release it only when the patient is completely immobilized on a long backboard.

Long Backboard Immobilization

All patients with suspected spine injury must be immobilized onto a long backboard. To immobilize a supine or prone patient, you must first roll the patient as a unit onto his side, slip the board under him, and then roll the

patient back onto the board. This procedure is called a **log roll** (Figure 24-7).

To perform a log roll safely, you need at least three rescuers (preferably four) who are trained in the procedure. One should stay at the head to maintain manual stabilization and to coordinate the move. The other two should position themselves along one side of the patient's body. With that in mind, follow these steps:

1. *Manually stabilize the patient's head and neck.* Continue to do so until the patient is completely immobilized.

2. *Apply a rigid cervical immobilization device.*

3. *Assess pulses, movement, and sensation* in all four extremities.

4. *Position the patient.* Place his arms straight down by his sides, if possible.

5. *Get in position yourselves.* At the signal of the rescuer at the head, the two at the side should reach to the far side of the patient. One rescuer should position his hands on the shoulder and the hip. The second rescuer should position his hands at the thigh and lower leg.

6. *On signal, simultaneously roll the patient onto his side.* Be sure all three rescuers move the patient as a unit. Note that this is a good time to assess the patient's posterior, if it has not been done already.

7. *Position the backboard.* A fourth person—another rescuer, a family member, or bystander—should push the board under the patient. If no one else is available, one of the rescuers at the side may lean over the patient, grab the backboard, and pull it under the patient.

8. *On signal, simultaneously roll the patient back down and onto the board.* If he is not in the middle of the board, gently pull him down and then up again until he is straight on the board. This is done at the shoulders and hips and by pulling in alignment with the long axis of the spine. Never push a patient over to the middle of the backboard.

9. *Reassess pulses, movement, and sensation* in all four extremities. Report any change to the incoming EMTs.

Once in place, pad the spaces between the patient and the board (Figure 24-8). For an adult, pad anywhere along the length of the body to maintain neutral alignment and provide comfort. For the infant and child, also pad under the shoulders. This is to keep the relatively larger head from flexing forward. Take care to avoid extra movement.

Your next step is to secure the patient to the long backboard. It should always be done in the following order (Figure 24-9): First, immoblize the torso. Then, immobilize the head. Finally, immobilize the legs.

The patient's head should always be secured after the torso to prevent movement of the neck during immobilization. While securing the head, take a great deal of care

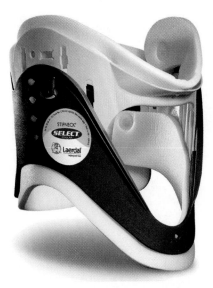

a. *STIFNECK® SELECT™ (Photography courtesy of Laerdal Medical Corporation)*

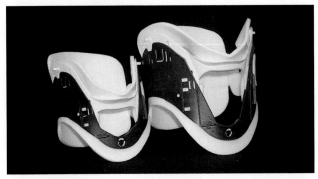

b. *Philadelphia Cervical Collar™ Patriol Adult and Pediatric. (Philadelphia Collar Corporation)*

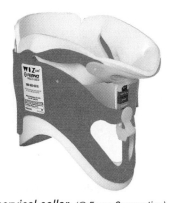

c. *WIZLOC cervical collar. (© Ferno Corporation)*

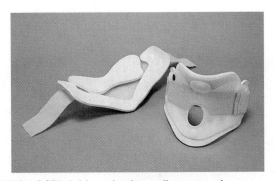

d. *NEC-LOC™ rigid extrication collar, opened.*

FIGURE 24-5 A variety of rigid cervical immobilization devices are available. Never use a "soft" collar in the field.

not to lock the jaw in place. If the patient should have to vomit, he must be able to open his mouth.

When immobilization to the long backboard has been accomplished, you may withdraw manual stabilization of the head and neck. Reassess pulses, movement, and sensation. Report any change to the incoming EMTs.

Short Backboard Immobilization

You can use a short backboard to help immobilize a seated patient. It minimizes the risk of further injury while the patient is being moved to a long backboard. Remember to maintain manual stabilization throughout the procedure and until the patient is completely immobilized.

To apply a short backboard to a seated patient (Figure 24-10):

1. *Maintain manual stabilization* of the patient's head and neck. If possible, hold his head and neck from behind.

2. *Apply a rigid cervical immobilization device.*

3. *Assess pulses, movement, and sensation* in all four extremities.

4. *Slide the short backboard in place behind the patient.* Slip it as far down into the seat as possible, but not below his coccyx. The top of the short backboard should be level with the top of the patient's head. The body flaps should fit snugly under his armpits. Try not to jostle the patient or the rescuer who is holding manual stabilization.

5. *Secure the patient to the backboard.* Strap up his torso first. If the device has leg straps, tighten those next. Finally, secure the patient's head. To make sure the head and neck remain in neutral alignment with the rest of the spine, you may need to pad behind them.

To move the patient to a long backboard, position it under or next to his buttocks. Rotate him until his back is in line with it. Then lower him onto the long backboard. Follow the instructions outlined above for securing the

SKILL SUMMARY   *Applying a Rigid Cervical Immobilization Device*

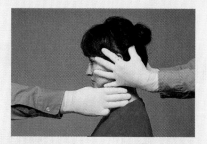

FIGURE 24-6A

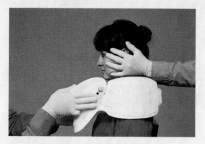

FIGURE 24-6B

SIZING. It is critical to select a collar of the correct size. Too tall can overextend the neck, force the jaw closed, and limit access to the airway. Too short can lead to inadequate immobilization. Too tight can impede blood flow. One way to measure collar size is to use your fingers to compare the neck size to the corresponding area of the collar.

NOTE: Do not use soft collars. Only use rigid cervical immobilization devices in the field. Also, do not use the chin piece as an anchoring point for the collar. This may cause hyperextension, which may injure the patient's cervical spine.

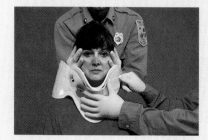

FIGURE 24-6C

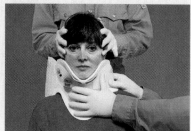

FIGURE 24-6D

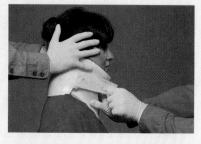

FIGURE 24-6E   *TIGHTENING. Grip the trach hole as you tighten the collar. Then check to see that the collar fits according to the manufacturer's instructions.*

SEATED APPLICATION. The patient's chin must be well supported by the chin piece. To accomplish this, slide the collar up the patient's chest wall. If the collar is pushed directly inward, it may be difficult to position the chin piece and, therefore, to apply the collar tightly enough.

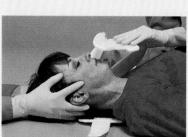

FIGURE 24-6F

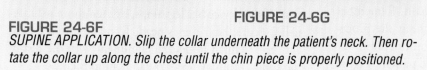

FIGURE 24-6G

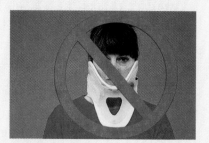

FIGURE 24-6H   *WARNING. Always check for neutral alignment and proper fit. Improper sizing or application may allow the patient's chin to slip inside the collar. This must be prevented.*

SUPINE APPLICATION. Slip the collar underneath the patient's neck. Then rotate the collar up along the chest until the chin piece is properly positioned.

SKILL SUMMARY *Performing a Three-Rescuer Log Roll*

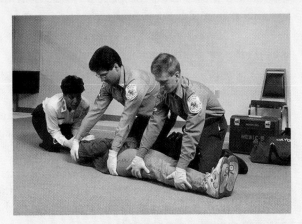

FIGURE 24-7A *Maintain the head and neck in a neutral, in-line position.*

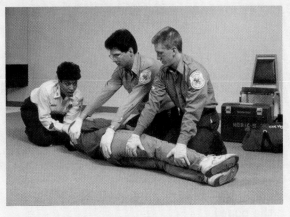

FIGURE 24-7B *Simultaneously roll the patient as a unit onto his side.*

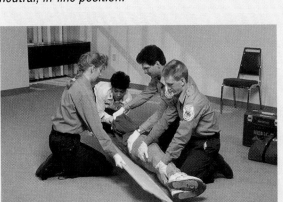

FIGURE 24-7C *A bystander or one of the three rescuers should move the long backboard into place.*

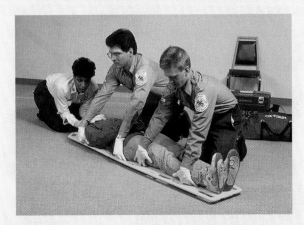

FIGURE 24-7D *On signal, simultaneously roll the patient back down and onto the board.*

patient. Release manual stabilization when the patient is completely immobilized.

Rapid Extrication

In general, rescuers should move a sitting spine-injured patient only after short backboard immobilization. However, in certain emergencies there is not enough time. A rapid extrication may need to be performed instead when any one of three conditions exists: the scene is not safe (for example, there is a threat of fire or explosion, a hostile crowd, or extreme weather conditions), life-saving care cannot be given because of the patient's location or position, or there is an inability to gain access to other patients who need life-saving care.

In general, a rapid extrication must be performed by a team of three or more rescuers. The objective is to move a sitting patient to a long backboard with only manual

stabilization of the spine. To perform a rapid extrication of a suspected spine-injured patient (Figure 24-11):

1. *Bring the patient's head into a neutral, in-line position.* This is best done from behind or to the side of the patient.

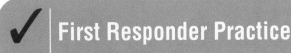

✓ **First Responder Practice**

Perform a rapid extrication only when there is an immediate threat to life. Unless such an emergency exists, the patient should not be moved and should receive instead manual stabilization of the head and neck, a cervical collar if possible, and immobilization to a short backboard.

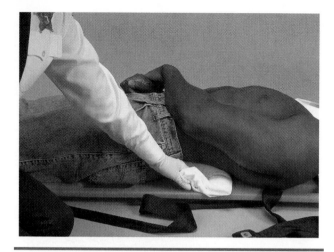

FIGURE 24-8 Pad the voids between the patient and the board.

2. *Apply a rigid cervical immobilization device.*

3. *Rotate the patient into position.* Do so in several short, coordinated moves until the patient's back is in the open doorway and feet are on the adjoining seat.

4. *Bring the long backboard in line with the patient.* It should rest against the patient's buttocks.

5. *Lower the patient onto the long backboard.* Then slide him into position in short, coordinated moves.

6. *Secure the patient to the long backboard.* Release manual stabilization only when the patient is completely immobilized.

Note that it may be necessary to hand off manual stabilization during the procedure to a rescuer outside the vehicle. Be sure it is maintained continuously until the patient is completely immobilized.

SKILL SUMMARY *Securing a Patient to a Long Backboard*

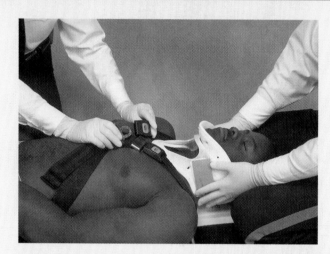

FIGURE 24-9A *Immobilize the patient's torso first.*

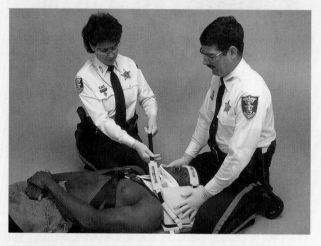

FIGURE 24-9B *Immobilize the head next.*

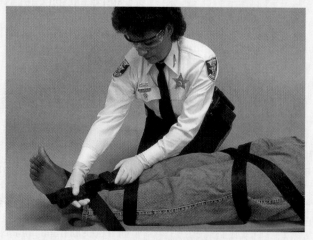

FIGURE 24-9C *Finally, immobilize the patient's legs.*

SKILL SUMMARY   *Securing a Patient to a Short Backboard*

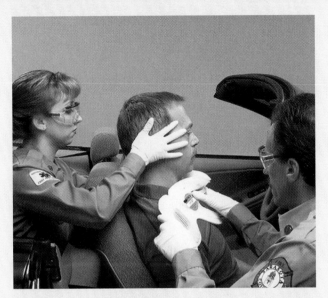

FIGURE 24-10A   *Manually stabilize the head and neck. Then apply a rigid cervical collar.*

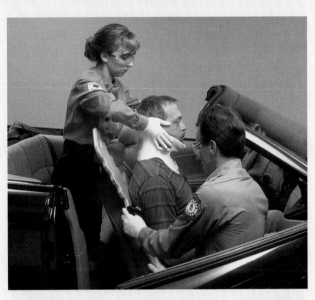

FIGURE 24-10B   *Position the short backboard behind the patient.*

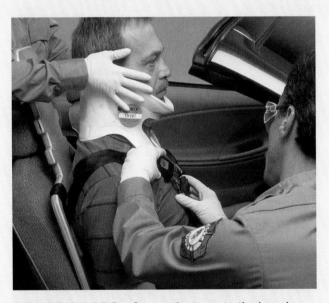

FIGURE 24-10C   *Secure the torso to the board.*

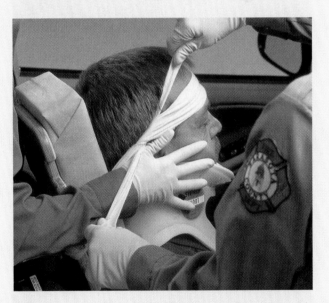

FIGURE 24-10D   *Pad behind the head and secure it to the board.*

Helmet Removal

There are two basic types of helmets: motorcycle helmets and sports helmets such as those worn for football. Typically, a sports helmet has an opening in front that allows easy access to the patient's airway. For many, the face shield can be unclipped or unsnapped for easy removal. A motorcycle helmet, however, may have a shield that prevents access to the patient's airway.

In general, if your patient can be properly assessed and the airway maintained, a helmet should be left in place. Do not attempt to remove a helmet alone. Wait for help.

If a helmet must be removed from a suspected spine-injured patient (Figure 24-12):

1. *Stabilize the helmet, head, and neck.* To do this, the rescuer at the head should hold each side of the helmet, while placing his fingers on the patient's lower jaw.

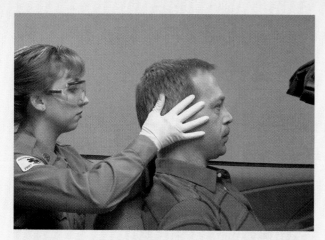

FIGURE 24-11A *Bring the patient's head into a neutral, in-line position.*

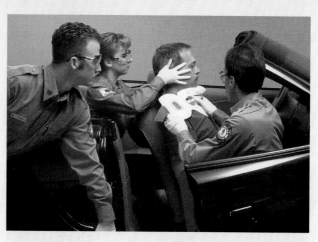

FIGURE 24-11B *Apply a rigid cervical immobilization device.*

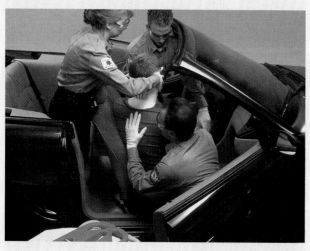

FIGURE 24-11C *Rotate the patient into position.*

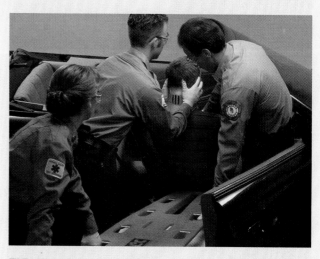

FIGURE 24-11D *Bring the long backboard in line with the patient.*

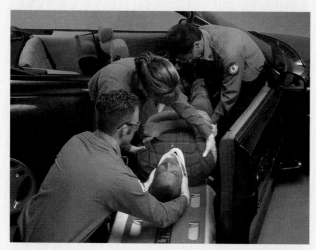

FIGURE 24-11E *Lower the patient onto the long backboard.*

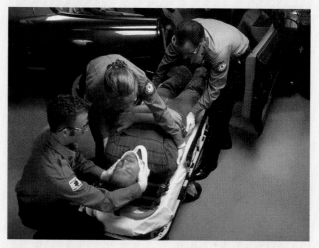

FIGURE 24-11F *Slide the patient into position in small steps, and secure the patient to the backboard.*

SKILL SUMMARY   *Removing a Helmet*

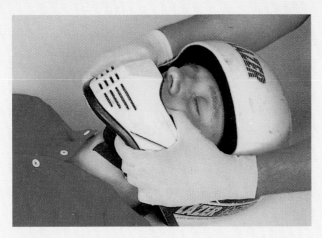

FIGURE 24-12A *Stabilize the helmet, head, and neck to prevent movement.*

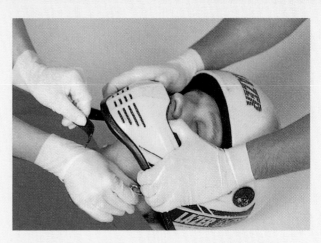

FIGURE 24-12B *Loosen the chin strap, while maintaining manual stabilization.*

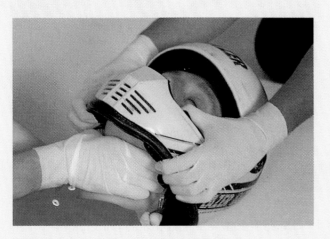

FIGURE 24-12C *Transfer stabilization.*

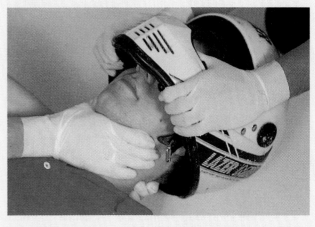

FIGURE 24-12D *Slip off the helmet about half way so your partner can maintain an in-line position of the head.*

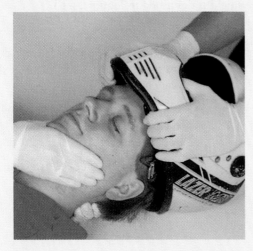

FIGURE 24-12E *When the helmet is completely removed, transfer manual stabilization to the rescuer at the head.*

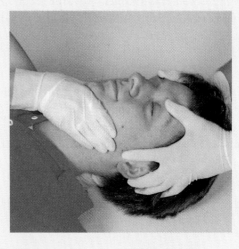

FIGURE 24-12F *Maintain manual stabilization until the patient is completely immobilized.*

SKILL SUMMARY   *Removing a Helmet—Alternative Method*

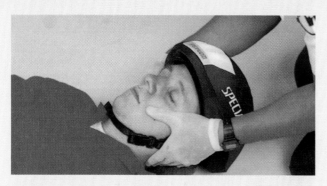

FIGURE 24-13A   *Stabilize the helmet, head, and neck to prevent movement.*

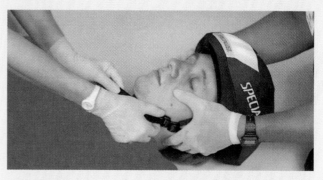

FIGURE 24-13B   *Remove the chin strap, while maintaining manual stabilization.*

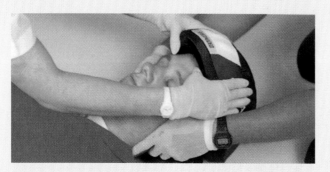

FIGURE 24-13C   *Full-face helmets will have to be tilted back to clear the nose.*

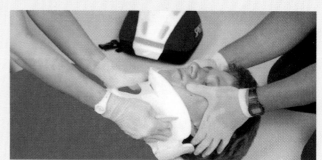

FIGURE 24-13D   *Apply a rigid cervical collar, and maintain manual stabilization until the patient is completely immobilized.*

2. *Loosen the chin strap.* While the rescuer at the head maintains manual stabilization, a second rescuer should loosen the helmet's chin strap.

3. *Transfer manual stabilization.* First, the second rescuer should place one hand anteriorly on the mandible at the angle of the jaw. He then should place his other hand at the back of the patient's head.

4. *Slip off the helmet about half way.* To do so, the rescuer at the head should spread the sides of the helmet so that it can clear the patient's ears. After the helmet has been pulled off about half way, the second rescuer should readjust his hands to maintain alignment of the patient's head.

5. *Remove the helmet completely.* The rescuer at the head should remove the helmet. He should then take over manual stabilization and maintain it until the patient is completely immobilized.

An alternative method for removing a helmet that has no face shield is described in Figure 24-13.

1. What are five emergencies for which your index of suspicion for spine injuries should be very high?

2. When should you begin manual stabilization of a patient's head and neck? When may you release it?

3. What is First Responder care for a suspected spine-injured patient?

▶▶ The Call Follow-up

At the beginning of this chapter, you read that First Responders were caring for a male patient—a college football player—with possible head and spine injuries. To see how chapter skills apply to this emergency, read the following. It describes how the call was completed.

Initial Assessment The trainer handed over manual stabilization to my partner, so that the trainer and I could work together to remove the patient's helmet. (The trainer had much more experience at helmet removal than we did.) When the helmet was removed, I used a jaw-thrust to open the patient's airway. It was clear of blood and secretions. Breathing was adequate but irregular. We applied 100% oxygen by nonrebreather mask, using a small portable oxygen tank. The patient's pulse was strong and bounding, and his skin was warm and dry. No bleeding was noted. We carefully applied a rigid cervical immobilization device.

Physical Examination The ETA of the ambulance was about three minutes. I began a physical exam as the team trainer carefully removed the patient's pads. My partner continued to hold manual stabilization and asked the coach about the patient's history. My first obvious finding was a deformity and swelling on the top of the patient's head. Clear fluid and blood seeped out of his ears. His facial bones all appeared to be intact.

Patient History The coach got the patient's medical history card from his pack at the sideline. It indicated that the player had no known allergies and that he did not take any medications regularly. His last physical by the team doctor was unremarkable. He had no other significant past medical history. The coach told my partner that the team players ate lunch about an hour before the game.

Ongoing Assessment We maintained manual stabilization. Since the patient was unresponsive and his respirations were somewhat irregular, we watched breathing carefully. We also checked his pulse again. We radioed for the ambulance to bring immobilization equipment and to drive right onto the field.

Patient Hand-off When the EMTs arrived, I gave them my report (see below). Then, while one EMT radioed the trauma center to report a possible neurosurgical emergency, we helped to log roll the patient onto a long backboard for head-to-toe immobilization.

Hand-off Report

"This is Henry Jones, 21 years old. He struck a steel goal post, cracking his helmet and sustaining a head injury. He was unresponsive upon our arrival and that hasn't changed. His respirations have been irregular but fast enough and deep. I suspect we'll have to assist his breathing soon. Pulse has dropped from 80 to 56. We also found blood and clear fluid coming from his ears. We assisted the trainer in removing the helmet and pads. We manually stabilized his head and neck the whole time. We have the patient on oxygen via nonrebreather, and a c-collar is in place. The coach has his history—nothing of note."

The Last Word *Head and spine injuries are among the most devastating injuries a patient can suffer. Always be alert to the possibility that an injury to the spine may have occurred. Then do everything you can to protect it from further harm. Remember, if the mechanism of injury suggests it, treat for it.*

Chapter Review

Focus on the EMS Team

One EMS instructor began a lecture on spine injuries by writing on the board, "Quadriplegia is forever." Quadriplegia (paralysis in all four extremities) can be caused by a spine injury—or by improper care of a spine injury. If the spine is injured, any movement of the spinal column can cause damage to the cord. You must stabilize the spine properly and protect it from moving until the EMTs/paramedics arrive. Preventing even a small movement can make a big difference.

Spinal precautions will be just as important to the patient when he is in the care of the EMTs. On the way to the hospital, they will maintain the spinal care you initiated. Nurses and physicians will, too, as they further assess and care for the patient. But remember, your ability to quickly recognize the potential for spine injury and to take immediate spinal precautions will begin the life-saving and spine-saving care so vital to your patient.

Summing Up

- The spine is divided into five regions—cervical, thoracic, lumbar, sacral, and coccygeal.

- The index of suspicion for a spine injury should be very high for motor-vehicle crashes; pedestrian-car crashes; falls; diving accidents; hangings; blunt trauma or penetrating trauma to the head, neck, or torso; any gunshot wounds; any speed sport accident; any unresponsive trauma patient.

- If the MOI suggests a possible spine injury, immediately upon completing scene size-up, manually stabilize the patient's head and neck. Then, assess the ABCs as you would any patient but use a jaw-thrust to open the airway and maintain manual stabilization throughout assessment. During the physical exam, assess pulses, movement, and sensation in all four extremities. If you have the proper training and enough assistance to do so safely, perform a log roll to examine the patient's back.

- First Responder care of a patient with a suspected spine injury is the same as for any other trauma patient, except spinal precautions should be taken and maintained until the patient is completely immobilized on a long backboard.

- Use a log roll when you must have access to the patient's back or in order to slip a long backboard under him. At least three rescuers trained in the technique are needed to perform a log roll safely.

- Immobilization techniques include:
  — *Rigid cervical immobilization device application.* After an initial assessment, apply the appropriate size collar to a supine or sitting patient. Continue to maintain manual stabilization of the head and neck during and after application.
  — *Long backboard immobilization.* All patients with suspected spine injury must be immobilized onto a long backboard.
  — *Short backboard immobilization.* Fitting the patient from neck to hip, this device is used to help immobilize a seated patient while he is being moved to a long backboard.
  — *Rapid extrication.* This technique is used to move a sitting patient to a long backboard with only manual stabilization of the spine. Use it only when the scene is not safe, life-saving care cannot be given because of the patient's location or position, or there is an inability to gain access to other patients who need life-saving care.
  — *Helmet removal.* If your patient can be properly assessed and the airway maintained, a helmet should be left in place. Do not remove it. If it must be removed from a suspected spine-injured patient, the head and neck must be maintained in its neutral, in-line position throughout the procedure.

Key Terms

cervical spine neck; formed by the first seven vertebrae.

coccygeal spine tail bone; formed by four fused vertebrae. *Also called* coccyx.

log roll a method of turning a patient without causing injury to his or her spine.

lumbar spine lower back; formed by five vertebrae.

rigid cervical immobilization device a device in the shape of a collar used to restrict movement of the cervical spine. *Also called* extrication collar.

sacral spine lower part of the spine; formed by five fused vertebrae. *Also called* sacrum.

thoracic spine upper back; formed by 12 vertebrae.

Knowledge Check

1. The cervical spine consists of ___ vertebrae.
   a. 3
   b. 5
   c. 7
   d. 9

2. To check a patient for sensation in a lower extremity, you should:
   a. assess the distal pulse.
   b. assess its skin temperature.
   c. ask the patient to wiggle her toes.
   d. ask the patient if she can feel your touch.

3. If the mechanism of injury suggests a spine injury in your patient, you should immediately:
   a. insert an oropharyngeal or nasopharyngeal airway.
   b. perform an initial assessment and treatment.
   c. stabilize the patient's head and neck.
   d. provide high-concentration oxygen.

4. To immobilize a patient on a long backboard, which part of the body should you immobilize first?
   a. head
   b. arms
   c. torso
   d. legs

5. You are called to an athletic field where a player has been injured and is complaining of neck and back pain. Since his helmet allows easy access to the airway, you are able to determine that the patient has no airway problems at this time. To continue First Responder care for this patient, you should:
   a. remove the helmet only.
   b. leave the patient's helmet in place.
   c. remove both the patient's helmet and shoulder pads.
   d. have the patient remove all of his protective gear.

6. A patient with an injury that has damaged the spinal cord would have loss of sensation or paralysis:
   a. in one extremity.
   b. on one side of the body.
   c. above the level of the injury site.
   d. below the level of the injury site.

7. You should open the airway of a suspected spine-injured patient by using a(n) ___ maneuver.
   a. log roll
   b. jaw-thrust
   c. in-line neutral
   d. head-tilt/chin-lift

8. In general, rescuers should move a sitting, spine-injured patient only after ___ immobilization.
   a. short backboard
   b. cervical collar
   c. long backboard
   d. rapid extrication

9. Securing a patient to a long backboard must be done in what order?
   a. torso, head, legs
   b. head, legs, torso
   c. legs, torso, head
   d. head, torso, legs

10. The thoracic spine has 12 fused vertebrae.
    a. True
    b. False

11. Rigid or hard cervical collars are designed to restrict movement of the head and neck by almost 100%, so no other restriction is necessary.
    a. True
    b. False

12. The term "neutral, in-line position" means the head is NOT flexed forward or extended back and the nose is in line with the navel.
    a. True
    b. False

13. Write the names of the regions of the spine in order from top to bottom.

_____

_____

_____

_____

_____

14. List six the emergencies in which your index of suspicion should be very high for spine injury.

_____

_____

_____

Scenario

You and your partner are at the scene of a car crash. The police are already patrolling traffic and are otherwise making the scene safe. Your patient was the driver. A police officer tells you that she ran a red light and, to avoid an oncoming vehicle, swerved into the curb and metal railing. He points to the badly damaged hood, front fender, and tires. Your patient's chief complaint is feeling "somewhat stunned." Your general impression is of a female in her 20s who has no obvious injuries but is pale and slow in responding to you.

a. Your patient is sitting in the driver's seat of her car, seat belt still on, steering wheel airbag deployed. How should you proceed with your initial assessment?

_____

_____

b. The ambulance ETA tells you that you have time to perform a physical exam of your patient. When you gently palpate the patient's neck, she complains of pain. What should you do?

_____

_____

c. What kind of an examination could tell you if the patient's nervous system (brain, spinal cord, nerves) has been injured?

_____

_____

_____

d. The EMTs have arrived and decided to move the patient from the car. What procedures would you expect them to use?

_____

_____

_____

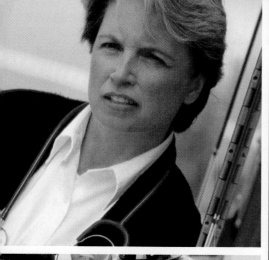
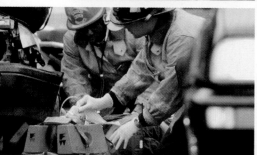
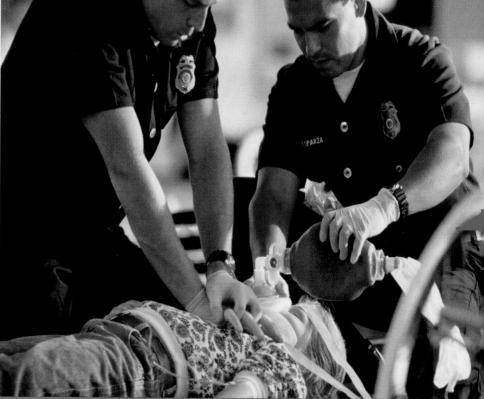

25 | Musculoskeletal Injuries

Objectives

From the U.S. Department of Transportation (DOT) 1995 "First Responder:
National Standard Curriculum." Material supplemental to the DOT curriculum
is listed under "Enrichment."

Cognitive

5-3.1 ▶ Describe the function of the musculoskeletal system. (p. 459)

5-3.2 ▶ Differentiate between an open and a closed painful, swollen, deformed extremity. (p. 460)

5-3.3 ▶ List the emergency medical care for a patient with a painful, swollen, deformed extremity. (pp. 461–463)

Affective

5-3.9 ▶ Explain the rationale for the feeling patients who have need for immobilization of the painful, swollen, deformed extremity. (pp. 461, 465)

5-3.10 ▶ Demonstrate a caring attitude towards patients with a musculoskeletal injury who request emergency medical services. (pp. 461, 465)

5-3.11 ▶ Place the interests of the patient with a musculoskeletal injury as the foremost consideration when making any and all patient care decisions. (pp. 461–463, 465)

5-3.12 ▶ Communicate with empathy to patients with a musculoskeletal injury, as well as with family members and friends of the patient. (pp. 461, 465)

Psychomotor

5-3.13 ▶ Demonstrate the emergency medical care of a patient with a painful, swollen, deformed extremity. (pp. 461–463)

Enrichment

▶ State the reasons for splinting. (p. 463)

▶ List the general rules of splinting. (p. 465)

▶ List the complications of improper splinting. (p. 465)

▶ Describe several different types of splints. (pp. 463, 465)

▶ Describe splinting of the upper extremities. (pp. 465–467, 468)

▶ Describe splinting of the lower extremities. (pp. 467, 469–471)

Introduction

Injuries to muscles, joints, and bones are some of the most common emergencies you will encounter in the field. They can range from a pulled muscle or twisted ankle to life-threatening breaks in a femur. Regardless of whether the injury is mild or severe, your ability to assess your patient and provide the appropriate emergency care can help prevent permanent disability and disfigurement.

Section 1 Injuries to Bones and Joints

The musculoskeletal system is made up of more than 200 bones and over 600 muscles. Together they give the body shape, protect internal organs, and provide for movement. Any time bones and muscles are injured, one of those functions is either temporarily or permanently impaired. (You may wish to turn to Chapter 4 to review system components now.)

Bones and muscles may be injured in four basic ways: a **fracture** (a broken bone), a **strain** (a muscle or a muscle and tendon are overextended), a **sprain** (a joint and ligament are injured), or a **dislocation** (a bone is moved out of its normal position in a joint and remains that way).

A mechanism of musculoskeletal injury may involve direct, indirect, or twisting forces (Figure 25-1). They can give you a good idea of how extensive an injury may be.

With a **direct force**, an injury occurs at the point of impact. For example, imagine that a patient is in a car crash. When he is thrust forward, one of his knees strikes the dashboard. The resulting broken kneecap is caused by that direct force, or direct blow.

THE CALL

Dispatch The temperature outside was dropping rapidly and snow flurries had already started. I was just sitting down for an evening of television, when the tones went out. "McKownville Fire/Rescue 360 and Ambulance 40 respond to an automobile crash, Route 20 and the entrance to the Northway."

Scene Size-up As my partner and I approached the scene, we could see several cars on the bridge, most off the road and against the guardrails. We were just stopping when we saw a police cruiser slide into a slow spin and glide past us. We exited our unit when the road was flared off and the scene was safe. The police then directed us to vehicle #3. It had been struck by another vehicle and had skidded into the guardrail.

Initial Assessment Our patient was a 19-year-old woman who was in the driver's seat. Her left thigh was bulging so much that we could see the deformity through her jeans. She was holding her leg tightly and appeared to be in a great deal of pain. My partner stabilized her head and neck, while I began the initial assessment.

Should these First Responders alter the patient assessment plan to address their patient's injury first? After all, one of the major arteries of the body is located in the thigh. What would your priorities be? Consider this patient as you read Chapter 25.

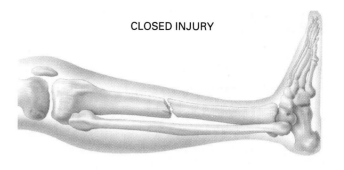

CLOSED INJURY

OPEN INJURY

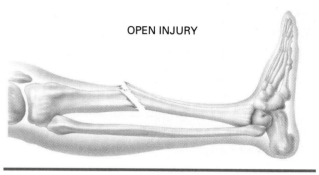

FIGURE 25-2 A closed injury vs. an open one.

✓ | **First Responder Practice**

An injury that causes pain, swelling, or deformity in an extremity may be the result of a fracture, sprain, strain, or dislocation. Because these injuries look so much alike in the field, you do not need to figure out which is which. Instead, always treat a painful, swollen, or deformed extremity as if it involved a broken bone.

With an **indirect force,** the energy of a blow travels along a path away from the point of impact. For example, think of a patient who falls onto her outstretched hand. The force of the blow can travel from her hand and wrist up through her arm and shoulder. The injuries caused by the indirect force could include broken arm bones and even a broken clavicle. So, look beyond the injury caused by a direct force when you examine a trauma patient. Additional injuries may be involved.

With a **twisting force,** one part of a limb remains stationary while the rest of it twists. An example would be the case of a jogger who steps into a hole and gets his foot caught. When he falls, the body would pull the leg one way, while the trapped foot would hold it firmly in its original position. That could twist the limb, causing any of its bones or joints to break. Again, suspect injuries beyond the most obvious one when you examine your patient.

In addition, a musculoskeletal injury is classified as either *closed* or *open* (Figure 25-2). In a closed extremity injury, the skin is not broken at the injury site. It remains intact. In an open extremity injury, the skin is broken, perhaps by protruding bone ends.

Note: Although bones may seem very solid, in fact they are not. The center of bones (commonly called *marrow*) is rich in blood vessels. This is why broken bones cause blood loss. When a large bone is broken or when there are multiple fractures, such blood loss can cause shock.

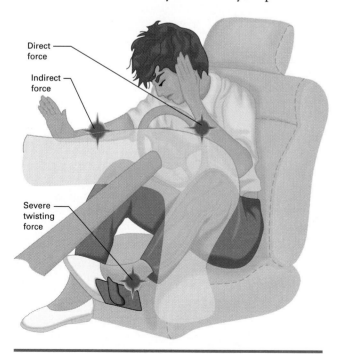

Direct force

Indirect force

Severe twisting force

FIGURE 25-1 Different types of forces can cause different types of injuries.

✓ | **First Responder Practice**

As you begin your assessment of a patient with musculoskeletal injuries, keep the following in mind:

- The mechanism of injury can alert you to hidden injuries.

- Broken bones can be serious. They bleed, and they cause shock. If there is a possibility that your patient has more than one broken bone, the potential for shock and other hidden injuries is very high.

- Perform a thorough physical exam. The head, neck, chest, and abdomen must be examined before the extremities because they contain the vital organs. Examine the extremities last.

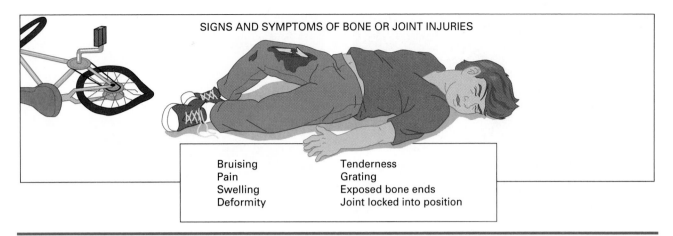

SIGNS AND SYMPTOMS OF BONE OR JOINT INJURIES

Bruising   Tenderness
Pain   Grating
Swelling   Exposed bone ends
Deformity   Joint locked into position

FIGURE 25-3 Bone and joint injuries can present with a variety of signs and symptoms.

Patient Assessment

As you conduct your scene size-up, consider the mechanism of injury and whether the forces involved were indirect, direct, or twisting forces. When you determine the scene is safe, perform an initial assessment and identify any life-threats. Do not be distracted by gruesome-looking injuries, especially when treating a patient with multiple trauma. Identify and treat life-threats first. Then perform a thorough physical exam of the patient, keeping the MOI and forces involved in mind.

Signs and symptoms of musculoskeletal injury include (Figure 25-3):

- Deformity or angulation (Figure 25-4). When compared to the uninjured limb, the injured one is a different size or has a different shape.
- Pain and tenderness.

- Crepitus (the sound or feeling of broken bones grinding against each other).
- Swelling.
- Bruising or discoloration.
- Exposed bone ends (Figure 25-5).
- Joint locked in position.

When examining a patient with a musculoskeletal injury, remember that he may be in a great deal of pain. Be careful not to move the injured limb or jar the body. Be gentle and reassuring to the patient and his or her family. ■

First Responder Care

Your priority is life before limb. Remain focused on treating the life-threats you identify in the initial assessment.

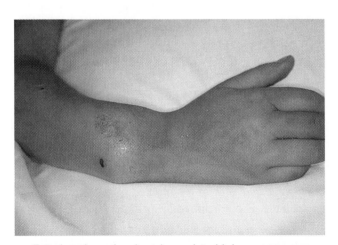

a. *Exterior view of a closed angulated injury. (Charles Stewart M.D. & Associates)*

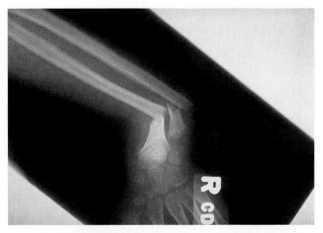

b. *X-ray of the same closed angulated injury. (Charles Stewart M.D. & Associates)*

FIGURE 25-4 An angulated injury gives a limb an abnormal size or shape.

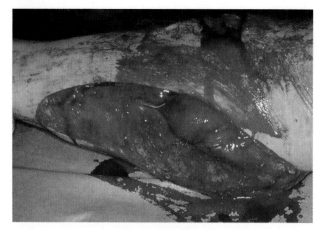

a. *Open injury.* *(Charles Stewart M.D. & Associates)*

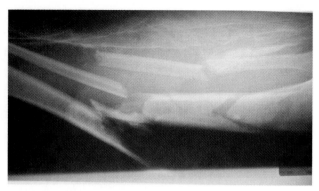

b. *X-ray of limb in photo to left, showing broken bones both above and below surface.* *(Charles Stewart M.D. & Associates)*

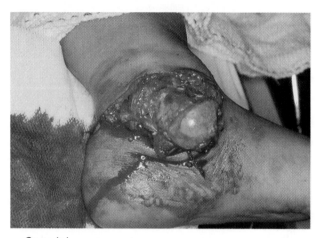

c. *Open injury.* *(Charles Stewart M.D. & Associates)*

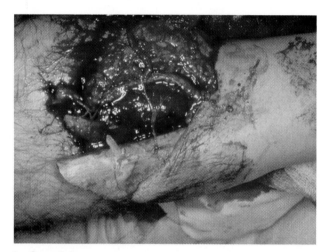

d. *Open injury.* *(Charles Stewart M.D. & Associates)*

FIGURE 25-5 In an open extremity injury, the skin is broken, sometimes by protruding bone ends.

Once that is done, you can turn to limb-threatening injuries, as follows:

1. *Maintain manual stabilization of the patient's spine,* if indicated, and continue to administer oxygen, if it is available.

✔ First Responder Practice

If ever you are tempted to dismiss an injured extremity as unimportant, don't! Musculoskeletal injuries are serious. They can cause significant bleeding, they have the potential to cause shock, and they often damage tissue and blood vessels under the skin. Your care for musculoskeletal injuries will not only help prevent shock in your patient, but it also will help prevent life-long disabilities.

2. *Stabilize the injured extremity after you have completed a physical exam.* Hold it manually above and below the injury site. Maintain stabilization until the limb is completely immobilized in a splint. It can prevent a closed injury from becoming an open one, and it can help reduce the patient's discomfort.

3. *Expose the injury site.* To avoid jarring the limb, you may cut away clothing. Remove jewelry, too.

4. *Treat any open wounds.* Control bleeding. Be careful to avoid applying any pressure to broken bone ends. Then dress open wounds with sterile dressings.

5. *Apply a cold pack to the injured area,* if you have one available. It can help reduce pain and swelling.

6. *Allow the patient to rest in a position of comfort* while you wait for the arrival of the EMTs. You also may wish to pad under the patient's injured limb to prevent discomfort.

7. *Continue to assess for pulse, movement, and sensation* below the injury site. Record any changes.

While you are stabilizing an injured limb, do not intentionally replace any protruding bones. Also, do not apply manual traction (pull the limb) in an attempt to straighten it or realign the bones, except when you are authorized to do so. Only trained medical personnel should attempt traction in the field. Be sure to follow all local protocols.

Maintain manual stabilization of an injured extremity until it is completely immobilized with a splint. Even if you find that you have to stay in an uncomfortable position for some time, maintain stabilization. The patient's best interests must be your foremost consideration. If you are trained and allowed to do so, splint the injured extremity after you have performed the steps described above. ■

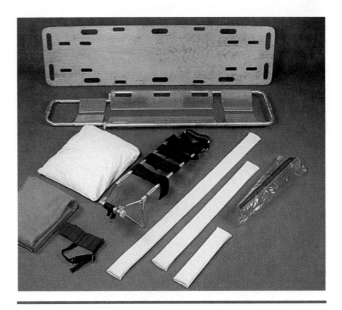

FIGURE 25-6 Examples of splints.

1. How many ways can a bone and muscle be injured? Name them.

2. What forces can be involved in a mechanism of musculoskeletal injury? Describe each one.

3. What are the signs and symptoms of a musculoskeletal injury?

4. What are the general guidelines for First Responder care of a patient with a musculoskeletal injury?

Section 2 Splinting Musculoskeletal Injuries

Any device used to immobilize a body part is called a **splint**. A splint may be soft or rigid. It can be commercially manufactured or it can be improvised from virtually any object that can immobilize a limb. (See Figure 25-6.)

There are five good reasons for splinting a musculoskeletal injury:

■ To prevent motion of bone fragments or dislocated joints.

■ To minimize damage to surrounding tissues, nerves, blood vessels, and the injured bone itself.

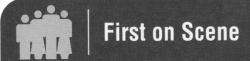

First on Scene

Do not let a musculoskeletal injury—even one that is gruesome—make you miss life-threats such as an open chest wound, severe bleeding, or shock. *Always treat conditions that are a threat to life first.*

■ To help control bleeding and swelling.

■ To help prevent shock.

■ To reduce pain and suffering.

Note that First Responders may not be allowed to immobilize musculoskeletal injuries in your EMS system. Make sure you follow all local protocols.

Types of Splints

Some common types of splints are *rigid splints, traction splints, circumferential splints, improvised splints,* and the *sling and swathe.* All are designed to accomplish the same task. They must immobilize an injured extremity.

Rigid Splints

Padded rigid boards, or rigid splints, are the most common type of splint. They may be made of wood, aluminum, wire, plastic, cardboard, or compressed fibers. Some are shaped specifically for arms or legs. Others are pliable enough to be molded to fit any appendage. Some come with washable pads. Others must be padded before being applied.

A rigid splint must be applied in line with the bone. Then it must be anchored to the limb with cravats secured with *square knots* (or straps or Velcro closures). Remember, never place a cravat across the injury site. It could cause further injury and pain.

Traction Splints

A **traction splint** is a mechanical device that provides a counter-pull to alleviate pain, reduce blood loss, and minimize further injury. It does not realign broken bones.

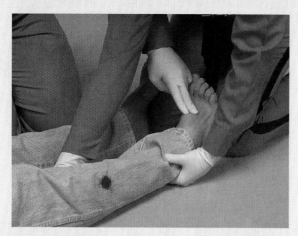

FIGURE 25-7A *Stabilize the limb, and assess pulse, movement, and sensation below the injury site.*

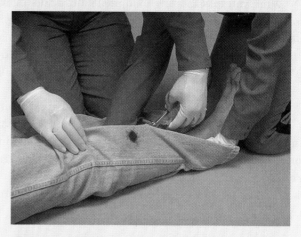

FIGURE 25-7B *Cut away clothing to expose the injury.*

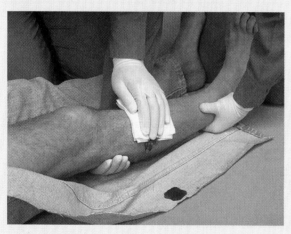

FIGURE 25-7C *After controlling bleeding, place a sterile dressing over open wounds, if any.*

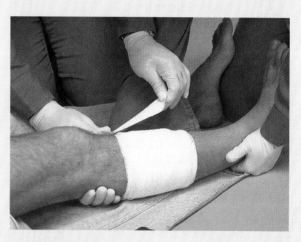

FIGURE 25-7D *If there is severe deformity, absence of pulse, or cyanosis in the extremity, align it with gentle traction. Maintain it until the limb is completely immobilized.*

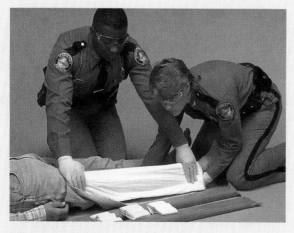

FIGURE 25-7E *Pad the splint.*

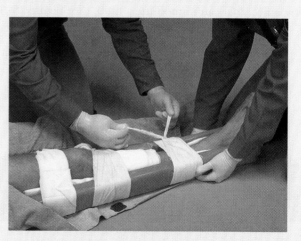

FIGURE 25-7F *Secure the limb to the splint, and reassess pulse, movement, and sensation.*

Several types of traction splints are available, and application procedures vary according to manufacturer. As a First Responder, you should use a traction splint only if you are specifically trained and allowed to do so. Follow local protocols.

Circumferential Splints

A **circumferential splint** completely surrounds, or envelopes, the injured limb. An example is an **air splint**. It can be inflated, either mechanically or manually, until it forms a semi-rigid sleeve around the injured limb.

Improvised Splints

An **improvised splint** is one made with materials found on hand. It can be made from a cardboard box, cane or walking stick, ironing board, rolled-up magazine, umbrella, broom handle, catcher's shin guard, or any similar object. It must be long enough to extend past the joints and prevent movement on both sides of the injury. It also should be as wide as the thickest part of the injured part.

A **self-splint** also may be effective. In fact, in some cases, a patient will not permit any other type of splint to be applied. In a self-splint, the injured limb is secured against the patient's body with a cravat or roller bandage. Voids between the limb and body are then padded with bulky dressings or similar material as appropriate.

Sling and Swathe

An injured arm can be supported by the **sling,** while a **swathe** keeps the limb protected and immobile against the body. When applying a sling, be sure to keep the knot off the back of the patient's neck. It can be very uncomfortable there.

General Rules of Splinting

Keep these general rules of splinting in mind (Figure 25-7):

- Be sure you have taken BSI precautions before splinting.
- Do not release manual stabilization of an injured extremity until it is properly and completely immobilized.
- Never intentionally replace protruding bones or push them back below the skin.
- You can't assess what you can't see. So cut away all clothing around the injury site before applying a splint. Also, remove all jewelry from the injury site and below it. Bag the jewelry and give it to the patient, a family member, or the police.
- Control bleeding and dress all open wounds before applying a splint.
- If a long bone is injured, immobilize it and the joints above and below it.

- If a joint is injured, immobilize it and the bones above and below it.
- If a limb is severely deformed by the injury, or if the limb has no pulse or is cyanotic below the injury site, align it back to anatomical position with gentle **manual traction** (pulling). If there is crepitus (pain or grating), stop pulling immediately. Perform this procedure only if you are specifically trained and allowed to do so. Follow all local protocols.
- Pad a splint before applying it to help keep the patient as comfortable as possible.
- Before and after applying a splint, assess pulse, movement, and sensation below the injury site. Reassess every 15 minutes thereafter and record your findings.

For all the obvious benefits splints provide, they also can cause complications if they are applied incorrectly. *Improper* splinting can compress nerves, tissues, and blood vessels under the splint, which can aggravate the injury and cause further damage. It can move displaced or broken bones, causing even further injury to nerves, tissues, and blood vessels. It can reduce blood flow below the injury site, risking the life of the limb. Finally, it can delay transport of a patient who has a life-threatening problem.

Remember that patients who have a painful, swollen, deformed extremity may be in considerable pain. They also may be concerned about regaining full use of the limb. So, as you provide emergency care, consider their feelings. Be gentle and reassuring.

Splinting the Upper Extremities

Clavicle

Often an injury to a shoulder will result in a fracture of a clavicle. When a clavicle is broken, the patient's shoulder may appear to have "dropped." The clavicle itself may look crooked and deformed. The best way to splint it is to apply a sling and swathe (Figure 25-8).

Shoulder

A dislocated shoulder is a common injury. Patients with one often have had the same injury many times before. The dislocated shoulder will appear to be deformed. You also may see a "hollow" in the upper arm below the clavicle. The patient frequently complains of severe pain and may refuse to let anyone touch the arm.

Attempt to apply a sling and swathe to the arm. Padding the void between the body and the arm may be helpful. Use a small pillow, towels, or even trauma dressings for padding.

In a shoulder dislocation, there is a danger of injuring nerves and arteries. So a great deal of care must be taken when applying the sling and swathe.

SKILL SUMMARY *Applying a Sling and Swathe*

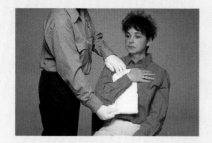

FIGURE 25-8A *Place a pad between the arm and chest.*

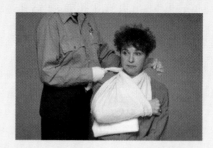

FIGURE 25-8B *Support the injured arm with a sling.*

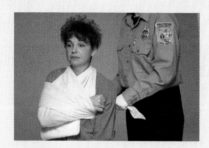

FIGURE 25-8C *Immobilize the arm with a swathe.*

Shoulder and Humerus

The bone that extends from the shoulder to the elbow is the humerus. It may break at midshaft or at the shoulder. It is thick and fairly strong. If it is injured, suspect other injuries nearby.

Manually stabilize the arm as soon as possible. Then check for pulse, movement, and sensation below the injury site. Apply a rigid splint to the outside of the arm, and pad the voids. Then, apply a sling and swathe (Figure 25-9). Do not forget to reassess pulse, movement, and sensation.

SKILL SUMMARY *Splinting the Shoulder and Humerus*

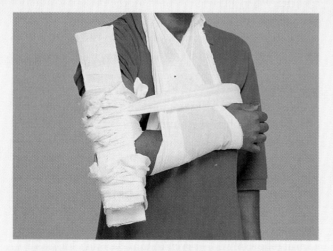

FIGURE 25-9A *Fixation or rigid splint with a sling and swathe.*

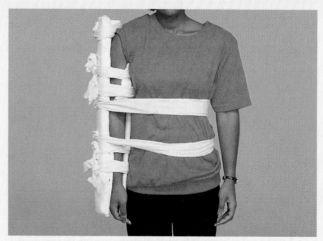

FIGURE 25-9B *Fixation or rigid splint with swathes.*

Elbow

The elbow should be splinted in the position in which it was found. Do not attempt to straighten it. If the arm is bent at the elbow, splint the injury with a sling and swathe (Figure 25-10a). However, if the deformity is severe, you may elect to use a large, flat pillow or even a blanket wrapped around the limb and secured to the chest with a strap.

If the elbow is straight, the entire arm should be splinted from the armpit to the fingertips on two sides (Figure 25-10b).

Forearm and Wrist

Forearm and wrist injuries are very common. They must be supported from the elbow to the fingertips. First, splint the injured area with a short arm board. Then, a sling and swathe should be applied (Figure 25-11a). If the injury is a closed one, a circumferential splint may be used instead (Figure 25-11b). Be sure the splint extends from the elbow to beyond the hand.

Hands and Fingers

If just one finger is injured, it may be taped to the uninjured finger beside it. This is called **buddy taping**. You may also use a tongue depressor as a splint (Figure 25-12a).

If more than one finger is involved, or if the hand injury is the result of a fight, the entire hand needs to be immobilized.

A hand must be splinted in the position of function. The easiest way to do that is to place a four-inch roll of bandage, a rolled hand towel, or a small ball inside the palm of the injured hand. Then, wrap the entire hand and place it on an arm board to immobilize the wrist (Figure 25-12b).

Splinting the Lower Extremities

Pelvis

Pelvis injuries can be life-threatening, because a large amount of blood can be quickly lost into the lower abdomen. So, suspect shock with any pelvis injury. Care includes placing the patient on a long backboard. Pad between the legs and consider putting a blanket on each side of the patient's hips. Then, secure the patient's whole body to the backboard. Keep the patient warm. If you suspect shock, the foot end of the backboard may be elevated slightly if it does not compromise the splinting.

Hip

The hip is actually the proximal end of the femur, where the femur fits into the pelvis. Fractures of the hip are most common in the elderly as the result of a fall. They also are common in patients involved in severe frontal car crashes.

Any femur fracture can be dangerous. The femoral arteries lie next to the femur and can be lacerated by broken bone ends. Bleeding in this location can be very difficult to detect. Sometimes the only outward sign is swelling in the thighs. With a broken hip, the leg on the injured side may be shorter than the other leg and rotated. The patient will complain of pain when the leg is moved or when the hips are gently compressed.

SKILL SUMMARY *Splinting the Elbow*

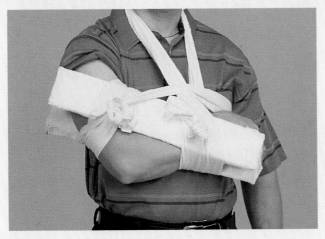

FIGURE 25-10A *Injured elbow immobilized in a bent position.*

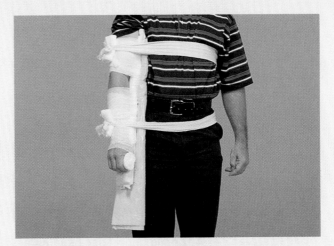

FIGURE 25-10B *Injured elbow immobilized in a straight position.*

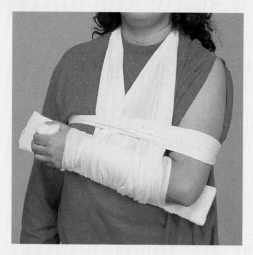

FIGURE 25-11A Immobilization of an injury to the forearm, wrist, or hand.

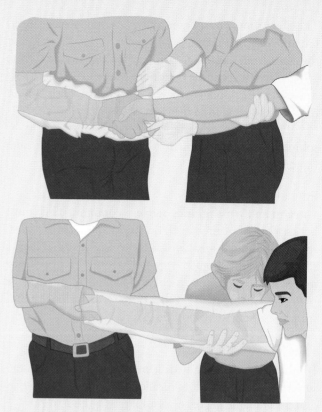

FIGURE 25–11B Applying and inflating an air splint.

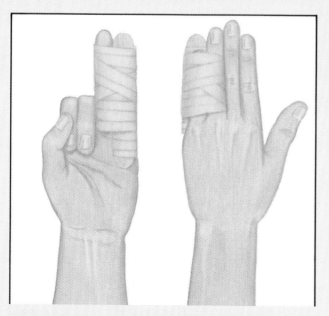

FIGURE 25–12A A tongue depressor used as a splint and then taped to an adjoining finger for stabilization.

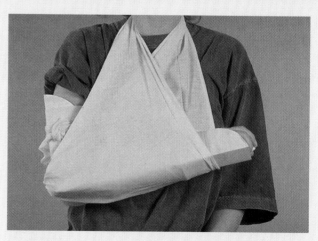

FIGURE 25-12B Cardboard splint of the forearm, wrist, or hand.

SKILL SUMMARY *Applying a Traction Splint*

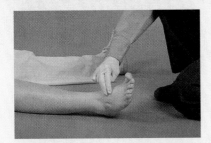

FIGURE 25-13A *Assess pulse, movement, and sensation below the injury site.*

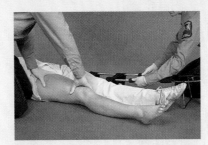

FIGURE 25-13B *Manually stabilize limb while second rescuer measures and adjusts splint.*

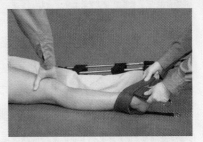

FIGURE 25-13C *Apply the ankle hitch.*

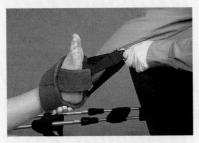

FIGURE 25-13D *Apply and maintain manual traction. Position the splint.*

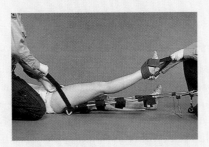

FIGURE 25-13E *Attach the ischial strap.*

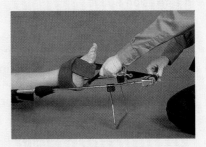

FIGURE 25-13F *Fasten the splint to the ankle hitch. Apply mechanical traction.*

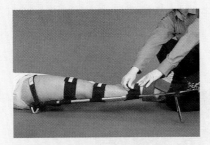

FIGURE 25-13G *Fasten leg support straps in place.*

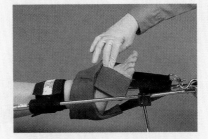

FIGURE 25-13H *Reassess pulse, movement, and sensation below the injury site.*

When you perform an initial assessment of a patient with a possible hip injury, be sure to assess and treat for life-threatening problems first, including shock. Then, stabilize the patient's hip. The best method is to immobilize the patient's whole body on a long backboard.

Femur

It takes a great deal of force to break the femur. Such an injury is not uncommon in sports such as sky diving and skiing. The result of a break is usually a marked deformity of the thigh, as well as a great deal of pain and swelling.

Emergency care consists of immobilizing the bone ends to prevent further injury.

The preferred method of immobilization is a traction splint (Figure 25-13). Remember, use a traction splint only if you are specially trained and allowed to do so.

Alternative care involves using two long boards to create a splint. The inner board must extend from the groin to below the bottom of the foot. The outer board must extend from the armpit to below the bottom of the foot (Figure 25-14). Pad the voids, then secure the boards to the patient with cravats at the shoulders, hips, knees, and ankles.

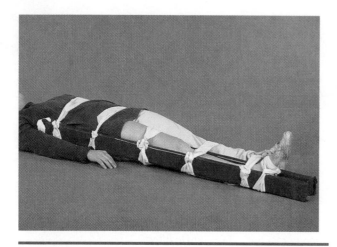

FIGURE 25-14   A high femur fracture immobilized in a fixation splint.

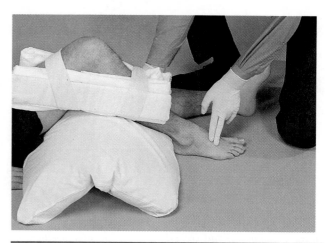

FIGURE 25-15   A splinted knee.

Knee

There are many types of knee injuries. Emergency treatment is basically the same. If you find the injured leg in a straight position, use two padded long boards to splint it in the position found. Place the first on the inner thigh so it extends from the groin to beyond the foot. Place the second on the outer thigh so it extends from the hip to beyond the foot. Then, secure the boards to the patient with cravats.

If you find the knee in a bent position, immobilize it in the position found. The bones above and below it should be splinted with two padded short boards. (See Figure 25-15.)

Tibia and Fibula

The two bones that extend from the knee to the ankle are the tibia and fibula. Open fractures of the tibia are common because only thin layers of skin protect it. Usually fractures of the fibula are not so readily apparent, since it is not a weight-bearing bone. Whichever one of the two bones is injured, the procedure for splinting remains the same.

Use two padded long boards (Figure 25-16). Place the first on the inner thigh so it extends from the groin to below the foot. Place the second on the outer thigh so it extends from the hip bone to below the foot. Then, secure the boards to the patient with cravats.

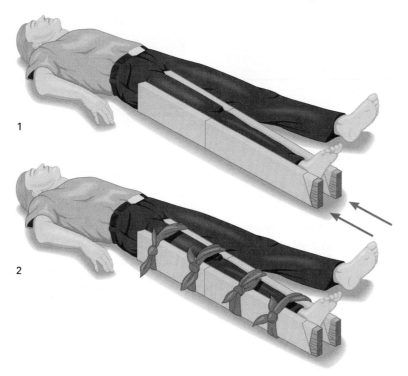

FIGURE 25-16   Fixation splint of the tibia/fibula using padded boards.

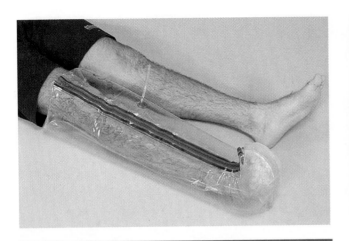

FIGURE 25-17 Air splint of the lower leg.

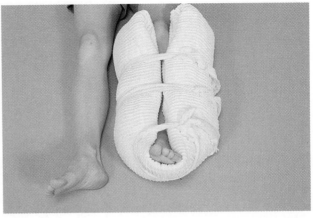

FIGURE 25-18 Blanket-roll splint of the ankle and foot.

An alternative method for a closed injury to the tibia or fibula is to use a circumferential splint. Make sure it extends beyond the knee and covers the entire foot (Figure 25-17).

Ankle and Foot

The foot is commonly injured by heavy objects falling onto it or twisting forces during a fall. The ankle bears so much weight, it does not take much movement in the wrong direction to make it unstable. No matter if the injury is to the ankle or foot, it is splinted in the same way.

Circumferential splints work well in these cases. However, the easiest splint may be a pillow. Simply wrap the pillow, or a blanket, around the foot. Then, secure it with cravats at the toes and the shin. The more cravats applied, the better (Figure 25-18).

1. What are the reasons for splinting a musculoskeletal injury?

2. What are five general rules of splinting?

3. What are some of the possible complications of improper splinting?

▶▶ The Call Follow-up

At the beginning of this chapter, you read that First Responders were caring for a patient who was involved in a car crash. She has a painful, swollen, deformed thigh. To see how chapter skills apply to this emergency, read the following. It describes how the call was completed.

Initial Assessment *(continued)* I didn't let the patient's injuries distract me. I proceeded with the initial assessment as I was trained to do. The patient was alert and cooperative. Her speech was clear. Her pulse was strong and fast, and her skin was cold and dry. There was no gross external bleeding. She had no trouble breathing, no chest pain, and no apparent injuries to her head. She did not have her seat belt on when the car crashed into the guardrail.

Physical Examination A quick physical exam revealed no other deformities, open injuries, tenderness, or swelling. At this point a police officer took manual stabilization of the femur above and below the injury site. I cut open the patient's jeans and saw that there was no obvious bleeding. The skin was unbroken.

Patient History During the interview, I asked the patient if she had heard a popping or snapping sound. "Yes," she answered. Then, I asked her to describe the pain on a scale of 1 to 10, with 10 being the worst. "10," she told us. She also said that she had consumed some alcohol, "two or three beers," but had not taken any medication.

Ongoing Assessment We monitored the patient carefully. We were especially concerned about shock because of the possible femur fracture. So we continued to check her pulse and respiration every five minutes. Her airway remained clear. Her respirations remained at 24 and adequate. Her pulse was 106 and strong.

Patient Hand-off When Ambulance 40 arrived, I gave a quick hand-off report (see below). The ambulance crew took over manual stabilization of the patient's femur and further medical care. It wasn't long before the patient was extricated, packaged, and on the way to the trauma center. We proceeded to keep our promise to contact her parents and tell them where she and her wrecked car were being taken.

 | **Hand-off Report**

"This is Lynn Solomon. She is 19 and was involved in a moderate-speed auto collision. Her chief complaint is pain in her left mid-thigh. She is awake, alert, and her airway is patent. Her breathing is rapid. She is not having trouble breathing. We put her on oxygen by nonrebreather mask. She is not bleeding externally. Her vital signs are respirations 24, pulse 100, blood pressure 120/90, and skin is cold and dry. She said she has had two or three beers."

The Last Word *Musculoskeletal injuries usually are painful and obvious. Even so, you should always* *assess for and treat life-threatening problems first. Remember, life before limb!*

Chapter Review

Focus on the EMS Team

Injuries to the musculoskeletal system require a lot of "hands." While some hands are tending to the patient's spine and ABCs, others will be needed to stabilize the injured extremity. Even more will be needed to prepare and secure a splint, as well as check distal pulses, movement, and sensation of the injured limb. As a First Responder, your hands will be the first. Be prepared, because after initial care, you may be asked to assist the EMTs while they are on the scene.

Summing Up

- Bones and muscles may be injured in four basic ways: fracture, strain, sprain, or dislocation. As a First Responder in the field, do not attempt to distinguish among these injuries. Instead, treat any extremity injury as a possible fracture.

- A mechanism of musculoskeletal injury may involve direct, indirect, or twisting forces. Be sure to look beyond an obvious injury or an injury caused by a direct force when you examine a trauma patient. Additional injuries may be involved.

- A musculoskeletal injury is classified as either closed or open.

- Assessment of a patient with bone and joint injuries includes identifying the MOI, identifying the forces involved, and assessing for signs and symptoms. However, remember "life before limb." Always assess for life-threats first.

- First Responder care for a patient with bone and joint injuries is the same as for any other trauma patient. In addition, manually stabilize an injured extremity after the physical exam. Maintain manual stabilization until the limb is completely immobilized in a splint.

- Reasons for manual stabilization of an injured limb include preventing further injury and helping to reduce pain.

- Reasons for splinting include preventing motion of bone fragments or dislocated joints; minimizing damage to surrounding tissues, nerves, blood vessels, and the injured bone itself; controlling bleeding and swelling; preventing shock; reducing pain and suffering.

- Some common types of splints are rigid splints, traction splints, circumferential splints (such as an air splint), improvised splints (including a self-splint), and the sling and swathe.

- General rules of splinting are: take BSI precautions; maintain manual stabilization of an injured extremity until it is immobilized; never intentionally replace protruding bones; expose the injury site, assess it, control any bleeding, and dress it before splinting; if a long bone is injured, immobilize it and the joints above and below it; if a joint is injured, immobilize it and the bones above and below it; pad a splint before applying it; before and after splinting and every 15 minutes thereafter, assess pulse, movement, and sensation below the injury site. If you are allowed by local protocol and are trained, use gentle traction to align a severely deformed limb, a limb with no pulse, or a limb with cyanosis below the injury site.

- Improper splinting can compress nerves, tissues, and blood vessels under the splint; move displaced or broken bones; reduce blood flow below the injury site; delay transport of a patient who has a life-threatening problem.

Key Terms

air splint a circumferential splint, which when inflated with air becomes rigid enough to help immobilize an injured limb.

buddy taping splinting an injured finger by taping it to the uninjured finger beside it.

circumferential splint a splint that completely surrounds, or envelops, an injured limb.

direct force a force that causes injury at the point of impact.

dislocation a bone is moved out of its normal position in a joint and remains that way.

fracture a broken bone.

improvised splint a splint made from the materials found on hand, such as a broom stick or a rolled-up magazine.

indirect force a force that causes injury along a path away from the point of impact.

manual traction pulling a body part to align it.

self-splint immobilizing an injured limb by securing it against the body with a cravat or roller bandage.

sling a large triangular bandage or other cloth applied to immobilize possible injuries to the upper extremities.

splint any device used to immobilize a body part.

sprain a joint and ligament are injured.

strain a muscle or a muscle and tendon are overextended.

swathe a large folded cloth usually used to secure a sling or rigid splint to the body.

traction splint a mechanical device that provides a counter-pull to alleviate pain, reduce blood loss, and minimize further injury.

twisting force a force that causes an injury when one part of a limb remains stationary while the rest of it twists.

Knowledge Check

1. The bone that extends from the shoulder to the elbow is called the:
   a. tibia.
   b. radius.
   c. patella.
   d. humerus.

2. A pulse distal to the femur is the _____ pulse.
   a. posterior tibial
   b. brachial
   c. femoral
   d. radial

3. When a long bone is injured, you should immobilize it and:
   a. nothing else.
   b. the joint above it.
   c. the joints above and below it.
   d. the same long bone in the opposite limb.

4. Which one of the bones listed below may be immobilized in a traction splint?
   a. tibia
   b. femur
   c. fibula
   d. humerus

5. You have splinted a patient's arm. After applying the splint, you find that the patient does not have a distal pulse in the injured extremity. (It had one before splinting.) The extremity also is cool to the touch. Which one of the following is most likely to be the cause?
   a. There is a hidden spine injury somewhere.
   b. The splint was applied too tightly.
   c. The patient has slipped into shock.
   d. The patient's arm "fell asleep."

6. Manually stabilize an injured extremity AFTER you have completed a physical exam.
   a. True
   b. False

7. If a limb is severely deformed by the injury, or if the limb has no pulse or is cyanotic below the injury site, align it with gentle manual traction.
   a. True
   b. False

8. List five reasons for splinting a musculoskeletal injury.

_____

_____

_____

_____

_____

9. List five common types of splints.

_____

_____

_____

_____

_____

Scenario

You are called to the parking lot of a local supermarket for a patient who has fallen. You arrive to find a 44-year-old male who tells you he wasn't paying attention and tripped on the curb. He states that he caught himself with his right arm. He complains of pain in the right wrist, which he is holding against his chest.

a. Does the mechanism of injury suggest other possible injuries? Explain your answer.

_____

_____

_____

b. Splinting requires immobilizing adjacent joints. What adjacent joints would be immobilized here?

_____

_____

_____

c. What type of splinting device would you use?

_____

_____

_____

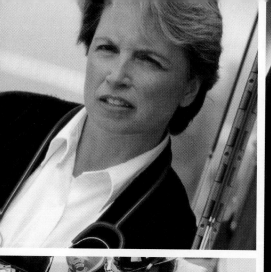
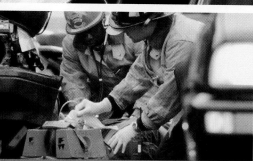
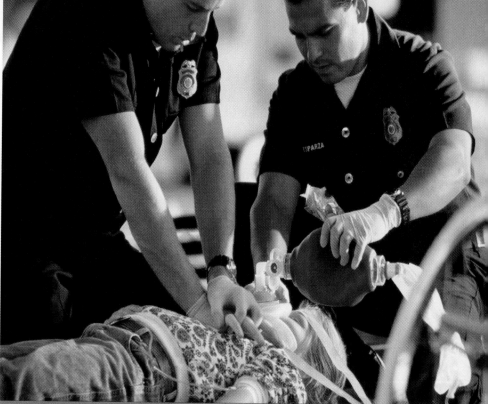

26 | Childbirth

Objectives

From the U.S. Department of Transportation (DOT)'s 1995 "First Responder: National Standard Curriculum." Material supplemental to the DOT curriculum is listed under "Enrichment."

Cognitive

6-1.1 ▶ Identify the following structures: birth canal, placenta, umbilical cord, amniotic sac. (p. 477)

6-1.2 ▶ Define the following terms: crowning, bloody show, labor, abortion. (pp. 477, 479, 486)

6-1.3 ▶ State indications of an imminent delivery. (p. 480)

6-1.4 ▶ State the steps in the pre-delivery preparation of the mother. (pp. 481–482)

6-1.5 ▶ Establish the relationship between body substance isolation and childbirth. (p. 481)

6-1.6 ▶ State the steps to assist in the delivery. (pp. 482–484)

6-1.7 ▶ Describe care of the baby as the head appears. (p. 483)

6-1.8 ▶ Discuss the steps in delivery of the placenta. (pp. 484–485)

6-1.9 ▶ List the steps in the emergency medical care of the mother post-delivery. (p. 485)

6-1.10 ▶ Discuss the steps in caring for a newborn. (p. 484)

Affective

6-1.11 ▶ Explain the rationale for attending to the feelings of a patient in need of emergency medical care during childbirth. (pp. 480, 481, 484)

6-1.12 ▶ Demonstrate a caring attitude towards patients during childbirth who request emergency medical services. (pp. 480, 481, 484)

6-1.13 ▶ Place the interests of the patient during childbirth as the foremost consideration when making any and all patient care decisions. (pp. 481, 482–484)

6-1.14 ▶ Communicate with empathy to patients during childbirth, as well as with family members and friends of the patient. (pp. 480, 481, 484)

Psychomotor

6-1.15 ▶ Demonstrate the steps to assist in the normal cephalic delivery. (pp. 480–484)

6-1.16 ▶ Demonstrate necessary care procedures of the fetus as the head appears. (p. 483)

6-1.17 ▶ Attend to the steps in the delivery of the placenta. (pp. 484–485)

6-1.18 ▶ Demonstrate the post-delivery care of the mother. (p. 485)

6-1.19 ▶ Demonstrate the care of the newborn. (p. 484)

Enrichment

▶ Describe emergency medical care of a patient who is suffering from the complications of pregnancy. (pp. 486–487)

▶ Discuss specific complications of pregnancy, including toxemia, spontaneous abortion, ectopic pregnancy, placenta previa, and abruptio placenta. (pp. 486–487)

▶ Describe emergency medical care of a patient who is suffering from the complications of childbirth. (pp. 487–488)

▶ Discuss specific complications of childbirth, including prolapsed umbilical cord, breech birth, limb presentation, multiple births, and premature birth. (pp. 487–488)

Introduction

A pregnant woman is too often rushed to a hospital, usually because the First Responder is afraid that the baby will be born before the mother can get there. In most cases there is no need for haste. Childbirth is a normal, natural process. Only in a few situations will you need to make sure the mother reaches the hospital quickly. First Responders are often called to help pregnant patients. So become familiar with the nature of childbirth and the emergency care of both the mother and the newborn.

Section 1 The Process of Childbirth

Anatomy of Pregnancy

The **uterus** is the organ that contains the developing fetus, or unborn infant. (See Figure 26-1.) A special arrangement of smooth muscles and blood vessels in the uterus allows for great expansion during pregnancy and forcible contractions during labor and delivery. After delivery, it also allows for rapid contractions, which help to constrict blood vessels and prevent excessive bleeding.

During pregnancy, the wall of the uterus becomes thin. The **cervix** (neck of the uterus) contains a mucous plug that is discharged during labor. The expulsion of this plug is known as the **bloody show** and appears as pink-tinged mucus in the vaginal discharge.

The **placenta** is a disk-shaped organ that develops during pregnancy on the inner lining of the uterus. Rich in blood vessels, it provides nourishment and oxygen to the fetus from the mother's blood. It also absorbs waste from the fetus into the mother's bloodstream. The mother's blood and the baby's blood do not mix. The placenta also produces hormones such as estrogen and progesterone that sustain the pregnancy.

After the baby is delivered, the placenta separates from the uterine wall and delivers as the **afterbirth.** It usually weighs about a pound or about one-sixth of the infant's weight.

The **umbilical cord** is the unborn infant's lifeline. It is an extension of the placenta through which the fetus receives nourishment. The umbilical cord contains one vein and two arteries. The vein carries oxygenated blood to the fetus. The arteries carry deoxygenated blood back to the placenta. When the baby is born, the cord resembles a sturdy rope about 22 inches long and one inch in diameter.

The **amniotic sac,** or *bag of waters,* is filled with a fluid in which the fetus floats. The amount of fluid varies. It usually ranges from 500 to 1,000 milliliters. The sac of fluid insulates and protects the fetus during pregnancy. During labor, part of the sac usually is forced ahead of the baby, serving as a resilient wedge to help dilate (expand) the cervix.

The **birth canal** is made up of the cervix and the vagina. The vagina is about 8 to 12 centimeters in length. It originates at the cervix and extends to the outside of the body. Its smooth muscle layer stretches gently during childbirth to allow the passage of the infant.

A full-term pregnancy lasts approximately 280 days. Toward the end, the baby usually is in a head-down position, which brings the uterus down and forward. Mothers often can feel the difference and say that the baby has "dropped." This position is most favorable for the baby's passage through the birth canal.

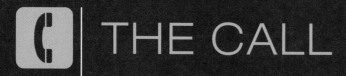

THE CALL

Dispatch A 28-year-old woman was in labor, and I was advised of a winter snow advisory with all roads hazardous for travel. A snow plow was being asked to respond to the ambulance station. As the deputy sheriff, I had access to a four-wheel drive and knew I could get to the scene. I informed dispatch that my ETA would be 5 to 10 minutes. She reported back that the ambulance could be 20 to 30 minutes. I found the OB kit, got my jacket on, and went out the door.

Scene Size-up I arrived at the residence, a farmhouse, and did a quick safety check of the area. I then advised the dispatcher of the road conditions and best access for the ambu-

lance. Once inside the house, the husband informed me that his wife was due in a few weeks but her "water broke" and she was in labor. I was led to the bedroom, where the wife was lying on the bed.

Initial Assessment The patient looked up at me and said, "The baby is coming. Now!"

Should the First Responder treat this patient the same way he treats patients with sudden illness or injury? What are his priorities for the mother and for the baby? Consider these questions as you read Chapter 26. How you would proceed?

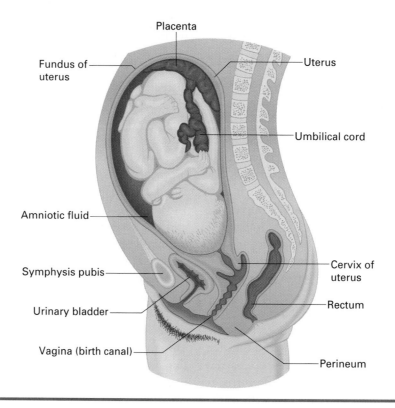

FIGURE 26-1 Anatomy of pregnancy.

Stages of Labor

Labor is the term used to describe the process of childbirth. It consists of contractions of the uterine wall, which force the baby and later the placenta into the outside world. Normal labor is divided into three stages: *dilation, expulsion,* and *placental* (Figure 26-2). The length of each stage varies greatly in different women and under different circumstances.

First Stage: Dilation

During this first and longest stage, the cervix becomes fully dilated (expanded). This allows the baby's head to progress from the uterus into the birth canal. Through uterine contractions, the cervix gradually stretches and thins until the opening is large enough for the baby to pass through.

The contractions may begin as an aching sensation in the small of the back. Within a short time, the contractions become cramp-like pains in the lower abdomen. These recur at regular intervals, each one lasting about 30 to 60 seconds. At first, the contractions usually occur 10 to 20 minutes apart and are not very severe. They may even stop completely for a while and then start again. Appearance of the mucous plug, or bloody show, may occur before or during this stage of labor. Also before or during this stage, the amniotic sac may rupture, resulting in a gush of fluid from the vagina. The patient may say something like "my water broke" when this occurs.

Stage one may continue for as long as 18 hours or more for a woman having her first baby. Women who have had a child before may only have two or three hours of labor. By the end of the first stage of labor, contractions are at regular three- to four-minute intervals, last at least 60 seconds each, and feel very hard. The patient may indicate that she is having a considerable amount of discomfort.

Second Stage: Expulsion

During this stage, the baby moves through the birth canal and is born. Contractions are closer together and last longer—45 to 90 seconds each. As the baby moves downward, the mother experiences considerable pressure in her rectum, much like the feeling of a bowel movement.

When the mother has this sensation, she should lie down and get ready for the birth of her child. The tightening and bearing-down sensations will become stronger and more frequent. The mother will have an uncontrollable urge to push down, which she may do. There probably will be more bloody discharge from the vagina at this point.

Soon after, the baby's head appears at the opening of the birth canal. This is called **crowning**. The shoulders and the rest of the body follow.

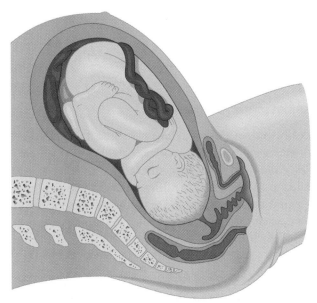

FIRST STAGE:
First uterine contraction to dilation of cervix

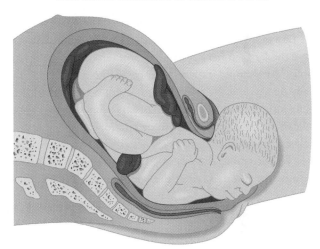

SECOND STAGE:
Birth of baby or expulsion

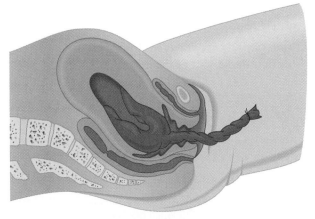

THIRD STAGE:
Delivery of placenta

FIGURE 26-2 Three stages of labor.

Third Stage: Placental

During this stage, the placenta separates from the uterine wall. Usually, it is then spontaneously expelled from the uterus.

Assisting in Childbirth

Ideally, childbirth should take place in a hospital, so calls for emergency childbirth are rare. Unlike other emergencies, childbirth is not an injury or illness. When you are called to a scene where the delivery of a baby is imminent, remain calm. Keep in mind that you are assisting a natural, normal process. And remember that you have two patients, the baby and the mother.

Patient Assessment

When you are called to the scene of a childbirth, perform a scene size-up and initial assessment and treatment as you would for any patient. Give the mother calming reassurance. Then, assess her condition to see if there will be time for transport to the nearest medical facility or if she will have the baby in her present location. Update EMS. Generally, you should expect to assist in the delivery of the baby on scene if the ambulance has not arrived; if the patient cannot reach the hospital or physician due to a natural disaster, bad weather, or some kind of catastrophe; or if delivery of the baby can be expected within five minutes.

To determine if delivery of the baby can be expected within five minutes, time the contractions. Follow these steps:

1. *Place your gloved hand on the mother's abdomen,* just above her navel. Feel the involuntary tightening and relaxing of the uterine muscles.

2. *Time these involuntary movements in seconds.* Start from the moment the uterus first tightens until it is completely relaxed.

3. *Time the intervals in minutes* from the start of one contraction to the start of the next.

 First Responder Practice

As a First Responder, your role in childbirth is largely supportive. Children have been born outside of hospitals for a long time. But when this happens today, it is usually unexpected and in unusual circumstances. Both the reassurance you can provide and your medical training will be quite valuable at the scene.

If the contractions are more than five minutes apart, the mother usually has time to be transported to a hospital safely, as long as traffic, weather conditions, or prolonged transport times are not a problem. If the contractions are two minutes apart, she probably does not have time. Prepare to help deliver the baby where you are.

If the contractions are between two and five minutes apart, you must make a decision based the factors listed below. The mother is usually nervous and apprehensive, so be gentle and kind. Show confidence and support. Ask these questions:

- Have you had a baby before? (The birth may take longer in a first pregnancy.) What is your due date? Have you seen a doctor during your pregnancy? Have you been told that you are having more than one baby or about any expected problems or complications?

- Are you having contractions? How far apart are they? Has the amniotic sac ruptured (or did your water break)? If so, when? What color was the fluid?

- Do you feel the sensation of a bowel movement? (If yes, the baby's head is pressing against the rectum and will soon be born. Do not let the mother sit on the toilet.)

- Do you feel like the baby is ready to be born?

Examine the mother. She should be on her back with knees bent and legs spread. Inspect the vaginal area, but do not touch it except during delivery and when your partner is present. Determine if there is crowning. If you can see bulging in the vaginal area, and either the head or other part of the baby is visible, prepare to deliver the baby where you are. Report your findings to EMS. ■

Supine Hypotensive Syndrome

Be alert to the possibility of a condition known as *supine hypotensive syndrome.* This condition may occur in the last few months of pregnancy when the patient lies on her back. The combined weight of the uterus and the fetus presses on the great vein (the inferior vena cava) that collects blood from the lower body and delivers it to the heart. That pressure can limit (decrease) the blood returning to the heart and circulating through the body. You may observe signs of shock in your patient, including reduced blood pressure, increased pulse, and pale skin color. Also be alert for fainting.

To avoid supine hypotensive syndrome, the patient should be in a sitting position, if appropriate, or lying on her left side. If you suspect the condition, position the patient on her left side and treat for shock. If the pregnant patient has experienced trauma, position her on the backboard with a pillow.

Preparation for Delivery

Always act in a professional manner. Be calm. Reassure the mother. Tell her that you are there to help with the delivery. Provide as much quiet and privacy for her as you can. Get rid of distractions. Hold her hand and speak encouragingly to her. Help the mother concentrate on breathing regularly with the contractions. Wipe the mother's face. Give her ice chips only if allowed by local protocol. (The mother should not eat or drink anything once labor starts.) The father or another rescuer can help.

At a minimum, the following materials and equipment should be included in your obstetrical (OB) kit:

- Sheets and towels, sterile if possible.
- One dozen four-inch square gauze pads.
- Two or three sanitary napkins.
- Rubber suction syringe.
- Baby receiving blanket.
- Surgical scissors for cutting the umbilical cord.
- Cord clamps or ties.
- Foil-wrapped germicidal wipes.
- Large plastic bags (one for the placenta and additional ones for waste).

All materials used during delivery should be sterile, or at least as clean as possible. This is to protect both the baby and the mother from contamination and infection.

In addition, because delivery results in exposure to a great deal of blood and other body fluids, you must take BSI precautions. Put on a face shield (or eyewear and face mask), protective gloves, a disposable gown, and shoe coverings if possible. Handle soaked dressings, pads, and linens carefully. Place them in separate bags that will not leak. Then seal and label the bags. Scrub your arms, hands, and nails thoroughly *before* and *after* the delivery, even if you wore gloves.

First Responder Practice

Never ask the mother to cross her legs or ankles. Never tie or hold her legs together to try to delay delivery. Never delay or restrain delivery in any way. The pressure could result in death or permanent injury to the infant.

Other guidelines include:

- Be prepared to provide basic life support to both the mother and the infant, including treatment for shock.
- Help the mother relax with each contraction. Inhaling causes muscles to tighten, so have her exhale with each contraction. Encourage her to keep her breathing slow but comfortable. Tell her not to strain or push during the first stage of labor.
- The amniotic sac may rupture, if it has not already done so. There also may be some blood-tinged mucus. These fluids increase as labor progresses. If you have a clean towel, place it under the mother's buttocks to absorb the fluids. Always wipe in a down-and-away direction to minimize contamination. Discard soiled towels or sheets used for this purpose. Replace them frequently with clean ones.
- If the patient feels more comfortable sitting, reclining, or in some other position during the first stages of labor, let her do so.
- As contractions become longer and closer together, the patient should lie down or get into a semi-sitting position on a flat, firm surface that she can push against. It is easiest for you if the mother is on an elevated surface. However, if the floor is the only firm surface available, use it. Pad it with folded sheets, towels, or blankets. Elevate the mother's buttocks about two inches with an additional pad of folded sheets or towels. The pad, which should extend about two feet in front of her, will help to support the slippery baby when he or she is born.
- When the mother is in position, her feet should be flat on the surface beneath her. Her knees will naturally spread apart because of the size of her abdomen. Do not pull them apart any further. Remove any constricting clothing, or push clothing above the mother's waist.
- Create a sterile field around the opening of the vagina. Place a sterile or clean sheet under the mother's hips. Touching only the corners of the sheet, have the mother lift her hips while you place one fold well under her hips. Unfold it toward her feet. If you have time, place another sheet or towel over the mother's abdomen and legs, leaving the vaginal area uncovered. Direct the best possible light toward the mother's genitals. Do not touch the vagina.
- During the second stage of labor, when the mother bears down, remind her not to arch her back. She should curve it and bring her chin to her chest to avoid excessive straining. Have her hold her breath for 7 to 10 seconds as she bears down. Holding the breath

longer will cause too much straining, broken blood vessels, and tearing of the vaginal area.

First Responder Care

To provide care to a patient who is ready to give birth (Figure 26-3):

1. *Place the palm of your hand gently on top of the baby's head,* avoiding the **fontanels** (the soft spots at the top of the head). When the head crowns, apply very gentle pressure to prevent an explosive delivery.

2. *Break open the amniotic sac* if it has not already broken. Tear it or pinch it open with your fingers and push it away from the infant's head and mouth. Note that the baby can safely inhale clear amniotic fluid. However, if

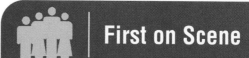

First on Scene

The presence of meconium (fetal bowel movement) is a serious condition. If you deliver the baby's head and see this green or brown fluid, be sure to report its presence to the EMTs who take over care.

there is **meconium staining** (greenish or brownish fluid), the baby has had a bowel movement, which could cause pneumonia if inhaled.

In the case of meconium staining, clean the area around the mouth and nose once the head is delivered.

SKILL SUMMARY   *Assisting in Childbirth*

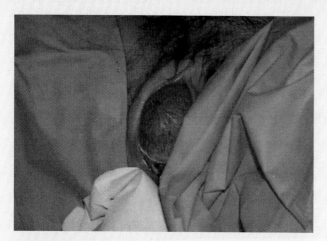

FIGURE 26–3A *Crowning.*

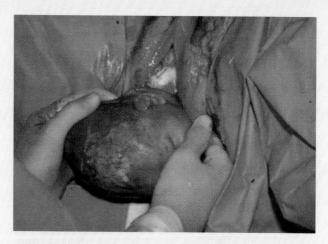

FIGURE 26–3B *Head delivers and turns.*

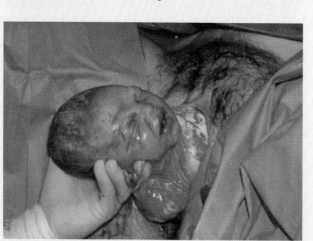

FIGURE 26–3C *Shoulders deliver.*

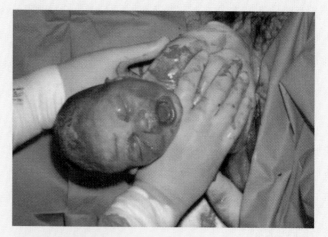

FIGURE 26–3D *Chest delivers.*

Suction the mouth first, and then the nose, with a rubber suction syringe. Expel all air from the suction bulb prior to placing it in the baby's mouth or nose. Release the bulb to create suction. Suctioning may need to be repeated to clear the airway. Note that meconium staining can be a life-threatening event. Consider requesting an advanced life support unit to assist.

3. *Determine the position of the umbilical cord.* When the baby's head delivers, check to see if it is around the baby's neck. If it is, use two gloved fingers to slip the cord over the shoulder. Only if you cannot dislodge it, attach two clamps a few inches apart. Then, cut between the clamps.

4. *Support the baby's head as soon as it appears.* Place one hand below it. Spread the fingers of your other hand gently around it. Avoid touching the fontanels. In most normal presentations, the baby's head faces down. It then turns so that the nose is toward the mother's thigh.

5. *Remove fluids from the infant's airway* with a rubber bulb syringe, mouth first and then the nose. Make sure you fully compress the syringe before you bring it to the baby's face. Insert the tip no more than an inch into the mouth, avoiding contact with the back of the mouth. Slowly release the bulb to allow fluid to be drawn into the syringe. If a syringe is not available, wipe the baby's mouth and then the nose with gauze.

6. *Support the baby with both hands as the rest of the body is born.* Once the shoulders are delivered, the rest of the body will appear rapidly. Note that you should never pull the baby from the vagina. Never touch the mother's vagina or anus. Handle the baby's slippery body carefully.

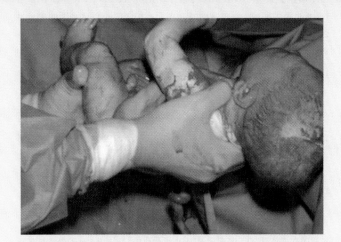
FIGURE 26–3E *Legs and feet deliver.*

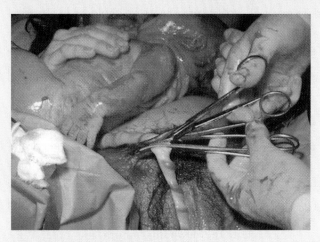
FIGURE 26-3F *Cutting of cord.*

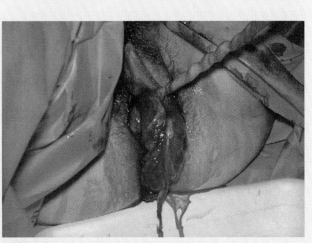
FIGURE -3G *Placenta begins delivery.*

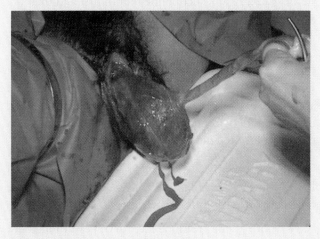
FIGURE 26-3H *Placenta delivers.*

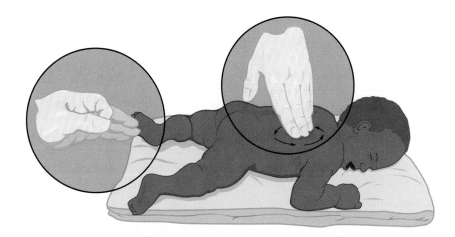

FIGURE 26-4 Stimulate breathing by gently rubbing the newborn's back or flicking the feet.

Do not put your fingers in the baby's armpits, because pressure on the nerve centers there can cause paralysis.

7. *Grasp the feet as they are delivered.* Be sure you don't pull on the umbilical cord.

8. *Position the baby level with the mother's vagina* until the umbilical cord is cut. The neck should be in a neutral position. Then, note the time of birth.

9. *Recognize that maternal bleeding is very common after childbirth.* (Care for the mother is described later in this chapter.) ■

Caring for the Newborn

Gently dry the infant with towels. Wrap him in a clean, warm blanket. Place the baby on his side, head slightly lower than the trunk. Turn the baby's head slightly to one side to allow mucus and fluid to drain from the nose and mouth. Only the face should be exposed.

Then clean the newborn's mouth and nose. Wipe blood and mucus from the baby's mouth and nose with sterile gauze. Again, suction the mouth first and then the nose. The infant should cry almost immediately.

If the baby is not yet breathing, provide tactile stimulation. Rub the back gently or slap the soles of the feet (Figure 26-4). Administer oxygen as soon as possible. Usually, placing an oxygen mask near the baby's face and allowing the oxygen to blow by is effective. Do not use oxygen tubing without a mask. The force of the oxygen coming out of the tube can be harmful.

Resuscitation of the Newborn

Perform artificial ventilation on the newborn if any of the following three conditions exist:

■ Newborn is not breathing after drying, warming, and tactile stimulation or there are gasping respirations.

■ Newborn's pulse rate is less than 100 beats per minute.

■ There is persistent central cyanosis, or bluish discoloration around the chest and abdomen after 100% oxygen has been administered.

The recommended rate for assisting a newborn's ventilations is 30–60 breaths per minute. Keep in mind that a baby's lungs are very small and require very small puffs of air. Never use mechanical ventilation on a newborn. A bag-valve-mask device may be used, but it must be the appropriate size for a newborn. Remember to observe for chest rise. Reassess after 30 seconds. For proper positioning of the head, a towel may be placed under the baby's shoulders.

If breathing and pulse are absent or if pulse rate is less than 60 beats per minute, or 60–80 beats per minute and not rising when oxygen is administered, start CPR. The rate of compressions is 120 per minute. The ratio of compressions to breaths for the newborn is 3:1.

Cutting the Umbilical Cord

Clamp, tie, and cut the umbilical cord when it stops pulsating, if your EMS system allows you to do so (Figure 26-5). Place two clamps or ties on it about three inches apart. Position the first clamp about four finger-widths (six inches) from the infant. Use sterile surgical scissors to cut the cord between the two clamps or ties. Periodically check the end of the cord for bleeding, and control any that occurs.

Caring for the Mother

Further First Responder care for the mother includes emotional support, assisting in the delivery of the placenta, and controlling vaginal bleeding.

Delivery of the Placenta

Observe for the delivery of the placenta. When it starts to separate from the uterus, the cord will appear to be longer. The uterus will also contract and feel like a hard,

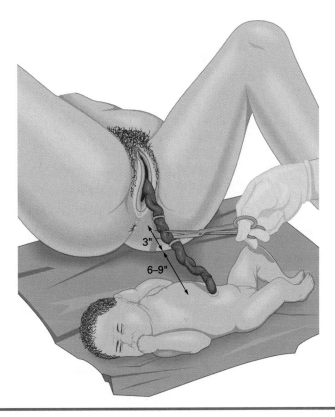

FIGURE 26-5 Cutting the umbilical cord.

grapefruit-size ball. Encourage the mother to bear down as the uterus contracts. It usually delivers within 10 minutes of the infant, and almost always within 30 minutes.

Normally, there will be some bleeding as the placenta separates. When the placenta appears, slowly and gently guide it from the vagina. Never pull. If you have not cut the cord, wrap the placenta in a sterile towel and place it next to the baby. Wrap the baby and the placenta in a third sheet or blanket. If the cord is cut, place the placenta in a plastic bag to be taken to the hospital where a physician can confirm the delivery is complete.

Controlling Bleeding After Birth

After the placenta delivers, check the mother's vaginal bleeding. Up to 500 cc (usually, less than a quart) of blood loss is normal and usually well tolerated by the mother. Place two sanitary napkins over the opening of the vagina. Touch only the outer surfaces of the pads. Do not touch the mother's vagina. Note that at this time, ask the mother if she plans to breastfeed the infant. If so, now is a good time to encourage the mother to start. Breastfeeding helps the uterus to contract, which decreases the size of the uterus and helps to stop bleeding.

Make sure that the mother and the baby are covered and warm. The mother as well as the infant can chill easily following birth. Activate the EMS system if you have not

already done so. The mother and the baby should be taken together to the hospital for evaluation by a physician.

If, after delivery of the placenta, bleeding appears to be excessive, treat the mother for shock and arrange for immediate transport. Then massage the uterus. That is, first place the medial edge of one hand horizontally across the abdomen, just superior to the symphysis pubis. Extend your fingers. Cup your other hand around the uterus. Use a kneading or circular motion to massage the area. It should feel like a hard ball. If bleeding continues to be excessive, check your massage technique.

Replace any blood-soaked sheets and blankets while waiting for transport. Place all soiled items in a marked infection-control bag and seal.

 1. What information must you have to decide if a birth is imminent?

2. How can you determine how fast and how close together contractions may be?

3. What can you do to assist a mother in delivery of the baby? Describe the process briefly.

4. When does the placenta usually deliver? What should you do with it when it does?

Section 2 Complications of Childbirth

Complications of Pregnancy

Toxemia of Pregnancy

About 5% of women develop toxemia (or "poisoning" of the blood) during pregnancy. This occurs most frequently in the last trimester (last three months). It often affects women in their twenties who are pregnant for the first time. Women with a history of diabetes, heart disease, kidney problems, or high blood pressure are at greatest risk.

Signs and symptoms of toxemia may include:

- High blood pressure (most common).
- Swelling in the extremities (most common).
- Sudden weight gain (two pounds or more per week).
- Blurred vision or spots before the eyes.
- Pronounced swelling to the face.
- Decreased urinary output.
- Severe and persistent headache.
- Persistent vomiting.
- Pain in the upper abdomen.
- Sudden seizures.

To provide First Responder care for toxemia of pregnancy, arrange for immediate transport. Position the patient on her left side to avoid compressing the inferior vena cava. Keep the patient calm. Administer oxygen, if you are allowed to do so.

If the mother suffers a seizure, monitor her breathing closely. When the seizure stops, elevate her head and shoulders and administer high-flow oxygen.

Spontaneous Abortion

Sometimes called a **miscarriage**, a spontaneous abortion is the loss of pregnancy before the twentieth week. It occurs naturally, unlike abortions deliberately performed in either legal or criminal settings. Signs and symptoms include vaginal bleeding that often is heavy, pain in the lower abdomen similar to menstrual cramps or labor contractions, and passage of tissue from the vagina.

To provide First Responder care, arrange for immediate transport. Treat the patient for shock. Save any passed tissue by packaging it in a sealed bag. The bag should then be transported with the patient for evaluation by a physician.

Ectopic Pregnancy

A woman has two **fallopian tubes.** Each one extends up from the uterus to a position near an **ovary.** Each month an egg is released from an ovary into a fallopian tube. The fallopian tube then conveys the egg to the uterus and sperm from the uterus toward the ovary.

In a normal pregnancy, a fertilized **ovum** (egg) is implanted in the uterus. In an ectopic pregnancy a fertilized ovum is implanted outside the uterus. It could be in the abdominal cavity, on the outside wall of the uterus, on the ovary, or on the outside of the cervix. In 95% of ectopic cases, the ovum is implanted in a fallopian tube.

An ectopic pregnancy is a severe medical emergency. The expanding fertilized ovum eventually causes rupture of a blood vessel and severe abdominal bleeding. It is the leading cause of death in pregnant women in their first trimester (first three months).

Signs and symptoms include:

- Sudden, sharp abdominal pain on one side. If bleeding is extensive, pain will become more diffuse.
- Pain under the diaphragm, or pain radiating to one or both shoulders.
- Tender bloated abdomen.
- Vaginal spotting or bleeding.
- Missed menstrual periods.
- Weakness when sitting.
- Signs of shock.

Suspect ectopic pregnancy in any woman of childbearing age when the above signs and symptoms are present. To provide First Responder care, arrange for immediate transport. Place the patient on her back with knees elevated. Keep the patient warm. Administer oxygen, if you are allowed.

Placenta Previa

Placenta previa occurs when the placenta is positioned in the uterus in an abnormally low position. When the cervix dilates (expands), the fetus moves, or labor begins, the placenta separates from the uterus and begins to bleed. This puts both the mother and the baby in danger.

Signs and symptoms include severe, usually painless bleeding from the vagina and signs of shock.

To provide First Responder care, arrange for immediate transport. Elevate the patient's legs. Maintain body temperature. If possible, administer 100% oxygen by mask.

Abruptio Placenta

Another major cause of bleeding during pregnancy is *abruptio placenta.* It is the leading cause of fetal death after blunt trauma. Life-threatening for both the mother and the baby, it needs to be recognized and treated rapidly.

There are several causes, including toxemia and trauma. Whatever the cause, the normally implanted placenta begins

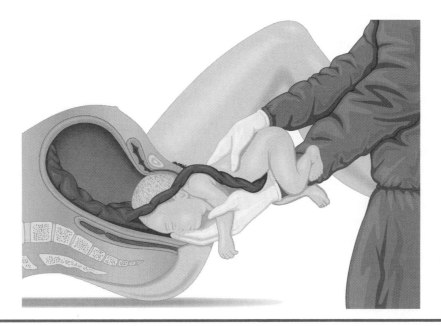

FIGURE 26-6 In breech birth, baby's feet or buttocks deliver first.

separating from the uterus sometime during the last three months of pregnancy. Bleeding begins, but it is often behind the placenta and the mother is unaware of it. Shock then develops in the mother, and the baby does not get enough oxygen.

Signs and symptoms include bleeding from the vagina but not usually in great quantities, severe abdominal pain, rigid abdomen, and signs of shock.

To provide First Responder care, arrange for immediate transport. Monitor vital signs carefully and treat for shock. Administer 100% oxygen by mask, if you are allowed.

Complications of Delivery

Prolapsed Umbilical Cord

In some situations, the umbilical cord comes out of the birth canal before the infant. When this happens, the baby is in great danger of suffocating. The cord is compressed against the birth canal by the baby's head, which cuts off the baby's supply of oxygenated blood from the placenta. Emergency care is extremely urgent. Arrange for immediate transport.

While you wait for medical help to arrive, position the patient. Have her lie down on her left side, if possible. Knees should be drawn to her chest, or her hips and legs should be elevated on a pillow. Administer high-flow oxygen. Next, free the umbilical cord. That is, with your gloved hand, gently push the baby up the vagina far enough so that the baby's head is off the cord. Place pressure around the outside of the head to avoid putting pressure on the anterior fontanel. (Another option recommended in some systems is to use two fingers between the baby's face and the cord to gently

lift the baby from the cord. Follow your local protocols.) Finally, cover the cord with a sterile towel moistened with clean water, preferably sterile. Do not try to push it back into the vagina.

Breech Birth

In a breech birth, the baby's feet or buttocks are delivered first (Figure 26-6). Whenever possible, the mother should be taken to the hospital for the birth. If that is not possible, prepare the mother for a normal delivery, letting the baby's buttocks and trunk deliver on their own. (Never try to pull the baby from the vagina by the legs or trunk.) Then place your arm between the baby's legs, letting the legs dangle astride your arm. Support the baby's back with the palm of your other hand. Let the head follow on its own, which usually occurs within three minutes.

If the head does not deliver within three minutes, the baby is in danger of suffocating when the head compresses the umbilical cord and prevents the flow of oxygenated blood from the placenta. To prevent that, clear the baby's face. That is, place the middle and index fingers of your gloved hand alongside the infant's face. Your palm should be turned toward the face. Form an airway by pushing the vagina away from the baby's face until the head is delivered. Hold the baby's mouth open a little with your finger so that the baby can breathe.

Limb Presentation

If the baby's arm or leg comes out of the birth canal first, it means that the baby has shifted so much in the uterus that a normal delivery is not possible. The baby will have to be delivered by a physician. Delay can be fatal. Never pull on the baby by the arm or leg. The mother must be taken immediately to a hospital. Transport without delay.

Multiple Births

Twins are delivered the same way as single babies, one after the other. In fact, since twins are smaller, delivery is often easier. Identical twins have two umbilical cords coming out of a single placenta. If the twins are fraternal (not identical), there will be two placentas.

The mother may not be aware that she is carrying twins. You should suspect them if one or more of the following conditions exists: the abdomen is still very large after one baby is delivered, the baby's size is out of proportion with the size of the mother's abdomen, or strong contractions begin again about 10 minutes after one baby is born. The second baby is usually born within minutes and almost always within 45 minutes.

To manage a multiple birth, follow these guidelines: After the first baby is born, clamp and cut the cord to prevent bleeding, which will affect the second baby. About one-third of second twins are breech. If the second baby has not delivered within 10 minutes, the mother should be transported to the hospital for the birth. After the babies are born, the placenta(s) should deliver normally. You can expect bleeding after the second birth.

Keep the babies warm. Twins are often born early and may be small enough to be considered premature. Guard against heat loss until they can be taken to a hospital.

Premature Birth

If a woman gives birth before the thirty-sixth week of pregnancy, or if the baby weighs less than five and one-half pounds, the baby is considered to be premature. Premature babies are smaller and redder. They have heads that are proportionally larger than full-term babies. Because they are very vulnerable to infection, special care must be taken:

- Keep the baby warm with a blanket. If you lack other supplies, use aluminum foil as an outer wrap.
- Keep the baby's mouth and nose clear of fluid by gentle suction with a bulb syringe.
- Prevent bleeding from the umbilical cord by clamping it securely. A premature infant cannot tolerate losing even a little blood without being at risk for shock.
- Administer oxygen, if you are permitted, by blowing it gently across the baby's face. Never blast oxygen directly into the face.
- Since premature babies are so vulnerable to infection, do not let anyone breathe into the baby's face. Do everything you can to prevent contamination.

1. What would you observe in a breech birth? A prolapsed cord?

2. How does a multiple birth differ from a single birth?

The Call Follow-up

At the beginning of this chapter, you read that a First Responder has just arrived on scene with a patient who announces that her baby is about to be born. To see how chapter skills apply, read the following. It describes how the call was completed.

Initial Assessment (continued) I introduced myself and assured the patient that I had been trained to handle this situation. As we talked, I determined that she was alert and oriented with a good airway and adequate respiration. Her pulse was strong and regular, and her skin warm and slightly sweaty. There was no bleeding. I moved next to her and explained that the ambulance was on the way. I told both parents what needed to be done and how they could help. I then updated dispatch.

Patient History The patient, Mrs. Frieda Whitney, told me that this was her second pregnancy and that there had been no problems with the first baby. The doctor had told her that this pregnancy was normal. She reported that her water broke 45 minutes before and contractions were two minutes apart with a 50-second duration. She said she felt pressure on her rectum, as if she had to move her bowels.

Physical Examination I asked Mrs. Whitney's permission to examine her for crowning and to prepare her

for delivery. She agreed. Acting quickly, I made sure I had on all appropriate personal protective equipment. The husband was next to his wife holding her hand and trying to reassure her. I discovered the baby's head had crowned, so I placed my hands gently on the head. The shoulders and the rest of the baby followed rapidly. Using the bulb syringe from the OB kit, I suctioned the mouth first and then the nose. The baby cried loudly. It was a boy. I wrapped him in a warm towel and placed him on his mother's belly. I then clamped the umbilical cord.

Ongoing Assessment Not long after the birth, Mrs. Whitney delivered the placenta. I placed it in a container for the paramedics to transport with the patients. Although the mother was tired, she was in good spirits and had no unusual complaints or distress. Her mental status was normal and vitals were stable. After being cleaned up a bit, the baby's color also appeared to be normal. His respirations were 48. Pulse was 146 and regular. He was actively moving around and had a good strong cry.

Patient Hand-off When the EMTs arrived, I gave them the hand-off report (see below). The EMTs quickly packaged the two patients and moved them to the ambulance. My heart was still racing as I watched them drive away.

 ## Hand-off Report

"This is Mrs. Frieda Whitney and her baby boy. The mother is 28 years old and this is her second child. Upon arrival, Mr. Whitney told me the baby was due in a few weeks, but his wife's water broke about two hours ago and within 20 minutes began to feel intense labor pains. Labor progressed rapidly, with frequent contractions. Our initial assessment found her to be alert with good vitals and no bleeding. A physical exam revealed that the baby's head had crowned, so we proceeded to assist in the delivery. It too progressed quickly and normally. The baby was born at 7:05 a.m. The placenta was delivered at 7:25 a.m. The baby's cord is clamped, and he has been suctioned, stimulated, dried, warmed, and placed on the mother's abdomen. The mother is stable with normal vitals. Baseline vitals for the infant are respirations, 48; pulse, 146 and regular; and he is actively moving with a good strong cry."

The Last Word *Childbirth is a rare and exciting event for a First Responder. Remember that birth is a natural process. You are there to assist the mother and then care for her and the baby after delivery. Your top priorities are the same as for any call. They are scene safety and the ABCs of your patients—both mother and child.*

Chapter Review

Focus on the EMS Team

For emergency childbirth, the EMS dispatcher provides initial instructions and reassurance. First Responders assess the emergency, provide life-saving care if necessary, and call for appropriate assistance. The EMTs provide more advanced care, if needed, and transport. But keep in mind that childbirth is a normal, natural event. In most cases, think of EMS personnel not so much as a team, but as coaches!

Summing Up

- The three stages of labor are dilation, expulsion, and placental. The length of each stage varies in different women and under different circumstances.

- Assessment of a patient in labor begins with a scene size-up and initial assessment and treatment, as you would for any patient. Then assess her condition to see if there will be time for transport to the nearest medical facility.

- To avoid supine hypotensive syndrome, the patient should be in a sitting position or lying on her left side. If you suspect the condition, position the patient on her left side and treat for shock.

- To prepare the mother for delivery, position her on a pad of folded sheets, towels, or blankets with a sterile or clean sheet under her hips and in front of her genital area. Her feet should be flat on the surface beneath her. Her knees will naturally spread apart. Place another sheet or towel over her abdomen and legs, leaving the vaginal area uncovered. Direct the best possible light toward the mother's genitals. Do not touch the vagina.

- When the baby's head is born, apply very gentle pressure to prevent an explosive delivery. Break open the amniotic sac, if it has not already broken, and check for meconium staining. If you see it, consider requesting an advanced life support unit, clean the nose and mouth, and suction the airway. Then check to be sure that the umbilical cord is not around the infant's neck. If it is, use two gloved fingers to slip the cord over the shoulder. If you cannot dislodge it, attach two clamps a few inches apart and cut between the clamps. Remove fluids from the infant's airway with a rubber bulb syringe, mouth first and then the nose. Support the baby with both hands as the rest of the body is born. Grasp the feet as they are delivered. Position the baby level with the mother's vagina until the umbilical cord is cut. Note the time of birth.

- Dry and wrap the baby and suction the airway again. The infant should cry almost immediately. If not, provide tactile stimulation and administer blow-by oxygen.

- Perform artificial ventilation on the newborn if he is still not breathing or there are gasping respirations; his pulse rate is less than 100 beats per minute; or there is persistent central cyanosis after 100% oxygen has been administered. The recommended ventilation rate is 30–60 breaths per minute. Reassess after 30 seconds. If breathing and pulse are absent or if pulse rate is less than 60 beats per minute, or 60–80 beats per minute and not rising when oxygen is administered, start CPR. The rate of compressions is 120 per minute. The ratio of compressions to breaths for the newborn is 3:1.

- Care for the mother includes assisting in delivery of the placenta, which usually occurs within 10 to 30 minutes of the infant. Help control bleeding by placing two sanitary napkins over the opening of the vagina. If bleeding appears to be excessive, treat the mother for shock and massage the area of the abdomen above the uterus.

- Complications of pregnancy and First Responder care include the following:
  - *Toxemia of pregnancy.* Arrange for immediate transport, position the patient on her left side, and administer oxygen.
  - *Spontaneous abortion.* Arrange for immediate transport, treat for shock, and save any passed tissue in a sealed bag, which should be transported with the patient.
  - *Ectopic pregnancy.* Arrange for immediate transport, position the patient on her back with knees elevated, and administer oxygen.
  - *Placenta previa.* Arrange for immediate transport, elevate the patient's legs, and administer oxygen.
  - *Abruptio placenta.* Arrange for immediate transport, treat for shock, and administer oxygen.

- Complications of delivery and First Responder care include the following:
  - *Prolapsed umbilical cord.* Arrange for immediate transport, position the patient on her left side with knees drawn to her chest or hips elevated on a pillow, administer oxygen, maintain pressure on the baby's head to keep the cord free until medical help arrives, and cover the cord with a moist sterile towel.
  - *Breech birth.* Arrange for immediate transport, place your arm between the baby's legs and support the baby's back with the palm of your other hand, and let the head follow on its own. If the head does not deliver within three minutes, form an airway by pushing the vagina away from the baby's face until the head is delivered and by holding the

baby's mouth open a little with your finger so that he can breathe.

—*Limb presentation.* The baby has to be delivered by a physician. Transport without delay.

—*Multiple births.* After the first baby is born, clamp and cut his cord. If the second baby has not delivered within 10 minutes, the mother should be transported to the hospital for the birth. After the babies are born, the placenta(s) should deliver normally.

—*Premature birth.* Treat the baby as you would a full-term infant, except be especially careful to keep him warm, to prevent bleeding from the umbilical cord, and to prevent anyone from breathing into the baby's face. Administer blow-by oxygen.

Key Terms

afterbirth the placenta, after it separates from the uterine wall and delivers.

amniotic sac the sac of fluid in which the developing fetus floats. *Also called* bag of waters.

birth canal an anatomical passage made up of the cervix and the vagina.

bloody show the plug of mucus that is discharged during labor.

cervix the neck of the uterus.

crowning the appearance of the baby's head or other body part at the opening of the birth canal.

fallopian tube one of two tubes or ducts that extend up from the uterus to a position near an ovary.

fontanel the soft spot between the cranial bones of the skull of an infant.

labor the term used to describe the process of childbirth.

meconium staining greenish or brownish color to the amniotic fluid, which means the unborn infant had a bowel movement.

miscarriage the natural loss of pregnancy before the twentieth week. *Also called* spontaneous abortion.

ovary one of two almond-shaped glands in the female that produce the reproductive cell (the ovum), as well as certain hormones.

ovum the reproductive cell, or "egg."

placenta a disk-shaped organ on the inner lining of the uterus that provides nourishment and oxygen to a developing fetus.

umbilical cord an extension of the placenta through which the developing fetus receives nourishment while in the uterus.

uterus the organ that contains the developing fetus.

Knowledge Check

1. **During pregnancy, the developing fetus is in the:**
   a. cervix.
   b. uterus.
   c. vagina.
   d. symphysis pubis.

2. **During which of the following does the infant's head progress from the uterus into the birth canal?**
   a. dilation stage of labor
   b. passage of the placenta
   c. expulsion stage of labor
   d. passage of the bloody show

3. **Contractions are two minutes apart. Which other indicator would signal an imminent delivery?**
   a. meconium staining
   b. a first pregnancy
   c. placental dilation
   d. urge to move bowels

4. Meconium is:

   a. a normal pregnancy.
   b. the covering of the placenta.
   c. a fetal bowel movement.
   d. the "bloody show."

5. When is the baby's actual time of birth?

   a. when the baby's head crowns
   b. after the umbilical cord is cut
   c. when the baby takes his or her first breath
   d. after the whole body, including the feet, deliver

6. Do not put your fingers in the newborn's armpits, because pressure on the nerve centers there can cause paralysis.

   a. True
   b. False

7. During the second stage of labor, the patient should hold her breath for about seven seconds as she bears down.

   a. True
   b. False

8. To avoid supine hypotensive syndrome, the pregnant patient should lie flat with legs elevated.

   a. True
   b. False

9. List three or four tips on how to use a rubber bulb syringe properly to remove fluids from a newborn's airway.

   _____

   _____

   _____

   _____

Scenario

You have responded to an emergency childbirth at the Rosario Ranch. Dispatch informs you that an ambulance is on the way, but it will take about 45 minutes to arrive on scene. You can be there in about 10 minutes.

a. When you arrive at the patient's side, you find her in a semi-sitting position on her bed. Your general impression is of a woman in her late teens or early 20s, full-term, and in labor. She appears sweaty, pale, tired, and in obvious discomfort. How should you proceed?

   _____

   _____

   _____

b. You must determine if delivery of the baby is imminent. Describe how to time the patient's contractions.

_____

_____

_____

_____

c. Your examination of the patient reveals the baby's head is crowning. You assist in the delivery, which progresses normally. When the baby is born, you position him level with his mother's vagina. But he is not breathing. What three steps can you take?

_____

_____

_____

d. You find that you have to assist the infant's ventilations. What is the recommended rate (breaths per minute)?

_____

_____

e. You have to provide CPR to the newborn. At what rates and ratios should you provide breaths and compressions?

_____

_____

f. The baby is finally breathing normally, and you turn your attention to the mother. What can you do to help control her bleeding?

_____

_____

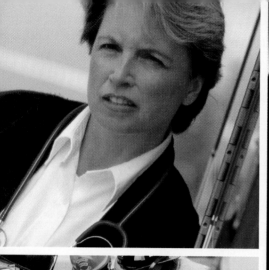
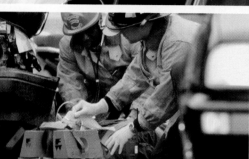
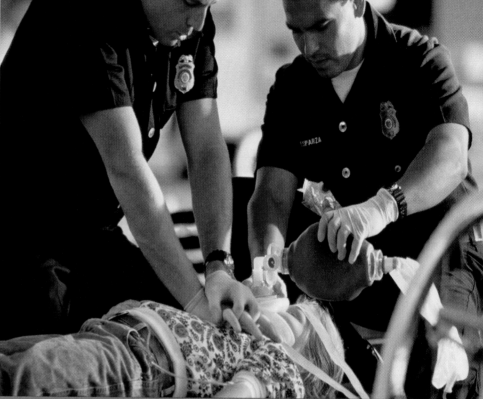

27 | Infants and Children

Objectives

From the U.S. Department of Transportation (DOT)'s 1995 "First Responder: National Standard Curriculum." Material supplemental to the DOT curriculum is listed under "Enrichment."

Cognitive

6-2.1 ▸ Describe differences in anatomy and physiology of the infant, child, and adult patient. (pp. 495–497)

6-2.2 ▸ Describe assessment of the infant or child. (pp. 499–507)

6-2.3 ▸ Indicate various causes of respiratory emergencies in infants and children. (pp. 509–511)

6-2.4 ▸ Summarize emergency medical care strategies for respiratory distress and respiratory failure/arrest in infants and children. (pp. 502–504, 509–511)

6-2.5 ▸ List common causes of seizures in the infant and child patient. (p. 512)

6-2.6 ▸ Describe management of seizures in the infant and child patient. (p. 512)

6-2.7 ▸ Discuss emergency medical care of the infant and child trauma patient. (pp. 507–509)

6-2.8 ▸ Summarize the signs and symptoms of possible child abuse and neglect. (pp. 513–515)

6-2.9 ▸ Describe the medical-legal responsibilities in suspected child abuse. (pp. 513–515)

6-2.10 ▸ Recognize need for First Responder debriefing following a difficult infant or child transport. (p. 515)

Affective

6-2.11 ▸ Attend to the feelings of the family when dealing with an ill or injured infant or child. (pp. 498, 499, 504, 516)

6-2.12 ▸ Understand the provider's own emotional response to caring for infants or children. (pp. 497, 515)

6-2.13 ▸ Demonstrate a caring attitude towards infants and children with illness or injury who require emergency medical services. (pp. 497, 506–507)

6-2.14 ▸ Place the interests of the infant or child with an illness or injury as the foremost consideration when making any and all patient care decisions. (pp. 496, 498, 507, 514–515, 517)

6-2.15 ▶ Communicate with empathy to infants and children with an illness or injury, as well as with family members and friends of the patient. (pp. 497, 498, 506–507)

Psychomotor

6-2.16 ▶ Demonstrate assessment of the infant and child. (pp. 499–507)

Enrichment

▶ Describe characteristics of infant and child development. (pp. 497–498)

▶ Describe the use of the pediatric assessment triangle. (pp. 499–500)

▶ Describe pediatric BVM ventilation. (pp. 502–504)

▶ Identify the signs and symptoms of shock (hypoperfusion) in cases of trauma or dehydration in infants and children. (pp. 508–509)

▶ Discuss the management of a patient with suspected sudden infant death syndrome (SIDS). (p. 513)

Introduction

This chapter focuses on the particular needs of children and how you can address those needs in emergency situations. It is meant to supplement the emergency care information found in the rest of the book.

Section 1 The Pediatric Patient

Anatomical Differences

The assessment and care of **pediatric patients** (infants and children) are very similar to that provided for an adult. However, there are differences. When you care for an infant or child, be aware of the following (Figure 27-1):

- Infants and small children have proportionately larger tongues than adults do. In other words, when you compare the size of the mouth and tongue in an adult to the mouth and tongue of an infant or small child, you will find that the tongue takes up more space in

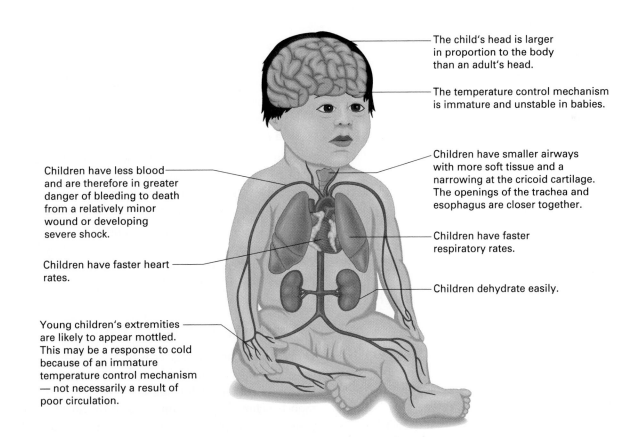

Children have less blood and are therefore in greater danger of bleeding to death from a relatively minor wound or developing severe shock.

Children have faster heart rates.

Young children's extremities are likely to appear mottled. This may be a response to cold because of an immature temperature control mechanism — not necessarily a result of poor circulation.

The child's head is larger in proportion to the body than an adult's head.

The temperature control mechanism is immature and unstable in babies.

Children have smaller airways with more soft tissue and a narrowing at the cricoid cartilage. The openings of the trachea and esophagus are closer together.

Children have faster respiratory rates.

Children dehydrate easily.

FIGURE 27-1 The anatomy and physiology of an infant or child is not exactly the same as an adult's.

THE CALL

Dispatch My partner and I responded to a child struck by a car in the 200 block of Martin Luther King Jr. Boulevard. The ambulance would be delayed.

Scene Size-up Police led us through the crowd to the scene of the incident. We saw that the child was out of the roadway on the grass. A very upset father was beside the child. While my partner tried to introduce herself to the father and calm him down, I questioned a witness. She told me that the car had been traveling at about 15 mph when it hit the child. She said the child appeared to glance off the left front of the vehicle, fall to the ground, and roll onto the grass. By that time my partner had calmed the father down and gotten consent to provide emergency medical care.

Initial Assessment The patient was on her side and not moving. She responded only to pain and had snoring respirations. She was little. Her father said she was six years old.

Consider this patient as you read Chapter 27. Will assessment of the six-year-old be any different from that of an adult? How about treatment? Will that be different or about the same?

the infant's or child's mouth. Therefore, when the pediatric patient's tongue relaxes, it can quite easily block the airway. Monitor an infant's or small child's breathing continually.

- Always support the head when you lift an infant. Before the age of nine months, an infant cannot fully support his or her own head. Sudden movement could cause injury.

- An infant has soft spots, or *fontanels,* between the cranial bones of the skull. The posterior fontanel ossifies (turns into bone) by the end of the first year, and the anterior fontanel ossifies by the end of the second year. So, whenever you must examine or care for the pediatric patient's head, do so very gently.

- Compared to an adult's head, the head of an infant or small child is larger in proportion to the rest of the body. It is also heavier, with less-developed neck structures and muscles. When you suspect an injury above the clavicles or when the mechanism of injury is unknown, provide in-line stabilization and, if possible, apply a cervical immobilization device.

- When there are suspected head, neck, or back injuries, make sure cervical immobilization devices fit correctly. Note that some children have very short necks. A commercially made device may not work on them. Use a rolled towel instead.

- Stop bleeding in a pediatric patient as quickly as possible. Blood loss comparatively small in an adult would be major in a child. Be alert to open fractures, which tend to bleed profusely.

- Injuries to the extremities can damage the growth plates, with long-term effects. When you assess extremities, be very gentle and careful not to cause any additional pain. Follow local protocols for splinting.

- A child's skin surface is large compared to body mass. This makes children more susceptible to dehydration and hypothermia. Response to burns also can be more severe. Watch for signs of shock.

Determining the Age of a Patient

Usually, a parent or caregiver is on scene to tell you the age of a young patient. However, there are times when determining age can be difficult. Even though age is a common benchmark for certain types of treatments, not all young patients physically mature at the same pace. Use your best judgment when the exact age of a patient is unknown.

TABLE 27-1 Childhood Development by Age

	Age	Characteristics and Behaviors
Infant	Birth to 1 year	Knows the voice and face of parents. Crying may indicate hunger, discomfort, or pain. Will want to be held by a parent or caregiver. It will be difficult for you to identify the precise location of an injury or source of pain.
Toddler	1–3 years old	Very curious at this age, so be alert to the possibility of poison ingestion. May be distrustful and uncooperative. Usually does not understand what is happening, which raises level of fear. May be very concerned about being separated from parents or caregivers. A stuffed toy may be helpful in gaining trust.
Preschooler	3–5 years old	Is able to talk, but still may not understand what is being said. Use simple words. May be scared and believe what is happening is own fault. Sight of blood may intensify response. Sometimes a Band-Aid® helps.
School Age	6–12 years old	Should cooperate and be willing to follow the lead of parents and EMS provider. Has active imagination and thoughts about death. Continual reassurance is important.
Adolescent	13–18 years old	Is able to provide accurate information. Modesty is important. Fears permanent scarring or deformity. May become involved in "mass hysteria." Be tolerant and do not get caught up in it.

Under normal circumstances most children will act as one might expect for their age. Yet, when children are in a stressful situation, they may act younger than they are. This can make it difficult for you to assess and provide care. So be aware that knowing a child's actual age may not always tell you how he or she will respond to you or handle the pain and stress of illness or trauma.

When possible, check with the parent or caregiver to find out if the child is reacting to the emergency normally or in what way he is reacting differently.

Developmental Characteristics

Knowing the characteristics of children at each age can help you in an emergency. You will have a good idea of what to expect from them and how best to communicate. (See Table 27-1 for a summary.)

As a First Responder, you will encounter pediatric patients when they are ill or injured. They are apt to be upset before you arrive. When you do get on scene, the presence of an unfamiliar person will add to what the patient already perceives as a frightening situation. This is a common and appropriate reaction to a stranger.

Children pick up on anxiety easily. It is very important for you to stay calm. Children, at any age, often take the lead from what they observe. So, if the adults on scene stay calm, a pediatric patient is likely to stay calm, too.

When dealing with younger children, it will help to get down to their eye level. Do not stare. Include them in your conversation. Do not make sudden movements when performing an assessment or providing emergency care. If a child is old enough to understand, ask permission to remove a piece of clothing or to touch his or her body. If a child holds out a hand or allows you to examine some part, seize the moment. The rule in pediatric care is to examine what you can when the opportunity presents itself.

With adolescents, it is important to be sensitive to their feelings of modesty. In many ways they are young adults. Permanent disfigurement may be a major concern. Also, they are very sensitive to peer pressure and may need to be reassured that what they tell you will be held in confidence. In fact, it may not be possible to get answers to sensitive questions when parents or friends are close by. That is okay. Most of the time, the patient's answers will not alter your care at the scene and can wait until the patient is in the hospital. Of course, you would still be required to include relevant information in your prehospital care report or in any report to emergency medical providers who have a need to know.

Dealing with Caregivers

With pediatric patients it is important to understand that caregivers, especially parents, may be very upset and concerned. In fact, when a child is ill or injured, the First Responder should view the situation as one that involves a family, not just the child. Anticipate a variety of responses from caregivers. A few of the more common ones are crying, emotional outbursts, anger, guilt, and confusion. Some of this emotion may be directed at EMS personnel. Do not take it personally. Caregivers need support and understanding.

As the assessment of the patient progresses, explain to the caregivers what is being done, and if time permits, tell them why. If appropriate, ask them to assist with emergency care. For example, a parent can hold an oxygen mask near the infant's face.

On occasion you may encounter a parent who will not let you help an ill or injured child. That parent may insist on remaining in control. Avoid becoming defensive. The parent's behavior has nothing at all to do with you. Remember, even though the parent may be coping in the only way he or she knows how, ultimately the child is the patient. Remember, if you were called, you must make sure the patient is not in need of emergency medical care.

The following techniques may help in situations where parents are especially anxious:

- Your first priority is to protect the health and safety of the patient. If parents are making unsafe demands, try an approach of reserved confrontation. Explain that your opinion and procedures are based on sound medical knowledge and their demands are obstructing what is considered appropriate and in the child's best interest.

- Realize that the parents may be correct. They usually know their children extremely well. A parent of a chronically ill child probably has a good grasp of what is going on.

- Regardless of how parents behave, treat them with courtesy, respect, and understanding. Avoid raising your voice. Tell them that you know they want help. Be as positive as you can, whenever it is appropriate to do so.

- Let parents stay as close to the patient as possible, as long as they are not interfering with care. If medically appropriate, a child can be held by a parent. Also, consider letting the parents do something for the child in order to help focus their attention away from you.

- Whatever you do, do not react with anger.

Using the Proper Equipment

Having the correct equipment in the correct size for the pediatric patient is extremely important to quality care. With children, one size does *not* fit all. It is very important for you to have a wide variety of sizes available to accommodate them. Equipment suited to fit the needs of each patient allows you to provide optimal care.

The following equipment has been recommended for emergency pediatric care by the National EMS for Children Resource Alliance:

Essential Equipment and Supplies

- Airway adjuncts in pediatric sizes.
- Bag-valve masks with oxygen reservoirs in appropriate sizes for pediatric patients.
- Oxygen masks in pediatric sizes.
- Nonrebreathing masks in pediatric sizes.
- Bulb syringe.
- Portable suction unit with regulator.
- Suction catheters, tonsil-tip and 6F to 14F.
- Cervical immobilization devices in pediatric sizes.
- Backboards in pediatric sizes.
- Extremity splints in pediatric sizes.
- Pediatric stethoscope.
- Blood pressure cuffs in pediatric sizes.
- Obstetric (OB) pack.
- Thermal blanket.
- Water-soluble lubricant.

Desirable Equipment and Supplies

- New, clean stuffed animal.
- Glasgow coma scale reference.
- Pediatric trauma score reference.

Q: 1. What are developmental characteristics and behaviors of pediatric patients? Name one for each of the following: infant, toddler, preschooler, school-age child, and adolescent.

2. What techniques might you use to deal with particularly anxious parents of a pediatric patient? Name two.

3. What types of EMS equipment are available in pediatric sizes?

Section 2 Pediatric Assessment

Although assessment of the pediatric patient follows the same basic plan as for an adult patient, there are some differences. For example, you already know that the normal ranges of vital signs are different. In this chapter, you also will learn that your very first observations of the child during scene size-up will be very important in your initial treatment decisions.

Scene Size-up

Many EMS rescuers say of a pediatric emergency, "90% of the assessment is done from the doorway." That is not really true. It is said only to make the point that pediatric assessment starts immediately upon entering the scene. Make sure you take a few seconds to get the big picture. In addition to your usual scene size-up, the observations you can make from "the doorway" include the interaction between the patient and parents, general appearance of the environment, and signs of possible **non-accidental trauma** (child abuse).

During scene size-up, see how caregivers are reacting and, if appropriate, consider how best to involve them in assessment and treatment of the patient. Note that you may be called to treat infant or child patients at a location other than where they were injured or became ill. It is not uncommon for adults to pick up a child in order to provide comfort or assistance. Understand they mean no harm. Ask caregivers specifically: Why was EMS called? What is the chief complaint? Has the child been moved? If so, where did the incident occur?

Be alert to the possibility of poison ingestion or some type of trauma, such as a fall. Consider the possibility that the ingestion or injury occurred somewhere else.

Initial Assessment

Pediatric Assessment Triangle (PAT)

One way to begin patient assessment quickly is to use the **pediatric assessment triangle (PAT)**. It can be a helpful

 First Responder Practice

Adults can usually tell you what is wrong. Children often cannot. Therefore, the visual appearance of a child is a valuable assessment tool. Pediatric patients who have obvious respiratory distress or who appear drowsy or lethargic should be immediately recognized as serious patients—even before you begin an initial assessment.

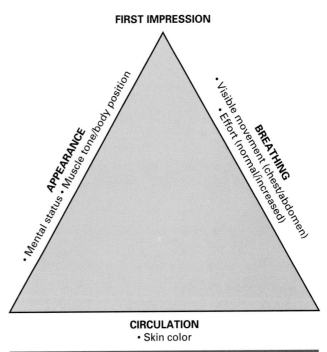

Pediatric Assessment Triangle

FIGURE 27-2 Apply the pediatric assessment triangle during scene size-up when you first see the patient. *(Used with permission of the American Academy of Pediatrics)*

tool. The PAT was developed to create a standard method of assessing children that accurately and easily identifies those in serious condition. Since calls involving children are rare, it is important to have an easy-to-remember but functional way to assess them.

PAT uses appearance, respiration, and circulation as key assessment findings. Apply it from "the doorway" to get a first impression of a pediatric patient and when you are performing initial assessment of the patient's ABCs (Figures 27-2 and 27-3). Table 27-2 provides details on how to interpret the PAT for respiratory emergencies. (Respiratory problems are among the most common causes of life-threatening medical emergencies in children.)

When you use the PAT and your findings are not normal for that child, consider starting emergency care immediately.

Assessing Responsiveness

To assess a pediatric patient's level of responsiveness, determine from the caregiver what is "normal." If a patient appears to be responsive but unable to recognize his or her own parents, consider this a serious medical emergency. Also, any child who cannot be consoled or calmed by a parent may have a significant medical problem.

Pediatric Assessment Triangle

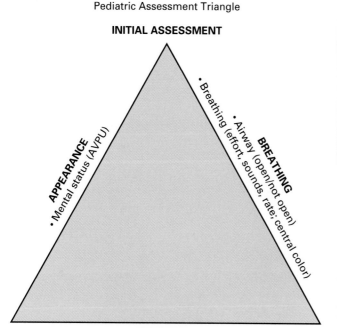

INITIAL ASSESSMENT

APPEARANCE
• Mental status (AVPU)

BREATHING
• Airway (open/not open)
• Breathing (effort, sounds, rate; central color)

CIRCULATION
• Pulse (rate/strength) • Skin color (extremities)/temperature
• Capillary refill time • Blood pressure

FIGURE 27-3 Apply the pediatric assessment triangle during your initial assessment. *(Used with permission of the American Academy of Pediatrics)*

Assessing the ABCs

Remember that an infant's or child's anatomy is not the same as an adult's (Table 27-3). However, assessment and treatment of the ABCs are as critical to the pediatric patient as they are to any other patient.

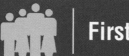

First on Scene

Most life-threatening problems in pediatric patients have to do with the airway and respiratory system. So ensure an open airway and adequate breathing in every pediatric patient you treat. Whether that is the first thing or the only thing you do, it is clearly the most important.

The single most important maneuver is to ensure an open airway. When trauma is suspected, always use a jaw-thrust to open the airway. Also, as you have read, the pediatric patient's head is large in proportion to the rest of the body. So when the patient is supine, the head can cause flexion of the cervical spine and airway compromise. One way to achieve a neutral position of head and neck is to place a folded towel under the patient's shoulders (Figure 27-4).

In infants and children, common signs of early respiratory distress are as follows (Figure 27-5):

- Noisy breathing, such as stridor, crowing, grunting.
- Cyanosis. (Early stages, seen in fingernails and around lips. Later, seen in the central part of the body.)
- Flaring nostrils.
- Retractions (drawing back) between the ribs or around the shoulders.
- Use of accessory muscles to breathe.
- Breathing with obvious effort.

TABLE 27-2 First Impression of Pediatric Respiratory Emergencies

Assessment	Respiratory Distress	Respiratory Failure	Respiratory Arrest
Mental status	Alert or agitated	Very agitated or sleepy	Unresponsive
Muscle tone/body position	Normal; able to sit	Somewhat limp	Completely limp
Breathing/visible movement	Present	Present	Slight or none
Breathing effort	Increased	Greatly increased with periods of weakness	Absent
Skin color	Pink or pale	Pale, mottled, or bluish	Blue
Actions	Work at moderate pace; help child into position of comfort; administer high-concentration oxygen without agitating patient.	Move quickly; open airway; suction; administer high-concentration oxygen; assist ventilations if needed.	Immediately open airway; suction; administer high-concentration oxygen; provide ventilations.

TABLE 27-3 Impact of Anatomical Differences on Assessment and Treatment

Anatomical Differences	Impact on Assessment and Treatment
Larger tongue	Can block airway.
Reduced size of airway	Can become easily blocked.
Abundant secretions	Can block airway.
"Baby" teeth.	Can easily dislodge and block airway.
Flat nose and face	Difficult to obtain good airway seal with face mask.
Proportionally large head	Must maintain neutral position to keep airway open and in-line stabilization of head and neck. Higher potential for head injuries in cases of trauma.
"Soft spots" on head	Bulging "soft spots" may indicate intracranial pressure; sunken ones may indicate dehydration.
Thinner and softer brain tissue	Consider head injury more serious than in adults.
Short neck	Difficult to stabilize and immobilize.
Shorter and narrower trachea, with more flexible cartilage	Can close off trachea with overextension of the neck.
Faster respiratory rate	Muscles fatigue easily, which can lead to respiratory distress.
Primarily nose breathers (newborns)	Airway more easily blocked.
Abdominal muscles are used to breathe	Difficult to evaluate breathing.
More flexible ribs	Lungs are more easily damaged. May be significant injuries without external signs.
Heart can sustain faster rate for longer period of time	Can compensate longer before showing signs of shock and usually decompensates more quickly than an adult.
More exposed spleen and liver	Significant abdominal injury more likely. Abdomen more often a source of hidden injury.
Larger body surface	Prone to hypothermia.
Softer bones	Can easily bend and fracture.
Thinner skin	Consider burns to be more serious than in an adult.

- Extreme respiratory rate (too slow or too fast).
- Altered mental status (agitation or less than alert).

Immediately provide oxygen if any of these signs are evident. Continually monitor for signs of respiratory distress. If an infant's respirations are less than 20 per minute or a child's are less than 10, assist ventilations.

Assess circulation by palpating the infant's brachial pulse. Palpate the unresponsive child's carotid or femoral pulse. Palpate the responsive child's radial or brachial pulse.

When you assess the pediatric patient's circulation, remember that inadequate oxygen can slow the heart. Provide oxygen and consider assisting ventilations as soon as you detect a slow pulse. Use a mask that is the correct size for the patient. When the patient is not breathing and has no gag reflex, an oropharyngeal airway should be inserted to assist in maintaining an open airway. *When an infant has a pulse below 60 beats per minute, perform CPR.*

Control external bleeding immediately. Remember that children have the ability to compensate for blood loss longer than an adult can. Decompensation (failure of the heart to maintain sufficient circulation of blood) is a very rapid process. It is imperative to monitor pediatric patients constantly.

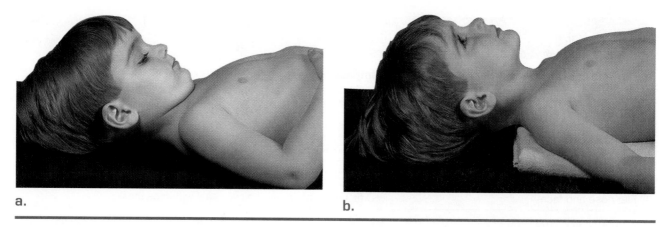

a.   b.

FIGURE 27-4 (a) When an infant or young child is supine, the head will tip forward, obstructing the airway. (b) To keep the airway aligned and open, place a folded towel under the shoulders.

After initial assessment and treatment, update EMS. Rapid transport is indicated for patients with significant airway problems, respiratory or cardiac arrest, or the possibility of shock.

Note: The most important care you can give a pediatric patient is done in the initial assessment. Never stop required airway care to perform a physical exam or gather a patient history.

Pediatric Bag-Valve-Mask Ventilation

Use bag-valve-mask ventilation when the pediatric patient is not receiving enough oxygen after opening the airway and applying supplemental high-concentration oxygen. Proceed as follows:

1. *Select the proper size mask.* It is critical to ensure a good seal, so choose a correctly sized mask—the smallest one that will cover the patient's mouth and nose without

SIGNS OF EARLY RESPIRATORY PROBLEMS

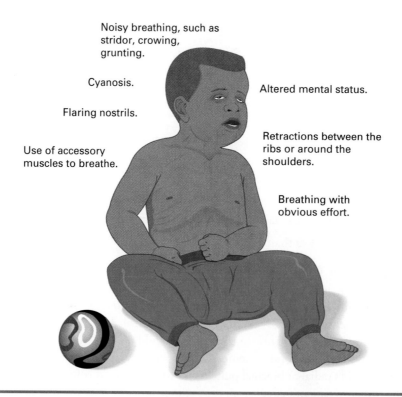

Noisy breathing, such as stridor, crowing, grunting.

Cyanosis.

Flaring nostrils.

Use of accessory muscles to breathe.

Altered mental status.

Retractions between the ribs or around the shoulders.

Breathing with obvious effort.

FIGURE 27-5 Early respiratory problems can present with a variety of signs.

pressing down on the eyes. When the mask is placed on the patient's face, the top should rest on the bridge of the nose and the bottom should reach the crease of the chin.

2. *Select the proper bag, attach the mask and tubing, and set the oxygen flow rate.* It should have a volume of at least 450 ml for newborns; 750 ml for infants, toddlers, and smaller children; and 1,200 ml for larger children and adolescents. The oxygen flow rate should be 10–15 LPM.

  Be sure to maintain an open airway by checking that the patient's head and neck are in the proper position. Insert an airway adjunct if needed.

3. *Apply the mask to your patient* using one of the following techniques:

One-Handed Mask Placement. If you are alone and you do *not* suspect trauma in your patient, use this one-handed or "E-C clamp" mask placement technique (Figure 27-6).

—Using your nondominant hand, apply the tips of your long, ring, and small fingers to the bony ridge between the chin and angle of the jaw. Your three fingers should form the "E."

—Keeping your fingertips in place along the jaw, gently rest the palm of your hand against the patient's temple.

—Place the clear plastic face mask with an inflatable rim over the patient's mouth and nose. Hold it in place by resting the tips of your thumb and index finger over the front of the chin and bridge of the

---

SKILL SUMMARY *One-Handed Mask Placement for the Pediatric BVM*

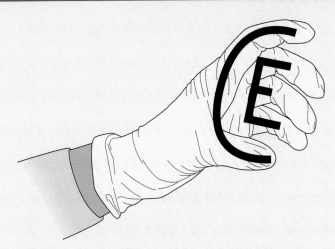

FIGURE 27-6A *This technique is referred to as the "E-C clamp" technique because, when it is properly performed, the rescuer's hand forms an "E" and a "C" with his or her fingers.*

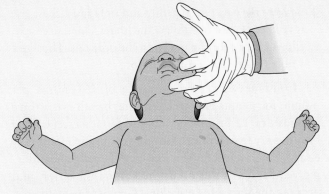

FIGURE 27-6B *First, rest your "E" fingers on the bony ridge of the patient's jaw.*

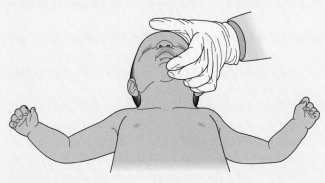

FIGURE 27-6C *Then, position your palm and "C" fingers to hold the mask in place.*

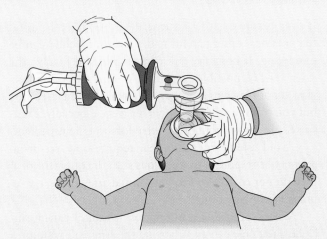

FIGURE 27-6D *Proper "E-C clamp" mask placement.*

nose. This will form the "C" part of the technique. To avoid damaging or obstructing the patient's airway, avoid pressing on the soft tissues of the face and neck.

Two-Handed Mask Placement. This technique requires two rescuers. It is the preferred technique if there is trauma or if the one-handed technique does not create an effective seal.

—If trauma is *not* suspected, the rescuer at the patient's head holds the mask on the patient's face with the thumbs and index fingers of both hands, using the other fingers to lift the chin. The rescuer at the patient's side squeezes the bag and watches for chest rise.

—If trauma *is* suspected, the rescuer at the patient's head performs a jaw-thrust maneuver, lifting the jaw into the mask while maintaining manual inline stabilization. The rescuer at the patient's side holds the mask in place, using the one-handed technique described above to squeeze the bag.

4. *Squeeze the bag.* Do so gently and only until chest rise is visible. Do not overinflate the lungs. Then, release it, allowing time for the patient to breathe out. The chest will fall back into resting position.

Continue ventilating at a rate of 20 breaths per minute for infants and children (one breath every three seconds), or 12 breaths per minute for adolescents (one breath every five seconds). Be prepared to suction, if necessary. Watch the abdomen for signs of enlargement during ventilation. If this occurs, reposition the airway and decrease the force of ventilations. Gently squeeze the bag while watching for chest rise.

Patient History

If time permits, gather a medical history. Keep in mind that anxious, upset parents and a screaming child can be unnerving. If possible, talk to the child and involve the caregivers. (A possible exception: You may need to interview an adolescent in a way that will prevent everyone but you from hearing his or her answers, especially if sensitive questions about "risk behaviors" are being asked.)

Avoid asking questions that require only yes-or-no answers. If responses to questions seem inconsistent or if they do not correspond to your initial assessment, try rephrasing the questions.

When you gather a history for a medical patient, include questions such as: When did the signs and symptoms develop? How have they progressed? Is the problem a recurring one? If so, has the child been seen by a physician? Is the specific diagnosis known? What treatment was received?

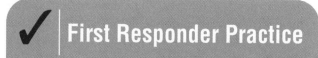

First Responder Practice

When assessing pediatric patients, it may be wiser to use a "toe-to-head" approach (the reverse of what you do for an adult). Starting at the child's feet will provide time for you to develop a rapport before assessing the head, face, and torso, areas that can make the child anxious.

When you gather a history for a trauma patient, include the details of the incident, such as the time it occurred, mechanism of injury, and emergency care already given.

Physical Examination

It is difficult to assess pain in children. They may lack the body awareness and vocabulary necessary to describe it. Children also may not be able to separate the fear they feel from their physical condition. Ask the parent, if possible, how the child usually responds to pain. This may give you some idea of how the present condition compares.

The bodies of infants and children can hide injury for some time. Only after their compensatory abilities fail will you see changes in vital signs. The changes may occur very quickly, and the patient's condition may deteriorate very fast. Take the vital signs of infants and children more frequently than you would for an adult. (See Table 27-4.) Also, pay attention to your overall impression of how the patient looks and acts. Your observations may tell you more about the status of the child than any one vital sign.

When you do assess a pediatric patient's vital signs, keep the following in mind:

- *Pulse.* Use the brachial pulse in an infant and the radial pulse in a child. If the radial pulse is not easily felt, check the brachial pulse. If the pulse is too rapid or too slow, immediately examine the patient for problems such as signs of respiratory distress, shock, or head injury.

  Rapid pulse may indicate oxygen deficiency, shock, or fever. It also may be normal in scared or overly excited children. A slow pulse in a child must first be presumed to be a sign of *hypoxia* (an insufficiency of oxygen in the patient's tissues). Other causes of slow pulse may include pressure in the skull, depressant drugs, or a rare medical condition. *Note: a pulse below 60 beats per minute in an infant requires CPR.*

TABLE 27-4 Normal Vital-Sign Ranges for Infants and Children

Normal Pulse Rates (beats per minute, at rest)

Newborn	120 to 160
Infant 0–5 months	90 to 140
Infant 6–12 months	80 to 140
Toddler 1–3 years	80 to 130
Preschooler 3–5 years	80 to 120
School age 6–10 years	70 to 110
Adolescent 11–14 years	60 to 105

Normal Respiration Rates (breaths per minute, at rest)

Newborn	30 to 50
Infant 0–5 months	25 to 40
Infant 6–12 months	20 to 30
Toddler 1–3 years	20 to 30
Preschooler 3–5 years	20 to 30
School age 6–10 years	15 to 30
Adolescent 11–14 years	12 to 20

Normal Blood Pressure Ranges

	Systolic	Diastolic
	Approx. 80 plus 2 × age	Approx. 2/3 Systolic
Preschooler 3–5 years	average 99 (78 to 116)	average 65
School age 6–10 years	average 105 (80 to 122)	average 69
Adolescent 11–14 years	average 114 (88 to 140)	average 76

Note: Blood pressure is usually not taken in pediatric patients under three years of age. In cases of blood loss or shock, a child's blood pressure will remain within normal ranges until near the end and then fail rapidly.

- *Respiration.* Children sometimes breathe irregularly. So monitor respirations for a full minute to determine rate. Do it frequently. (You also may need to place your hand on a "belly breather's" abdomen to get an accurate breathing rate.) Rates in children alter easily due to emotional and physical conditions. An increase over a previous rate can be significant.

  The quality of breathing also is important. Determine if it is adequate. Observe to see if the child is working to breathe and using accessory muscles. Look for retractions. Notice if breathing is noisy. Shortness of breath may indicate the need for you to assist ventilations.

- *Blood pressure.* A falling or low blood pressure in a pediatric patient can be a late indicator of shock. Be sure to use a blood pressure cuff that is the correct size for your patient. Use a pediatric stethoscope, if available. Do not take a blood pressure in children under three years of age.

- *Temperature.* Feel the arms and legs of infants and children to see if they are cold. The torso may be warm in comparison. Cold hands and feet may indicate shock, if your patient is not in a cold environment. Note that taking a rectal temperature and using a glass thermometer are not recommended for field use by First Responders.

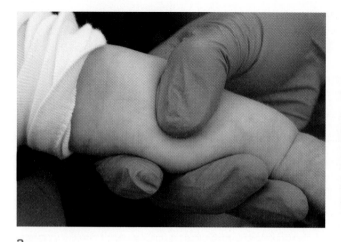
a.

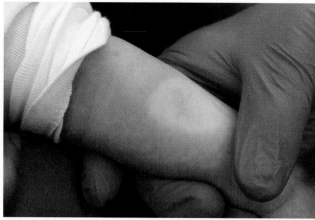
b.

FIGURE 27-7 Assess capillary refill in infants and children who are younger than six years of age.

- *Skin condition.* Always look at the pediatric patient's skin for signs of injury. Notice skin color. Though a newborn may have a mottled (blotchy) color on hands and feet, a child should not have a bluish discoloration. Stay alert.

- *Capillary refill.* Be sure to assess capillary refill (Figure 27-7). If it takes more than two seconds, the patient may be in shock. But a delayed capillary refill is not a stand-alone sign. In other words, if a pediatric patient has a delayed capillary refill, it is usually significant only if there are other signs of shock present. Also, it is difficult to get a reliable capillary refill determination when the child's extremities are cold.

Many children with head or spine injuries suffer nervous system damage as well. It is the cause of traumatic death a majority of the time. If the patient's history suggests trauma or if there is a significant mechanism of injury, then manually stabilize the infant's or child's head and neck immediately. Assess for damage to the nervous system as follows. (Remember that children do not have the same verbal skills as adults and their response to stimuli may be different. Parents may be able to describe a normal response.)

- Determine the level of responsiveness. If the patient appears to have an altered mental status, ask parents to describe what is normal.

- If the patient is not awake and alert, check to see if he responds to verbal or painful stimuli. To check painful stimuli, pinch the skin between the thumb and forefinger.

- Check the pupils. Find out if they are of equal size and, if practical, how they respond to light.

- Examine the head, neck, and spine for signs of injury.

- Check the ability to move arms and legs purposefully.

- Check for clear or bloody fluid draining from ears.

If you suspect damage to the nervous system, keep your patient as still and as calm as possible. Provide in-line stabilization of the patient's head and neck. Apply a cervical immobilization device, if you are allowed to do so. Do not allow untrained people to move the patient. Activate the EMS system, if it has not already been done, and continue to assess vital signs.

Following are tips for conducting a physical exam:

- If possible and appropriate, assess the child while he or she is on the parent's lap (Figure 27-8).

- Prepare yourself so you can radiate confidence, competence, and friendliness. Remember that children between one and six years old seldom like strangers.

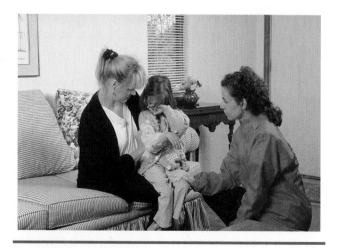

FIGURE 27-8 Having the child sit on a parent's lap can have a calming influence.

- Get as close as you can to a child's eye level. Sit next to the child if possible. When it comes time for a hands-on assessment, do it in the least threatening way. Consider starting at the toes and working your way up to the head.

- Describe to the parent and child what you are doing and why. Explain in terms a child can understand. Follow up on the child's questions. Maintain eye contact but do not stare. Speak calmly, using quiet tones in your voice. Even infants will respond to a calm voice, and an apparently unresponsive child may absorb much of what you say. Be calming, reassuring, and compassionate.

- Younger children tend to take statements literally. For example, if you say you want to take a pulse, they may think you mean to take something away from them. Watch your phrasing. Also older children do not like being talked about. Talk with them directly.

- Be gentle. Do everything you can to reduce the amount of pain that a child must endure. However, when there will be pain, be honest. "It will hurt when I touch you here, but it will last only a second. If you feel like crying, it's okay." Children can tolerate pain if they are prepared for it and are given adequate support. With children under school age, attempt to keep the most painful parts of the assessment for last. It will help if the child is kept on a parent's lap.

- Do not lie to a child. Always be honest. This does not mean you need to explain everything going on, but when you do answer questions or perform a procedure that could be uncomfortable, be candid.

- Sometimes children are reluctant to cooperate in a physical examination. Explain what you would like to do and ask the child for permission before looking or palpating. The parent can help by telling the child that what you are doing is okay. Also, if the child gives you an opportunity to examine something, like extending an arm to shake your hand, for example, seize the moment take a pulse, as the child may not be cooperative later.

- Separate a child from a parent only when emergency care is compromised.

- If a child is not calm enough to be treated, you may consider restraining him or her. However, be certain it is absolutely necessary to do so in order to provide essential care.

- A stuffed animal may help to win the confidence of a young child. It also may help to distract the child during assessment and treatment. Also, very shy children sometimes "talk through" a stuffed animal. For example, they may not tell you where they hurt but might tell where the animal hurts, thereby giving you information about themselves.

Ongoing Assessment

The ongoing assessment is the same for infants and children as it is for adults. It does not end as long as you are caring for the patient.

Patient Hand-off

Just as you would for adult patients, include in your infant or child hand-off report: age and sex of the patient; chief complaint; level of responsiveness (AVPU); airway, breathing, and circulation status; physical exam findings; patient history; treatment, interventions, the patient's response to them, and any changes in the patient's condition.

Q:
1. What is the single most important step in First Responder care of a pediatric patient?

2. Why should you take the vital signs of infants and children more frequently than you would for an adult?

3. How can you accurately determine a young child's level of responsiveness?

4. During patient assessment, what special conditions and situations due to the anatomy of an infant or child should you be aware of? Name three.

Section 3 Common Pediatric Emergencies

Trauma

Injuries are a leading cause of death in infants and children. Blunt injury is the most common. Basic life support and trauma management in pediatric patients is similar to care provided to adults. Remember to treat as you go. That is, as you assess the patient's ABCs, take care of any problem you find. Remember that children may take longer to go into shock, but when they do, it usually develops more rapidly than in adults. Time can be an important factor. Do not let a child's cries or behavior distract you from performing a complete assessment or providing appropriate care.

Always suspect trauma when infants and children are passengers in motor-vehicle collisions. Suspect unrestrained passengers of head and neck injuries. Suspect blunt trauma to the abdomen if the child was wearing a lap belt without a shoulder belt. Fully restrained passengers often have abdominal and lower spine injuries. The car seats in which infants ride are often fastened improperly. Suspect head and neck injuries in these patients.

First on Scene

Once children learn to move about on their own, they are more prone to injury. In fact, accidental trauma is a leading killer of children. When you arrive on scene and begin a size-up, make note of the mechanism of injury. Take c-spine precautions and use the pediatric assessment triangle for a quick general impression. These first-on-scene activities are crucial.

First Responder Practice

Initially, children can compensate well for blood or fluid loss. By the time a child's blood pressure drops from shock, he is near death. Anticipate shock. In cases where you would expect shock, do not wait for the signs to develop. Notify EMS immediately and arrange for transportation without delay.

In some EMS systems, you may be allowed to immobilize a child right in his or her car seat. This is done by applying a cervical immobilization device to the patient and placing padding between the child and seat to prevent movement. This procedure should not be used if the child has serious injuries or the potential for serious injuries, since the car seat may restrict the ability to control the airway and provide care. If you suspect any kind of damage to the car seat, do *not* use it for immobilization.

If a child is immobilized in a car seat, never tip the seat back. The position may impair breathing by putting pressure on the child's diaphragm. Always make sure that the seat remains upright.

If there is doubt that a child might require emergency care, remove him from the car seat before transport.

If a child riding a bicycle is struck by a car, suspect head, spine, and abdominal injuries. If the child was walking when struck, suspect head injury, abdominal injury, and pelvis or femur injury.

Children often get arms, legs, hands, feet, or heads trapped under or in rigid structures. The child is sometimes in pain and is almost always panicky. Try calming the child first. Then see if he or she can move independently. Lubricate skin surface with baby oil or a water-soluble lubricant. Make sure it is not applied near the patient's mouth, nose,

or eyes. If sawing or cutting is needed, make sure the child is protected with a heavy, fire-resistant cover. Someone can talk to the child to provide encouragement. After the child is freed, perform a complete patient assessment and provide care as required.

Shock

A major cause of shock in children is dehydration due to vomiting and diarrhea that may be related to infection. Another major cause is blood loss due to trauma.

Children tend to compensate more efficiently for shock. When they decompensate, it is a rapid process that can be devastating. Blood pressure may drop so far and so fast that the patient may go into cardiac arrest. You must constantly monitor the injured patient for signs and symptoms of shock. Take his or her vital signs constantly, including capillary refill.

Signs and symptoms of shock in the pediatric patient include (Figure 27-9):

- Altered mental status, from anxiety to unresponsiveness.

- Apathy or lack of vitality. This may present as the child's inability to identify a parent—an ominous sign.

- Delayed capillary refill.

SIGNS OF SHOCK

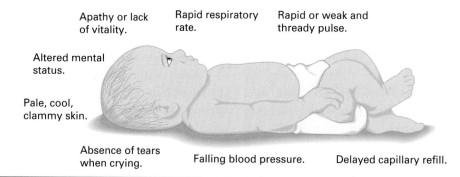

FIGURE 27-9 Shock in an infant or child can present with a variety of signs.

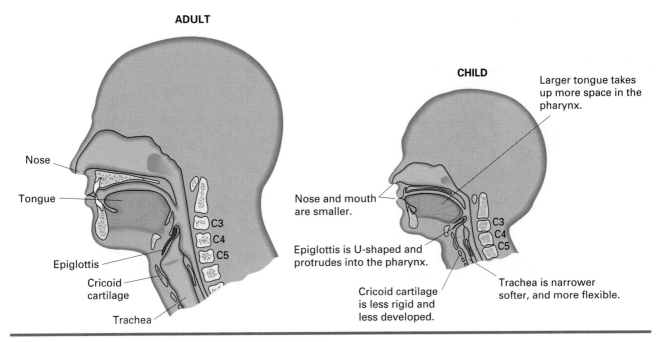

ADULT

Nose

Tongue

Epiglottis

Cricoid
cartilage

Trachea

C3
C4
C5

CHILD

Larger tongue takes
up more space in the
pharynx.

Nose and mouth
are smaller.

Epiglottis is U-shaped and
protrudes into the pharynx.

Cricoid cartilage
is less rigid and
less developed.

Trachea is narrower
softer, and more flexible.

C3
C4
C5

FIGURE 27-10 Comparison of the airways of an adult and an infant or child.

- Rapid or weak pulse (sometimes referred to as a thready pulse).
- Pale, cool, clammy skin.
- Rapid breathing.
- Falling or low blood pressure (a late sign).
- Absence of tears when crying.

Hypothermia can intensify shock in infants. They usually cannot shiver to warm themselves. So be sure to keep them warm. Remember especially to cover an infant's head.

While you are waiting for the EMTs to arrive on scene, try to have the patient lie flat. If that is not possible (due to the child's agitation or an infant's uncontrollable crying), make sure that the patient's position does not interfere with breathing. Be prepared to assist ventilations. Provide oxygen, if you are allowed to do so. Keep the patient warm and as calm as possible. Take vital signs often.

Remember that a relatively small blood loss in a pediatric patient can be very dangerous. For example, a newborn usually has less blood than the contents of a soda can. When there is significant visible blood loss or suspected internal bleeding, rapid transport and constant monitoring are essential.

Respiratory Emergencies

There is nothing more important than controlling the airway and ensuring adequate breathing in a pediatric patient. The National Pediatric Trauma Registry has reported that

30% of all pediatric trauma deaths are related to inappropriate management of the airway. The American Heart Association reports that more than 90% of pediatric deaths from foreign body airway obstruction occur in children younger than five years of age. Of those, 65% are infants. It is estimated that most could be saved by early detection.

Note that there are some differences in the way you manage a child's airway. They are as follows (Figure 27-10):

- Children are more susceptible than adults to respiratory problems. They have smaller air passages and less reserve air capacity. A child's airway can be compromised by less trauma or infection. Be especially attentive to ensure a clear and open airway.
- A child's airway structures are not as long or as large as an adult's. A child's airway can close off if the neck is flexed or extended too far. The best position is a neutral or slightly extended position. If the child is flat on the back, place a thin pad or towel under the shoulders to keep the head and neck properly aligned. Continually monitor signs of breathing.
- Because of immature accessory muscles, children use their diaphragms to breathe. If there are no reasons to prevent you from doing so, place a child in a position of comfort. That usually is a sitting position.
- Children have a large tongue that can block the airway. Make sure the tongue is forward. If a jaw-thrust maneuver is used, make sure your hand stays on the bony

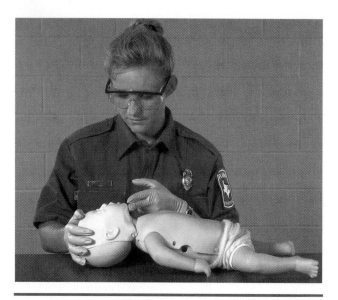

FIGURE 27-11 Airway obstruction may be relieved in an infant or child by keeping the head in a neutral or slightly extended position.

part of the chin (Figure 27-11). If it falls below, the tongue could be pushed back to block the airway.

- Infants and children tend to breathe through their noses. They also have abundant secretions. Be prepared to suction to keep the nose clear (Figure 27-12). Only suction for short periods of time (10 seconds for a child and 5 seconds for an infant). Provide oxygen before and immediately after each suctioning whenever possible.

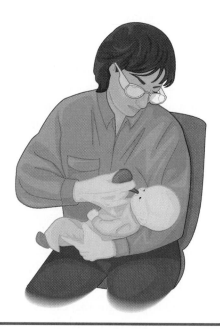

FIGURE 27-12 Use a bulb syringe for suctioning.

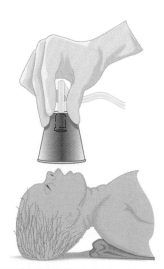

FIGURE 27-13 "Blow-by" oxygen using tubing and a paper cup. Never use a Styrofoam cup.

- Apply oxygen by way of a mask. Humidified oxygen is preferred, but never withhold or delay oxygen to have it humidified. If a child will not tolerate the mask, try the "blow-by" technique. Hold the mask or oxygen tubing two inches away from the patient's face. Some children respond well when the tubing is pushed through the bottom of a paper cup (paper, not Styrofoam), especially if the cup is colorful or has a picture drawn inside of it (Figure 27-13).

- If an infant or child is having a respiratory emergency, notify the incoming EMS unit and be sure an advanced life support (ALS) team is en route, if available.

- Even if the signs and symptoms of a respiratory emergency subside, it is still important for the child to be transported to a hospital.

For First Responder care of infants and children with respiratory emergencies, see Chapters 6 and 7. For more information about respiratory problems in all patients, see Chapter 14.

Croup

Croup is a common viral infection of the upper airway. It is most common in children between the ages of one and five. With croup, swelling progressively narrows the airway. As the child breathes, he or she may produce strange whooping sounds or high-pitched squeaking. There may be hoarseness, with the child's cough typically described as a "seal bark." Episodes of croup occur more commonly at night.

As the child gets worse, he or she may experience the following signs of respiratory distress: breathing with effort, including nasal flaring and **retractions** (pulling in of the sternum and ribs with each inhalation), rapid breathing, rising pulse, paleness or cyanosis, and restlessness or altered mental status.

Severe attacks of croup can be dangerous. About 10% of all children with croup need to be hospitalized. Treat a child with croup the same way you would treat any respiratory emergency. Arrange for transport to the nearest hospital as quickly as possible.

Epiglottitis

Epiglottitis is caused by a bacterial infection that inflames the epiglottis. It often resembles croup but is more serious. Thanks to vaccinations it does not occur often but, if left untreated, epiglottitis can be life-threatening. Signs and symptoms include occasional noise while inhaling; anxious concentration on breathing (the child may try to stay very still); sitting up and leaning forward, usually with chin thrust outward (tripod position); pain on swallowing and speaking; drooling; changes in voice quality; and high fever (usually above 102°F).

If you suspect epiglottitis, keep the child calm. Do not ask the child to open his or her mouth. Do not try to examine the child's throat or place anything in the mouth. Touching the larynx can cause the airway to close completely. Treat the child as you would for any respiratory emergency. If you must move the patient, move him as gently as possible. Arrange for transport to the nearest hospital as quickly as possible.

Asthma

Asthma is common among children, especially those with allergies. However, it should always be considered a serious medical emergency. Parents usually know the child's history and recognize an asthma attack. Determine if the child is taking medication.

An acute asthma attack occurs when the bronchioles spasm and constrict. This causes the bronchial membranes to swell and congest with mucus, which interferes with the child's ability to exhale. As a result, air gets trapped in the lungs, the chest gets inflated, breathing becomes impaired, and oxygen deficiency occurs.

Especially critical signs and symptoms include: rapid irregular breathing, especially in younger children; exhaustion; changes in level of responsiveness or sleepiness; cyanosis; rapid pulse and dropping blood pressure; signs of dehydration; **wheezing** (high-pitched breathing sounds usually heard when the child exhales); quiet or silent chest. In the late stages of respiratory distress, respirations may become so shallow that they no longer cause noise. Do not be fooled into believing that the child has gotten better. The condition has actually worsened.

First Responder care is the same as for any respiratory emergency. Be sure to monitor the airway and breathing constantly. Arrange for transport to the nearest hospital as quickly as possible.

Cardiac Arrest

Most cardiac arrests in infants and children result from airway obstruction and respiratory arrest. It is therefore extremely important to ensure an open airway and adequate breathing in your patients.

Signs and symptoms of circulatory failure in the pediatric patient are increased or decreased heart rate, unequal central (femoral) and distal pulse rates, poor skin color and delayed capillary refill, and altered mental status.

In cases of cardiac arrest in infants and children, provide CPR for one minute and then call for help if you are alone. Your goal is to keep your patient's brain alive. Remember that children have remarkable recuperative abilities. Cases of drowning, particularly cold-water drowning, and hypothermia may need an extensive resuscitation effort. Do not stop or interrupt CPR. Arrange for transport to the nearest hospital as quickly as possible. (CPR techniques vary for adults, children, and infants. See Chapter 8 for the details of emergency care.)

For use of an automatic external defibrillator (AED) on pediatric patients, follow the guidelines most currently recommended by the American Heart Association (AHA). Eligible pediatric patients are between one and eight years of age with no signs of circulation. Current AHA recommendations do not support the use of the AED in a patient less than one year of age. Ideally, an AED especially designed for pediatric patients should be used (Figure 27-14). The devices alter the energy level of the

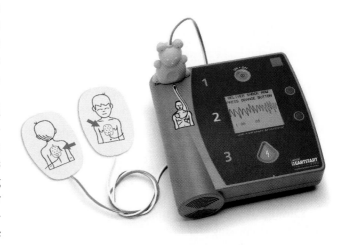

FIGURE 27-14 Example of a new AED for children.

defibrillations to account for the decreased weight in children. If the First Responder is the only rescuer on scene, it is recommended that one minute of CPR be performed before attaching the AED.

Seizures

Febrile seizures are seizures caused by a rapid rise in body temperature usually resulting in a high fever. They are the most common type of seizure in children. Some other causes include infection, poisoning, trauma, decreased levels of oxygen, epilepsy, hypoglycemia, inflammation to the brain, and meningitis. However, all seizures, including febrile seizures, should be considered potentially life-threatening.

During most seizures, a child's arms and legs become rigid, the back arches, muscles may twitch or jerk in spasm, the eyes roll up and become fixed, with dilated pupils, breathing is often irregular or ineffective, and bladder and bowels may lose control. The child may become completely unresponsive.

If the seizures last long enough, the child will show signs of cyanosis. The spasms will prevent swallowing. Saliva will be pushed out of the mouth, which will appear to be frothing. If saliva is trapped in the throat, the child will make bubbling or gurgling sounds. This may mean the airway needs suctioning when the seizure has ended. After the seizures, the child often appears to be extremely sleepy.

To obtain a patient history, ask the parents the following questions:

- Has the child had seizures before? How often? Is this the child's normal seizure pattern? Have the seizures always been associated with fever or do they occur when the child is well? Did others in the family have seizures when they were children?

- How many seizures has the child had in the past 24 hours? What was done for them?

- Has the child had a head injury, a stiff neck, or a recent headache? Does he or she have diabetes?

- Is the child taking a seizure medication? What has the doctor told you about the seizure disorder?

- Could the child have ingested any other medications?

- What did the seizure look like? Did it start in one part of the body and progress? Did the eyes go in different directions?

During the seizure, the tongue may relax and shift backward, decreasing the size of the air passage. To prevent this, as well as to encourage draining of mucus and frothing, place the patient in the recovery position. But do so only if there is no possibility of spine injury. Do not put anything in the patient's mouth.

Do not restrain the child during a seizure. Place him where he cannot fall or strike something. An open space on the floor with furniture and other objects moved away is fine. If the child is on a bed that does not have sides, move him to prevent a fall, if necessary. Loosen any tight and restricting clothing, especially around the neck or face.

After the seizure, make sure that the airway is open. The jaw may be relaxed, so consider gently pushing the mandible (the lower jaw bone) forward. This should help keep the airway open. Be prepared to suction.

Administer high-concentration oxygen if local protocol allows. Hold the mask slightly away from the patient's face until the seizure is completely over. If breathing is diminished or absent and the airway is clear, assist ventilations with a bag-valve mask (BVM) or pocket face mask with oxygen enrichment attachment. Follow local protocol.

Be sure to assess for injuries that may have occurred during the seizure.

If the seizure lasts longer than a few minutes and recurs without a recovery period, then the seizure may be *status epilepticus.* This condition is a true medical emergency. Notify the incoming EMS unit immediately. (See Chapter 15 for more information about seizures.)

Special Health-Care Needs

Children who have some type of physical or mental limitation have special health-care needs. In addition, a premature baby or a chronically ill child may be dependent on some type of mechanical device such as a ventilator. More and more of these children are receiving care that allows them to stay at home and attend school.

When responding to a call for such a child, as always focus on the patient's ABCs—airway, breathing, and circulation. If a child is on a ventilator and is having trouble breathing, it is more important to assist ventilations than to determine what might be wrong with the device. In these situations, disconnect the device and ventilate using a BVM with an oxygen reservoir. If oxygen is not available, ventilate with a BVM until oxygen can be brought to the patient.

Also, keep in mind that parents and caretakers can be very good resources for important information about the child's condition. They will probably know the child's baseline vital signs, medications, and how to operate the medical devices. In addition, they may have dealt with a similar problem previously and know what must be done. In many instances, the parents or caretakers may have initiated care before your arrival. Based on the circumstances, consider taking their lead and assist in providing care.

Sudden Infant Death Syndrome (SIDS)

Sudden infant death syndrome (SIDS) is defined as the sudden death of an infant in the first year of life. In the past it was more commonly known as "crib death" or "cot death."

SIDS cannot be predicted or prevented. In fact, it is still not completely understood. It almost always occurs while the infant is sleeping. The infant is typically healthy, born prematurely, and between the ages of four weeks and seven months when he or she suddenly dies. No illness has been present, though there may have been recent cold symptoms. There is usually no indication of struggle.

Managing the SIDS Call

Unless the infant has *rigor mortis* (stiffness), immediately initiate basic life support, even if other signs make the effort appear futile. Begin CPR, and have someone activate the EMS system if it has not already been done.

The extreme emotional condition of the parents makes them victims as much as the baby. They will be in agony from emotional distress, remorse, and feelings of guilt. Avoid any comments that might suggest blame. Help them feel that everything possible is being done but do not offer false hope. Follow local protocol.

When you can, obtain a brief medical history of the infant. This should not delay life-support efforts. If necessary, have other medical personnel find out the following: When was the child put in the crib? What was the last time the parents looked in on the baby? What were the circumstances concerning discovery of the infant? What was the position of the baby in the crib? What was the physical appearance of the infant and the crib? What else was in the crib? What was the appearance of the room and home? Is there medication present (even if it is for the adults)? What is the behavior of the people present? What is the general health of the infant, recent illnesses, medications, or allergies?

After ambulance personnel take over, encourage the parents to accompany their baby. Offer to stay with their other children until relatives arrive. Support the parents in any way possible. While the resuscitation efforts may seem futile to them, parents may receive comfort from knowing that everything that can be done is being done.

Note that it is very common for First Responders to experience emotions such as anxiety, guilt, or anger after a SIDS call. A debriefing or talking to a counselor, colleague, or spouse may be helpful. Remember that ignoring those feelings will not cause them to go away. Denying them could even have a serious, negative impact on your mental health.

Child Abuse and Neglect

The definition of **child abuse** is improper or excessive action so as to injure or cause harm. The term **child neglect** refers to giving insufficient attention or respect to a child who has a claim to that attention and respect.

Child abuse, or **non-accidental trauma,** occurs in all parts of our society. The estimated number of children who are abused or neglected in the U.S. is staggering. Estimates range from 500,000 to 4 million cases annually with thousands of abused children dying. In fact, child abuse has been the only major cause of infant and child death to increase in the past 30 years. These numbers are cause for alarm.

During an emergency call, the adult (usually a parent) who abuses a child often behaves in an evasive manner. He or she may volunteer little information or give contradictory information about what happened. However, a call for child abuse may be a call for help. Do not be judgmental. Focus on the child.

Some forms of abuse are difficult to recognize on scene. For example, broken bones at various stages of healing can be identified only at the hospital. However, you may be able to recognize some forms of abuse and neglect (Figure 27-15).

Signs and symptoms may include multiple bruises in various stages of healing; injury not consistent with the mechanism of injury described by the caregivers; patterns of injury that suggest abuse, such as cigarette burns, whip marks, or hand prints; fresh burns, such as scalding in a glove or dip pattern; burns not consistent with the history presented by the caregivers; and untreated burns.

Also suspect possible abuse when there are repeated calls to the same address, when the caregivers seem inappropriately unconcerned or give conflicting stories, and when the child seems afraid to discuss how the injury occurred. If an infant or child presents with unresponsiveness or seizure or signs of severe internal injuries but no external signs, suspect central nervous system injuries, or *shaken baby syndrome.*

Signs and symptoms of possible neglect include lack of adult supervision; appearance of malnourishment; unsafe living conditions; untreated chronic illness, such as no medication for asthma; and delay in reporting injuries.

If you suspect abuse or neglect, first and foremost make sure that the environment is safe for you and the patient. Provide necessary emergency care. As time permits, observe the child and the caregivers. Look for objects that

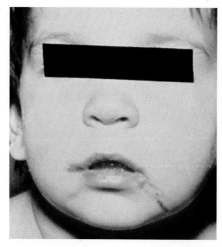

a. *Child abuse—gag bruise on mouth.*
(Robert A. Felter M.D.)

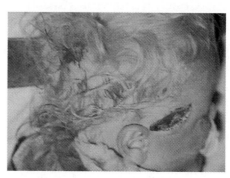

b. *Child physical abuse.*

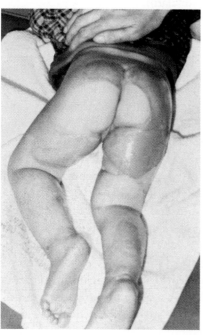

c. *Doughnut burns on buttocks.*
(Robert A. Felter M.D.)

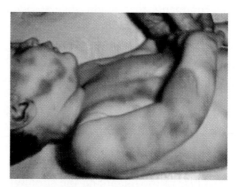

d. *Child-abuse death from multiple injuries.*

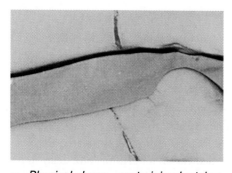

e. *Physical abuse—restraining by tying.*

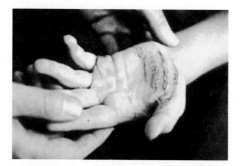

f. *Physical abuse—burns from hand held on an electric stove.*

FIGURE 27-15 Whenever you suspect abuse, report it to the proper authorities as per local protocols.

might have been used to hurt the child. Look for signs of neglect in the general appearance of the child. Sometimes abuse and neglect are well hidden.

If you find yourself in a position of giving emergency care to a possible victim of child abuse or neglect, follow these guidelines:

- Gain entry to the home and access to the child, if it can be done safely. If the parents placed the emergency call, you will probably get in without any difficulty. If someone else called, the parents may resist. You may need to call the police. Do not put yourself at undue risk.

- If you are asked to help the child, calm the parents. Tell them that if the child needs care, you will provide it. Tell them that is the only reason you are there. Speak in a low, firm voice.

- Focus attention on the child during emergency care. Speak softly. Use the child's first name. Do not ask the child to recreate the situation while parents are present.

- Do a full patient assessment. Treat as you go. Note any suspicious abrasions, bruises, lacerations, and evidence of internal injury. Look also for signs of head injury. Remember that you are there to provide emergency care, not to determine child abuse.

- Update EMS in the same way you would for any other child in need of care and transport.

- You are not expected to deal with child abuse issues on the spot unless the child is in danger. In all suspected cases, the child should be transported.

- Never confront parents with a charge of child abuse. Being supportive and nonjudgmental with parents will help them be more receptive to others providing emergency care.

- Accusations can delay transport and place the First Responder at risk. Instead, report objective information to the transporting unit's crew. Focus only on what you saw and what you heard. Be very cautious about providing subjective information (what you think). When transferring information, try to do it privately, away from the family and caretakers.

- Maintain total confidentiality regarding the incident. Do not discuss it with your family or friends.

You must always report your suspicions of child abuse to the proper authorities. It is critical for you to learn the reporting laws in your own state and the reporting protocols for your EMS system. Find out who must report the abuse, what types of abuse and neglect must be reported, to whom the reports must be made, what infor-mation a First Responder must give, what immunity a First Responder is granted, and criminal penalties for failing to report.

Taking Care of Yourself

Many children in the U.S. who die from accidents are pronounced dead either at the scene or at the hospital. The sudden and violent death of a child is emotionally wrenching, whether it occurs before you arrive or while you are giving care.

Recognize your reactions. Feelings of fear, rage, helplessness, anxiety, sorrow, and grief are common. It also is common for rescuers to feel shame and guilt, even if they did everything possible to help the child. These feelings are particularly intense if the child dies. Remember, some children will die despite your best efforts.

As a First Responder, you need to control your emotions while you are treating the child. In this way you can render the best assistance possible. After the call is over, however, you need to deal with your feelings. Talk them out. A critical incident stress debriefing (CISD) team may be helpful, but you can use other methods to discuss and deal with your feelings, including, for example, talking to a trusted friend. Do not delay!

Q:

1. When should you suspect trauma in infants and children who are in a vehicle collision?

2. What are major causes of shock in infants and children?

3. Why are infants and children more susceptible to respiratory problems than adults? Give two reasons.

4. What is First Responder care for pediatric patients with suspected croup, epiglottitis, or asthma?

5. What are the causes of most cardiac arrests in infants and children?

6. What are the signs of circulatory failure in infants and children?

7. What questions should you ask the parents of a pediatric patient who has a seizure emergency? List five.

8. What are the signs of possible child abuse? Of child neglect?

▶▶ The Call Follow-up

At the beginning of this chapter, you read that First Responders were on scene with an unresponsive six-year-old patient who had been hit by a car. To see how chapter skills apply to this emergency, read the following. It describes how the call was completed.

Initial Assessment *(continued)* We found the patient unresponsive with snoring respirations. My partner and I knew what we had to do in one word: airway. We got in position, applied manual stabilization, and turned her for better airway assessment and control. While my partner held her head and neck in line, I applied a cervical immobilization device. A jaw-thrust stopped the snoring. Further examination of the mouth showed that two baby teeth had been knocked out and there was blood in the mouth. Suction took care of it. Breathing appeared to be adequate. I applied oxygen by way of a pediatric nonrebreather at 10 liters per minute.

Just then dispatch informed us that the ambulance would be on scene in four to five minutes. We reported our general impression of the patient. "Six-year-old female was struck by vehicle. The airway is open, and she is breathing on her own. The patient is responsive to pain only." We advised the ambulance should continue to respond with red lights and sirens—priority one.

Physical Examination We covered the patient with a blanket to maintain body heat and decided to proceed with a head-to-toe exam. Our findings included swelling with discoloration on the left forehead above the eye. Pupils were reactive but sluggish. The lower left arm was observed to be deformed and swollen. We found her respirations were 12 and shallow, which was slower than our last assessment, so we assisted ventilations.

Patient History The father reported that the child was in good health and had no allergies.

Ongoing Assessment We continued to assist ventilations until the ambulance crew arrived.

Patient Hand-off When the paramedics got on scene, we gave them the hand-off report (see below). A few days later we went to the trauma center and asked about the little girl. We were told that her head injury required surgery, but she was doing well and was expected to make a full recovery. One of the doctors asked what had happened and we gave him all the details. He listened intently. When we were done, he said that opening the airway and alerting the paramedics to the slowing respirations may have made the difference in the patient's outcome.

Hand-off Report

"This is Tisa Kotto, six years old. She was hit by a car traveling approximately 15 mph about 20 minutes ago. We log-rolled her onto her back, applied a c-collar, and administered oxygen. She has an injury to the left forehead, two teeth knocked out, and a swollen deformed left arm. Her vitals are pulse 60, strong, regular; respirations 12 and shallow. We are assisting ventilations. There is no medical history of allergies."

The Last Word *Learn the unique aspects of providing First Responder care to pediatric patients. One of the most important is that you are not treating the patient only. A calm, professional, reassuring approach can help to minimize the impact of the emergency on both the patient and the family.*

Chapter Review

Focus on the EMS Team

Pediatric calls are not as common as calls involving adults. You will need the support of your partner and other EMS personnel to provide the best emergency medical care possible. However, that support should not stop when the call is over.

Dealing with the emotions involved in serious pediatric calls is no small matter. This is a time when EMS personnel should come together to support each other. That's what a team is for.

Summing Up

- All anatomical structures in the infant's or child's airway, including the mouth and nose, are smaller than an adult's and are therefore more easily obstructed. The tongue takes up proportionally more space in the mouth than the tongue of an adult. As a result, it can block an infant's or child's airway more easily. The trachea is narrower, softer, and more flexible, so tipping the head too far back or allowing the head to fall forward can close the trachea.

- Maintaining a good airway and ensuring quality breathing are the two most important concerns for a First Responder when dealing with a pediatric emergency. Remember: If you do *not* have an airway, you will *not* have a patient.

- When assisting ventilations in a pediatric patient, be sure to watch for chest rise. This is a good indicator of whether or not your breaths are effective.

- Administer oxygen to the pediatric patient for any type of respiratory problem. But if you do not have oxygen on scene, do not delay ventilations while you wait for it.

- The primary cause of cardiac arrest in infants and children is an uncorrected respiratory problem. Because the chest wall is softer, they tend to rely more heavily on the diaphragm for breathing. So watch for excessive movement of the diaphragm. It can alert you to respiratory distress in these patients.

- A word to the wise: with pediatric patients, all roads lead to the ABCs.

- Stop bleeding in a pediatric patient as quickly as possible. A comparatively small blood loss in an adult would be major for an infant or small child. In addition, they tend to compensate longer before going into shock. Be alert! They also decompensate very rapidly.

- When performing a pediatric patient assessment, take what you can when you can get it. For example, if a child holds out a hand, it is a good time to check the pulse or capillary refill.

- Infants and children are prone to hypothermia. Keep them warm. Cover the head whenever practical, since it is a major source of heat loss.

- A child's skin surface is large compared to body mass. This makes children more susceptible to dehydration and hypothermia. Response to burns also can be more severe.

- When the age of a child is unknown, use your best judgment based on the size of the child.

- In cases of suspected abuse or neglect, EMS personnel may be the only advocates a child has. Report as objectively as you can what you have seen and heard.

- When you treat an ill or traumatized child, you are treating a family.

- The interests of the infant or child must always be placed as the foremost consideration when making any and all patient-care decisions.

Key Terms

child abuse improper or excessive action so as to injure or cause harm to an infant or child.

child neglect insufficient attention or respect given to a child who has a claim to that attention and respect.

croup a common viral infection of the upper airway, most common in children between the ages of one and five.

epiglottitis a bacterial infection that inflames the epiglottis. It often resembles croup but is more serious.

non-accidental trauma injuries caused by abuse.

pediatric assessment triangle (PAT) a method of remembering the important components of pediatric assessment: appearance, breathing, and circulation.

pediatric patients patients who are infants or children.

retraction sucking in of the skin between the ribs, above the sternum, and above the clavicles.

wheezing a high-pitched breathing sound usually heard during an exhalation.

Knowledge Check

1. **When comparing a child's anatomy to an adult's, which one of the statements below is TRUE?**
   a. Children have the same heart rates as adults do.
   b. Children have faster breathing rates than adults do.
   c. Children and adults have the same blood volume.
   d. Children have wider airway passages than adults do.

2. **Which one of the following is NOT a sign of early respiratory problems in children?**
   a. cyanosis
   b. noisy breathing
   c. normal mental status
   d. breathing with obvious effort

3. **One sign of shock in children is:**
   a. warm and dry skin.
   b. normal mental status.
   c. slow respiratory rate.
   d. weak and rapid pulse.

4. **First Responder care of childhood seizures includes:**
   a. administering oxygen after the seizure.
   b. placing the patient in a supine position.
   c. restraining the patient during the seizure.
   d. placing a stick in the mouth to prevent biting.

5. **Which one of the statements below is MOST correct about an asthma emergency?**
   a. It is not a serious medical emergency.
   b. You should gather a medical history.
   c. The patient will be awake and alert.
   d. Breathing will be slow and regular.

6. **Which one of the following may be the BEST solution to a situation in which parents are especially anxious?**
   a. Raise your voice to distract them from their child's injuries.
   b. Keep them as far away as possible so they do not interfere with emergency care.
   c. Realize that they may be correct and could actually help you provide the proper care.
   d. Tell them that they are jeapardizing the life of their child and that you intend to report them.

7. **A child's skin surface is small compared to body mass. This makes children less susceptible to dehydration and hypothermia.**
   a. True
   b. False

8. **A comparatively large blood loss in an adult would be minor for a child.**
   a. True
   b. False

9. List six types of EMS equipment available in a variety of pediatric sizes.

_____   _____

_____   _____

_____   _____

Scenario

You are called to a "baby choking" at 4121 Fisher's Way early one evening. The dispatcher advises that a five-month old had apparently choked while eating. When you arrive on scene, the patient's father meets you at the door. "I'm glad you're here," he says. "We just started feeding Jason cereal and he choked. We thought he stopped breathing." He leads you into the residence, where you see a woman holding a baby. The baby appears to be calm, pink, not in any sort of respiratory distress, and responding to his mother.

a. Based on the concept of the pediatric assessment triangle, do you consider the patient in need of immediate action? Why or why not?

_____

_____

_____

b. The mother hands the baby to you to examine. The baby begins to scream. Is this a good sign or a bad sign? Explain your answer.

_____

_____

_____

c. The parents think that you should cancel the ambulance since everything appears to be okay. Do you agree? Why or why not?

_____

_____

_____

d. The parents believe they over-reacted. What do you tell them?

_____

_____

_____

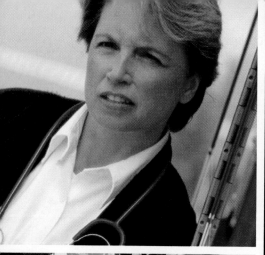

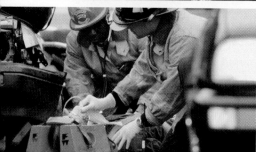

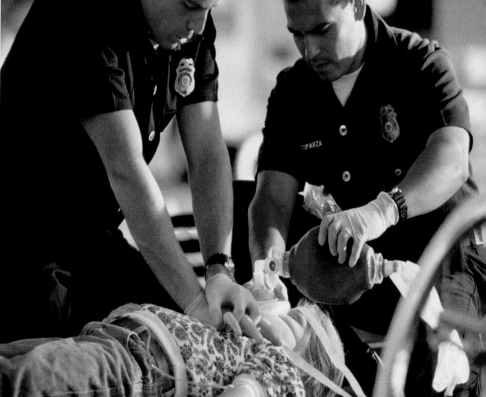

28 | Geriatric Patients

Objectives

From the U.S. Department of Transportation (DOT)'s 1995 "First Responder: National Standard Curriculum." Material supplemental to the DOT curriculum is listed under "Enrichment."

Cognitive

No objectives are identified by the DOT.

Affective

No objectives are identified by the DOT.

Psychomotor

No objectives are identified by the DOT.

Enrichment

▶ Relate the anatomical and functional changes of aging to illness and injury in the elderly. (pp. 521–524)

▶ Explain the reasons why an elderly person may be more seriously ill or injured than indicated by signs and symptoms and/or mechanism of injury. (pp. 525–527)

▶ Discuss the impact of social, psychological, and financial concerns on the health of the elderly. (pp. 524–525)

Introduction

In the U.S., the fastest growing age group is 65 years of age and older. Because they make up such a large segment of the population and because they are prone to a variety of illnesses and injuries, elderly patients may frequently rely on First Responders in emergencies.

Section 1 Changes in the Older Adult

Misconceptions

It is true that some conditions commonly occur with aging. That may lead some younger adults to believe that elderly people tend to be weak and sickly with decreased ability to hear, see, or remember things. They believe that most elderly people live in extended-care facilities or nursing homes. In fact, a majority of older adults experience good health, are independent, and live active lives (Figure 28-1).

Another misconception is older adults cannot understand or learn new information. This is most often not the case. So, be sure to explain procedures and give information to older adults as you would to younger patients. Do not assume that older patients are unable to accurately hear or answer questions about their own health. Seek information from family members or others only after you do so from the patient.

Older patients must be treated respectfully, and each one should be regarded as the unique, dignified individual he or she is.

Physical Changes and Problems

The most common theories about aging involve *genetic predetermination* (our genes make us do it), environment, and lifestyles. Whatever the underlying causes, the func-

tions of all of the body's systems decline with age. This general decline includes changes in the skin, sensory organs, respiratory system, heart and blood vessels, and the digestive, urinary, musculoskeletal, nervous, and immune systems. (See Table 28-1.)

The Skin

As people age, the skin develops more darkly pigmented areas, which are most noticeable in lighter-skinned individuals. These areas are sometimes called "age spots" or "liver spots." The skin secretes less oil, making it drier and flakier. Skin secretions also contain substances that help protect against infection. But as skin secretions decrease, so does the protection against infection.

Perspiration decreases, which is a contributing factor to heat-related emergencies in older adults. Some medications further inhibit perspiration, so that the elderly patient may not exhibit **diaphoresis** (excessive perspiration) when in shock.

Loss of fat and the weakening of the supportive structures within the skin cause it to become looser, thinner, and more fragile. The skin of older adults tears quite easily. It also causes older adults who cannot move around as much as they did to be prone to bedsores.

Sensory Organs

In general, aging leads to decreased sharpness of the senses. Visual changes include farsightedness, **cataracts,**

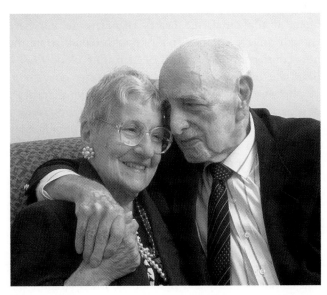

a.

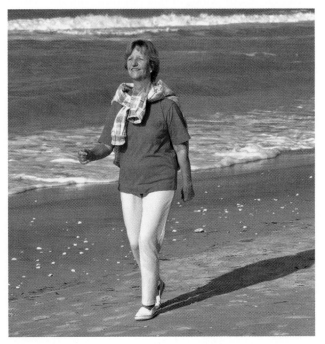

b.

FIGURE 28-1 Most older adults are healthy, active, and independent.

THE CALL

Dispatch A call for help from the St. Joseph Apartments is not unusual for our fire department. But besides a name and address, the only description of the emergency we had this time was that it was from an elderly female patient.

Scene Size-up There are many elderly people living in that location, and the potential for a serious medical emergency is always present. When we arrived, we found the superintendent of the building quickly, told him what was going on, and asked him to lead us to the apartment. On the way, he confirmed that the tenant's name is Mrs. Adele Washington, and he said, "She lives alone."

We knocked on the door with the super beside us. There was no response. He used a passkey to open up, and then he left to direct the paramedics to the scene.

The apartment seemed to be in order. We quickly determined that it was safe to enter. I called out, "Mrs. Washington?" Then I saw an elderly woman seated on the edge of her bed crying. She was well groomed and very pale.

Is the patient ill? Is she injured? How should the First Responders proceed? Consider this patient as you read Chapter 28.

---

yellowing of the lens of the eye, decreased night and peripheral vision, and less tolerance for glare. These changes can make it difficult to read directions on medication bottles or tell the color of one pill from another. Visual changes also contribute to many unintentional injuries, such as falls and vehicle crashes. However, attention to the environment of the elderly and reduction of potential hazards can reduce the likelihood of injuries.

Hearing becomes less acute, especially in picking up high-pitched sounds. The senses of taste and smell diminish, and there is less sensation in the skin. It is not difficult to imagine how an older adult could fail to hear a siren while driving, fail to smell a gas leak or spoiled food, or be unaware of trauma to the skin. The diminished senses of taste and smell also contribute to a decreased appetite and nutritional problems.

Respiratory System

Aging results in weakening of the chest muscles and stiffening of the cartilage of the rib cage, making breathing less effective. In addition, the lungs lose some of their capacity to provide oxygen to the blood. As a result, the elderly are less able to compensate when they need more oxygen, such as when there is blood loss. Because of other changes in the lungs and in the immune system, infections such as pneumonia are common.

Heart and Blood Vessels

The ability of the heart to contract with force declines with age. As a result, when the body demands increased blood flow, the heart will try to compensate by contracting more often. If too often, the heart's chambers do not have enough time to completely fill up with blood before the next contraction. So, instead of increasing blood flow, a heart rate that is too rapid may actually worsen circulation.

Because of the effects of certain medications, the heart of a patient with heart disease or high blood pressure is unable to beat faster. This means that the pulse rate may be normal in patients with blood loss, even when you would expect it to be rapid.

Many older adults have high blood pressure. This can lead to a heart attack or stroke. Significant blood loss will lead to a drop in blood pressure, but in a person whose blood pressure is usually high, a blood pressure in the normal range may actually represent a drop. Shock due to blood loss may go unrecognized because of this. Therefore, consider the mechanism of injury and monitor the elderly trauma patient's mental status. In such cases, a decrease in the level of responsiveness may be the first indication of shock.

In addition, genetic and lifestyle factors over time contribute to changes in the blood vessels, such as blockage or weakening of arteries to the heart and brain. Such problems can lead to heart attack or stroke.

TABLE 28-1 Physical and Functional Changes in the Older Adult

Body System	Changes	Complications
Skin	Decreased perspiration Decreased oil secretion Loss of fat and weakening of supportive structures beneath the skin	Heat-related illnesses Masks signs of shock Decreased resistance to infection Skin is easily torn Bedsores
Sensory Organs	Diminished vision Diminished hearing Diminished pain sensation Diminished taste and smell	Falls; vehicle crashes Unable to read directions for medication Unable to hear warnings such as smoke alarms or sirens May be unaware of injury or seriousness of injury Decreased appetite; malnutrition Unable to smell leaking gas or smoke
Respiratory System	Weakened chest muscles	Less able to compensate when the body needs more oxygen Less lung capacity
Heart and Blood Vessels	Decreased strength of heart contraction High blood pressure Blockage of blood vessels	Cannot meet higher demands for blood flow Heart attack, stroke, poor circulation to extremities Masks shock
Digestive System	Ulcers, tumors Dental problems	Gastrointestinal bleeding Malnutrition, choking on poorly chewed food
Urinary System	Incontinence	Catheterization may lead to infection
Musculoskeletal System	Diminished muscle strength Weakened bone structure	Minor falls or impacts can break bones
Nervous System	Fewer nerve fibers Alteration in chemical balance	Decreased sensory perception Depression Impaired sleep
Immune System	Less functional	Diminished ability to heal Infection Cancer

Digestive System

With age, the digestive system slows, producing fewer secretions for the breakdown of food. This, along with other changes, may lead to indigestion or heartburn, gas production, and constipation. Since the stomach empties more slowly, vomiting may occur during illness or injury.

The elderly may also suffer from ulcers or disorders of the intestinal tract, which can lead to bleeding. Such bleeding may be evident in vomit or from bloody or dark, tarry stools. Enough blood can be lost this way to result in shock.

Decreased taste and smell may lead to a decrease in appetite and dental problems. Fatigue may cause eating to be difficult. For these reasons—and others such as poverty and depression—the elderly may suffer from malnutrition. Malnutrition affects general health and makes existing medical problems worse.

Urinary System

Elderly men may suffer from blockage of urine flow due to enlargement of the prostate gland, making bladder and kidney infection more likely. Elderly women are also susceptible to infections of the urinary tract.

Elderly patients with urinary tract infections can be quite ill but not have specific complaints related to the urinary system. Overwhelming infection may occur, causing changes in circulation that lead to shock. This type of shock, called *septic shock,* should be suspected when the patient has signs and symptoms of shock without blood loss. First Responder treatment of this type of shock is the same as for shock due to blood loss.

Musculoskeletal System

Muscle strength and bone mass decrease with age. Muscles get fatigued more easily, contributing to falls and other injuries. Even minor falls commonly result in broken bones in the elderly. When a hip is broken, the decrease in mobility and tolerance for stresses to the body can lead to a rapid decline in the patient's overall health status.

Nervous System

Decreases in the number of nerve fibers and changes in the chemical balance of the brain may lead to decreased perception, changes in balance and coordination, and altered sleep patterns. These changes are factors that contribute to injuries among the elderly.

Although it is commonly believed that impairments in thinking and memory are normal processes of aging, this is not the case. When these events occur they indicate the presence of an abnormal condition. Sometimes confusion and agitated behavior among the elderly are temporary, caused by illness or the effects of medication.

Depression is not uncommon among older adults. It can lead to suicide or attempted suicide. Depressed patients may have poor hygiene, poor eating habits, and a disorderly living situation. In addition, frequent depression can lead to physical symptoms.

Immune System

Common illnesses, such as influenza, have a much higher fatality rate in the elderly. Though fever is often a sign of infection, it may not be present in the elderly. In addition, the increased risk of infection and decreased ability to heal make injuries and surgery more serious and more often fatal.

Response to Medication

The body's ability to respond to and eliminate medications also changes with age. This can result in patients having exaggerated responses to medications and more profound side effects compared to most younger patients. In addition, since older patients tend to be on several medications, life-threatening drug interactions can occur.

Psychosocial and Economic Factors

Many psychological, social, and economic factors impact the lives of the elderly. They include alcoholism, substance abuse, physical and psychological abuse, neglect, loneliness, and poverty. All of these factors have implications for the health of older adults. Being aware of these factors is a step toward developing empathy and compassion for your elderly patients.

Depression

Depression is common in the elderly. It may be a result of changes in the chemicals affecting the brain, or it may be the result of a variety of situational factors. Friends and relatives may have died, and the patient may be living alone and feeling isolated. Loss of independence and having to depend on others for help with daily activities may also be distressing. In some cases, the patient may feel shame, self-disgust, or embarrassment at loss of a body function or changes in appearance. Depression can be treated with therapy or medication, but it still is a factor in suicide among the elderly.

Substance Abuse

Health-care providers often fail to suspect alcohol and other substance abuse as a factor in the medical condition of the elderly. This may include dependence on prescription drugs, as well as the abuse of illegal substances. It may seem shocking to think of an older adult as having a substance-abuse problem, but a person who was in their 20s or 30s in the 1960s, a time when illicit drug use was popular, is now a person in his or her 60s or 70s.

Alcohol and substance abuse contributes to deterioration of physical health, may be a factor in altered mental status, and can contribute to injuries including those sustained in motor-vehicle crashes.

Elder Abuse and Neglect

Physical and psychological abuse of the elderly and neglect of dependent elderly are often first detected by EMS providers (Figure 28-2). There are several risk factors for abuse, regardless of whether the older adult lives with a spouse, his or her children, or in an extended-care facility. An older adult who requires assistance with daily activities, who has difficulty sleeping, who has lost bladder control, or who exhibits bizarre behavior due to altered mental status is more likely to be abused or neglected.

Abuse should be suspected when an injury seems inconsistent with the description of how it happened or there are multiple injuries in various stages of healing. The patient may be reluctant to discuss the nature of the injury in the presence of the abuser because of fear of punishment or because of feelings of shame or embarrassment. The neglected patient may be deprived of food and water, needed medications, and the assistance needed for activities such as bathing and changing clothing.

Do not confront the suspected abuser. Privately relate your suspicions to the arriving EMS crew. (Follow local protocol.)

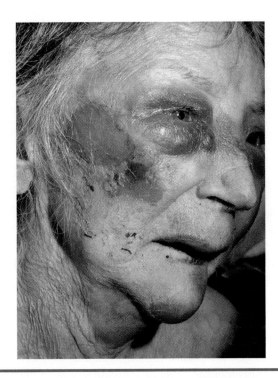

FIGURE 28-2 **Look for signs of elder abuse or neglect.**

Socioeconomic Concerns

Many older adults live on very limited incomes. As a result, the elderly may not have adequate shelter, safety, food, or medications. The elderly may not be able to secure their homes against crime, make necessary repairs, modifications, or upgrades to their homes, or otherwise maintain a safe environment. Lack of adequate heat or cooling of the environment can leave the older adult at risk of heat- and cold-related emergencies. Using alternative sources of heat, such as space heaters or an open oven, leads to burns, fires, and carbon monoxide poisoning.

The elderly with financial concerns also may not eat properly. They may take less medication than prescribed or may not take their medication at all in order to save money.

1. What are some common misconceptions about older adults? What is the truth?

2. Which of the body's systems are affected by aging?

3. What are some changes an aging adult might experience? Name three.

4. How does a limited income affect an elderly patient's health?

First on Scene

Don't forget about the possibility of a contagious disease in your geriatric patients. Any patient, even an elderly one, could have a disease that can spread to you. Not only can older patients have HIV or hepatitis, they also may be at higher risk for TB and other conditions. Remember: *take BSI precautions for all patients.*

Section 2 Illness and Injury in the Older Adult

Common medical complaints in the elderly include chest pain, difficulty breathing, fainting, and an altered mental status. Chest pain should always be considered serious. Difficulty breathing may occur due to lung or heart problems or because of airway obstruction (Figure 28-3). Fainting or near-fainting is common in the elderly. It may be due to a variety of causes, such as side effects of medication, heart problems, internal bleeding, or changes in the blood vessels that supply the brain with oxygen. When an older adult has an altered mental status, such as a change in personality or behavior, a family member or caregiver usually summons help.

The most common mechanisms of injury in the elderly are falls, burns, and vehicle crashes. These are usually due to effects of aging, such as diminished vision, hearing, and pain sensation, as well as loss of muscular strength, balance, and coordination. In addition, the physical changes

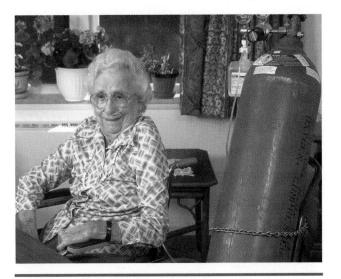

FIGURE 28-3 **Difficulty breathing is a common medical complaint in the elderly.**

associated with aging result in much less force being needed to produce injury than in younger people. In addition, the effects of some medications can mask the seriousness of an older adult's injury. Therefore, injuries may be more serious than they appear.

Scene Size-up

As with all calls, your first priority is your own safety and the safety of your crew. Size up the scene as you would for any emergency call. Keep in mind the following:

- An older adult with a substance-abuse problem, mental illness, or a condition such as Alzheimer's disease may become violent. Be prepared.

- Stay alert for conditions that suggest abuse, neglect, or the patient's lack of self-care.

- Be careful of potential hazards, such as loose or missing handrails on porches and stairs and clutter in the home.

- Look for poorly functioning or alternative heat sources to warn you of possible carbon monoxide poisoning.

When approaching the elderly patient, focus on him, rather than family members or caregivers who may be anxious to speak for him. This demonstrates respect for the patient, and it gives him more control over the situation. Make eye contact. Then, introduce yourself. Once you know the patient's full name, address the patient by that name—"Mr. Baker" or "Mrs. McFadden" for example. Do not address him or her as "honey," "dear," "sweetheart," or similar terms.

Take a position at the patient's eye level. It is less intimidating than towering over him. Offer a handshake to establish rapport and at the same time note the patient's skin temperature and ability to move and follow directions. At this point, establish the chief complaint by asking for the reason why EMS was called. Asking, "What is wrong?" may only result in a lengthy recitation of both medical and non-medical complaints.

Remember to be patient. Give the older adult the time he or she needs to answer your questions. Do not raise your voice. Instead, face the patient and speak clearly. If your patient has poor vision, it's a good idea for you to position yourself right in front of her where she has the best chance of seeing you. You might also put a hand on her arm to let her know where you are.

Speak louder than you usually do only if your first attempt to communicate is unsuccessful (Figure 28-4). Note that elderly people may find higher-pitched tones difficult to hear, so a person with a deeper voice may be more successful in communicating. If your patient has a hearing aid but is not wearing it, you may ask for it to be put it place.

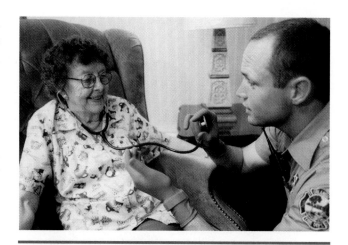

FIGURE 28-4 Do your best to be sure an elderly patient understands your questions. *(Craig Jackson/ In the Dark Photography)*

If your patient is not wearing his dentures (usually because they are uncomfortable), you may have a difficult time understanding what he is saying to you. If this is the case, you may ask him to put in his dentures.

Initial Assessment

Perform an initial assessment as you would for any patient. However, keep the following in mind:

- For your general impression, be sure to note whether or not the patient appears clean, well groomed, and cared for. Lack of good hygiene could indicate the patient is not tending to his medical needs.

- To address mental status, find out from the patient's family or caregivers if a behavior related to the emergency is usual for the patient or if the changes have occurred suddenly.

- Keep in mind that an elderly person who has had a stroke may have difficulty chewing, swallowing, or clearing the airway of secretions. In the unresponsive patient, dentures and other dental devices can cause airway obstruction.

- Correct positioning of the head and neck for airway care may be a challenge due to a curvature of the spine that occurs with aging. If it is difficult for you to tilt the patient's head or position the airway properly, you may need to perform a jaw-thrust maneuver.

- For artificial ventilation, it may be easier to form a seal with the mask if you leave dentures in place. They can help to support the facial structure.

- Bleeding control in the elderly may be more difficult if the patient is taking aspirin or other blood-thinning medications.

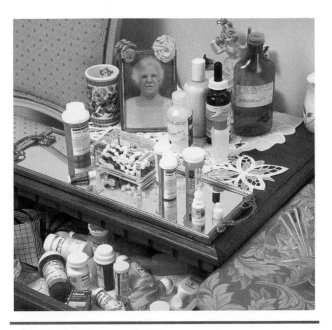

FIGURE 28-6 Make note of medications when you gather a patient history.

Physical Examination

Perform a physical exam, as you would for any patient who needs one. If one is required, keep in mind that many elderly patients wear several layers of clothing, which can make the assessment more difficult to perform. Also, remember to look for any medical identification devices, such as bracelets or pendants.

Patient History

Gather a patient history as you would for any patient with a similar emergency. Only if it becomes apparent that your patient is not a reliable source of information should you go to others (Figure 28-5).

It is important to note that elderly patients may deny symptoms of illness or injury. There are many reasons. They may fear leaving home, going to a hospital, or losing independence. They may have concerns about the cost of medical care, ambulance transport, and possible admission to a hospital. They also may be afraid to leave behind a spouse or sibling for whom they provide care. That companion may even be a pet. If at all possible, assist in finding a solution. Sometimes this is as simple as asking if there is someone the patient could telephone for help.

Another issue in obtaining the history of an older adult is that the patient may have only vaguely defined complaints, such as nausea or weakness. This can be true even with serious illness.

Many elderly patients take several medications (Figure 28-6). Ask where the medications are and then read the labels yourself. This is sometimes easier than asking the patient to remember and recite the name of each one.

Ongoing Assessment

The ongoing assessment is the same as for any other patient. However, note that an ill or injured elderly patient is likely to show a slow, steady decline, not a sudden change that would alert you to a deteriorating condition. Do not be lulled into complacency because you observe little or no significant change from one set of vitals to the next. Stay vigilant. Record all vitals and monitor them for any trends that may appear.

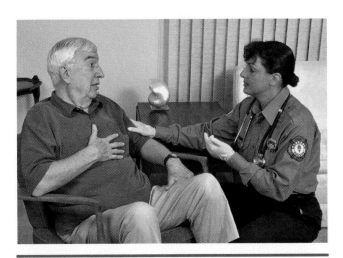

FIGURE 28-5 Just as with any other patient, speak to the elderly patient directly.

: 1. What are some complicating factors that affect the initial assessment of an elderly patient?

2. What are some complicating factors that affect gathering a pertinent past history of an elderly patient?

▶▶ The Call Follow-up

At the beginning of this chapter, you read that First Responders were on scene with a responsive elderly female with an unknown problem. To see how chapter skills apply to this emergency, read the following. It describes how the call was completed.

Scene Size-up *(continued)* "Hello, Mrs. Washington," I said. "My name is John Garcia. I'm from the fire department. What's wrong?" She just continued to sob. So I moved closer and asked again, "Can you tell me why you called 9-1-1, ma'am?" She heard me that time and responded. She said she was very dizzy and could not stand. Then she looked at me with real fear in her eyes and told me she could not tell if it was day or night.

I told her it was daytime, nine o'clock in the morning. As I did, I noticed about 10 bottles of pills on the nightstand by her bed. I wondered, could she have taken too few or too many?

Initial Assessment I continued to try to reassure her as I assessed her ABCs. She was breathing adequately and had a strong pulse. I told her an ambulance was on the way and that we would help her get to the hospital for the care she needed. I also started some oxygen.

Physical Examination I proceeded to take the patient's vital signs and had just started a head-to-toe exam when the paramedics arrived.

Patient History We didn't have time to gather much of a history.

Patient Hand-off I gave a hand-off report to the paramedics (see below). When the paramedics were ready to leave with the patient, Mrs. Washington reached over and asked me to phone her daughter. I wrote down the number she gave me. My partner and I helped the paramedics wheel the patient over the long distance to the elevator and then to the ambulance.

I called the patient's daughter as soon as I could and let her know that her mother had been taken to the hospital. I was glad to hear that she didn't live too far away and would be by her mother's side in a matter of a few hours.

Hand-off Report

"This is Mrs. Adele Washington. She is 75 years old. Her chief complaint is dizziness and confusion about whether it is night or day. She is slow to respond to questions, but she is doing so adequately. ABCs appear normal. We did not have time to perform a physical exam. Check out all of the medications on her nightstand. We also found an empty vial of Synthroid and both home blood-glucose and home blood-pressure testing devices. No interventions at this time."

The Last Word *When you are called to an emergency involving an elderly patient, rely on your patient assessment plan as you would for any patient. Try to be especially respectful and compassionate and keep in mind that an elderly patient's illness or injury may be much more serious than it appears to be.*

Chapter Review

Focus on the EMS Team

Caring for the ill or injured geriatric patient places the First Responder at the beginning of a spectrum of care that the patient will receive. The EMTs who follow you may provide care on scene and on the way to the hospital, where the patient may then receive further care, careful monitoring, and rehabilitation. Remember that your observations in situations such as depression, confusion over medications, the need for injury prevention, and others make your role vitally important.

Summing Up

- A misconception about the elderly is that they cannot live on their own. In fact, a majority of older adults experience good health, are independent, and live active lives.

- However, the functions of all of the body's systems do decline with age. Some important to First Responder assessment and care are:
  - *Skin.* A decrease in perspiration may be a contributing factor to heat-related emergencies. Diaphoresis, a sign of shock, may not occur.
  - *Sensory organs.* Changes in the senses contribute to many unintentional injuries, such as falls, burns, and vehicle crashes, which are the most common mechanisms of injury in the elderly. Changes sight, smell, and taste also contribute to a decreased appetite and nutritional problems.
  - *Respiratory system.* Breathing becomes less effective in the elderly, causing a decreased ability to compensate when they need oxygen.
  - *Heart and blood vessels.* Changes due to age plus medications can cause ill or injured elderly patients to appear to have a normal pulse and blood pressure, causing shock and other conditions to go unrecognized.
  - *Musculoskeletal system.* Even minor falls commonly result in broken bones in the elderly.
  - *Immune system.* Common illnesses, such as influenza, have a higher fatality rate in the elderly. Also, an increased risk of infection and decreased ability to heal make injuries more serious and more often fatal.
  - *Response to medication.* Changes in the elderly patient's ability to respond to and eliminate medications can result in more profound side effects, as well as life-threatening drug interactions. Because the effects of some medications can mask the seriousness of an older adult's injury, those injuries may be more serious than they appear.

- Patient assessment is the same for elderly patients as it is for any patient with a sudden illness or injury. However, there are differences in the general approach to the patient. Remember that the effects of aging and common medications can make the elderly less able to compensate for blood loss and less sensitive to pain. Those factors can mask signs usually associated with serious injury or illness. Be sure to continually reassess your elderly patients for any change in mental status and physical condition.

Key Terms

diaphoresis excessive perspiration.

cataracts opacity of the lens of the eye; the most common cause of blindness in adults.

Knowledge Check

1. Which one of the following factors does NOT contribute to the risk of injury in the elderly?

   a. weakened muscles
   b. diminished vision
   c. increased reaction time
   d. diminished coordination

2. Which of the following factors DECREASE an older adult's ability to compensate for bleeding?

   a. taking aspirin for arthritis pain
   b. taking medication for heart problems
   c. taking medication for high blood pressure
   d. all of the above

3. The elderly patient may underestimate the seriousness of injury because of:
   a. diminished pain sensation.
   b. specific complaints of pain.
   c. diminished sense of hearing.
   d. high fever with illness.

4. Which one of the following can contribute to the risk of injury in the home of an older adult?
   a. bright lighting
   b. throw rugs
   c. bathtub mats
   d. handrails

Scenario

Your First Response unit is called to an apartment complex for a "fall." You arrive to find an elderly male patient on the floor complaining of pain to his hip. The patient seems a bit confused when he tells you that his daughter checked on him "some days" ago. You see stains where he couldn't hold his bladder or bowels. It is a cool spring day, but it seems cold in the apartment.

a. What are some of the changes that occur with aging that may have contributed to this fall?

b. Why might this patient have the heat turned off even though it is cold in the apartment?

c. Is the patient at a higher risk of hypothermia because of his age? Why or why not?

d. What are some causes of falls in the elderly?

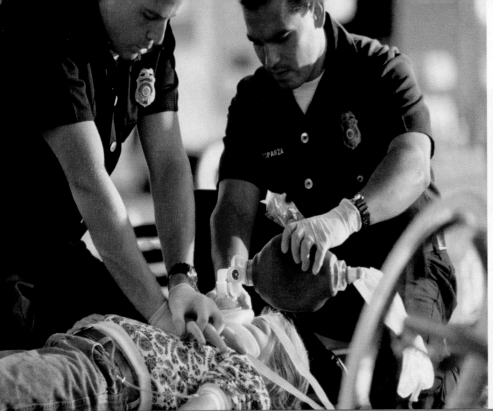
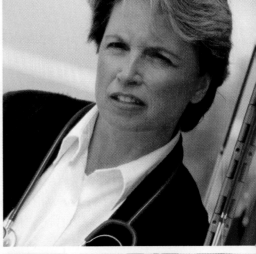
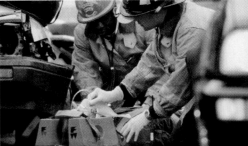

29 | EMS Operations

Objectives

From the U.S. Department of Transportation (DOT)'s 1995 "First Responder: National Standard Curriculum." Material supplemental to the DOT curriculum is listed under "Enrichment."

Cognitive

7-1.1 ▶ Discuss the medical and non-medical equipment needed to respond to a call. (pp. 532–533)

7-1.2 ▶ List the phases of an out-of-hospital call. (pp. 533–534)

Affective

7-1.11 ▶ Explain the rationale for having the unit prepared to respond. (p. 533)

Psychomotor

No objectives are identified by the DOT.

Enrichment

▶ Discuss ways of driving an emergency vehicle safely, including how to use seat belts, lights, and sirens properly. (pp. 535–537)

▶ Describe how to stay safe in traffic on foot and how to park, exit a vehicle, and channel traffic away from a scene. (pp. 537–538)

▶ Discuss safety tips for traveling in the passenger compartment of an ambulance, including how to brace oneself, secure a patient, secure equipment, and perform CPR. (pp. 538–539)

Introduction

The following chapter is meant to provide you with a brief overview of some operational aspects of out-of-hospital emergency care. Learn the six basic phases of an emergency response and become familiar with the medical and non-medical equipment used on scene. Even if you are not required to drive an emergency vehicle, become familiar with emergency vehicle safety. Because you may face situations where you are asked to travel in an ambulance, this chapter also provides related basic safety precautions.

Section 1 Recommended EMS Equipment

When you are on duty, you should have EMS equipment at your disposal. This equipment will include the following items (Figure 29-1):

- Equipment for airway and breathing:
  —Airway adjuncts.
  —Suction devices.
  —Pocket masks or bag-valve masks for artificial ventilation.
  —Automated external defibrillator (AED).

- Equipment for bleeding control and bandaging:
  —Dressings of various types and sizes.
  —Bandages of various types and sizes.
  —Materials to stabilize impaled objects.
  —Sterile saline.
  —Scissors.
  —Adhesive tape.

- Equipment for patient assessment:
  —Stethoscope.
  —Wristwatch with second hand.

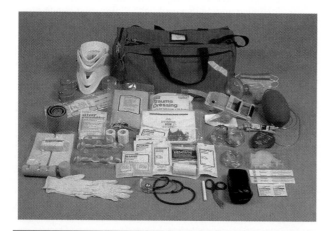

FIGURE 29-1 A basic First Responder jump kit.

  —Pen light.
  —Prehospital-care report forms.
  —Pen and notebook.

- Miscellaneous equipment:
  —OB (obstetric) kit.
  —Blankets.
  —Triage tags.
  —Chemical cold and heat packs.
  —Personal protective equipment for BSI precautions, such as disposable gloves, masks (including HEPA or N-95 respirator), eyewear, and gowns.
  —Antiseptic liquid or wipes, waterless handwashing solution, and bags or containers for contaminated materials.
  —Turnout gear, heavy-duty and puncture-proof gloves, shatter-resistant eye protection, and other clothing—such as waterproof and reflective clothing—that will protect you from environmental hazards.
  —Flares, cones, or reflective triangles for protection against traffic.
  —Fire extinguisher.
  —Flashlight and spare batteries.
  —Local street maps.
  —Latest edition of DOT's *Emergency Response Guidebook* for hazardous materials situations.
  —Personal flotation device.

- Optional equipment. Depending on the skills taught in your area, you may be trained to use some or all of the following:
  —Oxygen administration equipment.
  —Pulse oximeter.
  —Sphygmomanometer.
  —Splints.
  —Backboards.
  —Cervical collars.
  —Body armor.

Even when a First Responder is off duty, you may come upon the scene of an injury or illness. That is why so many First Responders carry personal protective equipment in

THE CALL

Dispatch Our EMS unit was dispatched to the interstate highway for a motor-vehicle collision. That stretch of highway has a reputation for some really bad collisions. We knew from experience that most crashes at this location are caused by lack of visibility. A light grade to the roadbed prevents drivers from seeing the road ahead. Cars go too fast and then can't stop for something in the road. This means that one crash usually turns into five or six.

Scene Size-up As we approached the scene, we saw a disheveled man standing at the top of the grade, waving oncoming traffic around the crash. We were far enough away and going slowly enough for this not to be a problem, but the man was definitely putting himself at risk.

Consider this call as you read Chapter 29. What can the First Responders do to keep the call safe for themselves, other rescuers, bystanders, and the patient?

their own vehicles and in their homes. Be sure you carry only equipment you are authorized to use.

Always use extra caution when off duty. You may not have radio contact or all the protective clothing you are used to having. You also may not be wearing clothing that identifies you as an EMS responder. Take extra time to explain to the patient who you are and that you are trained to help.

Q:
1. What equipment does a First Responder need for airway and breathing care?

2. What equipment does a First Responder need for bleeding control?

3. What BSI equipment does a First Responder need?

Section 2 Phases of a Response

There are six general phases of an EMS response: *preparation, dispatch, en route to the scene, arrival on scene, transfer of care,* and *post-run activities.*

Preparation

In the preparation phase of an EMS response you report for duty and remain available for calls. Obviously, this phase is not the most exciting part of your job, but it may

be the most important. That is because during this time you must check and ready your equipment for service (Figure 29-2). Supplies should be checked each day. They also should be restocked, cleaned, or maintained after each run.

If you drive an EMS vehicle while on duty, inspect it daily. Your employer or volunteer organization should have a clear protocol for performing regular service and maintenance, reporting vehicle problems, and taking vehicles out of service when they are unsafe. Legally, you may be liable for damage caused by a malfunctioning vehicle if you were aware of the problem. You also may be within your rights to refuse to use a vehicle you have reason to believe is unsafe.

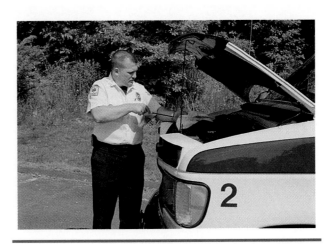

FIGURE 29-2 Check and ready your equipment.

Dispatch

Dispatch is the formal beginning of an EMS response. Dispatchers get important information from callers who report an emergency. That information includes:

- Nature of the call.
- Name, exact location, and call-back number of the caller.
- Location of the patient.
- Number of patients and the severity of the patient's problem.
- Any other special problems or considerations that may be pertinent.

As a First Responder, you may sometimes be the one who activates EMS by calling dispatch (Figure 29-3). Other times, a witness to the emergency will dial 9-1-1. He or she will provide the information to the dispatcher, who will in turn give it to you. Write the information down so you can refer to it en route. Use it to prepare yourself physically and mentally for the call. Do not hesitate to ask the dispatcher to repeat or restate information if anything is unclear.

Note that while you are en route to the scene, an emergency medical dispatcher may give to the caller specific, life-saving instructions to perform until you arrive.

En Route to the Scene

Traveling to the scene involves much more than speed. Responses also must be safe. Excess speed or carelessness will result in a crash, which will at least prevent you from helping the people who need it.

When responding, be sure you know the exact location of the emergency. Have a route planned for your response. Wear your seat belts at all times in moving vehicles. Notify the dispatcher when you have begun your response, so that other emergency teams will be aware you are responding and so that the time may be logged.

Arrival on Scene

Notify dispatch when you arrive on scene. Then approach cautiously. If you have driven to the scene, park your vehicle in a safe place. Then, complete your scene size-up in a rapid, organized, and efficient manner. Once you have determined the scene safe to enter, proceed with your patient assessment plan.

Transfer of Care

By the time the responding EMTs arrive on scene you may already be performing an ongoing assessment and beginning to package your patient. (The term **package** refers to getting the patient ready to be moved and includes procedures such as stabilizing impaled objects and immobilizing injured limbs.)

Be prepared to give a concise and accurate patient hand-off report (Figure 29-4). Also, be ready to assist the EMTs with packaging or lifting and moving, if they request your help.

Post-Run Activities

Report to dispatch when you return to your station. Then, after you turn in your prehospital care report, prepare for your next call. This means cleaning and disinfecting any equipment that may have become soiled as per your local protocols. Replace any disposable supplies. Change any soiled clothing. Fuel your vehicle, if necessary. Then notify dispatch that you are in service and ready for another call.

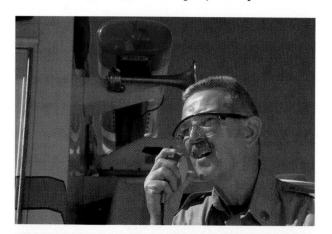

FIGURE 29-3 Dispatch is the formal beginning of an EMS response.

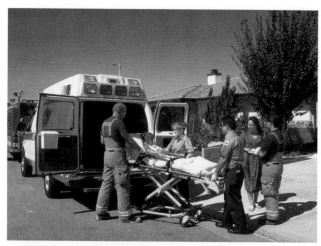

FIGURE 29-4 After hand-off, be prepared to assist the EMTs if you are asked to do so.

:

1. In which of the six phases of an EMS response do you check and ready your equipment?

2. Why should you notify dispatch that you have begun your response? During what phase of an EMS response should you do so?

3. What are your responsibilities during the phase called "transfer of care"?

Section 3 Emergency Vehicle Safety

Many rescuers spend a lot of time in traffic, both by driving and by moving around on foot at emergency scenes. If you have not had a basic safety course, check into the possibility of enrolling in one. It is a good idea to take advantage of refresher courses, too.

Driving Safely

Basic Safety Tips

Statistics show that haste is unnecessary in most emergency runs. The experts maintain that only about 3% to 5% of all runs are true life-or-death situations. Unless the situation is critical, travel at the posted speed limit. Excess speed makes an emergency vehicle less stable and poses a greater risk to you and others.

Much of driver safety depends on common sense and good judgment. The following basic tips can improve driver safety:

■ Learn all local and state guidelines related to driving emergency vehicles before you drive one. By law you

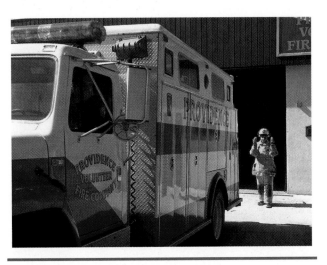

FIGURE 29-5 Travel in pairs. The rescuer who is not driving can help make sure patient and vehicle arrive safely.

must always exercise due regard for the safety of others, and that includes yourself.

■ When you can, travel in pairs. For example, the rescuer who is not driving can help the driver find the route, clear right-hand intersections, watch the road, and in case of litigation, act as a witness who can substantiate the record.

■ If you need to back up your vehicle, do so slowly and carefully. Use all available mirrors. Have your partner take a position near the rear of the vehicle to act as a spotter (Figure 29-5).

■ Know your territory. Take alternate routes whenever possible to avoid potential problems such as tunnels, bridges, and railroad crossings. Besides the obvious advantage of arriving on scene more quickly, when you know your territory you also can avoid collisions caused by trying to read a map while you drive.

■ Exercise extra caution when traveling in congested traffic, such as rush-hour traffic in urban areas or areas just around industrial centers at shift change.

■ Sudden braking is especially dangerous at high speeds. Remember that stopping time increases dramatically as speed increases. Plan for it.

■ If the nature of the emergency requires you to drive at increased speeds, practice special caution on curves and hills. Brake to a safe and comfortable speed before you enter a curve. Stay on the outside of the curve (Figure 29-6). Speed up carefully, gradually, and steadily as you leave the curve. When traveling down hills, use a lower gear instead of the brakes to maintain control of the vehicle.

 First on Scene

What factors influence EMS response times in your community? It is important for you to know and plan for them. For example:

■ *Time of day and day of the week.* In some towns and cities, weekdays have the heaviest traffic due to commuters. In resort areas, weekend traffic may be heavier. For your area, use a detailed map to mark trouble spots and plan alternative routes for peak traffic times.

■ *Temporary construction sites.* Road maintenance and building construction sites can seriously impede traffic flow. As soon as you learn of them, plan alternative routes or detours accordingly.

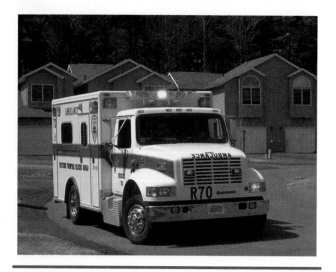

FIGURE 29-6 Use extra caution when on curves and hills.

Wearing Seat Belts

When in an emergency vehicle, always wear proper safety restraints, including lap and shoulder belts—whether or not you are required by law to do so. Fasten them before you start the ignition. Keep them on until you have turned off the ignition.

Never take off safety restraints as you approach the emergency scene. Research shows that the last two intersections before arriving on scene are especially dangerous to rescue drivers, who try to save time by disengaging restraints.

Using Lights and Sirens

Whenever you respond to an emergency in a vehicle, use headlights and emergency lights even during the daytime. They can help to alert other drivers in case emergency lights blend in with traffic lights, the tail lights of cars traveling in opposite directions, the color of buildings, or holiday decorations. Use minimal lighting in heavy fog. Turn off headlights when you park. If you need to alert oncoming traffic while parked, leave the emergency lights on.

Always use emergency lights and sirens as required by your local protocols. Note, however, that a siren has a bizarre effect on the driver of an emergency vehicle. Some drivers are easily hypnotized by a siren and lose the ability to negotiate curves and turns. A siren also can disorient or panic drivers. (Never pull up behind another driver and blast the siren.) Finally, a siren may not be effective, because often it is not heard. Insulation in newer vehicles can mask the sound of an approaching siren, as can a loud radio, conversation, pelting rain, thunder, dense shrubbery, trees, and buildings. To clear traffic quickly, use your vehicle's horn in conjunction with emergency lights and siren.

A significant safety advantage is to turn off your lights and siren as you approach the scene of an injury or illness. Lights and sirens attract crowds and can add to the chaos that already may exist. If hostile people are on scene, you can take the first step toward calming and controlling the scene by arriving discreetly.

Remember that once you turn off your lights and siren, you are no longer driving an "authorized" emergency vehicle. You are subject to all the laws meant to govern regular traffic.

Protecting Your Hearing

Chronic exposure to loud noises poses a danger to hearing. The trauma associated with repeated loud noise can cause permanent hearing loss. If your EMS system allows First Responders to drive or ride in emergency vehicles, take the following precautions to protect your hearing:

- Keep the windows closed while the siren is in use.
- Wear approved hearing-protection devices to protect your ears. Be aware that these devices may prevent you from hearing other emergency vehicles as they approach. Use caution and always follow local protocol.
- If you can, move the siren speakers from the top of the cab to the front grille. This move can reduce the decibel level by about 5%.

Avoid prolonged or repeated loud noise off the job, too. Protect yourself against loud music, high-volume radios and televisions, loud chain saws, lawn mowers, hydraulic tools, generators, and other noise.

Driving an Ambulance

As soon as a patient is loaded into an ambulance, the driver is responsible for at least three lives—his or her own, a partner's, and the patient's. In many cases there also may be multiple patients, family members, other helpers, or student riders. Most ambulances accommodate as many as six.

If your EMS system allows First Responders to drive ambulances, follow these guidelines to help ensure a safe trip:

- Except in the most critical situations, do not exceed the posted speed limit. Excess speed is unsafe for everyone in the ambulance, especially for the patient. Speed poses special hazards at intersections and on curves.
- Start and stop smoothly. Make the transition from one speed to another gradually to avoid aggravating the patient's illness or injury.
- Drive at a steady but safe speed. If you keep your speed even, you often can time your approach to intersections and travel through with the green light. Also avoid weaving through traffic. It can compromise the patient.

- Whenever you can, avoid rough dirt roads, potholes, and other hazards that can jostle the patient. The inner two lanes of a four-lane highway are the smoothest. The lane closest to the gutter on city streets is the roughest. If you see that you are going to drive over a bump, railroad tracks, or a stretch of rough road, warn those in the back so they can protect themselves.

As part of a driver-training program, many drivers are required to lie on the stretcher while the instructor drives the ambulance. Even at low to moderate speeds, the experience from the point of view of the patient is often enlightening. (Do not use the lights or sirens or drive at increased speeds for training purposes unless you are at an approved training facility.)

Staying Safe in Traffic on Foot

As soon as you get out of your vehicle on scene, you are at risk from oncoming traffic. Even while your focus is on the patient, or the scene itself, you must never compromise your own safety.

Parking for Maximum Safety

Turn off your headlights as soon as you park to prevent blinding oncoming drivers. If necessary, leave parking lights on or leave vehicle warning lights flashing to warn oncoming traffic.

Whenever you can, park on the shoulder of the road or in a driveway, in front of or behind the crash scene. Never park alongside a crash. If you are on a one- or two-lane road with no accessible parking areas, position your vehicle so that it blocks the entire roadway. This should prevent other vehicles from squeezing by. When the police are at the scene, follow their directions for vehicle placement.

An important part of ensuring your safety is to visually scan the scene as you approach. Notice areas of vulnerability or potential danger. Pinpoint places where you could seek concealment or protection. If you are with a partner, plan how you will approach before doing so. You may decide that your partner will go to the passenger who is still in the green car, for example, and you will go to the driver who is lying on the gravel.

Protect yourself from environmental hazards on scene by parking at a safe distance. Park at least 100 feet away from a burning vehicle and at least 2,000 feet from a scene involving hazardous materials. Whenever possible, park uphill and upwind of any hazardous material or fire. Avoid parking on or driving over spilled liquids and broken glass.

Exiting a Vehicle Safely

A specific transition takes place as soon as you leave your vehicle. You move from your "sanctuary" to someone else's

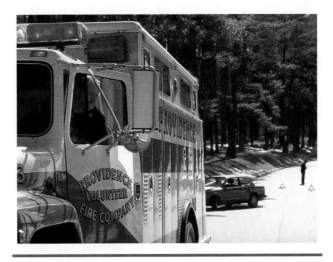

FIGURE 29-7 Slowly and cautiously open the door when exiting your vehicle.

turf, and that makes you vulnerable. Follow these tips for the greatest protection:

- Before you open the door, check the rear-view mirror to determine how much traffic is approaching from behind. If you can, wait a minute or two until traffic passes (Figure 29-7).

- Open your door slowly to alert passing motorists that you are getting out. Move carefully but quickly away from passing or oncoming traffic.

- If you have passengers in the rear compartment, have them get out through the rear doors instead of a side door, which might open into passing traffic.

- Be especially cautious about hazards at the scene, such as broken glass, twisted metal, or spilled gasoline. Immediately assess any crash involving trucks for hazardous materials.

- If the scene is safe to enter, walk purposefully to the patient. Running is a signal to others that you are out of control, and it causes your heart to race. The boost to your pulse and adrenaline levels can hinder your ability to effectively treat the patient.

Wearing Protective Equipment

Plenty of rescues take place outdoors in the dark and in bad weather. An essential for every rescuer is reflective clothing. That includes reflective tape at least, and a reflective vest or other gear if you have access to them. If you are channeling traffic away from the crash scene while waiting for police, it is essential that you wear as much reflective gear as possible. It will help you to be visible to drivers who may have pitted windshields, frayed windshield wipers, or drug or alcohol impairment.

Depending on the situation, consider the following protective gear:

- If there is any risk of falling debris, wear an impact-resistant protective helmet with reflective tape and a strap under the chin.

- In situations where splashing may occur (including splashing of blood and body fluids), wear safety goggles specified for work with power equipment. If you usually wear eyeglasses, get clip-on side shields.

- To protect yourself against the cold, wear gloves, a warm hat, long underwear, and several layers of medium-weight clothing.

Channeling Traffic Away from the Scene

While waiting for the arrival of law enforcement, you need to channel traffic away from the scene. This is not only for the safety of patients and bystanders but also for your own safety and that of other rescuers. Your goals should be:

- To channel the regular flow of traffic around the scene, preventing additional collisions and injuries.

- To monitor traffic to ensure minimal disruption.

- To clear the scene so that other emergency vehicles can reach the patients quickly.

Unless there is a distinct hazard that dictates otherwise, keep traffic moving. Even if the roadway is blocked, try to reroute traffic to an alternate road rather than bring traffic to a standstill. To effectively channel traffic you need additional rescue personnel and attention-getting devices such as flares, chemical lights, or reflective cones. Follow these general guidelines:

- Make sure all those who are channeling traffic are wearing adequate reflective clothing or tape so that they can be clearly seen by approaching drivers.

- Visual signals given by rescuers must be clear. Approaching drivers need to understand quickly and exactly what you want them to do.

- Place flares, chemical lights, or reflective cones 10 to 15 feet apart and approximately 100 feet toward the oncoming traffic.

If the collision is on a two-lane highway, the flares or cones should be placed in both directions. On a curve or hill, place them at the beginning of the curve or at the crest of the hill. They should direct motorists around the crash scene, at least 50 feet from wrecked cars. Use this general rule: the flares or cones should begin far enough from the scene so that a car can safely stop before it hits the scene, even if the driver did not notice the flares or cones from a distance.

Many EMS systems recommend the use of reflective cones instead of flares because of possible burns while lighting or using flares, the need to keep lighting new flares as old ones extinguish, the difficulty of keeping flares working in bad weather, and the possibility of toxins from the smoke. Follow local protocol.

The Patient Compartment

If you are part of an ambulance team or if you assist other EMS providers, you face tremendous hazards every time you climb into the patient compartment. It is normal and necessary to move around in the compartment as you treat the patient. However, too few rescuers remember to protect their own safety. Using appropriate restraints and learning to position yourself can help to prevent injury en route to the hospital.

Whenever you do not need to move around in the patient compartment, wear proper restraints such as a safety harness.

Hanging on and Bracing

The principle of hanging on is one borrowed from rock climbers. You have four possible points of contact with the ambulance: two hands and two feet. At any one time, you must maintain at least three-point contact for optimum safety and stability. In other words, you should never have more than one hand or one foot at a time off a stable surface in the patient compartment. Do not forget your fifth point of contact—the seat of your pants. Follow these tips:

- To maintain the greatest stability, keep a wide base of support. Keep your feet at about shoulder width. Do not place your hands too close together.

- If you need to reach for something, keep both feet planted firmly on the floor. Grasp a stable object, such as the overhead bar, with your free hand.

- If you need to walk, even a single step, hold on to a stable object with both hands. Slide your hands along as you walk instead of moving arm-over-arm. If you need equipment, try putting it down and sliding it.

- Even when you are sitting, hook your feet under the stretcher bar to give yourself increased stability.

Bracing means to exert an opposing force against two parts of the ambulance with your body (Figure 29-8). It provides additional stability and protection. You can use your hands, feet, knees, or any combination of hip, shoulder, knees, and hands. You can exert yourself against any solid surface in the patient compartment, such as the squad bench or an interior wall. For greatest stability and safety, keep your center of gravity low. For women, the center of gravity is the hips. For men, it is the shoulders.

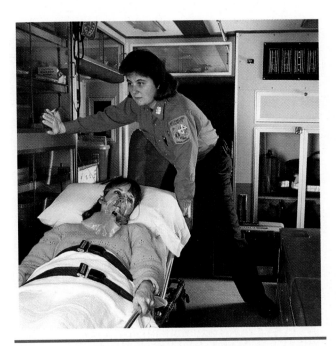

FIGURE 29-8 Hanging on and bracing help you to achieve optimum safety.

Securing the Patient

There are two reasons to firmly secure the patient in the compartment. First, you want to protect any patient from the risk of additional injury. Second, if the patient is hostile, you need to protect yourself and the patient from potential injury.

In the case of nonhostile patients:

- Secure anyone sitting with a seat belt.
- Place a pregnant woman in the captain's chair, since the lateral force from sudden stops is much less pronounced there than on the squad bench.
- If the patient is on a stretcher, use snug but comfortable straps across the lower chest (but not over the arms) and just above the knees. Then, secure the stretcher to the bar. If local protocol allows, use additional straps. If the patient's medical condition allows, elevate the head of the stretcher slightly to ease the patient's anxiety over sudden stops.

When assisting in the restraint of hostile patients, follow these guidelines:

- Never restrain a patient in a prone position. Use a supine position and be ready to protect the airway.
- Never apply restraints maliciously. Laws vary from one state to another about how and when restraints can be used. Use restraints only as a last resort to protect your safety. Document why they were necessary in your written report.

- Once you restrain a patient, never remove the restraints, even if the patient calms down. The patient should stay restrained until you arrive at the hospital.
- Whenever possible, use soft restraints. A quick and easy one is made by folding a gauze bandage in half, slipping it over your hand, and turning it over on itself. You can then loop these over the patient's wrists and ankles. Secure the ends in a bow-tie knot far enough from the patient's hands so they cannot be untied. Combine regular strapping over the chest and knees with soft restraints at the ankles and wrists.

Securing Equipment

If an ambulance is involved in a crash, especially a rollover, any unsecured piece of equipment could become a projectile that can injure you and the patient. As part of the clean up at the end of each ambulance run, secure all equipment. Stow it in appropriate storage areas, and secure doors shut with latches. Clamp heavy items to appropriate brackets. Use straps to secure portable gear. Devise hooks to keep bench tops closed.

Performing CPR in a Moving Ambulance

While you are performing CPR in an ambulance, you are in a risky position. You cannot maintain three-point contact. You cannot brace yourself adequately, and you cannot secure yourself in a seat belt. To improve your safety:

- Position your feet at least at shoulder width for the best possible base.
- Have someone sit on the squad bench and grasp the back of your belt. If the ambulance suddenly accelerates, the person hanging onto you can keep you from catapulting.
- Try for as much bracing as you can. Bend your knees into the side of the stretcher, wedge your feet against the squad bench, or brace one knee against the stretcher and the other against the squad bench.
- Do not brace yourself with your head. Your neck will not withstand the pressure.

 1. What are three basic tips for driving safely?

2. When should you take off your seat belt? Why?

3. How can a rescuer on foot stay safe in traffic?

4. What can you do to protect your own safety inside the patient compartment of an ambulance?

The Call Follow-up

At the beginning of this chapter, you read about a motor-vehicle collision at a place in the road known for its limited visibility. To see how chapter skills apply to this emergency, read the following. It describes how the call was completed.

Scene Size-up *(continued)* We placed the first response vehicle at the top of the grade so that it served as protection and an extra warning. At that time, we told the man who had been waving traffic away that his job was done and that we would take over from here. When we considered it safe, we exited our vehicle, watching our backs for traffic. Since we arrived before the state patrol, we immediately set up a pattern of flares and reflectors over 1,000 feet in front of the crash scene to protect ourselves. Then, we continued to size up the scene for other hazards, put on our gloves, and approached the crash vehicles. We saw a driver for each of the two vehicles present. They were standing by their cars. There were no passengers.

Initial Assessment My partner went to driver #1, and I went to driver #2. They both seemed alert. We led them over to the guard rail and out of traffic, introduced ourselves, and asked them what had happened. As we talked, we determined that airway and breathing were normal. We also saw no bleeding or any other obvious signs of injury.

Physical Examination The patients allowed us to check their vital signs and for possible injuries. Neither had any complaints. We could find no obvious signs of injury. However, we convinced them to stick around until the EMTs and the police got to the scene.

Patient History The ambulance arrived before we could get a history.

Ongoing Assessment We were only able to examine the patients once. They both refused any further assessments.

Patient Hand-off When the ambulance arrived, we told the crew what we had (see below). Neither of the patients wanted to be transported. We left our vehicle in position to protect the scene until the tire was changed and all other vehicles were cleared.

 ## Hand-off Report

"Patient #1 is Damen Merilli, 23 years old. He was changing his right front tire at the side of the road when the second car sideswiped his as it came over the grade. He reports no injuries. His baseline vitals are respiration 14 and pulse 66. The driver of the second car is Kyle Rau, 20 years old. He also reports no injuries. Baseline vitals are respiration 20, pulse 78. Both refused any further assessment."

The Last Word *Most basic training programs for rescuers teach how to react safely to a variety of dangers. However, the most common threat to safety is likely to be something as simple as oncoming traffic or the way an emergency vehicle is driven. Be prepared. Have the knowledge, equipment, and skills that allow you to meet the standards set by your EMS system for each phase of an emergency response.*

Chapter Review

Focus on the EMS Team

Simply stated, this chapter is about all of the things that must go on in order to make a call run smoothly. Things like preparation and driving to the scene may not seem to be as exciting as assessing or caring for a patient, but they are in fact essential. As a member of the EMS team, your responsibilities begin long before and continue long after patient care, and your fellow EMS team members depend on you to perform them well. Your preparation before a call, your response, and even your restocking after a call all set the foundation for the success of emergency patient care.

Summing Up

- EMS equipment you should have at your disposal includes equipment for airway and breathing care, bleeding control and bandaging, patient assessment, and BSI and other personal protective equipment. If authorized and trained to use them, you should also have: oxygen administration equipment, splints, backboards, and AEDs.

- There are six general phases of an EMS response:
  - *Preparation.* Report for duty and remain available for calls; check and ready your equipment; restock, clean, and maintain supplies. Also, service and maintain your emergency response vehicle.
  - *Dispatch.* Write down the information the dispatcher gives you. It should include the nature of the call; name of the caller, exact location, and call-back number; location of patient; number of patients and severity of problem; other considerations.
  - *En route to the scene.* Notify the dispatcher when you have begun your response. Travel safely on a route planned for your response.
  - *Arrival on scene.* Notify dispatch when you arrive on scene. Perform a scene size-up. Call for and wait for assistance if the scene is unsafe. Once safe, proceed with your patient assessment plan.
  - *Transfer of care.* Give a concise and accurate patient hand-off report to the EMTs who take over patient care. Assist them as requested.
  - *Post-run activities.* Report to dispatch when you return to your station. After you turn in your prehospital care report, prepare for your next call. Then notify dispatch that you are in service and ready for another call.

- Drive your emergency vehicle safely as per local and state guidelines. Always exercise due regard for the safety of others. When you can, travel in pairs. Know your territory and take routes appropriate for the time of day, weather, and so on. Wear your seatbelt! Always use emergency lights and sirens as required by your local protocols, even during the daytime.

- If you drive an ambulance, do not exceed the posted speed limit, except in the most critical situations. When possible, avoid any hazard that can jostle the patient.

- Park for maximum safety. Never park alongside a crash. Park uphill, upwind, and at least 100 feet away from a burning vehicle and at least 2,000 feet from a scene involving hazardous materials. Exercise caution when exiting a vehicle.

- Traffic control includes channeling traffic around the scene, causing a minimum of disruption in traffic flow, and clearing traffic so other emergency vehicles have access.

- Inside the ambulance patient compartment, maintain at least three-point contact for optimum safety and stability. Secure the patient, the patient's stretcher, all equipment, and passengers.

Key Terms

package refers to getting the patient ready to be moved; includes procedures such as stabilizing impaled objects and immobilizing injured limbs.

bracing exerting an opposing force against two parts of a solid surface, such as an interior wall of an ambulance, with your body.

Knowledge Check

1. Emergencies that are true life-or-death emergencies and require a very fast response make up roughly ___ of all EMS responses.
   a. 95%
   b. 50%
   c. 25%
   d. 5%

2. When EMTs from the ambulance arrive, you should be prepared to:
   a. leave the scene.
   b. notify dispatch.
   c. give a hand-off report.
   d. perform a scene size-up.

3. For traffic control, a First Responder's goal is to:
   a. protect the scene and keep traffic moving.
   b. surround the scene and stop traffic.
   c. clear the scene and maintain traffic.
   d. block the scene and slow traffic.

4. If a First Responder must restrain a hostile patient, the position the patient should be in is a(n) ___ position.
   a. fetal
   b. prone
   c. supine
   d. anatomical

5. Some 9-1-1 dispatchers are allowed to give emergency care instructions to callers while EMS is en route to the scene.
   a. True
   b. False

6. Driving with lights and sirens activated is more dangerous than routine driving.
   a. True
   b. False

7. List the equipment you should have at your disposal for bleeding control and bandaging.

_____   _____

_____   _____

_____   _____

8. List the equipment you should have at your disposal for patient assessment.

_____   _____

_____   _____

_____   _____

9. List the types of information you should receive from dispatch at the beginning of a call.

_____

_____

_____

_____

_____

Scenario

You are a volunteer in a community First Responder organization. You stop by the station at the start of your shift. The other member of your crew is there waiting for you. After talking together about what has happened since the last shift, you open the door to the truck to check your kits. "Oh come on," your partner moans. "The truck hasn't gone out for almost 48 hours. Why bother checking it?"

a. Why would you check the equipment?

_____

_____

_____

b. What would you say to your partner?

_____

_____

_____

c. What would happen if you responded to a call and you did not have a required piece of equipment?

_____

_____

_____

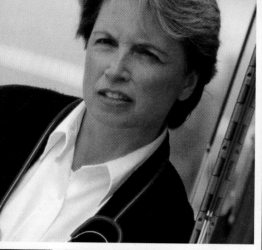
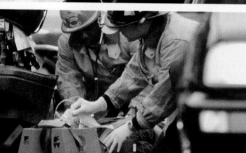
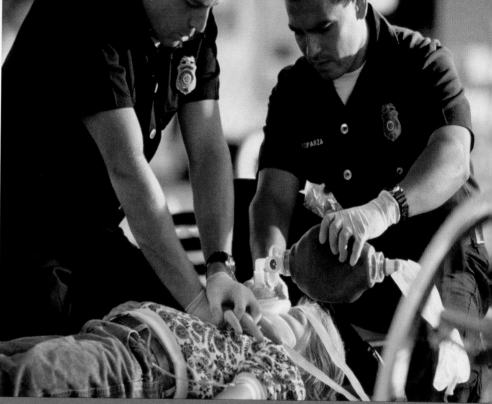

30 | Hazardous Materials Incidents and Emergencies

Objectives

From the U.S. Department of Transportation (DOT)'s 1995 "First Responder: National Standard Curriculum." Material supplemental to the DOT curriculum is listed under "Enrichment."

Cognitive

7-1.6 ▶ Describe what the First Responder should do if there is reason to believe that there is a hazard at the scene. (pp. 549–551)

7-1.7 ▶ State the role the First Responder should perform until appropriately trained personnel arrive at the scene of a hazardous materials situation. (p. 549)

Affective

No objectives are identified by the DOT.

Psychomotor

No objectives are identified by the DOT.

Enrichment

▶ Explain what hazardous materials are. (p. 545)

▶ Identify the training required to respond to a hazardous materials emergency. (p. 548)

▶ Discuss how to recognize the presence of a hazardous material at the scene of an emergency. (pp. 546–548)

▶ Describe the actions that need to be taken at the scene of a hazardous materials emergency. (pp. 549–551)

▶ Identify the resources that may be called upon once a hazardous materials incident is recognized. (p. 548)

Introduction

Over 50 billion tons of hazardous materials are made in the U.S. every year. To manage the risk to the public, our government has developed specific regulations. Unfortunately, hazardous materials still may be spilled or released accidentally. This chapter provides a brief overview of hazardous materials emergencies. As a First Responder, you are not required to deal with these materials. That takes specialized training and equipment. Instead, it is your job to recognize and report a hazardous materials emergency.

Section 1 Hazardous Materials

Hazardous materials are those that in any quantity pose a threat or unreasonable risk to life, health, or property if not properly controlled. They include chemicals, wastes, and other dangerous products. The principal dangers they present are **toxicity, flammability,** and **reactivity.** Hazardous materials commonly shipped in the U.S. are explosives, compressed and poisonous gases, flammable solids and liquids, oxidizers, corrosives, and radioactive materials.

Hazardous materials, or **hazmats,** may be transported directly to the user. Natural gas, for example, travels by fixed pipeline. However, most often they travel by rail and on local, state, and federal highways.

Hazardous materials also may be located in your community. For example, is there a hospital in your area that practices nuclear medicine? It will have radioactive materials and contaminated wastes. What about lawn and garden companies or farms? They usually stock fertilizers, insecticides, and pesticides. Businesses use a wide variety of hazardous materials for various purposes. Grocery stores, for instance, refrigerate produce with freezers cooled by ammonia. In addition, hazardous materials are used to manufacture products and are often the waste products of manufacturing.

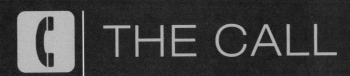

THE CALL

Dispatch I was working security, patrolling the lower level of the mall when I received a radio call: "Team A, respond to the lower entrance near the restaurant. Investigate a report of fumes and people with trouble breathing. Time out 22:03."

Scene Size-up As I approached the scene, I slowed my pace. Ahead I could see dozens of people streaming out of the restaurant. Many were bent over, trying to catch their breaths. Mike, the manager of the restaurant, ran over to me. He told me that the cleaning people were working in the kitchen. One of them mixed bleach, ammonia, and the "green stuff" together, which caused the problem.

I radioed communications. "We have a possible hazardous materials release. Please begin the Chemical Incident Plan. I will be incident command. Have emergency services respond to my location. Advise them that we have chemical fumes from a mixture of bleach, ammonia, and a green-soap solution." Scanning the area quickly, I added, "We have about 26 people with trouble breathing. Medical assistance is needed immediately."

Consider this situation as you read Chapter 30. What else may be done to ensure scene safety? Are all 26 people injured? How can they be treated appropriately and as fast as they need it?

Hazardous Materials Warning Labels

DOMESTIC LABELING

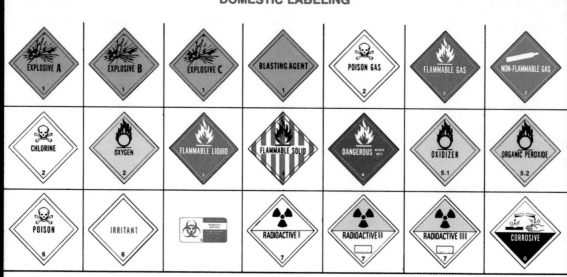

General Guidelines on Use of Labels
(CFR, Title 49, Transportation, Parts 100-177)

- Labels illustrated above are normally for *domestic shipments*. However, some air carriers *may* require the use of International Civil Aviation Organization (ICAO) labels.
- Domestic Warning Labels *may* display UN Class Number, Division Number (and Compatibilty Group for Explosives only) [Sec. 172.407(g)].
- Any person who offers a hazardous material for transportation MUST label the package, if required [Sec. 172.400(a)].
- The Hazardous Materials Tables, Sec. 172.101 and 172.102, identify the proper label(s) for the hazardous materials listed.

- Label(s), when required, must be printed on or affixed to the surface of the package near the proper shipping name [Sec. 172.406(a)].
- When two or more different labels are required, display them next to each other [Sec. 172.406(c)].
- Labels may be affixed to packages (even when not required by regulations) provided each label represents a hazard of the material in the package [Sec. 172.401].

**Check the Appropriate Regulations
Domestic or international Shipment**

Additional Markings and Labels

HANDELING LABELS

 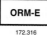

Cargo Aircraft Only 172.402(b) | ORM-E 172.316 | Package Orientation Markings 172.312(a)(c)

Bung Label 172.402(e) | INNER PACKAGES COMPLY WITH PRESCRIBED SPECIFICATIONS 173.25(a)(4) | Fumigation 173.9 | EMPTY 173.427

Here are a few additional markings and labels pertaining to the transport of hazardous materials. The section number shown with each item refers to the appropriate section in the HMR. The Hazardous Materials Tables, Section 172.101 and 172.102, identify the proper shipping name, hazard class, identification number, required label(s) and packaging sections.

Poisonous Materials

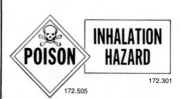

POISON 172.505 | INHALATION HAZARD 172.301

Materials which meet the inhalation toxicity criteria specified in Section 173.3a(b)(2), have additional "communication standards" prescribed by the HMR. First, the words "Poison-Inhalation Hazard" must be entered on the shipping paper, as required by Section 172.203(k)(4), for any primary capacity units with a capacity greater than one liter. Second, packages of 110 gallons or less capacity must be marked "Inhalation Hazard" in accordance with Section 172.301(a). Lastly, transport vehicles, freight containers and portable tanks subkject to the shipping paper requirements contained in Section 172.203(k)(4) must be placarded with POISON placards in addition to the placards required by Section 172.504 For additional information adn exceptions to these communication requirements, see the referenced sections in the HMR.

Keep a copy of the DOT Emergency Response Guidebook handy!

FIGURE 30-1 The DOT requires packages and storage containers to be marked with specific hazard labels.

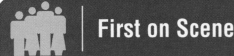

First on Scene

Hazardous materials can be found in more places than in tractor trailers. Remember that even household cleaners can cause a reaction as deadly as most you can find on the highway. Be prepared.

First on Scene

Never endanger yourself—or have others endanger themselves—in order to retrieve shipping papers from the scene of a hazardous materials incident. The risk does not outweigh the benefit.

Placards and Shipping Papers

The U.S. Department of Transportation (DOT) requires packages and containers to be marked with specific hazard labels. Placards are required on the outside of vehicles carrying hazardous materials. The driver of the vehicle also must have *shipping papers,* which identify the exact substance, quantity, origin, and destination. (See Figures 30-1 and 30-2.)

A **placard** is usually a four-sided, diamond-shaped sign. Many are red or orange. A few are white or green. Whatever the color, the placard contains a four-digit number and a legend. They identify the material as flammable, radioactive, explosive, or poisonous.

Shipping papers are sometimes called "manifests" or "waybills." They are another important means of

identifying hazardous materials. If you can locate them, shipping papers have the name of the substance, the danger it presents, and a four-digit identification number.

The National Fire Protection Association (NFPA) uses the NFPA 704 system (Figure 30-3). This system is generally used on fixed structures such as buildings. Its diamond-shaped symbol identifies danger with the use of color and numbers. The color blue indicates a health hazard. Red indicates a fire hazard. Yellow shows a reactivity hazard. White is used for information such as the need for protective equipment. Numbers used are 0 to 4. For example, 1 in a blue diamond and 4 in a red diamond mean the material presents a low health hazard but is very flammable.

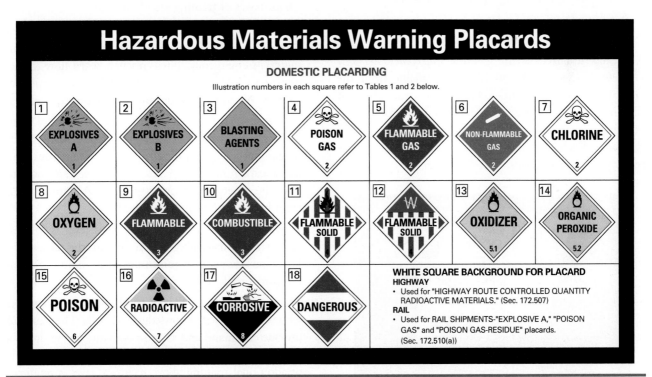

FIGURE 30-2 The DOT also requires display placards to be put on the outside of vehicles carrying hazardous materials.

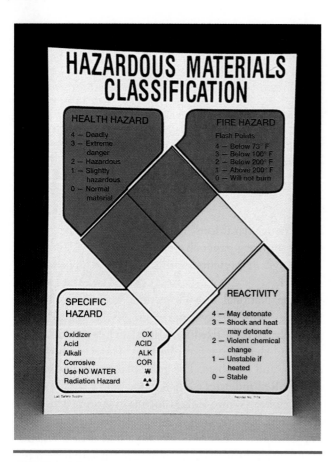

FIGURE 30-3 The NFPA 704 System helps you to identify health, reactivity, and fire hazards.

Available Resources

A special resource is the DOT's *Emergency Response Guidebook.* (See Figure 30-4.) It is available from the Government Printing Office. Carry it in your vehicle at all times. It includes a table of commonly used DOT labels and placards. That table is correlated with lists of chemicals. Each item in the lists is keyed to specific emergency action instructions.

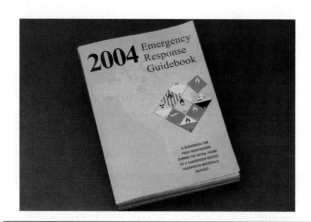

FIGURE 30-4 The DOT's *Emergency Response Guidebook.*

Material safety data sheets (MSDS) offer another resource. Under federal regulations, all employees working with hazardous materials have a right to know about the dangers of those materials. So, all manufacturers are required to provide MSDS on hazardous materials. These sheets generally name the substance, physical properties, and fire, explosion, and health hazards. Emergency first aid also is usually listed.

The Chemical Transportation Emergency Center (CHEMTREC) is a toll-free 24-hour emergency phone service provided by chemical manufacturers. They advise rescuers on the nature of a product and the steps to take to manage an incident. They also may contact the shipper, who will provide detailed information and field assistance. The CHEMTREC number is 1-800-424-9300.

Another important resource is the regional poison control center and your own system's medical direction. They can guide you in decontamination and treatment.

Training Required by Law

People can get hurt or lose their lives in hazmat emergencies. The Occupational Safety and Health Administration (OSHA) and the Environmental Protection Agency (EPA) have developed safety regulations. See the OSHA publication "29 CFR 1910-120—Hazardous Waste Operations and Emergency Response Standard (1989)."

Four levels of training are identified:

- *First Responder Awareness.* This level of training is for those who are likely to witness or discover a hazardous materials emergency. These rescuers learn how to recognize a problem and how to call for the proper resources. No minimum training hours are required.

- *First Responder Operations.* This level of training is for rescuers who initially respond to a hazmat emergency to protect people, property, and the environment. They learn how to keep at a safe distance and how to stop the emergency from spreading. A minimum of eight hours of training is required.

- *Hazardous Materials Technician.* This level is for rescuers who actually plug, patch, or stop the release of a hazardous material. A minimum of 24 hours of training is required.

- *Hazardous Materials Specialist.* This level is for rescuers who want advanced knowledge and skills. They learn to provide command and support activities at the site of a hazardous materials emergency. A minimum of 24 hours of additional training above technical level is required.

Note that the National Fire Protection Association (NFPA) has published Standard #473, which deals with competencies for EMS personnel at hazmat emergencies.

1. What are some hazardous materials commonly shipped in the U.S.?

2. What is the *Emergency Response Guidebook?* How is it organized?

3. What are four levels of hazmat training described by OSHA?

Section 2 Hazmat Emergency Guidelines

Many hazmat incidents are dispatched as vehicle collisions, poisonings, or unknown problem calls. Your initial actions build the crucial groundwork for the remainder of the incident. Your specific responsibilities include:

- Recognize the emergency as a hazmat incident.
- Position yourself in a safe location.
- Identify the hazardous materials.
- Establish command and control zones.
- Establish a medical treatment sector.

As always, your first priority is your own safety. *Never attempt a hazardous materials rescue unless you are properly trained and equipped.* If you have no training, radio immediately for help. While you are waiting, protect yourself and bystanders by keeping away from the danger. Avoid contact with any unidentified material, regardless of the level of protection offered by your clothing and equipment.

Recognizing a Hazmat Incident

Always consider the possibility of a hazmat incident. For example, if you are called to an unknown emergency, ask yourself: Is the call to the location of a previous hazmat incident? Is there an emergency plan for the location, which generally indicates that a risk exists? Use all the pre-arrival information available to you to decide on the best course of action.

As you approach the scene, use binoculars to begin to size it up (Figure 30-5). Identify any placards on vehicles, buildings, or containers (Figure 30-6). Proceed as always with caution. Too many First Responders discover a hazmat incident only after they are in the middle of it. Use all of your senses, coupled with a high index of suspicion. Visual clues can indicate a possible hazardous material:

- Smoking or self-igniting materials.
- Extraordinary fire conditions.
- Boiling or spattering of materials that have not been heated.

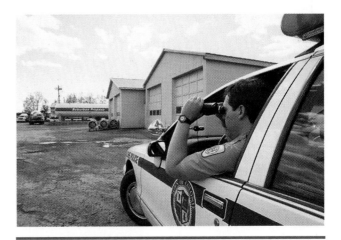

FIGURE 30-5 Use binoculars to identify hazmats from a distance.

- Wavy or unusual vapors over a container of liquid material.
- Colored vapor clouds.
- Frost near a container leak (may indicate a liquid coolant).
- Unusual condition of containers (peeling or discoloration of finishes, unexpected deterioration, deformity, or unexpected operation of pressure-relief valves).

Remember you may not be able to see or smell a hazardous material. Some are odorless and colorless. Others have properties that can deaden your senses. Always assume that the area surrounding a spill or leak is dangerous.

Identifying the Hazardous Material

After you identify an emergency as a hazmat incident, station yourself uphill and upwind of the scene. This vantage point should prevent the vapors from overwhelming

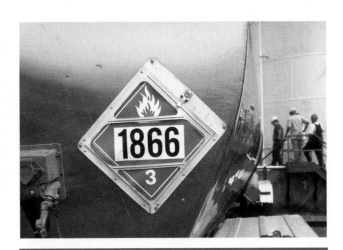

FIGURE 30-6 Hazmat placard displayed on a truck.

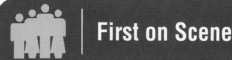

First on Scene

When you recognize a hazmat incident, restrain your natural impulse to take action. Never assume a scene is safe enough to enter. Assess the situation from a distance before you take action. Then, only those personnel trained to the Hazardous Materials Technician level or higher—and who are equipped with the proper personal protective equipment—should enter the scene.

you. Once stationed, report your position and the situation to dispatch. Your report should include:

- Nature and exact location of the incident.
- Description of the incident, including any potential for fire or explosion.
- Number of patients involved.
- Request for additional help, such as fire, police, EMS, and hazmat support.

Also suggest the best way other EMS responders can approach the scene. Include instructions for a **staging area** (the safe area where all responders should check in and get orders).

If possible, identify the hazardous materials and the severity of the situation. To do so, look for placards, NFPA numbers, or shipping papers. Then, refer to your *Emergency Response Guidebook* for the name, properties, and dangers of the material. Also determine the sizes, shapes, kinds, and conditions of the containers to see if there is imminent danger of the contamination spreading.

Although the hazmat team will be able to identify an unknown substance, you will be expected to make an initial identification.

Establishing Command

Your agency should have a plan ready in case of a hazmat incident. Before a hazardous materials emergency ever develops, all appropriate agencies need to know how forces will be mobilized to handle it. Generally, the plan addresses the worst possible scenario. That way, the community will be able to handle any emergency that arises. The following should be included:

- *One command officer* responsible for all rescue decisions at every stage of the incident. All rescuers should be aware of who the command officer is. If the command officer hands over the decision-making power

to someone else, all rescuers must be notified of the change.

- *Clear chain of command* from each rescuer to the command officer.
- *Established system of communications* used throughout the emergency. It should be one all rescuers are informed about, know how to use, and have access to.
- *Receiving facilities.* Choose facilities that can handle large numbers of patients, have surgical capacity and, if possible, have established decontamination procedures.

As the First Responder on scene, activate that plan and establish command. Stay in command until you are relieved by someone higher in the chain of command. The incoming incident command officer will want to know the following:

- Nature of the problem.
- Identification of the hazardous materials.
- Kind and condition of the containers.
- Existing weather conditions.
- Whether or not fire is present.
- Time elapsed since the emergency occurred.
- What has been done by people on scene.
- Number of victims.
- Danger of victimizing more people.

Once command has been transferred, be prepared to care for decontaminated patients or to support rescue personnel as directed.

Creating Control Zones

To prevent a hazmat incident from becoming worse, the danger area must be identified and isolated. That is usually done by designating three control zones (Figure 30-7):

- *Hot zone.* This is the most dangerous area. It can be entered only with the correct personal protective equipment. Initial or gross decontamination will be performed here.
- *Warm zone.* This is the area immediately outside the hot zone. Proper protective equipment must be worn here (Figure 30-8). Once the patient's immediate life-threats are managed, complete decontamination of the patient is performed here.
- *Cold zone.* This is the outer perimeter. All contaminated clothing and equipment must be removed before entering it.

Do not enter the warm zone unless you are trained and equipped to do so. Instead, patients should be brought to you for emergency medical treatment in the cold zone. Note

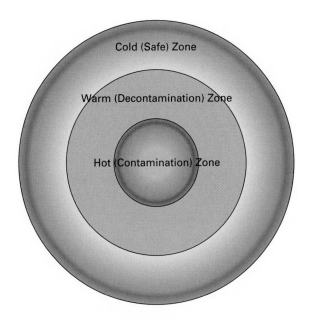

Hot (Contamination) Zone
Contamination is actually present.
Personnel must wear appropriate protective gear.
Number of rescuers limited to those absolutely necessary.
Bystanders never allowed.

Warm (Decontamination) Zone
Area surrounding the contamination zone.
Vital to preventing spread of contamination.
Personnel must wear appropriate protective gear.
Life-saving emergency care is performed.

Cold (Safe) Zone
Normal triage, stabilization, and treatment are performed.
Rescuers must shed contaminated gear before entering
the cold zone.

FIGURE 30-7 Three control zones.

that all people not necessary to the rescue should be kept
away from the zoned areas.

Establishing a Medical Treatment Sector

All EMS personnel and equipment must be staged in the
cold zone. The establishment of a definable perimeter
cannot be overstressed. In even relatively small incidents,
victims may scatter and spread the contamination with
them. The result can be an ever-increasing scene that
quickly becomes unmanageable. Note that anyone exit-

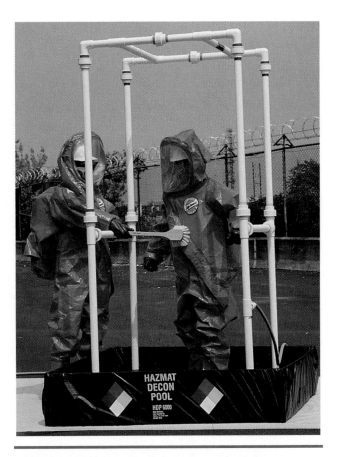

FIGURE 30-8 Rescuers in decontamination
process.

ing the hot zone should be considered contaminated until proven otherwise.

If the hazardous materials can be identified, follow the
treatment instructions given in your *Emergency Response
Guidebook* or by the regional poison control center.

1. What are your specific responsibilities at
   the scene of a hazmat incident?

2. Can you always see or smell a hazardous
   material? Explain your answer.

3. What are the three control zones usually
   designated at a hazmat incident?

▶▶ The Call Follow-up

At the beginning of this chapter, you read about a possible hazardous materials spill at a shopping mall restaurant, involving about 26 people with trouble breathing. To see how chapter skills apply, read the following. It describes how the call was completed.

Scene Size-up *(continued)* At this point, I realized I had a large number of people who could scatter, so I asked the other security guards to move the injured people to a safe non-contaminated area off the main corridor until help could arrive. If we let them wander, they would go to their cars and leave without treatment. Plus, EMS was staging in the parking lot right outside the nearest entrance. What with people leaving in droves and EMS responding, well, I was afraid things would get out

of hand. By the time law enforcement and fire rescue arrived, we had set up a 100-yard perimeter.

When the fire chief joined us, I gave him my report (see below). He immediately declared a hazardous materials incident and requested a hazmat team.

Triage and Transport After consulting with poison control, firefighters proceeded to administer high-flow oxygen to the patients and move them to a triage point. Some patients were having difficulty breathing, which caused others to panic. We assisted with assessment and care of the patients, as we were trained to do. All tolled, 10 patients were finally transported to a hospital. It is amazing how everyday cleaning fluids can cause so much harm.

 | ## Transfer of Command

"Chief, about 10 minutes ago, we had chemical fumes from the back kitchen of this restaurant from a mixture of cleaning fluids believed by the employees to be bleach, ammonia, and a green-soap solution. We have about 26 people with trouble breathing. According to the restaurant manager here, no one remains at the incident site. We set up a perimeter at 100 yards; the police have that now. People were starting to scatter, so I enlisted mall security to bring potential patients to a non-contaminated area, which can be accessed through that entryway. That's it. Do you have an assignment for us?"

The Last Word *A hazardous materials incident challenges the best in First Responders. Besides the usual patient-care issues, there are* *the additional safety problems. Be sure to learn and follow all of your local protocols for such emergencies.*

Chapter Review

Focus on the EMS Team

As a First Fesponder, you have several critical roles in the hazardous material incident. First and foremost is not becoming a patient yourself. Then, after recognizing an emergency as a hazmat incident, you are to safely identify the materials and establish command and control zones and a medical treat-ment sector. These initial actions build the crucial groundwork for the remainder of the incident and will affect the safety of other responders as well as patients and bystanders. Even if you aren't trained or equipped to deal with hazardous materials, your actions on scene as part of the EMS team are vital.

Summing Up

- Hazardous materials are everywhere. Not only do they travel through your community by rail and on highways, they also are used, stored, and discarded there.

- The U.S. DOT requires hazmat packages and containers to be marked with approved labels. Vehicles carrying hazardous materials must be marked with approved placards. The drivers of those vehicles must also have shipping papers.

- Always carry the latest edition of the DOT's *Emergency Response Guidebook* in your emergency vehicle. It lets you match a label or placard to a specific chemical and specific emergency action instructions.

- Another resource are the material safety data sheets (MSDS). Under federal regulations, all manufacturers are required to provide them to all their employees. The sheets name each substance, its physical properties, and fire, explosion, and health hazards. Emergency first aid also is usually listed.

- The Chemical Transportation Emergency Center (CHEMTREC) is a toll-free 24-hour emergency phone service that advises rescuers on the nature of a product and the steps that need to be taken to manage an incident.

- The levels of specialized training for rescuers are First Responder Awareness, First Responder Operations, Hazardous Materials Technician, and Hazardous Materials Specialist.

- Your specific responsibilities as the first to arrive at the scene are:
  - *Recognize the emergency as a hazmat incident.* Always consider the possibility, especially when called to an unknown emergency. If so, use binoculars to locate labels or placards and any other visual clues.
  - *Identify the hazardous materials.* Station yourself uphill and upwind of the scene. Report to dispatch the nature and exact location of the incident, a description, and the number of patients. Request the appropriate assistance. Give instructions for a staging area.
  - *Establish command and control (hot, warm, cold) zones.*
  - *Establish a medical treatment sector.* All EMS personnel and equipment must be staged in the cold zone.

Key Terms

flammability the degree to which a substance has the ability to ignite.

hazardous material a substance that in any quantity poses a threat or unreasonable risk to life, health, or property if not properly controlled. *Also called a* hazmat.

material safety data sheets (MSDS) manufacturers are required by law to give to their employees the name of hazardous materials, physical properties, and fire, explosion, and health hazards. Emergency first aid also is usually listed.

reactivity the degree to which a substance can change in response to other substances.

shipping papers drivers of vehicles carrying hazardous materials are required by law to carry these papers, which give the name of the substance, the danger it presents, and a four-digit identification number. *Also called* manifests *or* waybills.

staging area the safe area at an emergency scene where all responders should check in and get orders.

toxicity the degree to which a substance is toxic or poisonous.

Knowledge Check

1. **Your first priority before and during a hazmat incident is:**

   a. victim rescue.   b. personal safety.   c. decontamination.   d. substance identification.

2. When arriving at the scene of a possible hazmat emergency, your first step is to:
   a. call for additional rescuers.
   b. begin evacuation from the hot zone.
   c. gather information from a safe distance.
   d. establish command and set up control zones.

3. Decontaminated patients should be brought to EMS personnel, who are located in the ___ zone.
   a. cold   b. hot   c. warm   d. end

4. Once you establish command at a hazmat incident, you must remain in command until you are:
   a. notified that there are no people injured.
   b. called to another emergency by EMS dispatch.
   c. relieved by someone higher in the chain of command.
   d. sure the hazardous materials are properly contained.

5. When called to a hazmat incident, you should station yourself downwind and downhill of the scene.
   a. True   b. False

6. Always assume that the area surrounding a spill or leak is dangerous until proven otherwise.
   a. True   b. False

7. List three locations in your community where hazardous materials may be found.

_____

_____

_____

8. List three ways a First Responder can find out what hazardous material may be present.

_____

_____

_____

Scenario

You are called to a residence where a truck delivering some sort of fuel has rolled into the side of a house. You arrive to the vicinity of the scene and observe that the house's porch has collapsed on top of the vehicle.

a. How can you obtain information on the substance involved without going near the truck or residence?

_____

_____

b. When you are able to identify the hazardous substances involved, how do you find out additional information about the dangers they pose?

_____

_____

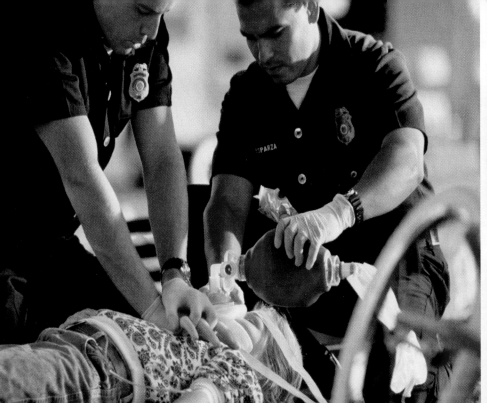
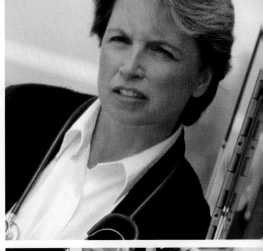
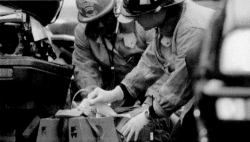

31 | Multiple-Casualty Incidents and Incident Command

Objectives

From the U.S. Department of Transportation (DOT)'s 1995 "First Responder: National Standard Curriculum." Material supplemental to the DOT curriculum is listed under "Enrichment."

Cognitive

7-1.8 ▶ Describe the criteria for a multiple-casualty situation. (p. 556)

7-1.9 ▶ Discuss the role of the First Responder in the multiple-casualty situation. (pp. 558–559)

7-1.10 ▶ Summarize the components of triage. (pp. 559–563)

Affective

No objectives are identified by the DOT.

Psychomotor

7-1.2 ▶ Given a scenario of a mass casualty incident, perform triage. (pp. 559–563)

Enrichment

▶ Describe the role of command in a multiple-casualty incident. (pp. 556–558)

▶ Identify the procedure for transferring command. (p. 559)

▶ Identify communications as a key component of any MCI. (p. 559)

▶ Describe the incident command system (ICS). (p. 556)

▶ Describe commonly used EMS sector functions. (pp. 556–558)

▶ Discuss the START triage system. (pp. 559–560)

▶ Identify a triage tag. (pp. 560–561)

▶ Discuss ways to reduce the psychological impact of disasters on patients and rescuers. (pp. 563–565)

Introduction

Multiple-casualty incidents range from a car crash to hurricanes, floods, earthquakes, and bombings. This chapter will introduce you to ways in which EMS systems respond to such emergencies. It also will give you an overview of your role as a First Responder, including how you can provide the best emergency care to the greatest number of patients.

Section 1 Incident Command System

One of the most challenging situations for a First Responder is a **multiple-casualty incident** or **MCI**. An MCI is any event where three or more patients are involved. Most communities have a plan in place for handling an MCI. However, for any plan to be effective, it must be flexible enough to work with a three-person car crash (the most common MCI) as well as a large-scale disaster involving 15 or more patients.

To meet the challenges of managing small- to large-scale incidents, the National Incident Management System (NIMS) has been developed by the U.S. federal government. Originating in California, it was first designed to handle large-scale fires involving multiple agencies. It now gives us a framework for all types of emergencies, from MCIs to hurricanes. In 2003 the president of the United States mandated that NIMS be adopted by local, state, and federal agencies if they receive federal preparedness and disaster funds.

The National Incident Management System (NIMS) is based on three main systems: the incident command system (ICS), multi-agency coordination system, and public information systems.

NIMS is a flexible plan that takes a "toolbox" approach to incident management. Only the necessary components of the system are used, depending on the size and scope of the incident. Components of the Incident Command System (ICS) are the elements most commonly used by police-fire-EMS responders.

How resources are used is basic to the incident command system (ICS). Not every MCI will need every community resource. In fact, most MCIs use only limited resources. The elements of ICS are like tools from a toolbox. Only the ones needed to handle a particular incident are used. That is, command is established at every incident. However, triage, treatment, transportation, and safety officers are designated only when the incident grows to the point where they are needed. At small-scale incidents, command assumes all functions under ICS.

As a First Responder, find out what your EMS system requires you to do in the first crucial minutes of an MCI. As the first medically trained rescuer on scene, you will set the stage for how the incident will be handled.

EMS Sector Functions

Command is established at all incidents (Figure 31-1). That person stays in command until command is transferred to someone else or until the incident comes to an end. If an

First on Scene

When most people think of multiple-casualty incidents, they think of plane crashes and commuter train wrecks. While these certainly qualify, the most common MCIs are two-car collisions with three injured passengers in each car. Most EMS systems would have to stretch resources to take care of these six patients. Learn what your EMS system expects of you.

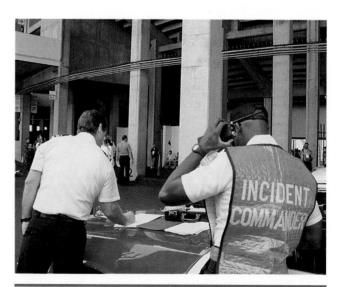

FIGURE 31-1 The incident commander directs the response and coordinates resources at an MCI.

THE CALL

Dispatch Shortly after checking out our EMS equipment and supplies, my partner and I were dispatched to an explosion with fire at a small factory.

Scene Size-up When we arrived at the address, we were told where to park our vehicle. I also was told by the incident commander to establish EMS command. My partner and I immediately donned our identification vests.

I wore the EMS command vest. She put on the triage sector vest. A plant security guard told me that nine people were working in the area when the explosion occurred. Eight escaped with their lives. One was still unaccounted for. I radioed this information to the incident commander.

Consider this situation as you read Chapter 31. What can be done to ensure that all patients get timely and appropriate emergency medical care?

incident is large or complex, command can designate sector officers to help (Figure 31-2). When needed, the EMS sector may include the following:

- *Triage officer.* This officer supervises patient assessment, tagging, and removal of patients to a designated treatment area.

- *Treatment officer.* This officer sets up a treatment area and supervises treatment. Generally, one EMS rescuer is assigned to each patient. The treatment and transportation officers make sure the most seriously injured are transported first.

- *Transportation officer.* This officer arranges for ambulances. He or she also tracks the priority, identity, and destination of all patients leaving the scene (Figure 31-3). The transportation and staging officers make sure resources are available as needed.

- *Staging officer.* This officer releases and distributes resources when they are needed. He or she also sees that "gridlock" does not occur in the transportation area.

- *Safety officer.* This officer maintains scene safety. He or she identifies potential dangers and takes action to prevent them from causing injury to patients and rescuers.

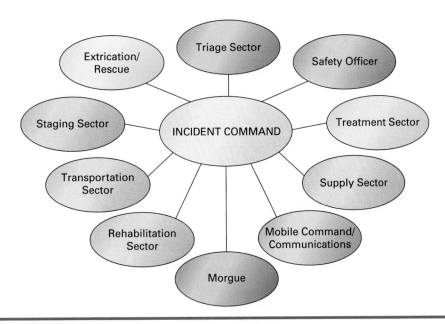

FIGURE 31-2 After an incident commander is identified, EMS sectors are established as needed.

THE COMMAND TOOLBOX

MULTICASUALTY RECORDER WORKSHEET

Ambulance Company	Ambulance ID Number	Patient Triage Tag Number	Patient Status	Hospital Destination	Off-Scene Time

FIGURE 31-3 Sample of a tracking sheet for the transportation officer at an MCI.

When many patients need special rescue or extrication from wreckage, an extrication sector should be established.

In large-scale operations where a great many resources are used for long periods of time, a *logistics officer* may be needed. This officer makes certain that medical supplies, communications equipment, transportation units, food, and any other supplies are available when needed. The logistics officer also may set up a rehabilitation sector where rescue personnel can go for evaluation and treatment as well as for food and water.

When there are deceased victims, a morgue may be set up. This sector should be overseen by the police along with a medical examiner or coroner.

First Responder's Role

The most senior First Responder arriving at an MCI is responsible for carrying out the MCI plan. Your major goals are then to establish command, size up the scene, request additional resources, and begin triage. (See Table 31-1 for a summary of command responsibilities.)

TABLE 31-1 Command Officer Responsibilities

- Assume an effective command mode and position. Provide continuing command until relieved by a higher-ranking official.
- Transmit a brief preliminary report to EMS dispatch.
- Rapidly evaluate the situation.
- Request additional resources.
- Quickly develop a safe management strategy.
- Delegate authority.
- Review and evaluate effectiveness of sector operations through frequent progress reports from sector officers.
- Modify sector operations as required.
- As incident winds down, return units to service and secure incident when appropriate.

Once you identify an incident as an MCI, resist the urge to jump in and provide treatment. And remember that patients with loud voices have open airways. Quiet patients may not be breathing.

During your scene size-up, identify the following:

- Scene safety.
- Number of patients, including the "walking wounded."
- Needs for extrication.
- Estimated number of ambulances needed.
- Other factors affecting the scene and resources, such as weather or terrain.
- Number of sectors needed.
- Area to stage resources.

Make an initial scene report to EMS dispatch. Keep it short and to the point. Be sure to give the information necessary for other rescuers to react to the MCI appropriately. For example:

> *"Firecom, this is Engine 405. We are on the scene of a two-car collision with entrapment of three priority-one patients. Dispatch a rescue company and three paramedic ambulances. Alert the trauma center. I will now be called Central Avenue Command. Police are needed to assist with traffic and crowd control ASAP. Approach from the north. Staging is on Central between Kennedy and 67th Street."*

Some MCI plans call for the command vehicle to have two traffic cones on top of it. Whatever method you use, make sure command can be identified easily. Bibs or vests should be worn by command personnel and sector officers for easy recognition.

Communication is a key component of any MCI plan. Keep calm when making radio transmissions. Use plain English and common terms. Try to keep radio traffic to a minimum. Encourage face-to-face communication.

When you are relieved by someone higher in the chain of command, report the following to him or her: nature of the problem, potential hazards, number of patients, time elapsed since the emergency occurred, and what already has been done.

If you respond to an MCI where command is already established, report immediately to the command sector. Identify the incident commander. Introduce yourself and your level of training and ask for instructions. Be prepared to care for patients or to support rescue personnel as directed.

Q:

1. What is a "toolbox approach" to incident command?

2. What should you determine during the size-up of an MCI scene?

3. As the first rescuer to establish command at the scene of an MCI, what should you report to the officer who relieves you?

Section 2 Triage and Emergency Care

Triage is a French word meaning "pick" or "sort." It is a process of classifying sick and injured patients first used by the military. During the Korean and Vietnam Wars, it resulted in a big improvement in the survival rates of the injured. Today, triage is used to determine the order in which patients receive medical care and transport.

Triage Systems

In triage, the most critical but salvageable patients are treated and transported first. Generally, triage systems identify three or more levels of care. Three-level systems are the most common (Figure 31-4). They sort patients into highest-priority, urgent-care, and lowest-priority categories. However, different areas may have their own ways of performing triage. Know what your EMS system expects of you. Follow all local protocols.

START

One popular method of triage is *Simple Triage and Rapid Transport (START)*. Triage should begin with the first on-scene unit using a public address or other system to ask patients who can move to do so. Patients should be instructed to go to a designated area where another rescuer from the unit can start to treat and identify injuries. When these patients move, they do several things, one of which is tell you by their actions that they are "walking wounded" and have minor injuries.

Providing direction to these patients helps prevent them from leaving the scene and getting transport to the closest hospital. This feeds into the MCI goals of not relocating the disaster and of doing the most good for the most patients. These patients do not have to be relocated to a serene pasture, but they should be moved to any easily locatable position or building where they can receive

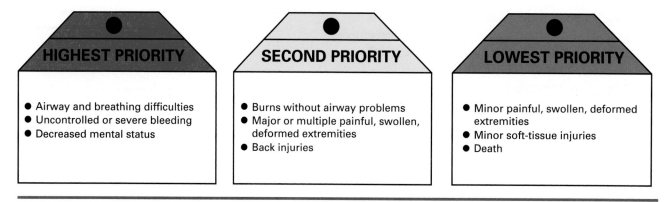

HIGHEST PRIORITY

- Airway and breathing difficulties
- Uncontrolled or severe bleeding
- Decreased mental status

SECOND PRIORITY

- Burns without airway problems
- Major or multiple painful, swollen, deformed extremities
- Back injuries

LOWEST PRIORITY

- Minor painful, swollen, deformed extremities
- Minor soft-tissue injuries
- Death

FIGURE 31-4 An example of a three-level triage system identified in the U.S. DOT's "First Responder: National Standard Curriculum."

basic medical care. These patients are immediately classified as "green."

When triaging patients, remember to work systematically to make sure that everyone is triaged. Keep triage time to a minimum; each patient encounter should last 15 to 30 seconds. Only the most basic care is performed during triage and is generally limited to opening airways and controlling major bleeding.

A critical note is to be accurate in your patient count. Many EMS systems will use colored surveyor's tape tied to patient's wrists to indicate that patient's triage status. One way of keeping track of a large number of patients is to then tear off another section of tape and place it in your pocket. At the conclusion of triaging your area, all these small pieces of triage tape will be in your pocket and will allow you to quickly divide them by color and provide command with an accurate count of patients in each category.

The START triage system is simple to use and relies on a condition-based classification, not an injury-based system of assessment. For instance, a badly burned patient might be triaged black, red, or yellow depending on how they fit into the criteria. This helps get treatment for the most seriously injured patients and allows resources to be managed more effectively.

After identifying the walking wounded, rescuers using START go on to check on the remaining patients. If a patient's airway is not open, the rescuer should open the patient's airway. If the patient is not breathing at this time, the rescuer should tag the patient "black" and move onto the next patient.

If the patient is breathing faster than 30 times per minute, tag the patient "red" and move on to the next patient. If the patient is breathing less than 30 times per minute, continue your assessment by checking for a radial pulse. If there is no radial pulse, tag the patient "red" and go to the next patient.

Some triage systems use capillary refill as a method of perfusion check, but this characteristic is falling from favor both because capillary refill is not always a reliable indicator of shock (because it is a late sign) and it can give false positives in cooler temperate environments.

If a radial pulse is present, ask the patient to follow a simple command. If the patient attempts to obey the command but is physically unable to complete it, tag the patient "yellow." If the patient cannot follow simple commands, tag him "red."

You will notice that patients tagged "red" are those with obvious signs and symptoms of shock. These patients require rapid transport to an emergency department or trauma center. In contrast, yellow-tagged patients are injured but can withstand a delay in care.

Triage Tags

After patients are assessed and sorted, they must be tagged for rapid identification. Triage tags come in a variety of sizes, shapes, and colors (Figure 31-5). Generally, use them only if more than 10 patients are involved in a single incident. Avoid tags that need a ball-point pen or carbons. Avoid tags that are too detailed. Be sure there is a method of securing the tags so that they do not come loose or drop off.

Once a patient is given a tag, do not remove it. If the patient changes status before being treated, draw a bold line through the original tag, note the time, and put a new tag on the patient. This procedure helps rescuers know that the patient has had a change in status.

One of the most popular tags is the *Mettag*. It uses symbols instead of words for rapid identification. It also is highly visible. With perforated divisions, it contains a strip for each of the categories: red (rabbit) for the highest priority, yellow (turtle) for second priority, green (ambulance with X through it) for those not in need of transport, and black (shovel and cross) for the dead. Rescuers simply tear off the strips not needed so that the applicable strip is on the outside edge.

Psychological Impact of an MCI

Psychological injuries can be severe, too. Almost all the people involved in an MCI experience fear. Many also feel shaky, perspire profusely, and become confused, irritable, anxious, suspicious, moody, restless, and fatigued.

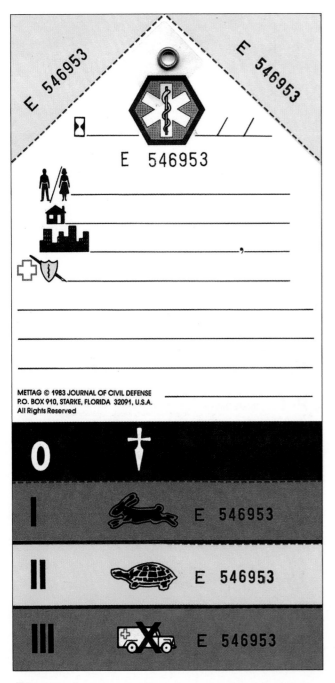

a.

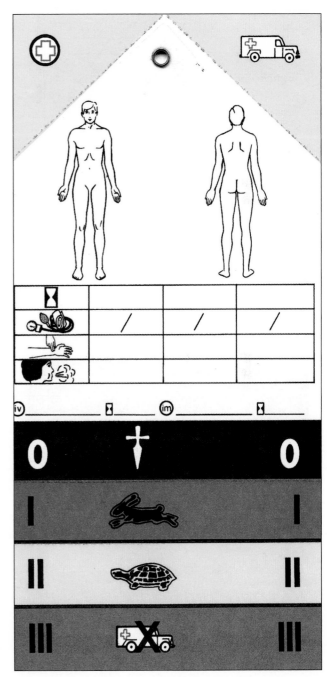

FIGURE 31-5 Example of a commonly used triage tag (front and back).

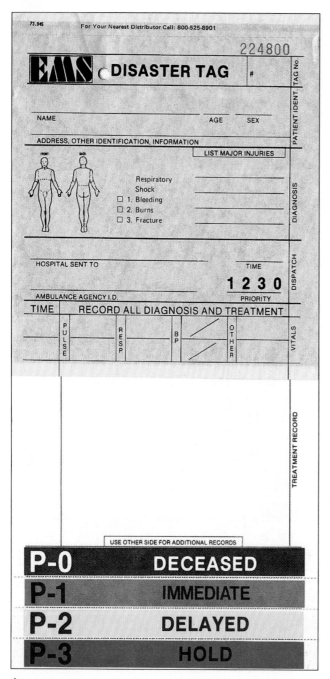

TREATMENT RECORD

TIME	RECORD ALL DIAGNOSIS AND TREATMENT

P-0	DECEASED	Expired Non-survivor
P-1	IMMEDIATE	Airway-respiratory, cardiac problems uncontrolled hemorrhage, open chest-abdomen severe head injury, shock, burns or medical.
P-2	DELAYED	Spinal cord injury, multiple-major fractures moderate burns, uncomplicated head injury.
P-3	HOLD	All minor & uncomplicated fractures, wounds, other injuries, burns & psychological problems.

b.

FIGURE 31-5 (continued) Example of an EMS disaster tag (front and back).

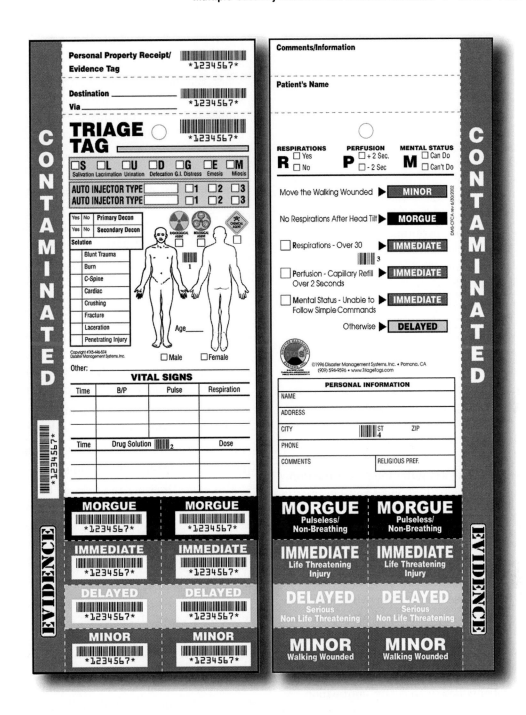

C.

FIGURE 31-5 (continued) Example of a contaminated patient tag (front and back). *(Disaster Management Systems, Inc., triagetags.com)*

Many will have sleep problems, concentration problems, depression, nausea, vomiting, and diarrhea. Survivors often experience anger, guilt, shock, denial, and feelings of isolation and vulnerability. All of these reactions are normal.

The reactions of children depend on age, disposition, and family and community support. Generally, preschoolers cry, lose control of bowels and bladder, become confused, and suck their thumbs. Older children suffer from extreme fears about their safety. They may show confusion, depression, headache, inability to concentrate, withdrawal, poor performance, and a tendency to fight with peers. Older children and adolescents may show extreme aggression. Their stress may be severe enough to disrupt their lives.

Others at risk for severe reactions are the elderly, those in poor physical or emotional health, the handicapped, and those who have unresolved past losses or crises.

Rescuers react, too. Often they react in the same way their patients do. Common reactions are fear about personal safety, crying, anger, guilt, numbness, preoccupation with death, frustration, and fatigue. Most reactions peak within about one week and then diminish. Some have dreams of the disaster for weeks or months afterward. In some cases, rescuers suffer long-term reactions.

Recognize that as a First Responder you can react in similar ways after being exposed to large-scale incident. If you do, seek help from a professional or through options made available through your employer or agency.

Managing Stress at an MCI

To start, do not let yourself become overwhelmed by the size of the emergency. Learn your local MCI plans well and follow them. They will help you keep calm and effective. General guidelines for managing the stress on patients and their families at any type of MCI are as follows:

- Families of patients deserve accurate information. As soon as possible, assign several workers to provide it to the properly authorized person only. That usually is the chief town executive, the public relations officer, or the incident commander.

- Reunite patients with their families as soon as possible. They will feel less stressed once they are together. Families also can provide medical histories that will increase your ability to care for patients. A separate area away from the scene, onlookers, and the press should be identified for this purpose.

- If the MCI involves a large number of patients, group them with their families ems neighbors. This will help reduce feelings of fear and isolation.

- Provide a structure. Tell patients exactly what is happening.

- Work can be therapeutic. Encourage the "walking wounded" to do necessary chores. Explain the tasks simply and clearly. Consider having the patients support each other until medical personnel are available.

- Help patients confront the reality of the disaster. Encourage them to talk about it and what they feel. If you sense that they are not facing reality or that their expectations are much worse than reality, help them adjust their views. If you engage a patient in this type of talk, make sure you have time to listen and respond.

- Do not give false assurances. If you do, patients may resist any further outside help. Honestly appraise the situation. Offer help where it is needed.

- Some patients will refuse help. There are many reasons why, including how they were brought up. Explain that accepting help is not admitting weakness. Make sure they understand help is only temporary and that as soon as things are under control they can help someone else.

- Arrange for a group discussion where patients can share ideas as soon as physical needs are taken care of.

- Encourage all those involved—including rescuers—to get good follow-up care and support.

Also consider using the help of the American Red Cross or a similar organization. They may be able to assist with psychological counseling and other support services to patients and families. Such organizations should be identified in the disaster plan and alerted as soon as possible in a large-scale MCI.

Reducing Stress in Rescuers

Once the rescue operation is underway, a new danger arises. Rescuers may begin to suffer from stress. If measures are not taken immediately, rescue workers can become inefficient and, at worst, become victims themselves. To help reduce stress, the following guidelines may be useful:

- Make sure rescue workers are fully aware of their exact assignments. Well-defined limits help to reduce stress.

- Assign rescue workers to tasks according to their skills and experience. If there are any questions, do not gamble. Give workers the tasks you are certain they can do.

- Tell rescuers to rest at regular intervals away from the hub of the disaster. They should sit or lie down, have something to eat or drink, and relax as much as possible. Have counseling available at the scene. If rest periods are effectively rotated, there will be enough workers to carry on disaster assistance.

- Have several workers circulate among rescuers to watch for signs of physical exhaustion and stress. If one worker appears to be having problems, he or she should rest for a longer period than usual. After rest, give him or her a less stressful task. If appropriate, trained psychological support personnel can evaluate rescuers if a high level of stress is suspected.

- Provide plenty of nourishing drinks and food. Encourage rescue workers to eat and drink to keep up their strength. Avoid foods high in fat, sugar, and caffeine.

- Encourage rescuers to talk among themselves. Talking helps to relieve stress. Discourage lighthearted conversation and joking. Some people may be offended, which can increase stress on scene.

- Make sure that rescuers have a chance to talk with trained counselors after the incident.

1. In the START system, which patients are treated and transported first?

2. Generally, when are triage tags used?

3. What are some ways to reduce the stress of rescuers at the scene of an MCI?

▶▶ The Call Follow-up

At the beginning of this chapter, you read that First Responders were on the scene of an MCI, an explosion with fire at a small factory. There are nine patients, one still unaccounted for. To see how chapter skills apply to this emergency, read the following. It describes how the call was completed.

Triage and Transport Jan, my partner, started triage. When another First Responder arrived, I assigned him to establish a transport sector and gave him a staging vest. I reminded him to make sure that he identified a safe area where ambulances could enter and exit quickly and safely.

Jan soon reported that two patients were Priority 1, three were Priority 2, and three were Priority 3. I updated the incident commander and requested seven ambulances, three of which were to be equipped for advanced life support (ALS). I also requested that he alert the trauma center.

A minute or so later it was confirmed that one patient was still inside the plant. We believed that patient to be a Priority 0. At that moment, the paramedic EMS supervisor arrived. I provided a full report (see below) and turned over EMS command to him. He then assigned me to assist in the treatment area.

Over the next half hour all eight patients were transported to a hospital. A police officer was assigned to guard the one dead body until the coroner arrived. Triage and transport for the injured patients had taken 45 minutes.

When EMS command was terminated, the incident commander told us that counselors would be available for all rescue personnel involved.

Transfer of Command

"We got here to find there had been an explosion with fire. Other than the fire, there are no additional hazards we are aware of. Initial reports indicated that there were nine employees involved—eight made it out. We've triaged eight patients, as you'll see here on the flow sheet, and have requested seven ambulances. We also notified the trauma center. They'll get back to us to let us know how many patients they can take. We set up a transport sector to prevent a traffic jam and things are moving. That's it. You've got EMS command. How can I help you?"

The Last Word *For you to be an effective member of EMS response to an MCI, you must learn your local plans and protocols. Review* *them often. Practice them whenever you are given the opportunity.*

Chapter Review

Focus on the EMS Team

The first providers at the scene of a multiple-casualty incident ensure scene safety and establish an orderly system of command. Then triage begins. Without it, there is no orderly way to treat a great number of patients efficiently. Finally, at some point in the incident, transport

of patients begins. Agency chief officers and more-senior members soon arrive on scene and take over command functions. But never forget that your action—the action of the First Responders—sets the foundation for a smooth-running and efficient MCI.

Summing Up

- The National Incident Management System (NIMS) is based on three main systems: the incident command system (ICS), multi-agency coordination system, and public information systems. Components of the Incident Command System (ICS) are the elements that are most commonly used by police-fire-EMS responders.

- EMS sector functions include triage, treatment, transportation, staging, safety and, where necessary, extrication. In large-scale operations where a great many resources are used for long periods of time, a logistics officer may be needed. When there are deceased victims, a morgue may be needed.

- Your role as the first rescuer on scene is to size up the scene, establish command, and initiate your ICS plan.
  — Determine scene safety, number of patients, needs for extrication, estimated number of ambulances needed, other factors affecting the scene and resources, number of necessary sectors, and area to stage resources. Report that information, plus the best approach to the scene, to dispatch.
  — When you are relieved by someone higher in the chain of command, report the following to him or her: nature of the problem, potential hazards, number of patients, time elapsed since the emergency occurred, and what already has been done.

- If you respond to an MCI where command is already established, report immediately to the command sector. Identify the incident commander. Introduce yourself and your level of training and ask for instructions. Be prepared to care for patients or to support rescue personnel as directed.

- Generally, triage systems identify three or more levels of care. Three-level systems are the most common. They sort patients into highest-priority, urgent-care, and lowest-priority categories. An example is the Simple Triage and Rapid Treatment (START) system, which sometimes also includes a no-care category.

- To perform triage at an MCI, you must assess each patient's condition, determine the urgency of the condition, and assign a priority for treatment. Then, place a tag on the patient for rapid identification. (You must learn and practice the triage system used in your area.)

- Most people involved in an MCI are under a great deal of stress. Children and the elderly are especially at risk for severe reactions. Things you can do to help manage that stress include provide accurate information, reunite families as soon as possible, and encourage all those involved—including rescuers—to get good follow-up care and support.

Key Terms

multiple-casualty incident (MCI) any emergency in which three or more patients are involved.

triage process of sorting patients to determine the order in which they will receive care and transport.

Knowledge Check

1. A multiple-casualty incident usually involves ___ or more patients.
   a. 20   c. 10
   b. 13   d. 3

2. What is the first priority of the first rescuer at the scene of an MCI?
   a. triage   c. treatment
   b. command   d. transportation

3. You are at a three-patient MCI with plenty of rescuers. A patient is found in cardiac arrest. That patient should be categorized as a priority number:
   a. green
   b. black
   c. red
   d. yellow

4. List all the possible functions of an EMS sector at an MCI.

   _____   _____

   _____   _____

   _____   _____

   _____   _____

5. You are the first rescuer at the scene of an MCI. List the information you must gather for your scene size-up.

   _____

   _____

   _____

   _____

   _____

   _____

Scenario

You are an EMS First Responder called to a "motor-vehicle collision on the highway." You don't receive any additional information, so you are quite surprised when you arrive on scene. There is a full-size bus on its side and 30 or 40 people milling around along side of it.

a. You are the only responder on scene. What hazards should you initially address in your scene size-up?

_____

_____

_____

_____

b. What is the difference between assuming command and performing triage?

_____

_____

_____

_____

c. In this incident, how would you begin triage?

_____

_____

_____

_____

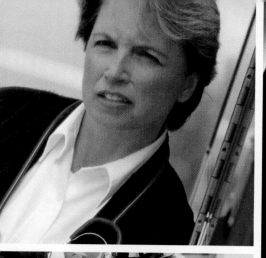
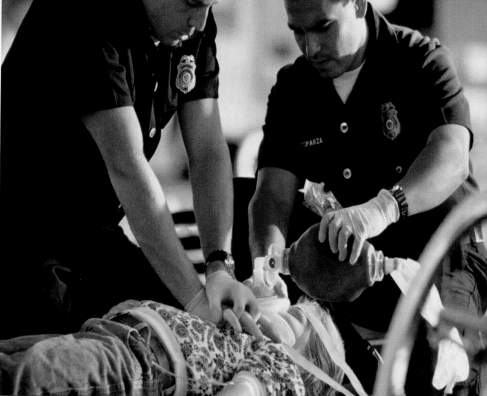
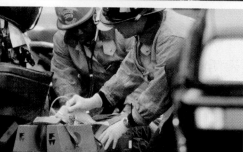

32 | Water Emergencies

Objectives

From the U.S. Department of Transportation (DOT)'s 1995 "First Responder: National Standard Curriculum." Material supplemental to the DOT curriculum is listed under "Enrichment."

Cognitive

> *No objectives are identified by the DOT.*

Affective

> *No objectives are identified by the DOT.*

Psychomotor

> *No objectives are identified by the DOT.*

Enrichment

- ▶ Understand how drowning and near-drownings occur. (pp. 571–572)
- ▶ Describe key components of scene size-up in a water emergency. (pp. 572–573)

- ▶ Discuss some of the difficulties of assessing a patient who is in the water. (p. 573)
- ▶ Describe emergency care of a near-drowning patient with no injuries to the spine. (pp. 573–574, 576)
- ▶ Describe emergency care of a near-drowning patient with suspected spine injuries. (pp. 573–574, 576)
- ▶ List the hazards commonly associated with fast-moving water. (pp. 576–577)
- ▶ Discuss the differences between warm-water and cold-water rescues. (pp. 571–572)
- ▶ Describe the assessment and emergency medical care of a patient with a diving emergency, including air embolism and decompression sickness. (pp. 578–580)

Introduction

Water is everywhere. Oceans, lakes, and streams are only the most obvious sites of possible water emergencies. Drownings also occur in home pools, which are numerous. Many industries have vats or pools large enough to drown several workers. Even bathtubs and toilets present a danger to small children. This chapter offers an overview of water rescue. It introduces you to the challenge of providing emergency care in water and to some of the common hazards.

Section 1 Water Rescue

Drowning and Near-Drowning

Drowning is defined as death from suffocation due to submersion. It is a leading cause of accidental death in the United States. After auto collisions, drowning is the most common cause of preventable death among children. It can be the result of cold, fatigue, injury, disorientation, intoxication, or limited swimming ability. (See Figure 32-1.)

"Wet" drowning occurs when fluid is aspirated (breathed into) into the lungs. "Dry" drowning occurs when a severe muscle spasm of the larynx closes it, preventing respiration and aspiration of water. About 10% to 40% of all drownings are estimated to be "dry." Autopsies

reveal that only a small percentage of patients who died from drowning aspirated a significant amount of water.

Survival from a near-drowning can depend on many factors, including whether the water is warm or cold. Unlike warm-water drownings, those that occur in cold water (below 68°F) have resulted in successful resuscitations, even up to an hour after submersion. Hypothermia and the "diving reflex" have something to do with this. Both slow down the body's metabolism and reduce the need for oxygen.

This is how the "diving reflex" works: When a person's face is submerged in cold water, breathing is inhibited, the heart slows, and blood vessels constrict. In this way, oxygen is sent only to where it is most needed to sustain life. In water at or below 68°F, the body's metabolic requirements are

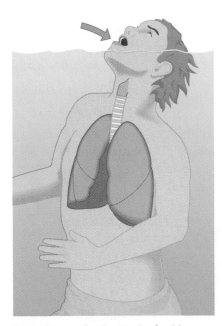

Drowning can be the result of cold, fatigue, injury, disorientation, intoxication, or limited swimming abilities.

a.

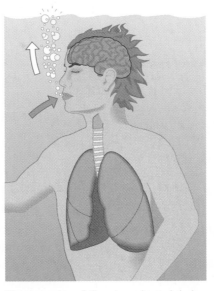

The drowning victim struggles to inhale air as long as possible. Eventually the victim inhales water or a muscle spasm of the larynx closes the airway.

b.

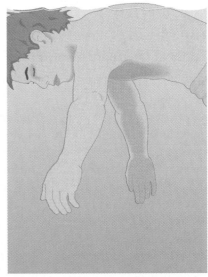

Loss of consciousness, convulsions, cardiac arrest, and death may follow.

c.

FIGURE 32-1 Drowning.

THE CALL

Dispatch I spend my summers working as a lifeguard at the town pool. I was doing my job, watching families and lots of children cool down in the water.

Scene Size-up I was on the stand keeping tabs on some youngsters using the low diving board, when I looked toward the middle of the pool. There I saw a young male floating face down. I knew him. It was Jimmy. I jumped in and swam over to him. Everyone was yelling. One bystander shouted that he had a seizure. I thought

quickly. I didn't see him dive. I didn't know if he'd been in a fight. All I knew was that he appeared to be unresponsive. I had to get his face out of the water, but I decided to move him as little as possible.

How can the First Responder provide emergency care in the water? Why wouldn't he want to move the boy out of the water immediately? Consider this patient as you read Chapter 32. What should be done to assess and treat his condition?

---

only about half of normal. The brain and heart remain oxygenated for some time and, as a result, death can be significantly delayed.

Unfortunately, when cold, muscles do not function properly. So it becomes difficult for the patient to keep afloat. The hypothermic patient also may be unable to follow directions or assist with the rescue. Note that cold water temperatures affect rescuers, too.

General Guidelines for Water Rescues

In a water-related emergency, you obviously need to reach the patient. However, you must do so with the utmost concern for your own safety. Remember that water can conceal many hazards. Holes, sharp drop-offs, and underwater entanglements, such as fallen trees and wire fences, may not be visible from shore. The force of moving water also can be very deceptive. Do not walk in fast-moving water over knee depth. It is not safe. Moving water in streams, rivers, even storm drains can push you over and hold you down.

Hazardous materials are also a concern in water emergencies. For example, a car in the water could leak oil or gas, which float on the surface. Such hazards pose a respiratory risk for both patients and rescuers. Floods can cause sewage to be released in normally safe waters. Risk of electrocution exists in flooded buildings or on flooded grounds. Severe bleeding of the patient also can pose the risk of infection to other patients and rescuers.

When determining how to respond to a water emergency, take into account the patient's condition, water conditions, and the resources on hand. Ask yourself the following questions:

■ *Patient condition.*
   —*Mental status.* Is the patient responsive and able to assist in the rescue? If so, reaching out with a pole or throwing a rope may be the safest method of rescue.
   —*Position.* Is the patient on the surface or is he submerged? If submerged, he may need basic life support immediately. He also may be difficult to locate.
   —*Injuries.* Does the patient have any obvious injuries? If so, you may have to extricate him from the water before beginning care.

■ *Water condition.*
   —*Visibility.* Can you see any potential hazards under the water? Can you see the patient and his injuries?
   —*Temperature.* For a cold-water drowning, you must continue resuscitation until the patient is rewarmed at the hospital. Note that even when the air is warm, the water may still be cold.
   —*Moving water.* Will the location of the patient change? Is it safe for you to enter the water?
   —*Depth of the water.* Can your feet touch the bottom so you can stand, or will additional equipment be needed?
   —*Other hazards.* Are there hazardous materials present, such as oil, gas, or sewage? Is there any risk of electrocution?

First on Scene

Never attempt a water rescue unless you are a good swimmer, specially trained in water rescue, wearing a personal flotation device, and accompanied by other rescuers.

■ *Resources on hand.* How many rescuers are on scene? Are they trained in water rescue? Can they all swim? Does each have a personal flotation device? Do you need any special rescue teams such as a dive team?

Never try a water rescue unless you are a good swimmer, specially trained in water rescue, wearing a personal flotation device, and accompanied by other rescuers. If you meet all four criteria, your patient is responsive and close to shore, and the emergency is occurring in open, shallow water that has a stable, uniform bottom, attempt a rescue.

Use the "reach, throw, row, and go" strategy in the following order:

■ *Reach.* Hold out an object for the patient to grab. Anything that will extend your reach will work. You can use a towel, shirt, backboard, or other strong object that will not break. Before holding out the object, make sure you have solid footing and will not slip in the water. Once the object is grabbed, pull the patient to shore.

■ *Throw.* If the patient is too far to reach, throw an object that floats (Figure 32-2). A thermos jug, a picnic

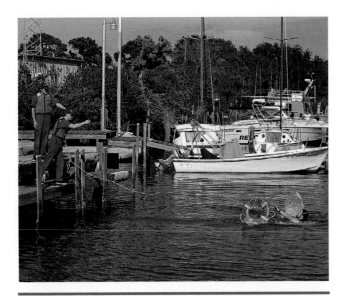

FIGURE 32-2 Tie a sturdy rope to an object that floats. Throw the object and pull the patient in.

cooler, or capped empty milk jug will do. This will give the patient support and give you more time to make the rescue. If possible, tie a rope to the object you throw. Toss the object to the patient, and pull on the rope to tow the patient in. Again, be sure of your own footing and stability.

■ *Row.* If the patient is too far to reach or throw an object to from shore, use a boat to get closer to the patient.

■ *Go.* If reaching, throwing, and rowing are not possible, swim to the patient but only if you are a good swimmer, specially trained in water rescue, wearing a personal flotation device, and accompanied by other rescuers.

Patient Assessment

If the water emergency is the result of a diving accident or if the patient has been struck by a boat, water skier, surfboard, or other object, suspect spine injury. Also suspect spine injury in any swimmer who is unresponsive, especially one in shallow, warm water.

Though any injury that can occur on land also can occur in water, note that it can be more difficult to detect injuries in water. Bleeding, for example, is easy to spot on land. In the water any bleeding that occurs may be immediately diluted and dispersed. So, not only may it be difficult to judge how severe the bleeding is, it also may not be possible to recognize that the patient is bleeding. Also, if the patient is wearing a wet suit, a large amount of blood can pool inside it before bleeding is recognized.

Broken bones, too, are difficult to identify in water. The water may be murky or dark. The surface of water can distort visual images. Limbs, for example, can appear angulated or straight when they are not, just by the refraction. One way to deal with this problem is to assume fractures until proven otherwise in any unresponsive patient.

The decision on whether or not to remove the patient from the water depends on several factors. (See next section for details.) ■

First Responder Care

To provide care to a patient with a water emergency, you first have to decide whether or not to remove him from the water. That decision depends on a number of factors, including the potential for spine injury, the patient's overall condition (including level of responsiveness), the temperature of the water, and the equipment and personnel available.

If the patient is responsive and you are sure there is no spine injury, he should be removed from the water. Then, administer high-flow oxygen and be prepared to suction.

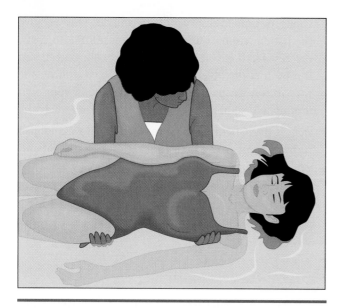

FIGURE 32-3 Hip and shoulder support.

Also, conserve the patient's body heat. To do so, remove wet clothing, place him on a blanket, and then cover him with another blanket. If possible, move the patient to a warm environment. Do not allow the patient to walk.

If your patient is unresponsive and in shallow, warm water, maintain the airway but do not move him. If the patient is breathing, keep him in a face-up position. Support the patient's back (Figure 32-3). If there is a second rescuer present, also stabilize the patient's head and neck (Figure 32-4).

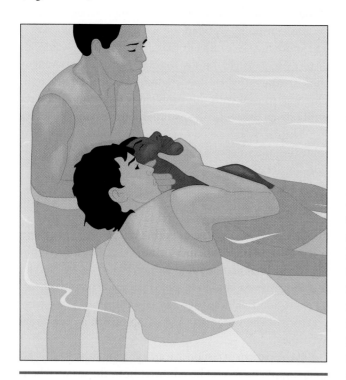

FIGURE 32-4 In-line stabilization with two rescuers.

If you find the unresponsive patient face-down in shallow water, you have to turn him. Use the head-splint technique to do so (Figure 32-5):

1. Get alongside the patient.

2. Extend the patient's arms straight up alongside his head. Press his arms against his head to create a splint.

3. If necessary, move the patient forward to a horizontal position.

4. Rotate the patient by bringing the farthest hand toward you and pushing away the hand that is closest. As you rotate the patient, lower yourself in the water until the water is at shoulder level.

5. Maintain stabilization of the patient's head. Do this with one hand by holding the patient's head between his arms. With your other hand, support the patient's lower back until help arrives.

If the unresponsive patient is in water that is unsafe (deep, cold, or moving) or if the patient needs CPR, qualified rescuers should position him on a backboard. Once immobilized, the patient should be removed from the water. Note that artificial ventilation can start in the water. Chest compressions cannot. Patients who need CPR must be removed from the water first.

To turn a patient to a face-up position in deep water, perform the head-chin support technique (Figure 32-6):

1. Position yourself alongside the patient.

2. Position one arm along the patient's spine, supporting his head with your hand. Place your other arm along the patient's chest in line with the sternum, supporting the mandible with your hand.

3. If necessary, move the patient forward to a horizontal position.

4. Then rotate the patient by ducking under his body.

5. Continue to maintain in-line stabilization until a backboard is used to immobilize the spine.

To immobilize a patient who is in the water, use a long backboard or other rigid support such as a water ski or surf board. Slide it under him. Let it float up until it is snugly against his back. Apply a rigid cervical immobilization device. Then, secure him to the backboard. Never try to support the patient's spine with anything that might bend or break, such as an air mattress or a Styrofoam float. As you are backboarding him, have enough rescuers helping. They need to make sure his face does not become submerged. After immobilization, lift the patient from the water head first. If he is wearing a personal flotation device, leave it in place. Pad under the patient's head to keep the spine in alignment.

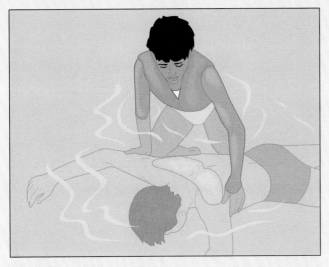

FIGURE 32-5A *Position yourself alongside the patient.*

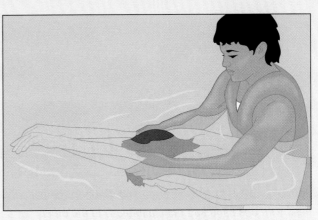

FIGURE 32-5B *Extend the patient's arms straight up alongside his head to create a splint.*

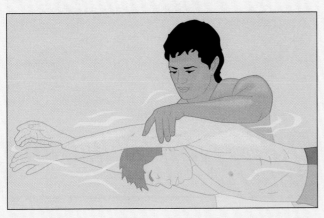

FIGURE 32-5C *Begin to rotate the torso toward you.*

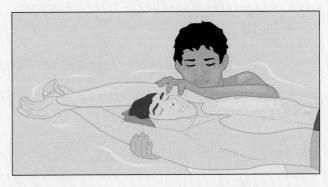

FIGURE 32-5D *As you rotate the patient, lower yourself in the water.*

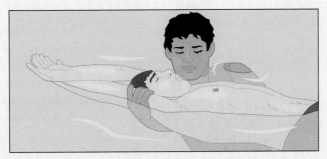

FIGURE 32-5E *Maintain stabilization by holding the patient's head between his arms.*

SKILL SUMMARY *Performing the Head-Chin Support Technique in Water*

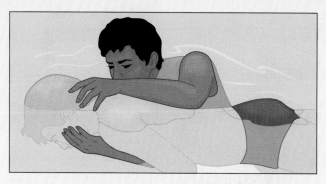

FIGURE 32-6A *Position yourself. Support the patient's head with one hand and the mandible with the other.*

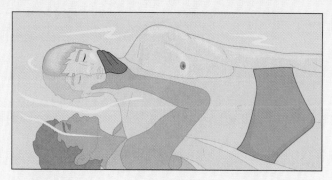

FIGURE 32-6B *Then rotate the patient by ducking under him.*

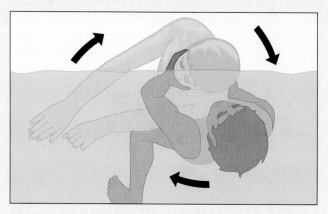

FIGURE 32-6C *Continue to rotate until the patient is face up.*

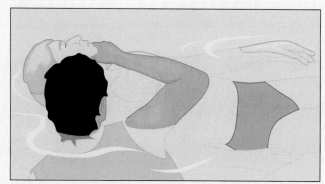

FIGURE 32-6D *Maintain in-line stabilization until a backboard is used to immobilize the spine.*

Note: Always have a near-drowning patient taken to a hospital, even if you believe the danger has passed. Complications can develop and may be fatal as long as 72 hours after the incident. ■

Moving-Water Rescue

Many people are drawn to moving water, or "white water," for recreation. Those who are trained and experienced know how to read moving water. They understand the hazards and manage them. It is all part of their sport. Moving-water incidents usually occur when someone unaware of the dangers gets into the water. This is true of both victims and rescuers.

The force of moving water is measured by its depth, width, and velocity. For example, a river that is 200 feet wide, 4 feet deep, and moving at 20 feet per second will move about 16,000 cubic feet per second. That is roughly equal to 550 pounds of force.

Fast-moving water is dangerous. Certain river features make it even more so. They include the following:

- *Strainers.* These are obstructions that allow water to pass through but catch people and other objects. Some of the most common are trees and branches. If a strainer catches a swimmer, the force of the water can hold the swimmer there until hypothermia sets in and he or she tires and drowns.

- *Obstructions.* Another problem is any type of obstruction in the river that a person can get pinned against, such as a bridge abutment. A person can easily become trapped against the object and be held there by the force of moving water. Again, hypothermia can set in and he or she can tire and drown.

- *Holes.* Not all the water in a fast-moving river flows downstream. When water flows over a large object, a recirculating current or "hole" may form. When this

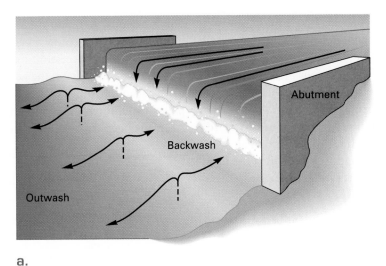

a.

Abutment

Backwash

Outwash

Boil line

b.

FIGURE 32-7 (a) A low-head dam can form (b) a large and uniform hole. If too close to the boil line, a boater can capsize and get pushed to the bottom.

happens, the current can keep recirculating a swimmer in its backwash until he or she tires and drowns. Holes are difficult to see from upstream. Large ones are very difficult to escape from.

- *Low-head dams* (Figure 32-7). These dams are only a few feet high. They are built from concrete and have vertical abutments on each side. They are very difficult to see from upstream and often tend to be very wide. Water that flows over these dams can form a very large and uniform "hole" that extends across the river. If a boater gets too close to the "boil line," he or she can get caught in the recirculating current and capsize. The person and the boat then can get pushed to the bottom and back to the surface again and again.

- *Entrapments* (Figure 32-8). Legs can get trapped between rocks or in other obstructions, especially in fast-moving water above a person's knees. Typically, this occurs to inexperienced folks who fall out of a boat and try to stand up. When this happens, the best thing to do is a back stroke with feet pointed downstream. Note that when an extremity gets caught, it must be extracted exactly in the same direction that it went in.

The basic, time-honored model for all water rescues is to reach, throw, row, and go. Remember, if you cannot easily effect a rescue using a simple shore-based technique (reach or throw), call for a team specializing in water rescue. *Do not enter the water.* Even special teams only try swimming or "live-bait" rescues as a last resort.

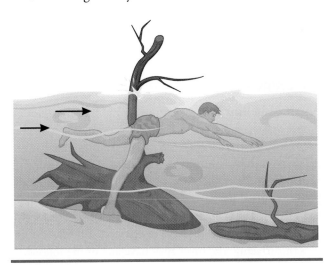

FIGURE 32-8 Entrapment in fast-moving water.

Ice Rescue

Judging the thickness of ice and overall safety is very tricky. The old rule-of-thumb—"one inch, keep off; two inches, one may; three inches, small groups; four inches, okay"—is *not* accurate. Many factors can alter the thickness of the ice over large and small areas. For example, underground springs cause water turbulence from beneath and thinner ice above. So do decaying plant matter, schools of fish, and so on.

The "reach, throw, row, and go" method is used for all water rescues, including ice rescue. However, you should note some differences :

- *Reach and throw.* As a drowning patient becomes more hypothermic, he will be less and less able to hold onto a rope. An alternative technique is to throw an inflated fire hose. By using modified end caps and air from a SCBA tank, a fire hose can be inflated quickly and pushed out to the patient.

- *Row.* A conventional boat may not be able to break the ice as it moves, unless the ice is very thin. An option may be to use a small inflatable craft with ropes to tether it and pull it from shore. Perhaps the best crafts for ice rescues are the air boat and hover craft. Either can be maneuvered over ice, water, or dry land.

- *Go.* When patients are too hypothermic to hang on, rescuers must go in to get them (Figure 32-9). This usually involves wearing a "dry" neoprene ice-rescue suit, which is tethered to shore. The rescuer then crawls, shuffles, or swims out to grab and pull the patient in.

When a person falls through ice, a First Responder must immediately call for a special ice-rescue team. Then,

don a personal flotation device and make reasonable attempts to reach or throw something to the patient from shore. If you are successful, the team can be canceled. If not, the team already on the way will have a chance to get to the scene in time to help the patient. Remember to prevent well-intentioned bystanders from going onto the ice. More people to save may lead to more lives being lost.

1. What is the difference between a "wet" and a "dry" drowning?

2. What makes a cold-water drowning different from a warm-water drowning?

3. Under what conditions should a First Responder attempt a water rescue?

4. If a First Responder qualifies and is properly equipped, what is the recommended strategy she should use for a water rescue?

5. What is First Responder care for a near-drowning patient who is responsive with no suspected spine injury? Unresponsive?

Section 2 Barotrauma

The term **barotrauma** refers to several conditions. It occurs when scuba or deep-water divers experience increasing underwater pressures or when they ascend in deep water improperly. Such patients may need both basic life support and transport to a treatment center that specializes in diving injuries.

Note that patients with diving emergencies require specialized medical knowledge and care. If needed, Duke University's "Divers Alert Network" is a source of free medical consultation services for dive-related emergencies. Their 24-hour emergency hotline number is 919-684-8111.

Air Embolism

An **air embolism** is one or more air bubbles that block a blood vessel. It occurs when a diver holds his or her breath during the ascent from a dive. Air in the lungs then expands rapidly, rupturing the alveoli and damaging nearby blood vessels. As a result, air bubbles enter the bloodstream. The most dangerous places for air bubbles to lodge are in the heart, brain, or spinal cord.

Signs and symptoms have rapid onset. Within 15 minutes of surfacing, the diver may have any of the following:

- Difficulty breathing.

- Blotching or itching skin.

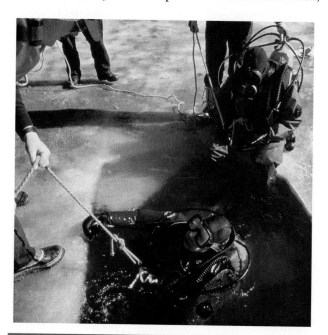

FIGURE 32-9 An ice rescue.

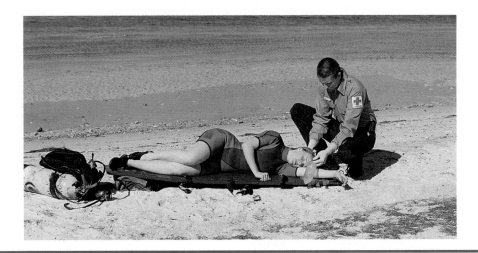

FIGURE 32-10 Proper positioning of a diving-accident patient.

- Frothy blood in the nose and mouth.
- Pain in the muscles and joints.
- Chest pain or pain in the abdomen.
- Swelling and a grating sound in the neck.
- Numbness or tingling in the extremities.
- General weakness, paralysis.
- Possible convulsions.
- Dizziness.
- Vomiting.
- Blurred or distorted vision.
- Loss or distortion of memory.
- Slurred speech, lack of coordination.
- Unresponsiveness.
- Cardiac or respiratory arrest.
- Behavioral changes (this may be the only sign).

The patient needs recompression treatment at the hospital. Be sure to arrange for transport as soon as possible. To provide First Responder care, treat all life-threats first. Ensure an adequate airway and administer 100% oxygen. If there is no sign of spine injury, position the patient on the left side with head and chest lower than the feet (Figure 32-10). Be prepared to provide ventilations or CPR.

Decompression Sickness

Decompression sickness, or "the bends," usually occurs when a diver comes up too quickly from a deep, prolonged dive. It can happen to anyone who is exposed to increasing pressure while breathing compressed air. It can range from mild to severe. It is more common than air embolism. The risk of decompression sickness increases if the diver flies within 12 hours of a dive.

Decompression sickness occurs when certain gases (usually nitrogen) are breathed by the diver over time. When the diver ascends, the nitrogen turns into tiny bubbles that lodge in the tissues throughout the body and eventually enter the bloodstream. The worst injuries occur when the nitrogen bubbles lodge in the brain, lungs, heart, or spinal cord. A burst lung is the most dire injury associated with this problem.

Signs and symptoms are gradual in onset. They usually occur 12 to 24 hours after the dive, but can occur up to 48 hours later. They include:

- Difficulty breathing, choking, or coughing.
- Chest pain.
- Itchy, mottled skin with a minor skin rash that can change in appearance.
- Swelling of tissues, with pits in the swelling.
- Severe, deep aching pain in the joints and muscles.
- Nausea and vomiting with abdominal pain.
- Fatigue, dizziness, collapse sometimes leading to unresponsiveness.
- Headache.
- Blurred vision.
- Hallucinations.
- Ringing of the ears or partial deafness.
- Staggering gait.
- Numbness, paralysis.
- Inability to urinate.

The patient needs to be taken to a facility with a recompression chamber for rapid treatment. Arrange for transport immediately. To provide First Responder care, treat life-threats first. Ensure an adequate airway, and administer 100% oxygen if you are allowed. Be prepared to provide CPR. If there is no sign of spine injury, position the patient on the left side with head lower than the feet. Slant the patient's entire body about 15 degrees to help prevent gas bubbles from injuring the brain or lungs.

The Squeeze

The "squeeze" and the "reverse squeeze" can involve any part of the body that is filled with air. When divers descend or ascend, air pressure must be equalized to maintain proper pressure in the body's air cavities. If proper pressure is not maintained, injury to the tissues of the air cavities results. If there is an air pocket in a tooth due to decay or a defective filling, the tooth may rupture. Divers are at increased risk of the squeeze and reverse squeeze if they have an upper respiratory infection or an allergy that obstructs the sinuses.

Signs and symptoms include:

- Mild to severe pain in the affected area.
- Blood or fluid discharge from the nose or ears.

- Bleeding from the tiny blood vessels in the eyes.
- Extreme dizziness, disorientation.
- Nausea.
- Ear pain (most common), ringing in the ears, possible deafness.

The patient needs to be cared for immediately at a medical facility to prevent permanent blindness, deafness, dizziness, or the inability to dive in the future. Arrange for transport immediately. To provide First Responder care, treat life-threats first. Suction to ensure an adequate airway. Administer oxygen if you are allowed. Keep the patient calm while waiting for medical help to arrive.

1. What are three emergencies that can occur in the diving environment?

2. What is the difference between an air embolism and decompression sickness?

▶▶ The Call Follow-up

At the beginning of this chapter, you read that a First Responder was on scene of a possible drowning at a public pool. To see how chapter skills apply to this emergency, read the following. It describes how the call was completed.

Initial Assessment I moved to Jimmy's head and carefully turned him over without stressing his spine. Then I opened his airway and checked to see if he was breathing. He wasn't. But he had a pulse.

We were pretty close to the side of the pool. Two other lifeguards arrived just above us, and one was quick enough to open the first-aid kit and hand me a pocket mask. She jumped in to help, while the other lifeguard went to call 9-1-1.

Even though I had never done it before on a real person, I put the face mask in place and started ventilations. It felt as if we were working on him for a while, but I guess it was only a minute or so when he started to cough. He brought up a little water, but not much. All of a sudden there was an ambulance crew above us.

Physical Examination The lifeguard who had jumped in the water to help me visually inspected the patient from head to toe. She reported that she found no signs of injury.

Patient History I knew Jimmy had had seizures before. He told me so. But I never actually witnessed one.

Ongoing Assessment The paramedics took over care before we had a chance to do anything but provide basic life support.

Patient Hand-off Our hand-off report was brief (see below). The paramedics then positioned a backboard under Jimmy, secured him, and lifted him from the water. He still wasn't wide awake, but we told him he was in good hands and that we'd contact his family.

 ## Hand-off Report

"The patient is Jimmy Rodriquez. He is about 14 years old. We found him face down in the water, unresponsive, and not breathing. We held manual stabilization of his head and neck while we turned him and during ventilations. We did not try to remove him from the water. Jimmy has a history of seizures and, according to an unknown bystander, he may have experienced one today. We could not rule out spine injury. We had performed artificial ventilation for about one minute, when he started to cough and breathe on his own."

The Last Word *Water-related emergencies pose a special challenge to First Responders. Patients in such emergencies often need immediate life-saving care. However, the same hazards that caused the emergency can endanger rescuers, too. Remember, your safety must come first. Do only what you are trained and equipped to do.*

Chapter Review

Focus on the EMS Team

Water emergencies can be surprisingly dangerous, even for good swimmers. Many people do not realize that the currents or water temperatures affecting the victim will affect them, too. And though television might portray water rescue as a simple matter of swimming out to and back with a grateful victim, in real life frantic victims can drown their rescuers.

Remember the basic rule of water rescue: Never attempt one unless you are a good swimmer, specially trained in water rescue, wearing a personal flotation device, and you are accompanied by other rescuers.

Summing Up

- When determining how to respond to a water emergency, take into account the patient's condition, water conditions, and the resources on hand.

- For any water emergency, use the "reach, throw, row, and go" method, even for an ice rescue.

- Suspect spine injury if a water emergency is the result of a diving accident or if the patient has been struck by a boat, water skier, surfboard, or other object. Also suspect spine injury in any swimmer who is unresponsive.

- If the patient is responsive, remove him from the water by any safe method possible as quickly as you can. Administer oxygen and conserve the patient's body heat.

- If the patient is unresponsive, do not attempt to remove him from the water until he is fully immobilized. Instead, maintain manual stabilization of the head and neck and support the back.

- Artificial ventilation can start in the water. Chest compressions cannot. Patients who need CPR must be removed from the water first.

- Always have a near-drowning patient taken to a hospital, even if you believe the danger has passed. Complications can develop and may be fatal as long as 72 hours after the incident.

- Unlike shallow water, fast-moving water hides dangers such as strainers, obstructions, holes, low-head dams, and entrapments. If you cannot easily effect a rescue using a simple shore-based technique (reach or throw), call for a team specializing in water rescue.

- Barotrauma occurs when scuba or deep-water divers experience increasing underwater pressures or when they ascend in deep water improperly. Such patients may need both basic life support and transport to a treatment center that specializes in diving injuries. If needed, Duke University's "Divers Alert Network" provides free medical consultation services for dive-related emergencies.

Key Terms

air embolism a type of barotrauma; occurs when one or more air bubbles block a blood vessel.

barotrauma refers to several conditions occurring when scuba or deep-water divers experience increasing underwater pressures or when they ascend in deep water improperly.

decompression sickness a type of barotrauma; occurs when a diver comes up too quickly from a deep prolonged dive.

drowning death from suffocation due to submersion.

Knowledge Check

1. You are at the scene of a person who appears to be drowning in a pond near shore. You should first:

a. row a boat to her.

b. jump in to save her.

c. throw floating objects at her.

d. reach out a pole for her to grab.

2. The patient has been successfully rescued from a near-drowning emergency and is cold, exhausted, and coughing up water. He is refusing medical attention, but you try to convince him to accept it because complications can develop as long as ___ hours after the incident.
   a. 72
   b. 36
   c. 24
   d. 12

3. Your patient has fallen out of a boat into swiftly moving waters that are just above her knees. She should:
   a. attempt to stand up and jump back into the boat.
   b. doggie paddle in the direction of the current.
   c. backstroke with feet pointed downstream.
   d. roll into a ball and hold her breath.

4. You are told that after diving into a pool, your patient was found face down in the water. You should suspect:
   a. near drowning.
   b. spine injury.
   c. heart attack.
   d. barotrauma.

5. The survival of a near-drowning victim depends on many factors, including whether the water is warm or cold.
   a. True
   b. False

6. For a cold-water drowning, you must continue resuscitation until the patient's body is cold.
   a. True
   b. False

7. Severe bleeding of the patient into the water can pose a risk of infection to others, including rescuers.
   a. True
   b. False

8. List the four criteria you must meet before attempting any water rescue.

   _____

   _____

   _____

   _____

9. List three hazards that may be found on or under water.

   _____

   _____

   _____

Scenario

You are called to a patient who was found unresponsive in an indoor pool. You are close and respond to the scene in your personal vehicle. Other people at the scene (who appear to have been drinking) say that the patient tried to dive from a tabletop into the shallow end of the pool. One person is in the pool and holding the patient afloat face-up. The bystanders do not appear to be a danger. You update incoming units and enter the shallow end of the heated pool.

a. What are your initial concerns about this patient?

_____

_____

b. Will you remove the patient from the pool? Explain your answer.

_____

_____

_____

_____

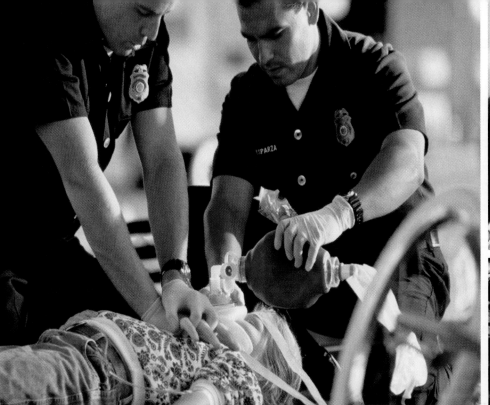
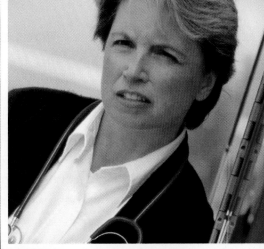
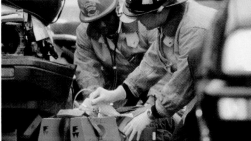

33 | Vehicle Stabilization and Patient Extrication

Objectives

From the U.S. Department of Transportation (DOT)'s 1995 "First Responder: National Standard Curriculum." Material supplemental to the DOT curriculum is listed under "Enrichment."

Cognitive

7-1.3 ▸ Discuss the role of the First Responder in extrication. (pp. 588, 590–591)

7-1.4 ▸ List various methods of gaining access to the patient. (pp. 588,590)

7-1.5 ▸ Distinguish between simple and complex access. (p. 588)

Affective

No objectives are identified by the DOT.

Psychomotor

No objectives are identified by the DOT.

Enrichment

▸ Describe the types of personal protective equipment recommended for rescue at the site of a vehicle collision. (p. 586)

▸ Discuss how to determine the number of patients at the scene of a vehicle collision. (p. 586)

▸ Describe basic goals of traffic control at the scene of a collision. (p. 587)

▸ State how a rescuer can recognize whether or not a vehicle is stable. (pp. 587–588)

▸ Describe the basic steps of stabilizing an upright vehicle and an overturned vehicle. (p. 588)

▸ List simple, basic tools that can be used in extrication. (p. 591)

Most of the time you will find your patients in safe, easily accessible locations where gaining access is no more than a knock on a door. However, there will be times when advanced rescue techniques must be used. By far the most common involve motor-vehicle collisions. You may find anything from an unhurt occupant in a stable vehicle to multiple vehicles with pinned occupants. This chapter provides an overview of how you can proceed safely and effectively. In practice, be sure to follow all local protocols.

Section 1 Scene Safety

Personal Protective Equipment

All EMS responders working in or around a wrecked vehicle and an extrication in progress must wear the following:

- *Eye protection.* Goggles or safety glasses with side shields are best to prevent flying metal shards from penetrating the eyes. Safety glasses with side shields also can be used to protect you from bloodborne pathogens. The flip-down shield on a firefighter helmet is not adequate protection for the eyes.

- *Hand protection.* Although firefighter gloves provide the best puncture protection, they allow for poor manual dexterity. A pair of snugly fitting leather work gloves provides less protection but is a good alternative.

- *Body protection.* A flame-retardant outer shell—such as firefighter turnout gear, brush-fire garment, or jumpsuit—provides some protection from fire and limited protection from sharp objects. All garments should have reflective trim to improve night recognition.

- *Foot protection.* With turnout pants, wear either short rubber or leather boots that have lug soles to prevent slippage. Boots should be above ankle height to prevent glass from dropping in.

In a vehicle collision—just as for every other type of emergency—ensure personal safety first.

First on Scene

At any crash scene, right from the beginning, safety must continually be your highest priority—to prevent injury to you and other rescuers and to help avoid additional injury to your patient.

Necessary Resources

To determine the resources you need on scene, find out how many patients are involved. It may be difficult to locate all of them at first, but it is critical that you do. Use a systematic approach:

- If it is safe to enter the scene, ask a responsive patient to tell you how many others were involved in the crash.

- Question witnesses to see if a victim walked away from the scene.

- In case of a high-impact crash, search the surrounding area carefully. Look in ditches and tall weeds.

- Look for tracks in the earth or snow. A person who could get free from wreckage may be wandering aimlessly.

- Search the vehicle itself carefully. A patient may be wedged under the dashboard, for example.

- Look quickly for items that give clues to unaccounted for children, such as a lunch box, diaper bag, or extra jacket.

Combine this information with your evaluation of scene safety. Are there enough rescue personnel on scene? If not, send for help immediately. Continue to evaluate the situation for the most efficient, safest ways to help patients and protect rescue teams.

If a car is on fire, decide if you can remove the passengers quickly enough or if you should fight the fire. If the passengers are not trapped, move them first. If they cannot be extricated quickly, deal with the fire. That is, safely do what you can within your training and with the available equipment.

Scene Control

The crash scene can involve environmental hazards as well as a great deal of confusion. Send for law enforcement and fire services to help control the scene. While you wait for them to arrive, begin scene control. Quickly deal with bystanders by having them move out of the danger zone.

THE CALL

Dispatch My partner and I are police officers with First Responder training. We were called to a vehicle collision involving multiple casualties. Time out was 10 p.m.

Scene Size-up As we approached, we saw a small red sports car sitting nose to nose with a large dump truck. The front of the little car was collapsed like an accordion under the truck's front axle. The front bumper of the truck was even with the windshield of the car. We saw a driver and a passenger in the truck, both appeared to be responsive. We also saw two motionless young people in the front seat of the car. There was a considerable amount of blood coming from multiple face wounds.

The next question the First Responders must ask themselves is this: "Is the scene safe to enter?" What do you think? Consider this emergency as you read Chapter 33. How would you proceed?

Spilled gasoline often is present at an auto crash. Allow no smoking on scene. Turn off all vehicle ignitions. If possible, get a fire crew with hoses to stand by during rescue.

Traffic Control

The basic goals of traffic control at the scene of a collision are:

- To channel the regular flow of traffic around the scene, preventing additional collisions and injuries.
- To monitor traffic to ensure minimal disruption.
- To clear the scene so that other emergency vehicles can reach the patients quickly.

Unless a distinct hazard justifies stopping all traffic, keep traffic moving. If the road is blocked, try to move traffic to an alternative route. Whatever you choose to do, make sure that motorists and pedestrians in the area know exactly what you want them to do. Keep rescue personnel well positioned along the roadway. If possible, rescuers should wear reflective clothing so they can be seen easily before and after dark. Use clear visual signals coupled with attention-getting devices such as flares or cones.

Fuses should be set 10–15 feet apart and extend 100 feet toward traffic. The pattern of fuses should lead traffic around the emergency. The danger zone includes at least a 50-foot radius around the wrecked cars. When the crash occurs on a curve, consider the start of the curve as the edge of the danger zone. On a hill, one edge of the danger zone should be the crest of the hill. If the highway has two lanes, position flares in both directions. If heavy trucks travel the road, extend the flare string, because trucks take much longer than cars to stop.

Vehicle Stabilization

After all possible outside hazards are controlled, make the rescue setting as safe as possible. Always suspect that a vehicle is unstable until you have made it stable. Assume the vehicle is not stable if:

- It is on a tilted surface such as a hill.
- Part of it is stacked on top of another vehicle.
- It is on a slippery surface such as ice, snow, or spilled oil.

First on Scene

Most cars are equipped with five-mile-per-hour bumpers designed to absorb low-speed front and rear-end collision damage. If the bumpers were involved in the collision, you may notice that the bumper shock absorber system is compressed, or "loaded." *Never stand in front of a loaded bumper.* If it springs out and strikes your knees, it could break your legs. Some rescue teams are trained to unload or chain the shock absorber to prevent an uncontrolled release.

- It is overturned.
- It rests on its side.

Basic to stabilization is **cribbing.** Cribbing is a system of wood or other supports used to prop up a vehicle. Wood is stacked in box-like squares and wedges to keep pressure uniform. To create a stable environment, the cribbing is arranged diagonally to the vehicle frame. Do not crib under wheels or tires, because the vehicle will tend to roll. Never stack cribbing higher than its own length. There should never be more than one or two inches between the cribbing and the vehicle.

Any vehicle that can be moved easily during extrication or patient care needs to be stabilized (Figure 33-1). Excess vehicle movement could prove fatal to a patient with severe spinal injuries and may injure the rescue team.

To stabilize a vehicle that rests on all four wheels, place the gear selector in park, or, if a standard shift, into reverse. Use blocks or wedges at wheels to prevent unexpected rolling. Chock wheels tightly against the curb when possible. To reduce the amount of movement even when you are using power tools, cut the tire valve stems so that the car rests on the rims.

To stabilize an overturned vehicle, place a solid object between the roof and the roadway. Use an object such as a wheel chock, spare tire, cribbing, or timber. If necessary, use a bumper jack to angle the vehicle against the solid object until it is stable. Hook a chain to the vehicle's axle. Then loop the chain around a tree or post.

Q:

1. Why should a First Responder wear goggles or safety glasses with eye shields at the scene of a collision?

2. What should you do to determine the number of patients involved in a collision?

3. What safety precautions should you take to control the scene of a collision?

4. What are your basic goals of traffic control at the scene of a collision?

5. When should you assume that a vehicle is unstable?

Section 2 Gaining Access and Extrication

Generally, emergency medical care is provided before patient extrication, unless a delay would endanger the life of the patient or rescuer. The role of the First Responder is to administer that care. The First Responder also is to make sure the patient is removed in a way that minimizes further injury.

In certain circumstances First Responders are required to take steps to gain access to the patient in a vehicle. Take only the steps you are trained to take. Call for additional assistance and rescue personnel if needed. In such cases, a chain of command should be established to ensure patient-care priorities.

Gaining Access

There are two basic ways a rescuer can gain access to a patient. **Simple access** is access that requires no tools. **Complex access** is access that requires tools and specialized equipment. Most emergencies do not present access problems. However, when you are confronted with one, quickly evaluate the situation and decide if a simple or complex access is needed. If complex access is needed, call for rescuers who have the training and equipment.

Get to the patient *safely.* A lot of emotion can be involved at a crash scene. Do not allow that to hurry you into a setting that is not safe to enter. Enter the wreck to administer emergency care only when the vehicle is stabilized and it is safe to do so.

Doors

A door is always the access of choice. This is because it is the largest uncomplicated opening in a vehicle. Always start by testing the door handles.

First, try to open the door nearest the patient. If the doors are locked, try to open the lock by either having the patient in the car do so or by using a coat hanger or other device between the door frame and window. Routinely unlock all other doors to allow access by other rescuers. If the doors cannot be opened, determine the best point of entry and proceed accordingly.

Since 1983 cars are made with a collision beam inside the door, which makes it tougher for a door to cave in. Beware that the beam can buckle after impact, and a sharp end may stick into the passenger compartment. As you try to gain access through a door, be sure that the angle of force does not propel the beam further into the vehicle.

Windows

If you can, remove a window without breaking it. To remove a fixed window installed in U-shaped black plastic or rubber, remove the rim first. Insert the point of a linoleum knife or similar tool into the molding at the

SKILL SUMMARY   *Stabilizing a Vehicle*

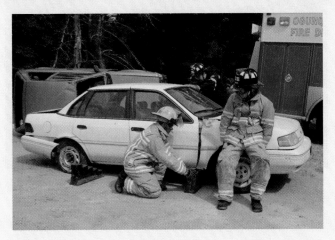

FIGURE 33-1A   *Stabilizing a car on its wheels with cribbing.*

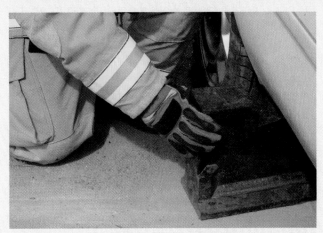

FIGURE 33-1B   *Placing a step chock.*

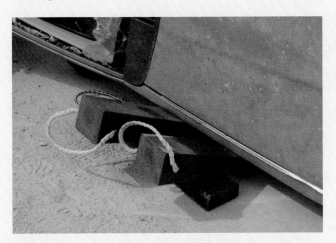

FIGURE 33-1C   *Stabilizing a vehicle on its side with cribbing.*

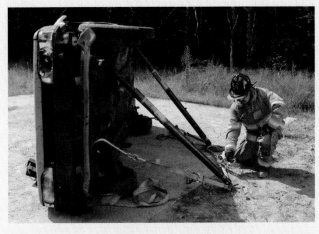

FIGURE 33-1D   *Stabilizing a vehicle on its side with struts.*

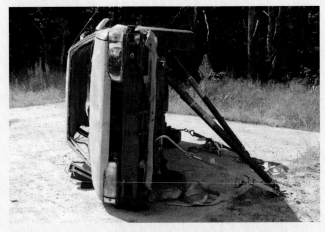

FIGURE 33-1E   *Stabilizing a vehicle on its side with cribbing and struts.*

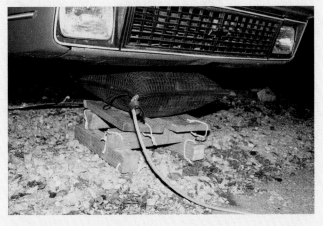

FIGURE 33-1F   *Stabilizing a vehicle on its roof with an air bag and cribbing.*

midpoint of the glass. Keep the blade as flat against the glass as you can. Draw the knife across the top and down the side. Repeat on the other side. Soapy water will keep the blade moving easily. Work the end of a short pry bar behind the glass and pry it loose from the top. The window will pivot on its bottom edge.

Car windows usually are made of tempered glass. Rear and side windows are designed to break into small granules. Fine particles can stay unnoticed in a deep wound and cause damage after it closes. So, if you must break a window, cover the patient with a heavy safety blanket first.

To break a window, locate the one farthest from the patient. Give a quick hard thrust in the lower corner with a spring-loaded punch, screwdriver, or other sharp object. If you can, put strips of broad tape or a sheet of contact paper over the glass to prevent broken pieces from spraying on the patient. Use your gloved hand to carefully pull the glass outside the vehicle. Clear all glass away from the window opening. Before you crawl in, drape a heavy tarp or blanket over the door edge and the interior of the car just below the window.

Windshield

Windshields usually are made of laminated safety glass, which cannot be broken safely. If the windshield is largely intact, pry up the chrome trim at the joints using a baling hook, pry bar, or screwdriver.

To remove the rubber seal that sets the windshield in the car, use a linoleum knife to slice the rubber bead. Drive the point into the channel and keep the blade flat against the glass. Then force a screwdriver behind the glass and simply pop out the windshield. For a Mastic-set windshield, remove the molding. Then use a Mastic cutter to free the windshield. The Mastic cutter may be obtained from an auto parts store or an auto windshield business.

Removal of a broken Mastic-set windshield may cause a great deal of splintering. Therefore, as with any extrication, you and the patient must be protected properly. Cover the patient with a safety blanket. Make sure each rescuer has full facial protection and wears a long-sleeved shirt and heavy gloves. Always consider using an alternative entry method before breaking or cutting glass.

Airbags

If the airbag has released (Figure 33-2), there may be some residue. This is not harmful and can be washed off. If the airbag was not triggered by the crash, disconnect the negative side of the battery and the yellow airbag connector. Do not cut the connector or its wires, since they

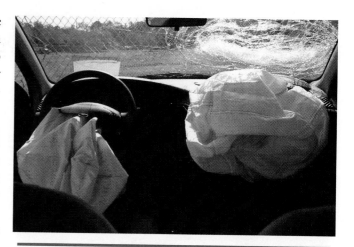

FIGURE 33-2 Discharged airbags. *(Stephen Bell Photographic Productions)*

keep the shorting bar activated and prevent accidental triggering.

Pinned Patients

Always summon a rescue unit when a patient is pinned beneath a vehicle. Use a sturdy jack to raise a vehicle, but do not use a jack on a completely overturned vehicle. A pry bar and blocks may be used. A large group of bystanders can assist in lifting the vehicle off a patient. Any time a vehicle is raised, be sure to shore it up with blocks or another non-compressible material so that it will not fall on the patient.

If a patient has a body part through a window, pad the extruded part well with bandaging material. Then carefully use pliers or a knife to break or fold away the glass. Once the body part is free, care for it.

If a patient is jammed or pinned inside the vehicle, consider the following simple procedures: Remove a shoe or other piece of clothing that may be pinning the patient. Move the front seat to give additional working space. Remove the back seat entirely. Cut off seat belts with shears or a knife, but support the dangling patient as you cut the belt.

Patient Assessment

During extrication, as in any emergency, your first priority is always your own safety. (You are no good to the patient if you become another casualty.) Be sure the scene is safe, the vehicle is stable, and you are wearing the appropriate personal protective equipment before you try to reach the patient. Once you do, stabilize the patient's head and neck. Complete an initial assessment. Be sure you have called for the necessary resources. If possible, perform a physical exam and gather a patient history. ■

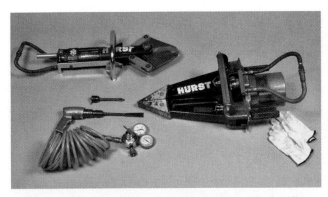

a. *Heavy rescue equipment: hydraulic cutter, hydraulic spreaders, air chisel.*

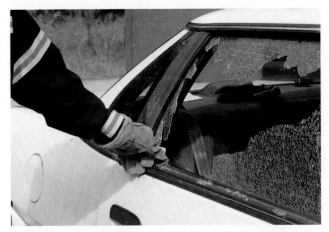

b. *Spring-loaded center punch to break windows.*

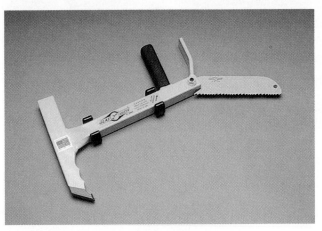

c. *Glas-Master saw for windshield removal.*

FIGURE 33-3 Be prepared with basic extrication tools in case a rescue square is not available.

First Responder Care

To care for a patient during extrication, maintain the manual stabilization of his head and spine. Maintain the ABCs and perform any critical interventions necessary. Remain with the patient during a complex extrication. Continually monitor his or her condition. If it begins to deteriorate, advise the rescue crew. They may be able to change the approach to the incident and get the patient out more quickly. During the process, be sure to protect yourself and the patient from the glass and flying debris. Use heavy blankets, a tarp, or even a solid object like a backboard.

Try to keep the patient calm during rescue. Even with an altered mental status, the patient may get very frightened. Keep him or her informed about what is being done to help. For example, let the patient know when a loud noise will occur and what is causing it.

Immobilize the patient's spine during rescue. (Follow the precautions and procedures described in Chapter 24, "Injuries to the Spine.") The only exception to this rule occurs when there is an immediate threat to life, such as fire, and an emergency move is required. ■

Extrication Tools

Where possible and appropriate, contact the local rescue squad immediately after a collision in which someone is trapped. They will be able to get to the patient and extricate him quickly and safely. However, it is important to be prepared in case a rescue squad is not available (Figure 33-3). Basic tools that can be used for extrication include hammer, screwdriver, chisel, crowbar, pliers, linoleum knife, work gloves and goggles, shovel, tire irons, wrenches, knives, car jacks, and ropes or chains. Ingenuity can put these tools to work in a safe and effective way.

Q:

1. What are the two basic ways a First Responder can gain access to a patient? Explain the difference between the two.

2. In case a rescue squad is not available, what are some basic tools a rescuer would need to extricate someone trapped in a wrecked vehicle?

The Call Follow-up

At the beginning of this chapter, you read that First Responders were on the scene of a two-vehicle head-on collision. There are four patients. To see how chapter skills apply to this emergency, read the following. It describes how the call was completed.

Scene Size-up *(continued)* This was a complex-access rescue situation. We immediately updated dispatch and requested specialized rescue crews and an ambulance for each patient. Then we positioned our vehicle about 100 feet from the wreckage to give the rescue units space to pull in.

As soon as we determined it was safe to approach, we saw that both vehicles had all four wheels on solid ground. They appeared to be stable. We made sure that both engines were turned off and the brakes were on. We also looked for any smoke or leaks.

Initial Assessment Next, we attempted to gain access to the mangled car. We couldn't open any of the doors and had limited access to the patients through windows. We updated dispatch to be sure heavy rescue was on the way. We did as much of an initial assessment as we could from the open windows of the sports car. We were able to keep the patients' airways open and maintain spinal stabilization but not more.

Physical Examination We could not do much of an assessment since our hands were tied up with the airway and c-spine stabilization. I could see that my patient had deformity to both legs and possible chest trauma. My partner's patient was starting to talk a bit and said his head hurt. We believed both were serious—just from the mechanism of injury. What we saw confirmed it.

Patient History Neither patient was able to provide a history. We scanned their necks and wrists for medical information devices and saw none.

Ongoing Assessment We were taking spinal precautions and attempting to maintain the airways of the patients when the first ambulance arrived. It had only been a few minutes but it seemed like along time.

Patient Hand-off We reported the number of patients and our initial observations to the EMTs (see below). While they proceeded to assess and care for the patients in the sports car, we went back to the patients in the truck, who did in fact have minor injuries.

It took a while for the patients to be disentangled from the wreckage. We assisted in every way we could—from redirecting traffic to holding manual stabilization of a patient's head and neck during extrication.

 ## Hand-off Report

"We have four patients: two patients with minor injuries in the truck and two seriously injured patients here in the sports car. My patient is unresponsive and has potential leg and chest injuries. His airway is clear and he is breathing adequately. This other patient was unresponsive but now will respond verbally. He complains of a head injury. That's about as far as we got."

The Last Word *As in all emergency situations, remember that your first priority is your own safety. Do not enter the scene of an emergency until you have determined that it is safe. Do not attempt a complex rescue unless you are trained and equipped to do so. Follow your local protocols.*

Chapter Review

Focus on the EMS Team

Rescue incidents involve almost every aspect of the EMS system from police and firefighters to First Responders, EMTs, and advanced life support personnel. The team concept is vitally important to a proper end result—the best extrication and care for the patient.

Every member of the team has a job. However, those jobs must be done in a specific order by trained people. For example, a First Responder may enter a vehicle through a window to hold stabiliza-tion of the patient's c-spine while the extrication team does its job. During that time, other First Responders and EMTs should not be near the vehicle for safety reasons. Once the patient is extricated, the extrication team will step back and the EMS team may begin emergency care.

It could be said that the rescue scene requires choreography. That is, it is a well-organized series of steps carried out by a well-orchestrated team.

Summing Up

- The most common emergency in which advanced rescue techniques must be used is the motor-vehicle collision. You must know how to proceed safely and effectively. Safely, because you would be no good to the patient if you were injured, too. Effectively, because you must gather accurate and appropriate information so that patient transport is not unnecessarily delayed.

- First, perform a size size-up. Identify the hazards and call for the appropriate assistance to control them. That may include law enforcement to control crowds and traffic, fire services for actual and potential fire hazards, hazardous materials crews, and extrication teams.

- After determining the number of patients, call for the appropriate number of ambulances. The incident command system should be used during incidents with multiple casualties or where numerous organizations must interface at the scene.

- Put on all necessary personal protective equipment before you enter the scene. All EMS responders working in or around a wrecked vehicle and an extrication in progress must wear goggles or safety glasses with side shields, firefighter or leather work gloves, a flame-retardant outer shell (turnout gear) with reflective trim, and ankle-high rubber or leather boots with lug soles.

- After all possible hazards have been controlled, the vehicle should be stabilized. Then gain access to the patient, enter the vehicle, and provide emergency care.

- Do not remove a patient from a crash vehicle unless he is in immediate danger.

- During extrication of a pinned patient, continue to provide care and ensure that no further harm is caused to the patient.

- To remove a patient from a vehicle, take all spinal precautions, including immobilization on a long backboard.

Key Terms

complex access the process of gaining access to a patient with the use of tools and specialized equipment.

cribbing a system of wood or other supports used to prop up a vehicle or other object.

simple access the process of gaining access to a patient without the use of tools.

Knowledge Check

1. Automobile side and rear windows are made of tempered glass, which will break into:
   a. long shards.
   b. large sheets.
   c. many small pieces.
   d. razor-sharp slivers.

2. After making sure the scene of a car crash is safe, the First Responder should:
   a. stabilize the vehicle.
   b. extricate the patient.
   c. gain access to the patient.
   d. treat the patient's wounds.

3. You have arrived at a car crash. The driver is trapped in the front seat, and the driver's door is jammed. You should try to:
   a. take out the windshield.
   b. pry the door open.
   c. open another door.
   d. break a window.

4. Generally, an airbag can be deactivated by disconnecting the yellow airbag connector and:
   a. locating the switch and turning it off.
   b. disconnecting the battery.
   c. deploying it.
   d. removing it.

5. To control traffic at a car crash, flares and cones should be set back at least ____ feet.
   a. 25
   b. 50
   c. 100
   d. 150

6. If the motor is off, a vehicle found in a parking space on a hilly street is considered STABLE.
   a. True
   b. False

7. During extrication, a First Responder's main responsibilities are to administer emergency care and to make sure the patient is not injured further.
   a. True
   b. False

8. List six examples of the personal protective equipment necessary for First Responders working at or around a wrecked vehicle.

   _____   _____

   _____   _____

   _____   _____

9. List three ways you can determine how many patients are at a collision scene.

   _____

   _____

   _____

Scenario

You are called to a motor-vehicle collision on a rural road in your town. You arrive to find a vehicle overturned in a ditch. The vehicle is on its roof and appears to be rocking, the hood and then the trunk striking the ground repeatedly. You hear at least one person moaning inside the vehicle.

a. Should you attempt to access any patients inside the vehicle? Why or why not?

_____

_____

b. What resources should be requested for this scene?

_____

_____

c. Is there any way to stabilize the vehicle prior to the arrival of specialized rescue units?

_____

_____

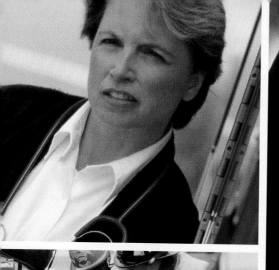
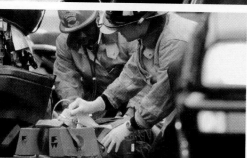
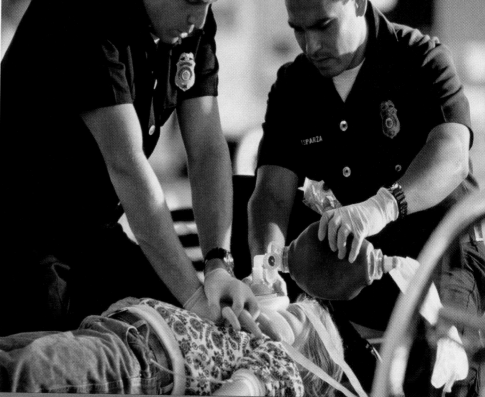

34 | Special Rescue Situations

Objectives

From the U.S. Department of Transportation (DOT)'s 1995 "First Responder: National Standard Curriculum." Material supplemental to the DOT curriculum is listed under "Enrichment."

Cognitive

    No objectives are identified by the DOT.

Affective

    No objectives are identified by the DOT.

Psychomotor

    No objectives are identified by the DOT.

Enrichment

▶ Describe some of the hazards involved in rescues of patients having confined-space emergencies. (pp. 597–598)

▶ Identify the role of the First Responder in a confined-space emergency. (pp. 597–598)

▶ Discuss the general guidelines for performing safe litter carries over distances on rough terrain. (p. 599)

▶ State the criteria for identifying a rescue as a low-angle or high-angle rescue. (p. 600)

▶ Describe the basic capabilities of a helicopter in rescue operations. (pp. 601–602)

▶ List the characteristics of a safe helicopter landing zone. (pp. 602–603)

▶ Describe the procedure for safely approaching a helicopter that has just landed. (p. 603)

Introduction

People who are drawn to public safety and emergency work tend to be very action-oriented. They almost always rather do something than just stand by and watch. The problem is that taking action in situations where you may be unaware of the hazards can result in serious injury or even death. This chapter will introduce you to some hazards of special rescue, hazards that could go unnoticed until it is too late.

Section 1 Confined-Space Emergencies

Most of the time we do not think about the air we breathe, unless it has a bad odor or it is irritating in some way. Unfortunately, not all hazards in the environment warn us away with odors. Confined spaces can be especially dangerous to rescuers as well as patients.

A **confined space** is defined as a place with limited access and egress that is not designed for human occupancy. Some examples of confined spaces are (Figure 34-1):

- *Silos.* Silos are used in agriculture to store solid materials. Some are designed specifically to limit the presence of oxygen. Hazards include poisonous gases emitted during the natural fermentation of crops, as well as engulfment and suffocation. Silos are perhaps the most common sites of confined-space emergencies.

- *Storage bins.* These include both grain bins and grain elevators. Like silos, they present the hazards of low oxygen levels and engulfment.

- *Underground vaults.* These include utility vaults for water, sewer, electrical power, telephone, and other communications cables. Hazards include poisonous gases and electrocution.

- *Wells, culverts, and cisterns.* These offer little oxygen and a high risk of drowning or entrapment.

A low oxygen level is a significant, common hazard in confined spaces. Also common are poisonous gases such as hydrogen sulfide, carbon dioxide, carbon monoxide, and methane. Note that some atmospheres are explosive as well as poisonous.

Safety Precautions

The U.S. Occupational Safety and Health Administration (OSHA) has taken an aggressive approach to safety for workers in confined spaces. Among its rules are the following:

- Atmosphere must be properly ventilated and monitored for oxygen, carbon monoxide, and hydrogen sulfide.

- Electrical systems must be locked and lagged out.

- Stored energy must be dissipated.

- Pipes must be disconnected or blanked out.

- Rescuers who plan to enter a space must use the appropriate respiratory protection, such as a self-contained breathing apparatus (SCBA) or supplied air breathing apparatus (SABA).

A call to a confined-space emergency is usually for a fall, medical problem, asphyxia, explosion, or machinery

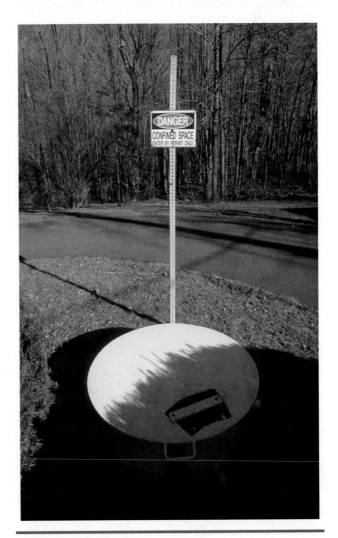

FIGURE 34-1 A confined space.

THE CALL

Dispatch My first response unit was dispatched for an automobile crash on County Route 402, the farthest part of our district. The report was that one car left the road and rolled over.

Scene Size-up We approached the scene. There were no signs of wires down, leaking gas, or hazardous materials. The car looked as if it had been bounced around a lot but somehow ended up on its wheels. There was one

passenger inside the vehicle. We put on our gear and gloves and approached. There was a star in the windshield where the driver hit his head. The steering wheel was bent. We soon discovered that we were unable to open the doors because the roof was pushed down on them. Rescue was notified.

How can these First Responders get to the patient? What kind of care can they provide until they do? Consider this emergency as you read Chapter 34. How would you proceed?

---

entrapment. As a First Responder, your responsibility is to recognize the emergency and call for the proper help as soon as possible. Do not enter a scene unless you know that it is safe. Only members of specialized teams trained and equipped for the emergency should enter.

When you are called to a confined-space emergency, proceed with scene size-up as follows: First, determine the nature of the emergency. That is, obtain a copy of the permit for the site and assess the type of work being done. Determine how many workers are inside the confined space and, without entering it, determine the hazards present in the space. Second, call for a specialized rescue team, as well as for emergency medical personnel and transport. Third, establish a perimeter and do not allow anyone to enter. Finally, when they arrive, assist medical or rescue personnel if you are trained to do so and if you can do so safely.

Cave-ins and Rescues from Trenches

Dirt may be too close to the top edge of a trench or ground vibration, water seepage, or an intersecting trench could cause one of the walls to give way. Therefore, OSHA requires **shoring** or a "trench box" in any trench deeper than five feet. Trench boxes are now commonly used all over the U.S. Unfortunately, a contractor or a do-it-yourselfer sometimes does not use one.

Most trench collapses occur at sites less than six feet wide and 12 feet deep. Usually, a worker was inside the trench when the walls collapsed, burying the worker either completely or partially. If someone jumps into the

trench to try to rescue the worker, a secondary collapse occurs and he or she gets buried, too (Figure 34-2).

Soil weighs about 100 pounds per cubic yard. That is, two feet of soil piled on top of a person's back or chest is equal to about a 1,000 pounds. So even if a person is only partially buried, the weight of the soil on his or her chest can cause respiratory difficulties. To rescue such a victim safely requires methodical and strenuous effort. It can be a slow process.

No matter how the cave-in occurs, if the trench is more than waist-deep, a specialized trench rescue team is needed. As a First Responder, your job is to secure the scene by establishing a perimeter. Do not allow anyone to enter the trench or its immediate area. Call for the rescue team as soon as possible. Remember, if a collapse has occurred, another one is very likely.

1. What is a "confined space"? Give three examples.

2. What personal protective equipment does OSHA recommend for workers in confined spaces?

3. What information should you gather during scene size-up of a confined-space emergency?

4. Why does OSHA require shoring in any trench deeper than five feet?

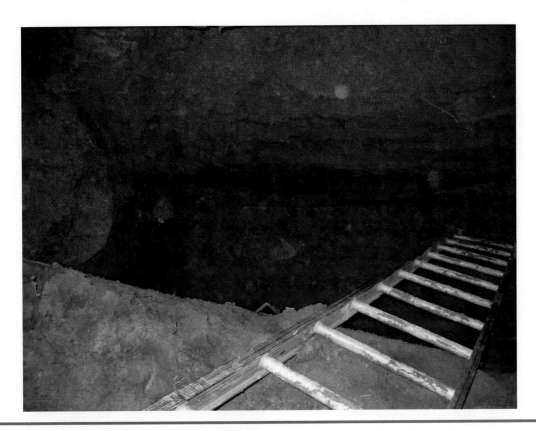

FIGURE 34-2 A worker is buried in a primary collapse; his back is barely visible. Sixty seconds after this picture was taken, a secondary collapse occurred burying the victim under another three feet of dirt. Had First Responders entered the trench, they too would have died. *(© Jon Politis)*

Section 2 Rough-Terrain Evacuations

More people are engaging in—and getting injured in—mountain biking, skiing, rock climbing, and other types of rough-terrain sports. As a First Responder, you may be required to assist in evacuation of these patients.

Litter Carries

It takes 18–20 people to carry a litter, or portable stretcher, for one mile. Wheels may be attached to some types of portable stretchers, but they work well only on fairly flat terrain.

To perform a litter carry over rough terrain for some distance, first select teams of four to six bearers each (Figure 34-3). Members of each team should be about

equal in height. After a team carries the portable stretcher a short distance, team members should change positions and then sides. After another short distance, a fresh team should rotate into position and take over.

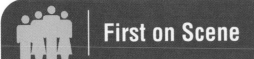

First on Scene

Become familiar with the emergency needs particular to your area, and plan for them. Being prepared and knowing what you can and should do are crucial to the success of special rescue situations.

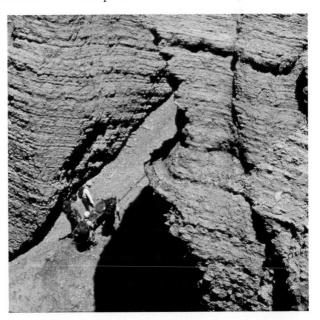

FIGURE 34-3 Litter carry over rough terrain. *(Howard M. Paul/Emergency Stock!)*

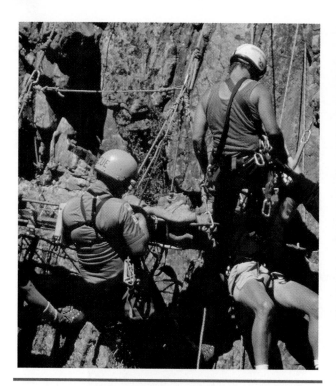

FIGURE 34-4 Rope system used for a high-angle rescue. *(Howard M. Paul/Emergency Stock!)*

High- and Low-Angle Rescues

When the angle of the terrain increases, the risk of falling and dropping a patient on a litter increases. One way to manage this risk is to use a rope system to lift or lower the stretcher while rescuers hold and guide it (Figure 34-4).

In most cases, a high-angle rescue is obvious. It would involve moving up or down a cliff, gorge, or side of a building, for example. If you have any doubt, a **high-angle rescue** team would be needed when:

- Slope forms more than a 40-degree angle.
- Slips or falls would likely result in serious injury or death due to the dangerous terrain below the slope.
- Terrain is so hazardous, it requires **rappelling** (getting down a slope by means of a secured rope).

A **low-angle rescue** generally does not need a rope system. You can identify a low-angle rescue by the following conditions:

- Slope forms less than a 40-degree angle.
- Hands are not needed for balance or scrambling.
- Slips or falls would not likely result in serious injury or death.

As soon as you recognize a low- or high-angle emergency, call immediately for specialized personnel to perform the rescue. Follow your local protocols.

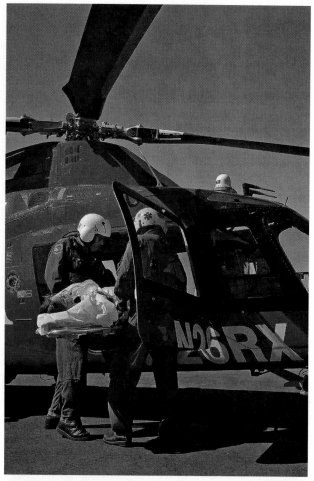

a.

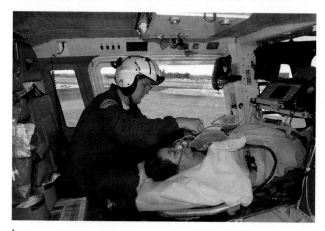

b.

FIGURE 34-5 Helicopter rescue.

1. How many people does it take to carry a portable stretcher for one mile? How many teams?

2. How should rescuers lift or lower a patient's stretcher in a high-angle rescue?

Section 3 Helicopters in Rescue Operations

A helicopter's ability to hover, land in small places, and carry people and equipment make it a logical rescue platform. Over the years, search-and-rescue operations have come to depend on helicopters (Figure 34-5). However, ground-based rescue efforts should never wait for air support. Weather conditions or other aircraft limitations can result in significant delays. So when calling for air support, make sure you have a back-up plan in case air rescue is delayed or impossible. (See Table 34-1 for guidelines for when to request air support.)

Helicopter Capabilities

Weather Limitations

An aircraft can take off and land either visually or by way of instruments. However, *instrument flight rules (IFR)* are used only to fly from one airport to another. Sometimes they are used to guide a pilot to safety when weather suddenly turns bad.

Visibility is crucial to rescue operations. The pilot and crew must be able to see the ground team for flight instructions. Since visibility is needed, an aircraft would not be able to launch if the weather is below minimum standards. A good rule of thumb to follow to estimate visibility at the rescue site is:

Day—500-foot cloud ceiling and one mile of visibility.

Night—1,000-foot cloud ceiling and three miles of visibility.

Altitude also plays an important role. The ability of a helicopter to hold a hover is key to a rescue operation. As the altitude of a craft increases, air density decreases. In addition, the warmer the air, the less dense it is. As air density decreases, more power is needed for the aircraft to hold a hover. At some point, altitude or air temperature may make it impossible to accomplish a mission.

Control Systems

Piloting a helicopter is complex. The pilot must be able to operate three main control systems. The "collective" system controls the angle of the main rotor blades. It also controls the vertical motion of the craft. By using the collective and a great deal of power, the aircraft can lift off the ground. The "cyclic" system tilts the spinning rotors and produces the forward, backward, and side movements of the craft. Finally, the "rudder pedals" control the pitch of the tail rotor and the rotation of the aircraft.

During takeoff, the helicopter pilot must increase the power and rotor speed. Then, he or she uses the collective to increase the angle of the rotor blades and lift off. The cyclic is moved forward to make the transition from vertical lift to forward flight. As the aircraft moves forward, additional air speed is needed for more lift. Once the craft is at the proper altitude, the need for power is reduced. Because of the engine power needed, take-offs and landings are dangerous times.

The controls of the helicopter are very sensitive. A small movement of one of them can mean a major change in the attitude of the craft. To pilot a helicopter during a hover is especially strenuous and stressful. It has been compared to rubbing your belly, patting the top of your head, and reciting the Gettysburg address all at once.

In addition, when in a hover, the pilot cannot see the target below. The crew chief watches the spot and verbally guides the pilot. The pilot also needs to spot a reference point. Normally, this is tricky. At night or in low-light conditions, it can be very difficult.

TABLE 34-1 When to Call for a Helicopter

Operational Reasons	Medical Reasons
Normal ground travel to the appropriate medical facility would take more than 30 minutes.	The patient has a life- or limb-threatening condition.
Extrication will be prolonged or location of the emergency is at a remote site.	The patient's condition is unstable (shock, head injury with altered mental status, chest trauma with respiratory distress, penetrating injuries to body cavity, amputations, burns over 15% of the body or to the face).
Patient needs paramedic-level care.	There is a serious mechanism of injury (fall of 15 feet or more, blow from a vehicle traveling over 20 mph, ejection from vehicle, a rollover without restraints, major deformity to passenger compartment or to vehicle's front end, death of one of the car passengers).

Space and Load

Some crafts are large enough to carry a whole squad of people. Others are small and cannot hold many more than a pilot, patient, and one crew member. In general, helicopters are very weight sensitive.

When the capacity of a craft is listed, it usually does not take into account the fuel load, crew, equipment, altitude, and air temperature. All of these factors have a major influence on the performance of the craft. If a craft is heavily weighted, for example, it may be able to land in a tight spot, but it may not be able to take off without getting rid of unnecessary gear or crew.

Special Tactics

One of the main reasons to choose a helicopter for rescue is its ability to pick up and extract people without landing. That involves hoisting, rappelling, and flying with external loads. All of these tactics are risky. Because of the danger and stress of hovering, special tactics are almost always aimed at reducing hover time.

Hoisting

Some aircraft are equipped with mechanical hoists. They are made to insert or to extract people from the ground. They are most commonly found on military craft and on some public safety aircraft.

Hoisting operations require hover time, which will vary depending on the speed of the hoist and the amount of cable out. Operations also are limited by the safe working load of the cable and the number of duty cycles of the system.

If you work around helicopters that have hoists, become familiar with the ground safety procedures. One that applies to all hoist cables relates to static electricity. When a cable is lowered, it must touch the ground to allow its electrical charge to dissipate. If the cable is touched before that happens, the first person who touches it will get an electrical jolt.

SPIE Line

The use of a special insertion and extrication (SPIE) line is called the "short-haul technique." It was developed by mountain rescue teams in Europe and by Parks Canada. It involves flying beneath the helicopter as an external load. It is commonly used with light duty aircraft without hoists to both insert and extract rescuers and patients.

Generally, a weighted and backed-up rope system is attached to the cargo hook or belly band of a helicopter. At the other end of the rope, rescuers in flight helmets with communications and harnesses are clipped in. When the helicopter ascends, they dangle beneath the craft as they are flown to the target area and gently lowered to the ground.

To extract, the craft flies into position and the ground team clips the litter or patients into the SPIE line. They are then flown back to a staging area and gently lowered into position.

Both insertion and extraction are risky operations. They should be undertaken only by specialized rescue teams. Note that if an external load becomes destabilized during flight or if an emergency occurs where the helicopter and crew are in jeopardy, an external load may be jettisoned.

Landing Zones

The helicopter landing zone should be at least 100 feet by 100 feet square (Figure 34-6). The landing zone (LZ) should be flat or have no more than an eight-degree slope. The LZ also should be (Table 34-2):

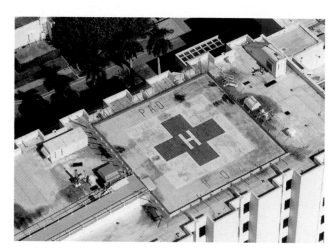

a.

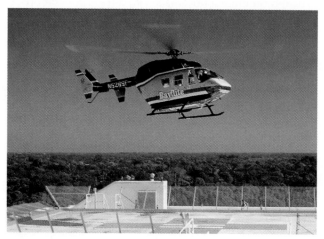

b.

FIGURE 34-6 Aeromedical transport is an important part of the EMS system for transporting critically ill or injured patients to the hospital. *(Maria A. H. Lyle)*

TABLE 34-2 **Landing Zone Guidelines**

- Approximately 100 × 100 foot area.
- Free of all obstructions.
- Clear of wires, towers, vehicles, people, and loose objects.
- Firm ground with less than 8° slope.
- Markers on all four corners.
- All emergency red lights should be on.
- No white lights, spotlights, or blue lights directed toward the helicopter or landing zone.
- No smoking.

■ *Free of obstructions.* This includes wires, trees, buildings, and other obstructions. If it is surrounded by obstructions, the pilot will be forced into a vertical take off, which takes tremendous power and is very dangerous. If there are any obstructions near the LZ, inform the pilot by radio.

■ *No loose objects.* Anything loose on the ground will blow around in the 100-mile-per-hour rotor wash of the helicopter. Stones, dirt, and other objects are easily picked up and blown into people and vehicles causing both injury and property damage.

■ *Scene lighting.* Keep emergency lights on to help the pilot locate the scene. Also place markers on all four corners of the LZ. Chemical light sticks or small strobe lights work well. Avoid shining spotlights on the helicopter because they can blind the pilot.

■ *Traffic control.* The LZ must be absolutely secure. There should be no traffic within 100 feet of the aircraft.

Both the main and tail rotors on a helicopter are extremely dangerous. Do not approach the craft until the pilot or crew chief signals you to approach or escorts you to the ship. Never approach from the rear. The tail rotor is spinning so fast, it is nearly invisible and it can kill. In addition, the main rotor may be lower than it appears to be. Depending on the grade of the LZ, the spinning blade may be no more than a few feet above the ground.

If you are signaled to approach the helicopter, maintain eye contact with the pilot or crew chief. Approach only from the front. Stay low. Avoid carrying anything above your head. Avoid wearing anything loose that can be blown away by the rotor wash.

 Q:
1. What are some operational reasons for calling for a helicopter rescue?
2. What are the characteristics of a safe helicopter landing zone?

▶▶ The Call Follow-up

At the beginning of this chapter, you read that First Responders were in a remote location at the scene of a car crash. To see how chapter skills apply to this emergency, read the following. It describes how the call was completed.

Initial Assessment The patient was moaning. He seemed to know who we were but he wasn't alert. He was moving air and had no airway obstructions. We didn't see any obvious bleeding. The man's skin was pale and moist. My partner stabilized his head and neck, and I checked his pulse. It was 110 and weak.

We were concerned about the mechanism of injury and the signs of shock. I radioed for the MedFlight helicopter. They were available and had an ETA of less than 20 minutes.

Physical Examination We couldn't get the man out of the car, so we continued stabilization. I began an assessment. He appeared to have a chest injury and a contusion to his forehead. His level of responsiveness had diminished somewhat from the time we arrived. We had oxygen with us, so we applied it via nonrebreather mask.

Patient History We were unable to obtain a history.

Ongoing Assessment We monitored the patient closely until the EMTs arrived.

Patient Hand-off We reported what little we knew (see below). The EMTs then began emergency care. I went across the street to a level area and checked out a landing zone for the helicopter. I radioed dispatch with the exact location. There were wires on our side of the road so I wanted them to be careful.

Rescue soon began to extricate the patient. It didn't take that long once they got there. The helicopter arrived just as the EMTs, with help from my partner, performed a rapid extrication since the patient was unstable. They turned him over to the crew from the helicopter. The travel time to the hospital was about 10 or 12 minutes. It would have been at least 30 minutes for us.

The patient survived. I called the other day. It was close, they said. He almost didn't make it to surgery. The helicopter saved time—and his life.

Hand-off Report

"We were first on the scene and found this man, in his 20s, pinned inside the vehicle. The car seems stable and we didn't see other hazards. We had one First Responder climb into the car to hold stabilization immediately. We found the patient to be breathing adequately with a pulse of 110 and weak. His color is bad. There is a star on the windshield and the steering wheel is bent. No air bags. Definitely an unstable patient. We can keep our responder inside for stabilization while he is extricated."

The Last Word *Know the area you are assigned to. Find out how people live, work, and play there. Then learn about the hazards common in your community and the resources available to handle them.*

Chapter Review

Focus on the EMS Team

One of the reasons you have decided to become a First Responder may be the variety of situations you will encounter or your desire to help other people. In any case, people will always need rescue from dangerous and unusual circumstances.

This chapter has discussed some of the most dangerous and unusual rescue situations you could encounter. Rescue technology and procedures have kept up with the challenges you face today. One thing is certain. The First Responder is a vital part of the response to any type of unusual circumstance or rescue scene. Your actions at the scene—including early notification of the appropriate response teams—are vital.

Summing Up

- Among the locations where a confined-space emergency may occur are silos, storage bins, underground vaults, wells, culverts, and cisterns. A low oxygen level is a significant, common hazard in confined spaces, as are poisonous gases, which may result in an explosive atmosphere. When you are called to a confined-space emergency, determine the nature of the emergency. Then call for a specialized rescue team, emergency medical personnel, and transport. Establish a perimeter and do not allow anyone to enter. Assist rescue personnel when they arrive, if you are trained and equipped to do so.

- If a trench is more than waist-deep and has collapsed on one or more workers, request a specialized trench rescue team immediately. Establish a perimeter and do not allow anyone to enter. Remember, if a collapse has occurred, another one is very likely.

- It takes 18–20 people to carry a litter for one mile over rough terrain. Have teams of four to six bearers carry a stretcher, changing positions and sides and rotating teams periodically as appropriate.

- When the angle of the terrain increases, the risk of falling and dropping a patient on a litter increases. One way to manage this risk is to use a rope system. So, as soon as you recognize a low- or high-angle emergency, call immediately for specialized personnel to perform the rescue.

- Follow local protocols for appropriate times to call for helicopter rescue. However, make sure you have a back-up plan in case air rescue is delayed or impossible.

- When you call for helicopter rescue, you must prepare a landing zone. It should be at least 100 feet by 100 feet square; free of all obstacles; clear of wires, towers, vehicles, people, and loose objects; on firm ground with a less than eight-degree slope; with markers on all four corners and emergency red lights turned on. There should be no smoking and no white or blue lights directed toward helicopter or landing zone.

- Follow all related safety procedures when involved in a helicopter rescue, including staying away from it until the pilot or crew chief signals you to approach. Maintain eye contact with the pilot or crew chief. Approach only from the front. Stay low. Avoid carrying anything above your head. Avoid wearing anything loose that can be blown away by the rotor wash.

Key Terms

confined space a place with limited access and egress that is not designed for human occupancy.

high-angle rescue a rescue involving a rope system to move a patient up or down a slope of 40 degrees or more.

low-angle rescue a rescue involving a move of a patient up or down a slope of less than 40 degrees, where hands are not needed for balance, and falls would be unlikely.

rappelling a special technique of getting down a slope by means of a secured rope.

shoring a system of beams or timbers propped against a structure to provide support.

Knowledge Check

1. The main danger in confined spaces is:
   a. lack of oxygen.
   b. electrocution.
   c. engulfment.
   d. explosion.

2. For a one-mile evacuation over rough terrain where a litter must be carried, there should be at least ___ rescuers.
   a. 6
   b. 12
   c. 18
   d. 24

3. Low-angle litter evacuation generally involves moving over angled terrain of ___ degrees or less.
   a. 20
   b. 30
   c. 40
   d. 80

4. You have called for a helicopter to evacuate a trauma victim. The landing zone area should be flat, without obstructions, and at least ___ feet.
   a. 50 × 50
   b. 75 × 75
   c. 100 × 100
   d. 200 × 200

5. You have been ordered to approach a helicopter by its crew chief. Generally, you should avoid approaching near which section of the aircraft?
   a. tail rotor
   b. side doors
   c. pilot's door
   d. front

6. OSHA requires the confined spaces in which people work to be properly ventilated and monitored for oxygen, carbon monoxide, and hydrogen sulfide.
   a. True
   b. False

7. OSHA requires shoring or a "trench box" in any trench deeper than five feet.
   a. True
   b. False

8. List the characteristics of terrain that would require a high-angle rescue.

_____

_____

_____

9. List six characteristics of a helicopter landing zone.

_____   _____

_____   _____

_____   _____

Scenario

You are called to a local residence for several people who are "sick." The dispatcher believes that one or two may be unresponsive and three others report "scratchy throats" and difficulty breathing. You arrive at a single-family residence and find a woman and child sitting on the lawn outside the house. The woman tells you that her mother was mixing something to clean the floors when she passed out. There are three people, including an infant, inside the residence.

a. Should you go inside to check the other patients? Why or why not?

_____

_____

b. What additional assistance should you call for?

_____

_____

c. Does this qualify as a multiple-casualty incident? Why or why not?

_____

_____

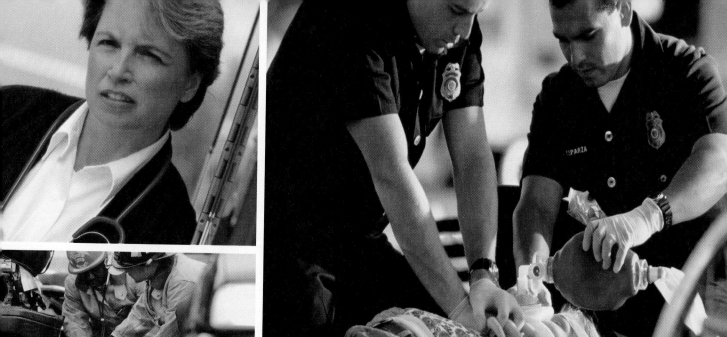

Appendix | First Response to Terrorist Incidents

Objectives

Material supplemental to the DOT curriculum is listed under "Enrichment."

Enrichment

▶ Define the terms "terrorism" and "weapons of mass destruction." (p. 609)

▶ List four types of weapons that may be used by terrorists to cause harm or destruction. (p. 609)

What Is Terrorism?

Terrorism is the use of violence or the threat of violence to provoke fear and influence behavior for political, social, religious, or ethnic goals. It can be committed by a single person, a small group of individuals, or a cluster of organizations. Whether the perpetrators use bombs, guns, or chemicals, the intent is meant to have a psychological impact.

Terrorist incidents can happen anywhere. Their weapons can be anything from fertilizer bombs (similar to those used in the 1993 bombing of the Alfred Murrah Building in Oklahoma City) to sarin gas (a nerve gas released into the Tokyo subway system in 1995) to commercial airliners (as in the 2001 attack on the World Trade Center in New York City and the Pentagon in Washington, DC) (Figure A-1).

The term **weapons of mass destruction** generally refers to weapons that have the ability to kill and injure in numbers much greater than the weapon's actual physical size might indicate. Such weapons include:

- *Chemical weapons.* These include chemicals such as phosgene and chlorine gas, hydrogen cyanide, mustard and sarin gas, and nerve agents.

- *Biological weapons.* Spores and germs that can be used include anthrax, botulism, smallpox, Ebola or Marburg viruses, or West Nile encephalitis.

- *Radiological weapons.* These injure people by exposure to radioactive rays, including gamma radiation. Exposures to cesium-137, iridium-192, and cobalt-60 are all known to be dangerous.

- *Nuclear weapons.* These can range in size from artillery shells to "suitcase bombs." They use highly enriched uranium, weapons-grade plutonium, or simple radioactive dust.

While First Responders may feel ill prepared to meet these challenges, an important fact to note is that between 1980 and 1999 the FBI found that more than 70% of terrorist activity involved bombs or other explosive devices.

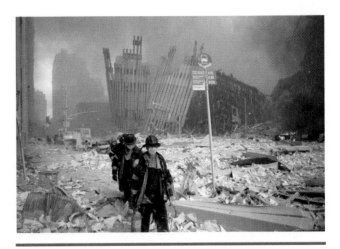

FIGURE A-1 The Twin Towers of the World Trade Center in New York City were destroyed and thousands were killed on September 11, 2001, when terrorists flew hijacked jetliners into them. *(Corbis/Sygma)*

Although chemical, biological, or nuclear weapons could be used, historically they have not.

Preparing for a Terrorist Incident

When responding to emergency situations, First Responders should suspect terrorism when the incident involves the following elements: unusual or unexpected events; high-interest targets, such as water treatment facilities, power plants, and military bases; psychologically important dates; greater than usual numbers of patients; and reports of unusual signs and symptoms in groups of people.

For EMS personnel and other rescuers, terrorism is a deadly combination of a multiple-casualty and a hazardous materials incident. A plan of action can help rescuers meet the challenge. One way to start the planning is by using the "Five Ss" as a guide:

S—Self.
S—Size up.
S—Send info.
S—Set up the medical group.
S—Stabilize.

Self

"Self" refers to your own safety. Be prepared. If there is a particularly vulnerable potential target in your area, such as an airport or a major pharmaceutical manufacturer, become familiar with it. Learn how many people could be affected and what hazardous materials might be involved. Then determine what you will need to protect yourself and your crew in a response. Remember: Never become part of the emergency.

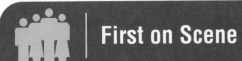

First on Scene

Terrorism is a new facet of our everyday lives. Using systems already in place for multiple-casualty incidents, hazmats, and natural disasters can blunt the psychological impact on a community as well as save lives.

Size Up

Scene size-up is always your first step in any emergency. As you approach the scene, observe for indications of the type of emergency. For example, look to see if people are running away from a building where an obvious explosion has occurred, or are they all on the ground seizing? Ask the same questions you would normally ask. That is, after you ensure your own safety and identify the mechanism of injury or nature of illness, you must determine the necessary resources. Find out the number of patients involved, if any hazardous materials are on scene, and if specialized rescue teams should be called in. Size-up should also include determining the correct address or location of the incident, establishing command, and evaluating the probable "hot zone."

Send Info

The third "S" is "Send Info." It refers to getting your size-up information to the appropriate agencies and personnel as quickly as possible. It is important to spread the facts of an actual or potential terrorist attack to the appropriate agencies as soon as you can. Many can and will assist you. They include the FBI, which has a National Domestic Preparedness Office that can streamline federal services to localities that suffer terror attacks.

At a regional level, state law enforcement, environmental agencies, and public works will need to be mobilized quickly. At a local level, additional EMS, fire, and police personnel may also be called in. Local hospitals must be warned so they can prepare for the number of patients and their injuries. They, too, will need to call in additional staffing and key personnel. Finally, expert hazmat crews or other technically trained teams will need to be activated to confront the emergency.

Set up the Medical Group

Setting up the medical group, or EMS sector, will be very important. (The incident command system and EMS sector functions are discussed in Chapter 31.) The earlier command is established and a multiple-casualty response is in place, the more successful the response is likely to be. Triage will be important, but even before First Responders arrive on scene, the lowest-priority patients will probably leave and travel to hospitals in their own vehicles. Second priority patients may be rescued by bystanders or other victims. The highest-priority patients will likely be in the "hot zone" waiting for rescue.

First on Scene

The incident command system (ICS) is used at terrorist incidents just as it would be in any fire scene, hazmat, or major highway collision. However, there are a few differences. Terrorist acts involve crimes and are intentionally designed to affect large numbers of people. Although rare, terrorist incidents can also involve nuclear or biological contamination, which affects triage and treatment of patients. Finally, since these are acts of violence, be alert for secondary attacks that detonate or occur after the initial event. They are designed to cause more casualties—especially to rescuers.

Stabilize

The scene should be stabilized as soon as possible. Otherwise, people will be running toward it, trying to rescue loved ones and friends, and people will be running away from it toward safety. Such chaos does not make the scene any safer or easier to work in. Communications must be established quickly, and the first arriving rescue personnel must move ambulatory ("walking wounded") patients to a designated area for triage and decontamination purposes.

1. What is "terrorism"?

2. What are "weapons of mass destruction"? Give some examples.

3. When should a First Responder suspect terrorism?

Answers to Knowledge Check

Page numbers offered below are references to textbook pages on which answers may be found.

Chapter 1

1. c (pp. 4–5, 7)
2. a (pp. 8–9)
3. b (p. 4)
4. d (p. 9)
5. b (p. 9)
6. b (p. 7)
7. d (p. 4)
8. b (pp. 8–9)
9. b (pp. 4, 8–9)
10. a (p. 8)
11. Maintain up-to-date knowledge and skills. (p. 9)
12. On-line is person-to-person at the time of the emergency; off-line is by way of standing orders and written protocols. (p. 9)
13. Any three of the following: Protect your own safety and the safety of your crew, the patient, and bystanders. Gain access to the patient. Assess the patient to identify life-threatening problems. Alert additional EMS resources. Provide care based on assessment findings. Assist other EMS personnel. Participate in record keeping and data collection as required. Act as liaison with other public safety personnel. (pp. 8–9)
14. Any three of the following: trauma centers, burn centers, pediatric centers, perinatal centers, poison centers. (p. 7)
15. Answers will vary. (pp. 8–9)

Chapter 2

1. d (p. 26)
2. b (pp. 17–18)

3. c (pp. 8, 23)
4. b (pp. 27–29)
5. a (pp. 26–27)
6. a (p. 28)
7. a (p. 19)
8. If the First Responder becomes a victim, he won't be able to help the patient and, by forcing other EMS personnel to rescue him, may be placing them in jeopardy as well. (pp. 8, 23)
9. Many other diseases can be transmitted during a call, including other forms of hepatitis. BSI precautions can prevent that from happening. (pp. 16–22)
10. Denial, anger, bargaining, depression, acceptance. (p. 26)
11. Any three of the following: Never wipe away blood. Touch only what you need to touch to provide patient care. Move only what you need to move to protect the patient and to provide proper care. Do not use a telephone unless the police give you permission to do so. Observe and document anything unusual at the scene. Do not cut through holes in the patient's clothing. Do not cut through any knot in a rope or tie. If the crime is rape, do not wash the patient and discourage the patient from doing so. Do not allow the patient to change clothing, use the bathroom, or take anything by mouth. (pp. 24–25)
12. Gloves and face shield (or protective eyewear and mask). (pp. 16–22)

Chapter 3

1. c (pp. 39, 41)
2. a (p. 35)

3. b (p. 36)
4. d (pp. 39, 41)
5. a (p. 41)
6. d (pp. 36, 37–39)
7. a (pp. 36, 37–39)
8. a. Any EMS provider may be called to testify in court, even years after an emergency call. Be prepared. Always make sure you document your calls properly.
9. The First Responder had a duty to act, there was a breach of duty, the patient was injured physically or psychologically, and the First Responder caused the injury. (pp. 39, 41)
10. Standard of care is the care that would be expected to be provided to the same patient under the same circumstances by another First Responder who had received the same training. (p. 42)
11. No, because you made sure the patient was in the care of EMS personnel with the same or more expertise and training than you have. (pp. 39, 41)
12. Explain the risks in language he can fully understand. Write down what you tell him. Then have the patient read it aloud to see if he understands. Consult medical direction as required by local protocol. (pp. 37–39)
13. Yes. Risk to you includes charges of assault and battery. Risk to the patient depends on his condition. (pp. 37–39)
14. No, because the patient is a competent adult. (pp. 36–37)
15. Yes, since he is probably under the influence of drugs and therefore not competent. (pp. 36–37)

Chapter 4

1. c (p. 50)
2. b (p. 50)
3. a (p. 50)
4. d (p. 50)
5. a (p. 50)
6. d (p. 58)
7. c (p. 62)
8. a (pp. 59, 61)
9. c (p. 56)
10. b (p. 51)
11. b (p. 54)
12. d (p. 61)
13. b (p. 58)
14. a (p. 54)
15. a (pp. 59, 61)
16. a (p. 53)

17. a (p. 51)
18. a (pp. 61–62)
19. b (pp. 56, 61–62)
20. g, i, h, a, c, b, f, d, e, j (pp. 53–56)
21. Liver, kidney, colon, pancreas, gallbladder, colon, small intestines, ureter, appendix. (pp. 52, 54)

Chapter 5

1. c (pp. 76–77)
2. d (pp. 78–79)
3. c (pp. 75–76)
4. a (pp. 82–83)
5. b (pp. 87–89)
6. c (pp. 78–79)
7. d (pp. 78–79)
8. c (pp. 79–82)
9. b, a, d, c (pp. 83–88)
10. Emergency move, because the patient is in immediate danger of being run over by oncoming vehicles. (pp. 78–79)

Chapter 6

1. a (p. 95)
2. b (p. 109)
3. d (p. 109)
4. c (p. 103)
5. a (pp. 103, 106, 113–114)
6. a (pp. 102–103)
7. It is highly recommended that two rescuers operate a BVM, because it is too difficult and tiring for one rescuer. If alone, a rescuer should use a pocket face mask instead. (pp. 112–113)
8. 3, 1, 2 (p. 107)
9. a (pp. 102–103)
10. a. Monitor patient. Provide oxygen by nonrebreather mask at 10–15 liters per minute. (pp. 102–103, 106, 115)
    b. The patient is breathing inadequately. Assist ventilations with a pocket face mask or BVM with supplemental oxygen. Monitor and suction as necessary. (pp. 102–103, 106, 115)
    c. Administer oxygen via nonrebreather mask at 10–15 liters per minute. Monitor the patient carefully in case inadequate breathing develops. (pp. 102–103, 106, 115)
    d. This patient is breathing inadequately. Assist ventilations with a pocket face mask or BVM with supplemental oxygen. Monitor the patient in the event that respirations cease or suction is needed. (pp. 102–103, 106, 115)

Chapter 7

1. a (p. 127)
2. c (pp. 136–137)
3. d (pp. 102–103, 128–129)
4. d (pp. 127–128)
5. c (pp. 102–103, 106, 113–114, 128–129)
6. a (p. 138)
7. a (p. 102)
8. a. 44% (p. 128)
   b. 90% (p. 129)
   c. Without supplemental oxygen, close to 16%, which is the percentage of oxygen in exhaled air. With supplemental oxygen, perhaps a bit more. (p. 103)
   d. 100% (p. 112)
9. A mild obstruction allows enough air for the patient to be able to speak and cough—and live. A severe obstruction allows a very limited amount of air into the body, which allows the patient only slight noises and minimal—or absent—air exchange. (p. 136)
10. a. Roll the patient onto his side and suction his airway. If suction is not available, sweep what you can out of his mouth without the risk of getting bitten by the patient. (pp. 100–101, 125–127)
    b. No. This patient requires ventilatory assistance, since his own respirations are inadequate. Use a pocket face mask or BVM with supplemental oxygen to ventilate the patient. (pp. 102–103, 128)
    c. Provide artificial ventilation at the rate of 10–12 breaths per minute. Check the patient's pulse frequently because his heart also may stop. Notify incoming EMS units. (pp. 103, 106–107)
    d. Roll the patient onto his side and suction him. Ventilations that are too rapid or forceful may contribute to vomiting. Ventilate carefully. (pp. 107, 125–127)

Chapter 8

1. a (pp. 149, 158)
2. b (p. 158)
3. c (p. 152)
4. d (pp. 154, 160)
5. c (pp. 151–152)
6. d (p. 158)
7. b (p. 158)
8. a (p. 156)
9. If your fingers rest against the chest wall during compressions, chances of separating and injuring the patient's ribs increase. (p. 151)

10. a. May fracture ribs and cause lacerations to lung and liver. (p. 159)
    b. May fracture ribs and cause lacerations to lung and heart. (p. 159)
    c. May crack sternum. (p. 159)
    d. May break off xiphoid process and lacerate the liver. (p. 159)
11. a. EMS must be activated. Someone must get the AED. CPR must be performed. (p. 152)
    b. The answer to these two questions would depend somewhat on the level of training of other employees. However, generally, you would begin CPR while delegating one or more people to activate EMS and retrieve the AED. (pp. 152–153)

Chapter 9

1. c (pp. 149, 167)
2. b (p. 169)
3. c (pp. 169–170, 173)
4. d (p. 171)
5. a (p. 171)
6. c (p. 169)
7. b (p. 169)
8. a (p. 171)
9. d (p. 173)
10. a (p. 167)
11. b (p. 173)
12. It is believed that there is enough oxygen left in the system in the first few minutes after the heart stops, so that when a shock is delivered, the body is able to function. If the patient has been down longer (four to five minutes), the cells may need oxygen in order to successfully respond to defibrillation. (pp. 169–170, 173)
13. Defibrillation. CPR chest compressions can only provide artificial circulation. They cannot transmit a shock that is powerful enough to correct a lethal heart rhythm, as defibrillation has the potential to do. (p. 170)
14. a. Stop CPR, so that you can check the patient's pulse and respirations. (p. 171)
    b. Stop CPR, instruct everyone to clear the patient, press the "analyze" button. (p. 171)
    c. Perform CPR for two minutes and then reanalyze the heart rhythm. (p. 171)
    d. Post-resuscitation care includes the following: Monitor the pulse carefully, and ventilate the patient as necessary. Place him in a recovery position when pulse and respirations are adequate. Administer high-concentration oxygen. (p. 173)

Chapter 10

1. b (p. 179)
2. d (p. 182)
3. c (pp. 183–185)
4. b (pp. 186–187)
5. a (p. 190)
6. c (pp. 180–182)
7. d (pp. 180–182)
8. a (pp. 179–180)
9. a (pp. 182–183)
10. b (pp. 187–188)
11. Call for two ambulances, one for each of the potentially serious patients. Also call for fire services for extrication, police for traffic control and collision investigation, and the utility company to deal with the wires. (p. 191)
12. a. Hazards from unstable sections of scaffolding, parts of the building under construction, which may be loose, and items such as building materials falling from the scaffolding. (p. 189)

    b. Call for two to three ambulances, depending on the potential seriousness of the injuries. You may also need fire department resources for disentanglement. (pp. 189, 191)

    c. Consider the height of the fall, the surface landed on, parts of the patient that had contact with the ground and if anything broke the fall or was struck by the patient on the way down. For the patient who was on the ground, consider the part of the body that was struck by debris and the type of object that struck the patient. (p. 189)

Chapter 11

1. a (pp. 201–202)
2. b (pp. 205–207)
3. d (pp. 202–203)
4. c (p. 203)
5. a (p. 201)
6. d (pp. 205–207)
7. d (pp. 201–202)
8. b (pp. 204–205)
9. a (pp. 205–207)
10. a (pp. 203–204)
11. b (pp. 203–204)
12. Scene size-up, initial assessment, physical examination, patient history, ongoing assessment, patient hand-off. (p. 198)
13. Sight—observing for scene safety, patient's level of distress. Hearing—listening to patient's complaints and answers to your questions, listening to determine adequate breathing, listening for pulse through stethoscope. Touch—palpating the patient to feel for abnormalities or to elicit a response. Smell—identifying odors that can give clues to the patient's condition. (pp. 197–198)
14. A medical patient is ill. A trauma patient is injured. (p. 199)
15. a. First, make sure the scene is safe to enter. Look for hazards, such as electricity (is there water near the power source?), chemicals (do you smell odd odors or see containers the patient may have been using?), possible violence, or other hazards such as bees or snakes. If no mechanism of injury is apparent and the caller cannot give you any information about possible injury, consider nature of illness. (Chapter 10)

    b. Since there are no signs of injury, the patient is most likely suffering from an illness. Therefore, you should gather a patient history first. Then, if there is time, conduct a thorough physical exam. (pp. 198–200)

Chapter 12

1. a (pp. 214–221)
2. b (p. 215)
3. d (p. 227)
4. b (p. 223)
5. c (p. 227)
6. b (p. 229)
7. c (pp. 219–221)
8. a (p. 219)
9. c (p. 227)
10. a (p. 227)
11. b (pp. 214–221)
12. a (p. 215)
13. a. radial; b. radial or brachial; c. brachial; d. carotid; e. carotid or femoral; f. brachial (p. 219)
14. approximate age, sex, chief complaint, airway and breathing status, circulation status (pp. 220–221)
15. a. General impression, which should include the chief complaint of each patient, their age and sex, and a brief immediate assessment of the environment in which the emergency has taken place. (pp. 214–221)

    b. Immediately open the airway. Inspect it for blood, vomit, and secretions. Look for loose teeth or other foreign matter that could cause an obstruction. Clear the airway using suction or a gloved finger. If there is no gag reflex, insert an oral airway. (pp. 217–218)

c. Notice if the responsive patient can speak clearly. Listen for gurgling or other sounds that could indicate something like teeth, blood, or other matter is in the airway. Also make sure the patient can speak full sentences. (pp. 217–219)

Chapter 13

1. b (p. 237)
2. c (pp. 238–239)
3. a (pp. 240–243)
4. d (pp. 240–243)
5. d (pp. 239–240)
6. a (pp. 237–238)
7. a (pp. 238–239)
8. Any three: speak slowly and clearly; push the "push to talk" button one second before speaking; listen before you transmit; avoid broadcasting personal information about a patient; bring your portable radio with you on scene. (pp. 238–239)
9. Any three: infectious disease exposure, injury to EMS personnel, conflicts between agencies, multiple-casualty incidents. (p. 243)
10. a. Unit identifier and the fact that you are a First Responder; patient's age, sex, and chief complaint; brief, pertinent history of the events leading to the injury or illness; your observations on the patient's condition; the fact that the family refuses consent for assessment and care; and the reason why you are calling, which in this case is to convince the family not to move the patient until the paramedics arrive on scene. (pp. 238–239)
    b. The patient appears to have a significant mechanism of injury, which suggests a possible spine injury. The patient needs to be immobilized before being moved. (Chapters 10 and 12)

Chapter 14

1. b (p. 258)
2. d (p. 252)
3. b (Chapter 9)
4. b (p. 261)
5. a (p. 257)
6. a (pp. 252, 258)
7. a (p. 254)
8. Any six: physical inactivity, cigarette smoking, obesity, high serum cholesterol and triglycerides, diabetes, age (incidence increases over 30 years of age), hypertension (blood pressure above 140/90), family history of coronary artery disease under age 60. (p. 251)

9. Normal rate, effortless, regular in rhythm, free of unusual sounds, adequate and equal chest expansion, adequate depth. (p. 257)
10. a. Size up the scene and take all necessary precautions. (Chapters 2 and 10)
    b. You should ask her if she is the person who called EMS and, if so, why (patient's chief complaint). (Chapters 10 and 12)
    c. Conduct an initial assessment. Ensure an open airway, adequate breathing, and adequate circulation. (Chapter 12)
    d. Update EMS and request advanced care. (Chapter 12)

Chapter 15

1. b (p. 270)
2. b (pp. 269–272)
3. d (pp. 274–276)
4. a (p. 281)
5. c (pp. 272–274)
6. b (pp. 268–269)
7. b (pp. 274–276)
8. b (pp. 268–269, 270–272)
9. c (pp. 279–280)
10. a (pp. 269–272)
11. b (pp. 274–276)
12. b (p. 269)
13. a (p. 270)
14. Dilute some sugar in a glass of water or juice or give her a fruit juice. (pp. 271–272)
15. Facial droop, arm drift, and speech. (pp. 272–274)
16. Ensure scene safety and take BSI precautions. Ensure an open airway, adequate breathing, and adequate circulation. Gather a patient history as soon as possible. Monitor the patient's airway and breathing closely. If the patient is not injured, place him in the recovery position. Administer high-flow oxygen if the patient is breathing adequately. If breathing is inadequate, assist ventilations. (pp. 268–269)
17. a. The same as for any other patient; that is, assess the airway, breathing, and circulation and provide the appropriate care for any life threats, including suction and oxygen. Assist ventilation if necessary. (Chapter 12)
    b. No, since the patient's level of responsiveness is only painful (on the AVPU scale) and, therefore, may not be able to control his own airway. (pp. 269–272)
    c. Yes. Altered mental status changes in a patient—in this case responsive only to pain with a history

of diabetes—is enough to consider the emergency serious and the patient unstable. (Chapter 12)

Chapter 16

1. b (p. 292)
2. c (p. 292)
3. b (p. 293)
4. c (pp. 295–296)
5. c (pp. 294–296)
6. d (p. 294)
7. b (p. 292)
8. a (p. 292)
9. c (pp. 297–298)
10. a (p. 298)
11. b (p. 298)
12. Shivering, apathy and decreased muscle function, decreased level of responsiveness, decreased vital signs, death. (p. 290)
13. High heat, high humidity, sweating during strenuous activity, age, medical condition, and the use of certain drugs and medications. (pp. 294–295)
14. Any 10: warm, tingling feeling in the mouth, face, chest, feet, and hands.; itching, hives, and flushing; swelling of the tongue, face, neck, hands, and feet; tightness in the throat or chest; cough, hoarseness; rapid or labored breathing; noisy breathing, stridor, wheezing; increased heart rate; decreased blood pressure; itchy, watery eyes; headache; runny nose; sense of impending doom; decreasing mental status. (pp. 297–298)
15. a. Size up the scene. Determine if there is any danger. (Chapter 10)
    b. Muscle cramps; weakness, exhaustion; dizziness, faintness; rapid pulse rate that is strong at first, but becomes weaker; headache; loss of appetite, nausea, vomiting; altered mental status; moist, pale, and normal-to-cool skin. For a serious heat emergency, hot and dry or hot and moist skin. (pp. 295–298)
    c. Call for help. You also could have removed her backpack, loosened her clothing, had her lie down in the shade, and cooled her by fanning. If she remained alert and there was no nausea, you could have encouraged her to drink some water or sport drink. If necessary, you could have provided basic life support. (p. 296)

Chapter 17

1. c (pp. 313–314)
2. a (pp. 316–317)

3. d (p. 313)
4. b (pp. 319–320)
5. d (p. 319)
6. a (p. 318)
7. b. Once you have responded to a behavioral emergency, the patient's safety is legally your responsibility until someone with more training arrives on scene. (p. 315)
8. Answers will vary, but may include weapons or items that could be used as weapons; overturned furniture or other signs of chaos; a history of being aggressive or combative; witnesses report the patient was violent at the scene; if the patient's body language or words are threatening. (pp. 314–315)
9. Rephrasing or repeating part of what is said; asking questions to show you are paying attention; using gestures such as a nod of the head or verbal responses such as "I see" or "Go on." (pp. 315–316)
10. a. Your immediate goals are to protect your own safety, maintain the patient's airway, and manage life-threatening conditions. (pp. 319–320)
    b. Your top priority is your patient's airway. Quickly establish an open airway. Turn the patient's head to the side for drainage, and suction to clear the airway of anything that might obstruct it. (pp. 319–320)
    c. Monitor mental status and vital signs frequently. Be prepared to provide basic life support if needed. Maintain the patient's body temperature. Comfort, calm, and reassure the patient. Attempt to get the patient's medical history from the college. Give any medications or drugs you find on scene to the transporting EMS personnel. (pp. 319–320)

Chapter 18

1. a (p. 330)
2. c (p. 327)
3. a (pp. 335–337)
4. d (pp. 328, 330)
5. b (pp. 330, 332)
6. d (p. 337)
7. a (p. 327)
8. b (p. 330)
9. b (pp. 335, 337)
10. c (p. 330)
11. a (p. 330)
12. Any four: Keep all of the patient's open wounds covered with dressings. Never touch your mouth, nose, or eyes during emergency care. Never handle food during emergency care. Wash your hands

properly after every patient. Decontaminate or properly dispose of any item that has been in contact with the patient's blood or body fluids. (p. 327)

13. Any 10: a mechanism of injury that suggests it; scrapes and bruises, swelling, deformity, or impact marks; penetrating wounds to the skull, chest, or abdomen; unexplained shock; discolored, tender, swollen, or hard tissue; increased respiratory and pulse rates; pale, cool, clammy skin; nausea and vomiting bright red blood or blood the color of dark coffee grounds; thirst; changes in mental status including anxiety, restlessness, or combativeness; dark, tarry stools or stools that contain bright red blood; tender, rigid, or distended abdomen; weakness, faintness, or dizziness. (p. 334)

14. a. No matter what the emergency might be, your patient assessment plan is always the same: scene size-up, initial assessment, physical exam, patient history, ongoing assessment, and hand-off report. (Chapters 9 and 12)

   b. Conduct an initial assessment. That is, assess airway and breathing. Then look at the wound. If it is still bleeding, apply direct pressure, elevate the foot and, if necessary, apply pressure to the femoral pulse point. Dress and bandage the wound properly once bleeding is under control. Since the patient looks "sick," treat for shock (administer oxygen, get him in a supine position with both legs elevated, and keep him warm). (pp. 330, 337–338)

Chapter 19

1. c (pp. 350–353)
2. d (p. 357)
3. b (pp. 358–359)
4. a (pp. 353–355)
5. d (p. 353)
6. c (p. 353)
7. d (p. 355)
8. c (p. 355)
9. a (pp. 353–355)
10. b (pp. 348–349)
11. a (p. 349)
12. Any five: controls bleeding, prevents further contamination and damage to the wound, keeps the wound dry, stabilizes the wound site, enhances healing, and adds to the comfort of the patient. (p. 358)
13. Infection, severe discomfort and, in rare cases, loss of a limb. (p. 358)
14. f, b, e, c, e, d, g (pp. 348–353)

15. a. Who is in charge of the scene? How many patients are there? Where are they? What exactly is the problem? What assistance has been requested? Is the scene safe to enter? (Chapters 9 and 12)

   b. Ask the patient to state his chief complaint. Observe his response to give you some idea of his mental status and the status of his airway and breathing. Look for bleeding and any signs of shock. Treat all life-threats immediately. Have your partner gather a patient history from the mother. (Chapter 12)

   c. Expose the entire bite site and the claw wounds. Clear the areas of blood and debris with sterile gauze. Check for any tooth fragments. Apply dry sterile dressings that cover each wound entirely. Check distal pulses and secure the dressings with bandages. After bandaging, check distal pulses again. Be comforting, calming, and reassuring to both the patient and his mother until the EMTs take over patient care. (pp. 353, 357–358)

Chapter 20

1. c (pp. 372–373)
2. b (pp. 370)
3. d (pp. 374–375)
4. c (p. 372)
5. a (p. 377)
6. d (pp. 377–378)
7. a (p. 379)
8. a (pp. 370–371)
9. a (pp. 370–371)
10. a. With the patient lying down on her back, knees flexed and supported, check for DOTS, watch how the abdomen moves as the patient breathes, and gently palpate all four quadrants, the most painful last. Take spinal precautions, if warranted. (Chapter 12 and p. 377)

   b. As with any patient, your top priorities for a patient with abdominal injuries are airway, breathing, and circulation. Once the ABCs are assessed and treated, update or activate EMS immediately to arrange for transport. Also, place the patient in the position most comfortable for him. If you suspect a pelvic fracture, prevent movement. Immobilize the patient on a long backboard if possible. (pp. 377–378)

Chapter 21

1. c (p. 387)
2. c (p. 387)
3. b (pp. 386–389)

4. d (p. 386)
5. c (p. 385)
6. a (p. 385)
7. b (p. 385)
8. a. 18%
   b. 18%
   c. 1%
   d. 9%
   e. 9%
   f. 18% (p. 387)
9. a. 18%
   b. 18%
   c. 1%
   d. 18%
   e. 9%
   f. 14% (p. 387)
10. a. Scene safety is the first priority. The First Responder must call Dispatch for the immediate assistance of law enforcement, the fire service, and the power company. Law enforcement will move all onlookers away from the scene and the dangers it poses. Fire service will address all fire hazards, and the power company will stabilize the pole and handle any electrical hazard it may pose. (Chapter 10)
    b. As with all patients, perform an initial assessment and treat any life-threats first. The mechanism of injury (the car crash) suggests head and spine injury, so take spinal precautions immediately. During the initial assessment, be especially alert to the patient's airway and breathing status. Then, after life-threats are treated, perform a physical exam, during which you can determine the severity of the burns and look for any other injuries caused in the crash. (Chapters 10 and 12)
    c. 27% BSA. (pp. 387, 389)
    d. Stop the burning process; after life-threats have been identified and treated, administer oxygen; dress all open wounds including burns; keep the patient warm; be prepared to provide basic life support if needed. (pp. 389–392)
    e. Stop the burning process in this patient by pouring water over his burns, using caution not to get it in the airway. A moist nonfibrous dressing may be dabbed on the face to help stop burning. (pp. 389–390)
    f. Use dry dressings. (pp. 389–392)

Chapter 22

1. c (p. 402)
2. d (pp. 402–403)
3. b (pp. 402–403)
4. c (Chapters 9 and 12)
5. a (p. 406)
6. a (p. 410)
7. b (pp. 411–413)
8. Answers will vary, but may include: hazardous materials, machinery accidents, confined space emergencies, trench emergencies, aerial or high-angle emergencies. (pp. 411–413)
9. Answers will vary, but may include: tractors, power takeoff (PTO) shafts, combines, augers, corn pickers and snapping rolls, hay balers. (pp. 406–409)
12. a. You should not approach this patient until the tractor has been stabilized. This will be done by the incoming rescue team. (p. 402)
    b. You can monitor the patient's airway and stabilize his spine. If available, oxygen may be administered to the patient. You may also assess visible parts of the patient and take vital signs. Update incoming units and prepare any equipment (such as backboards). Reassure the patient while you are with him. (pp. 402–403)
    c. Based on the mechanism of injury, you should suspect severe injuries. Expect fractures to the pelvis and lower extremities. Spinal injuries are also likely. The patient has the potential for serious blood loss and shock as well. (Chapters 18 and 19 and p. 406)

Chapter 23

1. a (pp. 419–421)
2. d (p. 421)
3. d (pp. 423, 425)
4. c (pp. 423, 425)
5. c (p. 419)
6. b (p. 419)
7. a (p. 419)
8. Manually stabilize the head and neck, use a jaw-thrust maneuver to open the airway, identify the need for suction, apply oxygen, ventilation when breathing is inadequate or absent. (p. 421)
9. Any five: an eye injury should always be examined by a physician; patch both eyes, even if only one is injured; follow local protocol on flushing of eyes; do not put salves or medications in the injured eye; do not remove blood or blood clots from the eye; never attempt to remove embedded material; remove contacts only when there has been a chemical burn to the eye or when it is medically necessary; do not try to force the eyelid open unless you have to flush out chemicals; do not let a patient with an

eye injury walk without help, especially up or down stairs; do not allow the patient with an eye injury to eat or drink. (p. 428)

10. a. Safety first. Find out if the scene is safe. Ask: Are any specialized teams required to make the scene safe? Has the lumber been moved and stabilized? Has the crane been shut down and stabilized? (Chapters 10 and 21)

    b. If there is an obvious head injury, if the mechanism of injury suggests a head or spine injury, or if a trauma patient is unresponsive, you must immediately stabilize the patient's head and neck. Then perform an initial assessment. (Chapters 10 and 12 and pp. 419–421)

    c. A blow to the head that is forceful enough to cause unconsciousness in a patient should be considered significant. Skull fracture, injuries to the brain (some of which can develop slowly), and concussion are all possible, even in a closed injury to the head. So, you should attempt to convince the patient to go to the hospital for an examination or at least to let the EMTs or paramedics take a look at him. (pp. 419–423)

Chapter 24

1. c (p. 439)
2. d (p. 442)
3. c (pp. 440, 442)
4. c (pp. 444–445)
5. b (p. 449)
6. d (p. 442)
7. b (p. 440)
8. a (pp. 445, 447)
9. a (pp. 444–445)
10. b (p. 439)
11. b (pp. 442, 444)
12. a (p. 440)
13. Cervical, thoracic, lumbar, sacral, coccygeal. (p. 439)
14. Any six: motor-vehicle, including motorcycle, crashes; pedestrian-car crashes; falls; diving accidents; hangings; blunt trauma or penetrating trauma to the head, neck, or torso; any gunshot wounds; any speed sport accident, such as roller blading, bicycling, skiing, surfing, or sledding; any unresponsive trauma patient. (p. 440)
15. a. Even if the patient has no obvious injuries, a crash is a potentially serious MOI. Tell the patient not to move and take spinal precautions immediately. You or your partner should climb in behind her

to manually stabilize head and neck. Once that is done, proceed with the initial assessment. Be sure to use a jaw-thrust to open and inspect the airway if necessary. (pp. 440, 442)

    b. Stop. Do not continue palpating the painful area. Continue the assessment by examining other areas of her body. (p. 442)

    c. Inspecting and palpating the limbs would help you discover any obvious injuries. An assessment of the patient's pulses, movement, and sensation in all four extremities would tell you if the patient's nervous system has been affected. (p. 442)

    d. They would probably apply a rigid cervical immobilization device first. Then they would apply a short backboard to the sitting patient, so that they could move her onto a long backboard for head-to-toe immobilization. The whole time, manual stabilization of the patient's head and neck would be maintained. (pp. 442, 444–445, 447)

Chapter 25

1. d (Chapter 4)
2. a (Chapters 4 and 12)
3. c (p. 465)
4. b (p. 469)
5. b (p. 465)
6. a (p. 462)
7. a (p. 465)
8. To prevent motion of bone fragments or dislocated joints; to minimize damage to surrounding tissues, nerves, blood vessels, and the injured bone itself; to help control bleeding and swelling; to help prevent shock; to reduce pain and suffering. (p. 463)
9. Rigid splints, traction splints, circumferential splints, improvised splints, and the sling and swathe. (pp. 463–465)
10. a. The patient should be checked along the length of the arm to the shoulder and his neck. He should be asked about any other pain or injury. Obtain a description of the fall from the patient and bystanders. (pp. 459–460)

    b. The elbow would be immobilized. The bones of the hand and fingers distal to the injury would be immobilized by the splint. (p. 467)

    c. Rigid boards or Velcro splints are common choices for immobilizing the wrist and forearm. If the arm was straight, these could immobilize the elbow. Since the wrist is bent and held against his chest, short splints combined with a sling would provide immobilization. (p. 467)

Chapter 26

1. b (pp. 477–479)
2. a (pp. 477–479)
3. d (pp. 479, 480)
4. c (p. 482)
5. d (pp. 482–484)
6. a (p. 484)
7. a (pp. 481–482)
8. a (p. 480)
9. To use the syringe, fully compress it before bringing it to the baby's face. Insert the tip no more than an inch into the mouth, but do not make contact with the back of the mouth. Slowly release the bulb to allow fluid to be drawn into the syringe. Suction the mouth first, and then the nose. (p. 483)
10. a. First take BSI precautions. Then perform an initial assessment and treat any life threats. Once that is accomplished, you must assess her condition to see if there will be time for transport to the nearest medical facility or if she will have the baby in her present location. (p. 480)
    b. Place your gloved hand on the mother's abdomen, just above her navel, in order to feel the involuntary tightening and relaxing of the uterine muscles. Time these involuntary movements in seconds. Start from the moment the uterus first tightens until it is completely relaxed. Time the intervals in minutes from the start of one contraction to the start of the next. (p. 480)
    c. Step one: dry the baby, wrap him in a clean blanket, position him, and suction the airway. The infant should cry almost immediately. If not, then go to step two: provide tactile stimulation and administer blow-by oxygen. If the baby still doesn't breathe, step three is: perform artificial ventilation. (p. 484)
    d. The recommended rate for assisting a newborn's ventilations is between 30–60 breaths per minute. (p. 484)
    e. The rate of compressions is 120 per minute. The ratio of compressions to breaths for the newborn is 3:1. (p. 484)
    f. Place two sanitary napkins over the opening of the vagina, and massage the area on the abdomen that is just superior to the symphysis pubis. You might also ask the mother if she plans to breastfeed the infant, this would be a good time to start because it, too, can help stop the bleeding. (pp. 484–485)

Chapter 27

1. b (p. 495)
2. c (pp. 500–501)
3. d (pp. 508–509)
4. a (p. 512)
5. b (p. 511)
6. c (p. 498)
7. b (p. 501)
8. b (pp. 508–509)
9. Any six: airway adjuncts, BVMs with oxygen reservoirs, oxygen masks, nonrebreathing masks, cervical immobilization devices, backboards, extremity splints, blood pressure cuffs. (p. 498)
10. a. No. All indications point toward a patient who is not in immediate danger. (pp. 499–502)
    b. A good sign. It indicates a normal mental status. A bad sign would be no response to you, a stranger. (p. 497)
    c. No. Let the EMTs respond to assess further and document patient refusal. (Chapter 3)
    d. That it must have been frightening to see the baby choking. It is never a problem to call. Call any time. You are glad that the baby is doing well. (Chapter 3 and p. 498)

Chapter 28

1. c (p. 525)
2. d (p. 526)
3. a (pp. 522, 523)
4. b (p. 525)
5. a. The patient's eyesight, balance, and coordination may be diminished. Fatigue plus reduced muscle mass and bone strength can cause falls as well as make the falls more serious when they do occur. (pp. 521–525)
    b. Many older patients are on a fixed income and keep the heat turned down. Heavy sweaters and layers of clothing are worn to compensate for the low temperature. (pp. 525, 527)
    c. Although the patient may wear layers because of the cold, long periods of inactivity while in contact with a cool surface such as a floor is a recipe for hypothermia. It is important to remember that while you may not feel as if you would be hypothermic, the elderly patient with reduced ability to retain and regulate temperature may be hypothermic at temperatures just below a common room temperature. (Chapter 16 and pp. 521–525)

d. In addition to weaker bones and muscles, the elderly may have reduced vision, which can cause missteps and subsequent falls. Many causes of falls are preventable. They include loose throw rugs, shoes with slippery soles, and lack of handrails around stairs. (pp. 521–525, 526)

Chapter 29

1. d (p. 535)
2. c (p. 534)
3. a (p. 538)
4. c (p. 539)
5. a (p. 534)
6. a (p. 535)
7. Dressings, bandages, materials to stabilize impaled objects, sterile saline, scissors, adhesive tape. (p. 532)
8. Stethoscope, wristwatch, pen light, sphygmomanometer, prehospital care report forms, pen and notebook. (p. 532)
9. Nature of the call; name, exact location, and call-back number of the caller; location of the patient; number of patients and the severity of the patient's problem; any other special problems or considerations that may be pertinent. (p. 534)
10. a. Regardless of how many times the truck has or has not been out, you should check your equipment at the start of every shift. If the crew before you used something on a call in the middle of the night and did not replace it, you could find yourself needing it—and not being able to find it—on your next call. (p. 533)
    b. (Answers will vary. One example follows:) Just tell your partner that it is always a good idea to check the equipment. If all is okay, it won't take long.
    c. If an important piece of equipment were to be missing, it could hinder your ability to help your patient. It could also lead to liability if you were not able to do everything necessary for patient care. (p. 533)

Chapter 30

1. b (p. 549)
2. c (p. 549)
3. a (p. 550)
4. c (p. 550)
5. b (p. 550)
6. a (p. 549)
7. Answers will vary.

8. Any three: labels and placards, shipping papers, material safety data sheets, NFPA numbers. (pp. 545–548)
9. a. You should carry binoculars to look for placards safely from a distance. If the driver of the truck was able to exit it, call him to you (be sure he is not contaminated) to obtain further information. (p. 549–550)
    b. The DOT's *Emergency Response Guidebook* will provide safety information. It will give advice on safe distances, evacuation guidelines, and chemical information. (p. 548)

Chapter 31

1. d (p. 556)
2. b (p. 558)
3. a (pp. 559–560)
4. Triage, treatment, transportation, staging, safety, special rescue or extrication. (pp. 557–558)
5. Scene safety; number of patients, including the walking wounded; needs for extrication; estimated number of ambulances needed; other factors affecting the scene and resources, such as weather or terrain; number of sectors needed; area to stage resources. (Chapter 10 and p. 559)
6. a. Make sure that traffic does not pose a danger; that is, make sure no other vehicles crash into the scene and patients don't wander onto the highway. Also determine whether the bus is stable or if it could move and cause further harm. Calling for fire rescue would likely be beneficial. (Chapter 10 and p. 559)
    b. EMS command is responsible for oversight of the incident from an EMS perspective; triage establishes treatment priorities and is focused on that one task. In a major incident, the First Responder would most likely establish command to deal with big-picture issues first. However, if you were to come upon a two-vehicle MCI with four patients, you could start triage immediately after addressing hazards. (pp. 558–559)
    c. You should use a vehicle speaker or shout to get all patients who can walk to gather at a location away from the scene and away from the highway. This helps to ensure their safety, identifies and clears out the "walking wounded," and allows the triage officer to look around the bus for those who may be more seriously injured. However, only enter the bus if it is stabilized. (pp. 559–560)

Chapter 32

1. d (p. 573)
2. a (p. 576)
3. c (p. 577)
4. b (p. 573)
5. a (pp. 571–572)
6. b (pp. 571, 572)
7. a (p. 572)
8. You must be a good swimmer, specially trained in water rescue, wearing a personal flotation device, and accompanied by other rescuers. (p. 573)
9. Answers will vary, but may include strainers, obstructions, holes, low-head dams, entrapments, and hazardous materials such as oil, gas, or sewage. (pp. 572–573, 576–577)
10. a. You will need to take spinal precautions and determine if the patient is breathing and breathing adequately. (pp. 573–574)
    b. If the patient is breathing adequately, you may choose to leave the patient in the pool. The pool is heated, so hypothermia is not an immediate concern. However, if you are unable to maintain his airway or ventilate, you may be forced to remove him from the pool. The ETA of additional rescuers and equipment you have on hand are also a consideration. (pp. 573–574)

Chapter 33

1. c (p. 590)
2. a (pp. 587–588)
3. c (pp. 588, 590)
4. b (p. 590)
5. c (p. 587)
6. b (pp. 587–588)
7. a (p. 588)
8. Answers will vary, but should include BSI equipment, goggles or safety glasses with side shields, firefighter gloves or leather work gloves, a type of flame-retardant outer shell for body protection, and short rubber or leather boots with lug soles. (p. 586)
9. Any three: ask a responsive patient to tell you how many others were involved in the crash, question witnesses to see if a victim walked away from the scene, search the surrounding area carefully including in ditches and tall weeds, look for tracks in the earth or snow, search the vehicle itself for patients who may be wedged or otherwise hidden, look for clues such as a lunch box or extra jacket. (p. 586)

10. a. No. Do not approach or enter an unstable vehicle. This vehicle is clearly unstable. (pp. 587–588)
    b. Make sure the police have been called. You will need at least one ambulance—but it may be safer to request two in the event another (possibly unresponsive) person is found inside the vehicle after it is stabilized. You will need fire and rescue to stabilize the vehicle and perform any additional extrication that is necessary. (Chapter 10 and p. 586)
    c. Many emergency units equipped for extrication carry wood blocks or cribbing to stabilize vehicles such as this one. If you don't have these materials, you could search the area for wood that could be used as makeshift cribbing. It would have to be solid and there should be enough pieces to create a full and firm platform. (pp. 587–588)

Chapter 34

1. a (p. 597)
2. c (p. 599)
3. c (p. 600)
4. c (pp. 602–603)
5. a (p. 603)
6. a (p. 597)
7. a (p. 598)
8. Slope forms more than a 40-degree angle; slips or falls would likely result in serious injury or death due to the dangerous terrain below the slope; terrain is so hazardous, it requires rappelling. (p. 600)
9. Answer should include: at least 100 feet by 100 feet square; free of all obstacles; clear of wires, towers, vehicles, people, and loose objects; on firm ground with less than an eight-degree slope; with markers on all four corners and emergency red lights turned on. Answer may also include: there should be no smoking at the site and no white or blue lights directed at the helicopter or landing zone. (pp. 602–603)
10. a. No. The scene inside may be hazardous. Even though it appears to be a household incident involving cleaning supplies, all signs point to a dangerous hazardous-material incident. You may want to go in and attempt a rescue—especially if an infant is inside. But don't. It is not safe. (Chapter 30)
    b. With a total of five patients, some of whom are believed to be unresponsive, you should call for

at least three ambulances, perhaps more. In a worse-case scenario, you could have five patients who require aggressive care. (Chapter 10)

c. Yes. Any time the emergency exceeds resources, it is an MCI. It doesn't have to be 10 or 20 or even 100 patients. In addition, experienced providers know that incidents such as this can catch First Responders off guard. Don't let that happen to you. Don't rush in and don't wait until it is too late to call for help. (Chapter 31)

Glossary

A

abandonment a legal term referring to discontinuing medical care without making sure that another health-care professional with equal or a higher level of training has taken over patient care.

ABCs short for airway, breathing, and circulation.

abdominal cavity the space below the diaphragm and continuous with the pelvic cavity.

abdominal thrusts See *Heimlich maneuver.*

abrasion an injury caused by scraping, rubbing, or shearing away of the outermost layer of skin; a type of open wound.

abuse improper or excessive action so as to injure or cause harm.

absorption a route of exposure whereby a poison enters the body upon contact with the skin.

accessory muscles additional muscles; in regard to breathing, these are the muscles of the neck and the muscles between the ribs.

activated charcoal a finely ground charcoal that is very adsorbent (binds with harmful substances) and may be used as an antidote to some ingested poisons.

acute having a sudden onset; severe.

advance directive a patient's instructions, written in advance, regarding the kind of resuscitation efforts that should be made in a life-threatening emergency.

advanced cardiac life support (ACLS) prehospital emergency care that involves the use of intravenous fluids, drug infusions, cardiac monitoring, manual defibrillation, intubations, and other advanced procedures.

afterbirth the placenta, after it separates from the uterine wall and delivers.

agonal respirations reflex gasping with no regular pattern or depth; related to death or dying.

air embolism a type of barotrauma; occurs when one or more air bubbles block a blood vessel.

air splint a circumferential splint, which when inflated with air becomes rigid enough to help immobilize an injured limb.

airway adjunct an artificial airway.

altered mental status a change in a patient's normal level of responsiveness.

alveoli air sacs of the lungs. Singular *alveolus.*

amniotic sac the sac of fluid in which the developing fetus floats. *Also called* bag of waters.

amputation an injury that occurs when a body part is severed from the body; a type of open wound.

analgesic a medication that relieves pain.

anaphylactic shock an acute allergic reaction with severe bronchospasm and vascular collapse, which can be rapidly fatal. *Also called* anaphylaxis.

anatomical position the position in which a patient is standing erect with arms down at sides and palms front.

anatomy the structure of the body.

anecubital space the hollow, or front, of the elbow.

angina pectoris pain in the chest, occurring when blood supply to the heart is reduced and a portion of the heart muscle is not receiving enough oxygen.

anterior toward the front.

apical pulse an arterial pulse point located under the patient's left breast.

arterial bleeding recognized by bright red blood that spurts and pulsates from a wound.

arteries blood vessels that take blood away from the heart.

arterioles the smallest arteries.

arteriosclerosis a condition that causes the walls of the arteries to become thick and hard.

artificial ventilation a technique used to help maintain lung function in a patient who is either breathing inadequately or not breathing at all. *Also called* pulmonary resuscitation *or* rescue breathing.

asphyxia a lethal condition caused by an insufficient intake of oxygen; in extreme cases, convulsions, unconsciousness, and death may result. Also called *suffocation.*

aspirate to inhale material into the lungs.

assault an act that unlawfully places a person in apprehension of immediate bodily harm without his consent.

asthma a condition in which the bronchioles constrict, causing a reduction of airflow and creating congestion.

atria the two upper chambers of the heart. Singular *atrium.*

auscultation a method of examination that involves listening for signs of illness or injury. Taking a blood pressure by auscultation refers to listening for the systolic and diastolic sounds through a stethoscope.

automated external defibrillator (AED) an electrical apparatus that can detect fatal heart rhythms and deliver a shock through the patient's chest.

autonomic nervous system the part of the nervous system that handles involuntary activities.

AVPU memory aid for the four categories, or levels, of responsiveness: alert, verbal, painful, unresponsive.

avulsion an injury characterized by a torn flap of skin or soft tissue either still attached to the body or pulled off completely; a type of open wound.

B

bag of waters amniotic sac.

bag-valve mask (BVM) an aid for artificial ventilation; consists of a self-inflating bag, one-way valve, face mask, and oxygen reservoir.

bandage any clean material used to hold a dressing in place.

barotrauma refers to several conditions occurring when scuba or deep-water divers experience increasing underwater pressures or when they ascend in deep water improperly.

base station a stationary radio located in a dispatch center, station, or hospital.

basket stretcher designed to surround and protect the patient, this stretcher is used to move a patient from one level to another or over rough terrain. *Also called* Stokes stretcher.

battery the unlawful touching of another individual without his consent.

behavior the manner in which a person acts or performs.

behavioral emergency a situation in which a patient exhibits abnormal behavior, or behavior that is unacceptable or intolerable to the patient, family, or community.

birth canal an anatomical passage made up of the cervix and the vagina.

blanching losing color from.

blood pressure the amount of pressure surging blood exerts against arterial walls.

bloody show the plug of mucus that is discharged during labor.

blunt trauma an injury caused by an object not sharp or forceful enough to penetrate the skin.

body armor a garment made up of a synthetic material that resists penetration by bullets.

body mechanics the safest and most efficient methods of using the body to gain a mechanical advantage.

body substance isolation (BSI) a strict form of infection control based on the premise that all blood and body fluids are infectious.

bounding a term used to characterize a pulse that is unusually strong.

brachial pulse point the location where an arterial pulse can be felt on the inside of the arm between the elbow and the shoulder.

bracing exerting an opposing force against two parts of a solid surface, such as an interior wall of an ambulance, with your body.

bronchi the two main branches of the trachea, which lead to the lungs. Singular *bronchus*.

buddy taping splinting an injured finger by taping it to the uninjured finger beside it.

C

capillaries the smallest blood vessels through which the exchange of fluid, oxygen, and carbon dioxide takes place between the blood and tissue cells.

capillary bleeding recognized by dark red blood that slowly and evenly oozes from a wound.

capillary refill the time it takes for capillaries that have been compressed to refill with blood.

cardiac arrest the cessation of circulation.

cardiac dysrhythmias abnormal heart rhythms that follow a heart attack; generally caused by injury to the heart's electrical conduction system.

cardiopulmonary resuscitation (CPR) heart-lung resuscitation procedure; combined compression and ventilation techniques that maintain circulation and breathing in a patient.

carotid pulse point the location where an arterial pulse can be felt on either side of the neck.

cataracts opacity of the lens of the eye; the most common cause of blindness in adults.

catheter a hollow tube that is part of a suction device. *Also called* tonsil tip *or* tonsil sucker.

cc cubic centimeters.

central nervous system the brain and the spinal cord.

cerebrospinal fluid (CSF) a cushion of fluid that helps to protect the brain and spinal cord from injury.

cerebrovascular accident (CVA) See *stroke*.

cervical spine the neck; formed by the first seven vertebrae.

cervix the neck of the uterus.

chain of survival term used by the American Heart Association for a series of interventions that provide the best chance of survival for the cardiac-arrest patient.

chief complaint the reason that EMS was called, stated in the patient's (or the caller's) own words.

child abuse improper or excessive action so as to injure or cause harm to an infant or child.

child neglect insufficient attention or respect given to a child who has a claim to that attention and respect.

chronic of long duration.

chronic bronchitis a condition characterized by inflammation, edema, and excessive mucus in the bronchial tree; one of the most common chronic obstructive pulmonary diseases.

circumferential splint a splint that completely surrounds, or envelops, an injured limb.

cleaning the process of washing a soiled object with soap and water. See also *disinfecting* and *sterilizing.*

closed wound an injury to the soft tissues beneath unbroken skin.

coccygeal spine tail bone; formed by four fused vertebrae. *Also called* coccyx.

colicky pain cramps that occur in waves.

compensatory shock the first stage of shock, during which the patient's body is still able to maintain perfusion.

competent a competent adult is one who is lucid and able to make an informed decision about medical care.

complex access the process of gaining access to a patient with the use of tools and specialized equipment.

concussion a temporary loss of the brain's ability to function as a result of a blow or fall.

confined space a place with limited access and egress that is not designed for human occupancy.

congestive heart failure the failure of the heart to pump efficiently, leading to excessive blood or fluids in the lungs, body, or both.

consent permission to provide medical care. See *expressed consent* and *implied consent.*

constrict get smaller.

contusion a bruise; a type of closed wound.

COPD chronic obstructive pulmonary disease.

coronary artery disease the narrowing of one or more places in the arteries of the heart.

crepitus a sound or feeling of broken bones grinding against each other.

cribbing a system of wood or other supports used to prop up a vehicle or other object.

cross-finger technique a method of opening an unresponsive patient's clenched jaw.

croup a common viral infection of the upper airway, most common in children between the ages of one and five.

crowing a breathing sound similar to the cawing of a crow; may indicate that muscles around the larynx are in spasm.

crowning the appearance of the baby's head or other body part at the opening of the birth canal.

crush points two large objects come together to cause a crushing action.

cyanosis bluish discoloration of the skin and mucous membranes; a sign that body tissues are not receiving enough oxygen.

D

deadspace the areas of the respiratory system that hold the portion of inhaled air that does not participate in gas exchange.

decompensated shock the second stage of shock, during which the patient's body can no longer maintain perfusion. Without medical intervention, further decline occurs.

decompression sickness a type of barotrauma; occurs when a diver comes up too quickly from a deep prolonged dive.

deep remote, or far from the surface. Opposite of *superficial.*

defibrillation the process by which an electric shock is applied to the chest of a patient to correct fatal heart rhythms.

dehydration excessive loss of body fluids.

dermis the second layer of skin.

diaphoresis excessive perspiration.

diastolic pressure the result of the relaxation of the heart between contractions.

dilate enlarge.

direct force a force that causes injury at the point of impact.

direct medical control refers to an EMS medical director or other physician giving orders to an EMS rescuer on scene via telephone, radio, or in person.

disinfecting the process of cleaning plus using a chemical, such as alcohol or bleach, to kill many of the microorganisms on an object.

dislocation a bone is moved out of its normal position in a joint and remains that way.

distal distant, or far away from the point of reference, which is usually the torso. Opposite of *proximal.*

do not resuscitate (DNR) order document that relates the wish of the chronically or terminally ill patient not to be resuscitated.

dorsalis pedis pulse an arterial pulse point that can be felt at the top of the foot on the side of the great toe.

DOTS   memory aid used to recall what signs to look for during a physical examination: deformities, open injuries, tenderness, and swelling.

dressing   a sterile covering for a wound.

drowning   death from suffocation due to submersion.

drug abuse   the self-administration of one or more drugs in a way that differs from approved medical or social practice.

duty to act   the legal obligation to provide emergency care to a patient who requires it.

E

ecchymosis   black-and-blue discoloration of the skin; a type of closed wound.

edema   swelling resulting from a buildup of fluid in the tissues.

emancipated minor   a minor who is married, pregnant, a parent, in the armed forces, or financially independent and living away from home with the permission of the courts.

embolism   a thrombus, or clot of blood and plaque, that has broken loose from the wall of an artery.

emergency medical services (EMS) system   a network of resources linked together to provide emergency care and transport to victims of sudden illness or injury.

emergency move   a move made when there is an immediate danger to the patient.

emphysema   a condition in which the lungs suffer a progressive loss of elasticity; one of the most common chronic obstructive pulmonary diseases.

EMT-Basic   an emergency medical technician trained to the next level above the EMS First Responder. *Also called* EMT-B.

EMT-Intermediate   an emergency medical technician trained to a higher level than the First Responder and EMT-Basic. *Also called* EMT-I.

EMT-Paramedic   the most highly trained emergency medical technician in EMS. *Also called* EMT-P *or* paramedic.

enhanced 9-1-1   a type of 9-1-1 service in which the EMS dispatcher can see the caller's address and phone number on a computer screen. *Also called* E-9-1-1.

epidermis   the outermost layer of skin.

epiglottis   a leaf-shaped structure that prevents foreign objects from entering the trachea during swallowing.

epiglottitis   a bacterial infection that inflames the epiglottis. It often resembles croup but is more serious.

ETA   estimated time of arrival.

evisceration   the protrusion of internal organs from an open wound; a type of open wound.

expressed consent   permission that must be obtained from every responsive, competent adult patient before medical care may be rendered.

external   outside. Opposite of *internal.*

external bleeding   bleeding that occurs on the outside of the body.

extremities   the limbs of the body.

F

fallopian tube   one of two tubes or ducts that extend up from the uterus to a position near an ovary.

FBAO   foreign body airway obstruction.

femoral pulse point   the location where an arterial pulse can be felt in the groin area in the crease between the abdomen and thigh.

finger sweeps   technique used to remove a foreign object from the mouth.

First Responder   the first person on scene with EMS training.

flail chest   a closed chest injury resulting in the chest wall becoming unstable.

flushed   redness of the skin.

fontanel   the soft spot between the cranial bones of the skull of an infant.

fracture   a broken bone.

frostbite   freezing or near freezing of a specific body part. *Also called* local cold injury.

full-thickness burn   a burn that extends through all layers of skin and may involve subcutaneous tissue, muscles, organs, and bone.

G

gangrene   localized tissue death.

gastric distention   inflation of the stomach.

geriatric patients   patients who are elderly.

glucose   a simple sugar.

Golden Hour   a term trauma experts use to refer to the belief that severely injured patients have the highest survival rates when they are on the operating table within 60 minutes of injury.

grieving process   the process by which people cope with death and dying.

H

hand-off report   a verbal report of the patient's condition and the care given, made to the EMS personnel who take over patient care.

hazardous material   a substance that in any quantity poses a threat or unreasonable risk to life, health, or property if not properly controlled. *Also called a* hazmat.

head-tilt/chin-lift maneuver a manual technique used to open the airway of an ill (uninjured) patient.

heat cramps common term for muscle cramps in the lower limbs and abdomen, associated with fluid loss and possibly salt loss while active in a hot environment.

heat exhaustion prolonged exposure to heat, which creates moist, pale skin that may feel normal or cool to the touch.

heat stroke prolonged exposure to heat, which creates dry or moist skin that may feel warm or hot to the touch; associated with elevation of core body temperature.

Heimlich maneuver a technique used to dislodge and expel a foreign body airway obstruction. *Also called* subdiaphragmatic abdominal thrusts *or* abdominal thrusts.

hematoma a lump with bluish discoloration caused by a large collection of blood under the skin; a type of closed wound.

hemoglobin the iron-containing pigment of red blood cells that carries oxygen from the lungs to the tissues.

hemothorax the accumulation of blood in the pleural space.

HEPA respirator a high-efficiency particulate air respirator; a mask designed to filter out small particles in the air, including bacteria.

herniation the displacement of body tissue through an opening.

high-angle rescue a rescue involving a rope system to move a patient up or down a slope of 40 degrees or more.

hives slightly elevated red or pale areas of the skin that also may be itchy.

hoarseness losing the voice.

hyperglycemia increased blood sugar.

hyperthermia fever or raised body temperature.

hyperventilation a condition characterized by rapid breathing.

hypoglycemia low blood sugar.

hypothermia an overall reduction of body temperature.

hypoxia an insufficiency of oxygen in the patient's tissues.

I

immobilize to make immovable.

impaled object an object embedded in an open injury.

implied consent the assumption that in an emergency a patient who cannot give permission for medical care would give it if he or she could.

improvised splint a splint made from the materials found on hand, such as a broom stick or a rolled-up magazine.

incontinent unable to retain; loss of control, especially of urine or feces.

indirect force a force that causes injury along a path away from the point of impact.

indirect medical control refers to EMS system design, standing orders and protocols, education for EMS personnel, and quality management.

infectious disease a disease that can spread from one person to another.

inferior toward, or closer to, the feet. Opposite of *superior.*

ingestion a route of exposure whereby a poison is introduced into the body by way of the mouth.

inhalation a route of exposure whereby a poison is introduced into the body by way of the respiratory system.

initial assessment a component of patient assessment, conducted directly after the scene size-up, in which the rescuer identifies and treats life-threatening conditions.

injection a route of exposure whereby a poison enters the body by way of an object that pierces the skin.

inspection a method of examination that involves looking for signs of injury or illness.

insulin a hormone secreted by the pancreas to metabolize sugar; a medication used by people with diabetes to perform the same function as the hormone.

internal inside. Opposite of *external.*

internal bleeding bleeding that occurs inside the body.

interventions actions taken to correct a patient's problems.

irreversible shock the last stage of shock, during which the body's cells are dying. Even with treatment, damage to vital organs is permanent.

J

jaw-thrust maneuver a manual technique used to open the airway of an unresponsive patient who is injured or of any patient who has a suspected spine injury.

L

labor the term used to describe the process of childbirth.

laceration a break of varying depth in the skin; a type of open wound.

larynx the voice box.

lateral toward the left or right of (away from) the midline of the body.

lateral recumbent position position in which the patient is lying on the left or right side.

level of responsiveness   mental status; usually categorized as alert, verbal, painful, or unresponsive. See *AVPU.*

local cold injury   freezing or near freezing of a specific body part. *Also called* frostbite.

log roll   a method of turning a patient without causing injury to his or her spine.

long backboard   a rigid device, about six to seven feet long, that can help stabilize a patient's entire body.

low-angle rescue   a rescue involving a move of a patient up or down a slope of less than 40 degrees, where hands are not needed for balance, and falls would be unlikely.

lumbar spine   lower back; formed by five vertebrae.

M

manual traction   pulling a body part to align it.

material safety data sheets (MSDS)   manufacturers are required by law to give to their employees the name of hazardous materials, physical properties, and fire, explosion, and health hazards. Emergency first aid also is usually listed.

mechanism of injury (MOI)   the force or forces that cause an injury.

meconium staining   greenish or brownish color to the amniotic fluid, which means the unborn infant had a bowel movement.

medial   toward the midline of the body.

medical director   the physician legally responsible for the clinical and patient-care aspects of an EMS system.

medical patient   a patient who is ill, not injured.

metabolism   all the physical and chemical changes that occur in the body, including digestion.

minor   any person under the legally defined age of an adult; usually under the age of 18 or 21.

miscarriage   the natural loss of pregnancy before the twentieth week. *Also called* spontaneous abortion.

mottled   many colors or discolorations.

mouth-to-barrier device ventilation   technique of artificial ventilation that involves the use of a barrier device such as a face shield to blow air into the mouth of a patient.

mouth-to-mask ventilation   technique of artificial ventilation that involves the use of a pocket face mask with one-way valve to blow air into the mouth of a patient.

mouth-to-mouth ventilation   technique of artificial ventilation that involves a rescuer using his mouth—with no protective barrier—to blow air into the mouth of a patient.

multiple-casualty incident (MCI)   any emergency in which three or more patients are involved.

myocardial infarction (MI)   a heart attack.

N

N-95 respirator   a mask used by medical personnel to filter out harmful bacteria.

nasal cannula   oxygen delivery device characterized by two soft plastic tips, which are inserted a short distance into the nostrils.

nasopharyngeal airway   an artificial airway positioned in the nose and extending down to the larynx. *Also called* NPA *or* nasal airway.

nature of illness (NOI)   the type of medical condition or complaint a patient may be suffering.

neglect   refers to giving insufficient attention or respect to someone who has a claim to that attention and respect.

negligence   carelessness, inattention, disregard, inadvertence, or oversight that was accidental but avoidable; emergency care that deviates from the accepted standard of care and results in further injury to the patient.

9-1-1   a phone number by which the public can access EMS and, in some areas, other emergency services. *Also called* universal number.

non-accidental trauma   injuries caused by abuse.

non-emergency move   a move made by several rescuers usually after a patient has been stabilized. *Also called* non-urgent move.

non-9-1-1 system   a system that uses a regular seven-digit phone number (or numbers) for emergency services.

nonrebreather mask   oxygen delivery device characterized by an oxygen reservoir bag and a one-way valve.

O

occlude   block, close up, or obstruct.

occlusive dressing   a dressing that can form an airtight and sometimes watertight seal.

open wound   an injury that has broken the skin. *Also called* open injury.

OPQRRRST   memory aid used to help get a good description of pain from the patient; letters stand for onset, provocation, quality, region, radiation, relief, severity, and time.

oropharyngeal airway   an artificial airway positioned in the mouth and extending down to the larynx. *Also called* OPA *or* oral airway.

ovary   one of two almond-shaped glands in the female that produce the reproductive cell (the ovum), as well as certain hormones.

overdose   an emergency that involves poisoning by alcohol or other drugs.

ovum   the reproductive cell, or "egg."

P

pacemaker   a device that emits electrical discharges to the heart in order to trigger contractions.

package   refers to getting the patient ready to be moved; includes procedures such as stabilizing impaled objects and immobilizing injured limbs.

palmar surface method   a way of estimating the amount of body surface area involved in a burn by considering the palm of the patient's hand as 1% of total body surface area. *Also called* rule of palms.

palpate   feel; sense by touch.

palpation   a method of examination that involves feeling for signs of injury or illness.

palpitations   a sensation of throbbing or fluttering of the heart.

paradoxical breathing   a condition in which a segment of the chest moves in the opposite direction to the rest of the chest during breathing; typically seen with a flail segment.

partial-thickness burn   a burn that involves both the epidermis and dermis.

patent airway   an airway that is open and clear of obstructions.

pathogens   microorganisms such as bacteria and viruses.

patient assessment   the gathering of information to determine a possible illness or injury. A First Responder's patient assessment plan includes scene size-up, initial assessment, physical examination, patient history, ongoing assessment, and patient hand-off.

patient history   facts about the patient's medical history that are relevant to the patient's condition. See *SAMPLE.*

pediatric assessment triangle (PAT)   a method of remembering the important components of pediatric assessment: appearance, breathing, and circulation.

pediatric patient   a patient who is an infant or child.

pelvic cavity   space bound by the lower part of the spine, the hip bones, and the pubis.

pelvis   the hip bones.

penetrating injury to the chest   an injury that occurs when an object passes through the chest wall and into the chest cavity.

penetration/puncture wound   the result of a sharp, pointed object being pushed or driven into soft tissues; a type of open wound.

perfusion   refers to the circulation of blood and delivery of oxygen throughout the body's organs and other structures.

peripheral nervous system   the nerves; portion of the nervous system that is located outside the brain and spinal cord.

personal protective equipment (PPE)   equipment used by a rescuer to protect against injury and the spread of disease.

pharynx   the throat.

physiology   the study of how the body works.

pinch points   two objects meet to cause a pinching or pulling action.

placenta   a disk-shaped organ on the inner lining of the uterus that provides nourishment and oxygen to a developing fetus.

plasma   the fluid that surrounds the blood cells.

pleural space   the area between the lungs and the walls of the chest cavity.

pneumonia   a term used to describe a group of illnesses characterized by lung infection and fluid- or pus-filled alveoli.

pneumothorax   an accumulation of air in the pleural space.

portable stretcher   commonly made of an aluminum frame and canvas, this cot has no wheels. It is valuable when there is not enough space for a standard stretcher or when there are multiple patients.

positional asphyxia   suffocation caused by the position a patient is in, usually face-down; associated with hog-tie or hobble restraints.

posterior   toward the back. Opposite of *anterior.*

posterior tibial pulse   an arterial pulse point that can be felt behind the medial ankle bone.

posturing   a condition in which a patient's limbs exhibit an abnormal flexion or extension either spontaneously or in response to a painful stimulus.

power grip   a technique used to get maximum force from the rescuer's hands while lifting and moving.

power lift   a technique used for lifting that helps prevent injury to rescuers and provides a stable move for the patient.

prehospital care report (PCR)   documentation of an emergency call; usually includes run data, patient information, and a narrative.

prone position   a position in which patient is lying face down on his or her stomach.

protocols   developed by the medical director, these are lists of steps to be taken in certain situations.

proximal close to or near the point of reference, which is usually the torso. Opposite of *distal.*

psi pounds per square inch.

public access defibrillation (PAD) the availability of fully automated external defibrillators in public and/or private places where large numbers of people gather or people who are at high risk for heart attacks live.

pulse oximeter an electronic device that measures the percentage of hemoglobin bound with oxygen (oxygen saturation or SpO_2).

pulse the wave of blood propelled through the arteries as a result of the pumping action of the heart.

pustules raised areas on the skin that are filled with pus.

R

radial pulse point the location where an arterial pulse can be felt on the palm side of the wrist.

rape sexual intercourse performed without consent and by compulsion through force, threat, or fraud.

rape trauma syndrome a reaction to rape that involves four general stages: acute (impact) reaction, outward adjustment, depression, and acceptance and resolution.

rappelling a special technique of getting down a slope by means of a secured rope.

reasonable force refers to the amount of force needed to keep a patient from injuring himself or someone else.

recovery position lateral recumbent position; used to allow fluids to drain from a patient's mouth instead of into the airway.

relative skin temperature an assessment of the skin temperature obtained by touching the patient's skin.

repeaters devices that receive a low-power radio transmission and rebroadcast it with increased power.

respiration passage of air into and out of the lungs.

respiratory arrest the cessation of spontaneous breathing.

retraction a pulling inward, a shortening; the condition of being drawn back; sucking in of the skin between the ribs, above the sternum, and above the clavicles.

rigid cervical immobilization device a device in the shape of a collar used to restrict movement of the cervical spine. *Also called* extrication collar.

rule of nines a way of estimating the amount of body surface area involved in a burn that considers each of 11 regions of the body equal to 9%.

rule of palms See *palmar surface method.*

run data bare facts of an EMS response; include the date, time, unit involved, location of the call, and the names of the crew members.

S

sacral spine lower part of the spine; formed by five fused vertebrae. *Also called* sacrum.

SAMPLE memory aid for gathering a patient history; the letters stand for signs and symptoms, allergies, medications, pertinent past history, last oral intake, and events that led up to the emergency.

scene size-up an overall assessment of the emergency scene, consisting of ensuring personal safety, identifying the mechanism of injury or nature of illness, and determining necessary resources.

scoop stretcher this cot splits in two or four sections, so it can be used where larger stretchers cannot fit. *Also called* orthopedic stretcher.

scope of care the actions that are legally allowed to be provided by the First Responder.

seizure a convulsion caused by a sudden discharge of electrical activity in the brain.

self-splint immobilizing an injured limb by securing it against the body with a cravat or roller bandage.

septum a wall that divides two cavities; an example is the wall dividing the two nostrils.

sexual assault any touch that the victim did not initiate or agree to and that is imposed by coercion, threat, deception, or threats of physical violence.

shear points two objects move close enough together to cause a cutting action.

shipping papers drivers of vehicles carrying hazardous materials are required by law to carry these papers, which give the name of the substance, the danger it presents, and a four-digit identification number. *Also called* manifests *or* waybills.

shock a life-threatening progressive condition that results from the inadequate delivery of oxygenated blood throughout the body. *Also referred to as* hypoperfusion.

shoring a system of beams or timbers propped against a structure to provide support.

short backboard three to four feet long, this device can help stabilize a patient down to the hips. It is used for patients with suspected spine injuries who are in a sitting position.

shoulder girdle the clavicles (the collarbones) and the scapulae (shoulder blades) that attach the upper extremities to the skeleton.

sign   any injury or medical condition that can be observed in a patient.

silent myocardial infarction   a heart attack without pain.

simple access   the process of gaining access to a patient without the use of tools.

sling   a large triangular bandage or other cloth that is applied to immobilize possible injuries to the upper extremities.

soft-tissue injury   an injury to the skin, muscles, nerves, and/or blood vessels.

sphygmomanometer   an instrument used to determine arterial blood pressure.

spinal precautions   methods used to protect the spine from further injury. For First Responders, this usually refers to manual stabilization of the head and neck until the patient is fully immobilized.

splint   any rigid device used to immobilize a body part.

sprain   a joint and ligament are injured.

sputum   substance expelled by coughing or clearing the throat; may contain mucus, blood, pus, cellular debris, and microorganisms.

stabilize   to hold firmly and steadily.

staging area   the safe area at an emergency scene where all responders should check in and get orders.

stair chair   a lightweight folding device that is used to safely move patients up or down stairs.

standard of care   the care that would be expected to be provided to the same patient under the same circumstances by another First Responder who had received the same training.

standard stretcher   a cot with wheels. It may also have a collapsible undercarriage that makes it possible to load it into an ambulance.

standing orders   a policy issued by a medical director that authorizes EMS personnel to perform particular skills in certain situations.

status asthmaticus   a severe, life-threatening, prolonged asthma attack.

sterile   free of all microorganisms and spores.

sterilizing   a process in which a chemical or other substance, such as superheated steam, kills all of the microorganisms on an object.

sternum   the breastbone.

stethoscope   an instrument used to listen to sounds within the body.

stoma   a permanent, surgically created opening that connects the trachea directly to the front of the neck.

stored energy   the potential for movement even after machinery has been shut down.

strain   a muscle or a muscle and tendon are overextended.

stridor   a harsh, high-pitched sound made during inhalation, which may mean the larynx is swollen and blocking the upper airway.

stroke   a sudden loss of neurological function caused by an interruption of blood flow to a portion of the brain. *Also called* cerebrovascular accident (CVA) *or* brain attack.

subcutaneous tissue   the layer of fat beneath the skin.

sucking chest wound   an open wound to the chest that bubbles or makes a sucking noise.

suctioning   using negative pressure created by a commercial device in order to keep a patient's airway clear.

superficial   near the surface. Opposite of *deep*.

superficial burn   a burn that involves only the epidermis.

superior   toward or closer to the head. Opposite of *inferior*.

supine position   position in which the patient is lying face up on his or her back.

swathe   a large folded cloth usually used to secure a sling or rigid splint to the body.

symptom   any injury or medical condition that can only be described by the patient.

systolic pressure   the result of a contraction of the heart, which forces blood through the arteries.

T

tension pneumothorax   a severe buildup of air that compresses the lungs and heart toward the uninjured side of the chest.

thoracic cavity   space above the diaphragm and within the walls of the thorax. *Also called* chest cavity.

thoracic spine   upper back; formed by 12 vertebrae.

thorax   the rib cage. *Also called* the chest.

thready   a term used to characterize a pulse that is weak and rapid.

tourniquet   a constricting band used as a last resort on an extremity to apply pressure over an artery in order to control bleeding.

trachea   the windpipe.

traction splint   a mechanical device that provides a counter-pull to alleviate pain, reduce blood loss, and minimize further injury.

transient ischemic attack (TIA)   a kind of stroke that resolves within 24 hours, but may be a warning sign of an impending larger stroke. *Also called* mini-stroke.

trauma patient   a patient who is injured, not ill.

triage   process of sorting patients to determine the order in which they will receive care and transport.

trimester a three-month period.

tripod position a position in which the patient is sitting upright, leaning forward, fighting to breathe.

twisting force a force that causes an injury when one part of a limb remains stationary while the rest of it twists.

U

ulcer a patch of skin or mucous membrane marked by redness, possible infection, and loose dead skin.

umbilical cord an extension of the placenta through which the developing fetus receives nourishment while in the uterus.

uterus the organ that contains the developing fetus.

V

veins blood vessels that carry blood back to the heart from the rest of the body.

venous bleeding recognized by dark red blood that flows steadily and slowly from a wound.

ventricles the two lower chambers of the heart.

venules the smallest veins.

vertebrae the 33 bone segments of the spinal column. Singular *vertebra*.

vesicles small blisters.

vital signs signs of life; assessments related to breathing, pulse, skin, pupils, and blood pressure.

W

wheal a raised, round, red mark.

wheezing a whistling or high-pitched breathing sound usually heard during an exhalation.

withdrawal refers to the effects on the body that occur after a period of abstinence from the drugs or alcohol to which the body has become accustomed.

wound a soft-tissue injury.

wrap points an aggressive component moves in a circular motion.

X

xiphoid process lowest (inferior) portion of the sternum.

Index